Introduction to
Health Services

For N. Williams, the memory of D. Williams,
and J., C., J.C., and N. Torrens

Introduction to Health Services

Sixth Edition

Edited by

Stephen J. Williams, Sc.D.
Professor of Public Health
Head, Division of Health Services Administration
Graduate School of Public Health
San Diego State University
San Diego, California

Paul R. Torrens, M.D., M.P.H.
Professor of Health Services
School of Public Health
University of California, Los Angeles
Los Angeles, California

DELMAR
THOMSON LEARNING ™

Australia Canada Mexico Singapore Spain United Kingdom United States

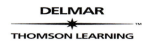

DELMAR

THOMSON LEARNING

Health Care Publishing Director:
William Brottmiller

Executive Editor:
Cathy L. Esperti

Acquisitions Editor:
Marie Linvill

Developmental Editor:
Patricia A. Gaworecki

Editorial Assistant:
Jennifer Frisbee

Executive Marketing Manager:
Dawn F. Gerrain

Project Editor:
Mary Ellen Cox

Production Coordinator:
Anne Sherman

Art and Design Coordinator:
Jay Purcell

For permission to use material from this text or product, contact us by
Tel   (800)730-2214
Fax   (800)730-2215
www.thomsonrights.com

Library of Congress Cataloging-in-Publication Data

Introduction to health services/edited by Stephen J. Williams, Paul R. Torrens.—6th ed. p.cm.
    Includes bibliographical references and index.
    ISBN 0-7668-3611-8 (alk. paper)
    1. Medical care—United States. 2. Health services administration—United States.
I. Williams, Stephen J. (Stephen Joseph), 1948- II. Torrens, Paul R. (Paul Roger), 1934-

RA395.A3 I495 2001
362.1'0973—dc21   2001037292

NOTICE TO THE READER

INTRODUCTION TO THE SERIES

T his series in Health Services is now in its second decade of providing top quality teaching materials to the health administration/public health field. Each year has witnessed further strengthening of the market position of each of the principal books in the series, while also reflecting the continued excellence of the products. Each author, book editor, and contributor to the series has helped build what is widely recognized as the top textbook and issues collection of books available in this field today.

But we have achieved only a beginning. Everyone involved in the series is committed to further expansion of the scope, technical excellence, and usefulness of the series. Our goal is to do more for you, the reader. We will add new books in important areas, seek out more excellent authors, and improve the physical attributes of the books to make them easier for you to use.

We thank everyone, the authors and users in particular, who have made this series so successful and so widely used. And we promise that this second decade will be dedicated to further expansion of the series and to enhancement of the books it contains to provide still greater value to you, our constituency.

Stephen J. Williams
Series Editor

DELMAR SERIES IN HEALTH SERVICES ADMINISTRATION

Stephen J. Williams, Sc.D., Series Editor

Ambulatory Care Management, third edition
   Austin Ross, Stephen J. Williams, and Ernest J. Pavlock, Editors

The Continuum of Long-Term Care, second edition
   Connie J. Evashwick, Editor

Health Care Economics, fifth edition
   Paul J. Feldstein

Health Care Management: Organization Design and Behavior, fourth edition
   Stephen M. Shortell and Arnold D. Kaluzny, Editors

Health Politics and Policy, third edition
   Theodor J. Litman and Leonard S. Robins, Editors

Motivating Health Behavior
   John P. Elder, E. Scott Geller, Melbourne F. Hovell, and Joni A. Mayer, Editors

Really Governing: How Health System and Hospital Boards Can Make More of a Difference
   Dennis D. Pointer and Charles M. Ewell

Strategic Management of Human Resources in Health Services Organizations, second edition
   Myron D. Fottler, S. Robert Hernandez, and Charles L. Joiner, Editors

Financial Management in Health Care Organizations
   Robert A. McLean

Principles of Public Health Practice
   F. Douglas Scutchfield and C. William Keck, Editors

The Hospital Medical Staff
   Charles H. White

Essentials of Health Services, second edition
   Stephen J. Williams

Essentials of Health Care Management
   Stephen M. Shortell and Arnold D. Kaluzny, Editors

Essentials of Human Resources Management in Health Services Organizations
   Myron D. Fottler, S. Robert Hernandez, and Charles L. Joiner, Editors

Health Services Research Methods
   Leiyu Shi

CONTENTS

PART ONE   **Overview of the Health Services System 1**

Chapter 1	**Historical Evolution and Overview of Health Services in the United States**	2
Chapter 2	**Overview of the Organization of Health Services in the United States**	18
Chapter 3	**Medicine and Technology**	47
Chapter 4	**Patterns of Illness and Disease and Access to Health Care**	61

PART TWO   **Financing and Structuring Health Care 91**

Chapter 5	**Financing Health Services**	92
Chapter 6	**Managed Care: Restructuring the System**	124
Chapter 7	**Private Health Insurance and Employee Benefits**	140

PART THREE   **Providers of Health Services 161**

Chapter 8	**The Evolution of Public Health: A Joint Public-Private Responsibility**	162
Chapter 9	**Ambulatory Health Care Services**	177
Chapter 10	**Hospitals and Health Systems**	202
Chapter 11	**The Continuum of Long-Term Care**	234
Chapter 12	**Mental Health Services**	280

PART FOUR   **Nonfinancial Resources for Health Care 309**

| Chapter 13 | **Pharmaceuticals** | 310 |
| Chapter 14 | **Health Care Professionals** | 326 |

PART FIVE   **Assessing and Regulating Health Services 351**

Chapter 15	**Health Policy and the Politics of Health Care**	352
Chapter 16	**Assessing and Improving Quality of Care**	373
Chapter 17	**Ethical Issues in Public Health and Health Services**	392

ACKNOWLEDGMENTS

Data tables presented throughout this book for which specific sources are not contained within the table itself were obtained from the National Center for Health Statistics, Health, United States, 2000, Hyattsville, MD: 2000. U.S. Government websites, especially those of the National Center for Health Statistics, provide current data for many tables. The authors wish to thank Debbie Doan, Cathy Pugh, and Teresa Laughlin for their assistance in the preparation of this manuscript.

FOREWORD

When the first edition of *Introduction to Health Services* was published in 1980, the Foreword was provided by the two deans of the Schools of Public Health at the University of Washington and the University of California, Los Angeles. It is not surprising that the deans introduced this now popular textbook because, at that time, it was written and edited exclusively by faculty from their own institutions. Twenty years later, as a former faculty member of the University of Washington and as the new Dean at UCLA, I am pleased to provide the Foreword to the sixth edition and to continue the association of this text with these two institutions and their present or former colleagues.

As the former Director of the National Institute for Occupational Safety and Health, I am also grateful for this opportunity to reflect from the vantage point of the workplace on the rapidly changing forces and challenges facing the United States health care system. In the face of lost opportunities to assure universal access to health care, the albeit imperfect underpinnings of the "system"—namely, voluntary employer-provided insurance—are unraveling. Despite the wish of some politicians to characterize the uninsured as those outside the economic and social mainstream, it is abundantly clear that not only is the problem of access to health care mounting, but that workers and their families are predominant victims. Many employers across all sectors of the economy are ceasing to provide health insurance in whole or in part. This trend is perhaps demonstrated most dramatically in small and medium-sized companies, those employers of the bulk of the American working population. And the decreased participation of employers in providing insurance does not fall equally within these company size strata, but disproportionately affects the young, the lesser educated, those in lower paying jobs, and workers of color. Given that this erosion of employer-sponsored insurance occurred during the economic "best of times," one must worry about the future as we now face an economic slowdown or worse.

The Institute of Medicine report on medical errors, released in 2000, drew an unexpectedly large media response and significant congressional attention and action. With the estimate of perhaps as many as 100,000 fatalities per year attributed to medical errors (a large number even if critics are correct that some events characterized as errors were more accurately inevitable adverse outcomes), the role of the health professional workforce was little noted. Many of us concerned with workplace health and safety had evolved to appreciate that protecting workers was not only a value in itself, but could reliably be related to a company's bottom line and to productivity and quality of the product made. (For example, a healthier workforce turned out a better made car.) Similarly, there was emerging evidence that would link the well-being of the health care workforce to productivity and quality of patient care (and hence reduced medical errors). So, as the health care system tackles systematic approaches to reducing medical errors, it would be a tremendous lost opportunity to ignore the increasingly stressed and overburdened workforce in the process.

In addition to these challenges arising from a new understanding of the United States workplace, other challenges (what optimists might call "opportunities") are emerging from the rapidly expanding scientific understanding of disease and its causation, not to mention new diagnostic and therapeutic technologies. As I write this Foreword, the human genome "map" has recently been published. This new information and what will soon follow will create extraordinary opportunities for understanding human disease. Medical advancements will also engender remarkable challenges to the health system, such as profound ethical dilemmas and even greater financial stresses than those that already plague the system.

Introduction to Health Services has had an impressive history of charting the progress of health care in the United States over the past twenty years and has contributed greatly to the preparation of health care professionals of all types. It is my sincere hope that this textbook will continue to fulfill this important function, and that some future Foreword writer will be able to describe how our system has met its old challenges and how it is looking ahead to addressing new issues.

Linda Rosenstock, M.D.,M.P.H.
Dean
School of Public Health
University of California, Los Angeles
Los Angeles

PREFACE

The rate of change in our nation's health care industry has accelerated since the last edition of this book was published. Significant changes in market forces, including the apparent failure of the managed care initiative to substantially reduce health care costs, combined with continuing pressures to address the issues of the uninsured, the underinsured, the need to update the Medicare program, the increasingly complex debate concerning the role of government in all aspects of health care, and other public policy concerns continue to mount. At the same time, phenomenal developments in biomedical research and clinical practice, as well as in the application of information technology to health care, augers for a complete revolution in the provision of health care and its potential accomplishments in improving health status and function for our nation.

The benefits from years of biomedical research are only beginning to be realized as we increase our understanding of the molecular nature of health, illness, and disease, and apply that knowledge to fundamental, scientific discovery to control, or in many instances, cure disease. Information technology is revolutionizing the delivery, control, and assessment of health care services. In the future, these technologies will improve efficiency and enhance the quality of care for all Americans. The sixth edition of *Introduction to Health Services* enters the scene as we face some of our most daunting challenges in the health care arena.

This edition includes a number of new chapters in response to these challenges. Other chapters make a repeat appearance, brought up to date utilizing current knowledge and data sources.

This edition is published as our nation's health care system appears to be in the early stages of an new era. This era should be one in which we will finally satisfactorily resolve long-standing public policy issues and concerns while making available to all Americans the results of our investment in biomedical knowledge and health care delivery infrastructure.

Part One provides an introductory section to set the stage. Chapter 1 presents an historical overview of the nation's health care system, setting the stage for the detailed analyses that follow in subsequent chapters. The chapter also provides context and a starting point for the reader's assessment of the complex components of the nation's health care system and their interaction.

Chapter 2 is new and presents an analytical overview of the health care system. Three case studies set the stage for examining our nation's health care system by illustrating the situation that exists in three geographical locations of the country. The first two case studies in this chapter focus on health care delivery in Boston, Massachusetts and in Orange County, California. The third and last section of this chapter provides a prospective on examining health, disease, illness, and mortality in Los Angeles, California.

Chapter 3, also new, focuses on a discussion of biomedical technology and clinical medicine. Because the complexity of medicine today precludes a comprehensive overview of all aspects of medicine, this chapter utilizes illustrative technologies that are both innovative and forward-looking to provide a valuable perspective on the nature of our current developments in biomedical knowledge and their implications for health care delivery and clinical practice.

Chapter 4 provides a comprehensive perspective on historical and current patterns of disease and of access to health care services in the United States. This chapter presents a fundamental assessment of the underlying factors associated with the causes and characteristics of health care utilization and the translation of such characteristics into actual access to health care—a recurrent theme in this book.

Part Two focuses on the financing of health care in the United States and the impact that financial changes are having on the organizational structure of the system. Chapter 5 reviews the sources and uses of financial resources for health care in the United States. Chapter 6 focuses on the dominant role of managed care in the health care delivery system. Although several other chapters in the book address issues related to managed care, Chapter 6 presents a philosophical and logical overview of the role, structure, and mechanisms inherent in managed care, as well as our successes and failures in restructuring the nation's health care system using managed care principles.

Finally, Chapter 7 describes the evolution and current status of the private health insurance industry in the United States. This chapter also addresses the interaction of private health insurance with other key financing and organizational trends, including managed care.

Part Three examines provider organizations and settings through which health care services are offered. The first chapter in this section, Chapter 8, addresses the role of health promotion and disease prevention activities in improving the health of the public through public health services and agencies. This chapter includes an historical perspective and stresses the key role of the public/private partnership for public health that has emerged in the United States and whose focus is on protecting the health and well-being of populations as opposed to individuals.

Chapter 9 addresses the central role of ambulatory care services in the provision, coordination, and control of health care. The expansion of group practices and other key ambulatory care providers is also addressed.

Chapter 10 examines the radically changing role of hospital and health systems and the evolution of the hospital from being solely a provider of in-patient services to an integrator of comprehensive delivery systems. Chapters 11 and 12 focus on the provision of long-term care and mental health services, both key areas that have experienced dramatic changes. Each of these areas presents very complex challenges for the future.

Part Four deals with the key nonfinancial resources used in the provision of health care services in the United States. Chapter 13 addresses the role of the pharmaceutical industry in meeting the health care needs of our nation. Chapter 14 examines the human resources used in providing health care services, particularly the professionals necessary for the successful functioning of the health care system.

Part Five asks how our health care system can be evaluated, regulated, monitored, and assessed. Chapter 15 looks at the role of government in the health care industry. It reviews how public policy in health care has developed over the years and examines its current status and outlook. Chapter 16 focuses on the measurement and evaluation of health care services, particularly addressing clinical assessment issues. Finally, Chapter 17 discusses the many ethical issues associated with providing health care services. Ethical issues have become increasingly important, particularly in the development of public policy as our biomedical capability has increased over the years and as cost pressures, managed care, and issues of uninsured and underinsured individuals have presented themselves to policymakers.

Over the past two decades, our nation's health care system has adopted a market-driven focus with the objective of increasing efficiency and reducing redundancy. At the same time, issues of life and death, of access to health care, and of making available proven technologies to improve the health of individuals and populations are still the fundamental objectives of the nation's health care delivery system. The challenges and the opportunities have never been greater. Our potential to provide longer, higher quality lives is greater now than ever in our nation's history. At the same time, the challenges of costs, access, politics, and ethics are also greater than ever.

Today we have more at stake in our nation's health care system than ever before. The promises generated by technological advances are mind-boggling. At the same time, we are challenged to address such fundamental issues as providing adequate access to essential health services to all Americans, and assuring a comfortable and healthy retirement for our older population. The problems that exist in such areas as long term care and mental health services sometimes appear to be overwhelming. In addition, the social challenges that our nation faces—environmental concerns, economic problems, social disruptions, and criminal activity—continuously impinge on the smooth functioning of the nation's health care system.

Here in the United States, we have invested more human and fiscal capital in health care than any other nation in the history of humanity. We seek to improve our physical and mental well-being through a health care system that often seems inadequate and unstable. We also recognize the tremendous resources that our nation has available to improve the lives of all Americans through a financially realistic and operationally efficient health care system.

As in previous editions of this book, a multidisciplinary, empirical approach is used throughout. The emphasis is on the practical application of an increasingly sophisticated body of knowledge and research.

We continue to owe a debt of gratitude to the many students and practitioners who provide us with guidance as this book evolves. We are profoundly grateful to our contributors, our editors, our colleagues, and to all others involved in the production of this book. We hope that it will contribute in some small measure to a better health care system for all Americans.

Stephen J. Williams
Paul R. Torrens

CONTRIBUTORS

A. E. Benjamin, Ph.D.
Professor
Department of Social Welfare
School of Public Policy and Social Research
University of California, Los Angeles
Los Angeles, California

Lester Breslow, M.D., M.P.H.
Professor and Dean Emeritus
School of Public Health
University of California, Los Angeles
Los Angeles, California

William L. Dowling, Ph.D.
Professor of Health Services
Chairman, Department of Health Services
School of Public Health and Community Medicine
University of Washington
Seattle, Washington

Connie J. Evashwick, Sc.D., F.A.C.H.E.
Endowed Chair and Professor
Center for Health Care Innovation
California State University, Long Beach
Long Beach, California

Alma L. Koch, Ph.D.
Professor of Public Health
Graduate Program in Health Services Administration
Graduate School of Public Health
San Diego State University
San Diego, California

Philip R. Lee, M.D.
Professor Emeritus
Department of Medicine and Senior Advisor to the Dean
School of Medicine
University of California, San Francisco
San Francisco, California

Stephen S. Mick, Ph.D.
Arthur Graham Glasgow Professor of Health Administration and
Chair
Department of Health Administration
Virginia Commonwealth University
Richmond, Virginia

Mary Richardson, Ph.D.
Professor
Department of Health Services
School of Public Health and Community Medicine
University of Washington
Seattle, Washington

Ruth Roemer, J.D.
Adjunct Professor Emerita
School of Public Health
University of California, Los Angeles
Los Angeles, California

Sharyne Shiu-Thornton, Ph.D.
Department of Health Services
School of Public Health and Community Medicine
University of Washington
Seattle, Washington

Paul R. Torrens, M.D., M.P.H.
Professor of Health Services
School of Public Health
University of California, Los Angeles
Los Angeles, California

Pauline Vaillancourt Rosenau, Ph.D.
Professor, Management & Policy Sciences
Center for Society and Population Health
UT-Houston School of Public Health
The University of Texas
Houston Health Science Center
Houston, Texas

Scott Weingarten, M.D., M.P.H.
Director, Health Services Research
Cedars-Sinai Medical Center
Associate Professor of Medicine
University of California, Los Angeles
School of Medicine
Los Angeles, California

Gary Whitted, Ph.D., M.S.
Vice President
United HealthCare
Portland, Oregon

Stephen J. Williams, Sc.D.
Professor of Public Health
Head, Division of Health Services Administration
Graduate School of Public Health
San Diego State University
San Diego, California

PART
1

Overview of the Health Services System

CHAPTER

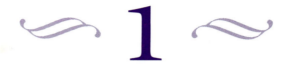

1

Historical Evolution
and Overview of Health Services
in the United States

Paul R. Torrens

Chapter Topics

- Historical Evolution of Health Services in the United States
- Predominant Health Problems of the American Population
- Technology Available to the American People
- Social Organization of Health Care in the United States
- Involvement of the People in Their Health and Health Care

Learning Objectives

Upon completing this chapter, the reader should be able to:

- Understand the major stages in the development of the nation's health care system
- Appreciate the many forces affecting the development of health services in the United States
- Realize the key role of technology in shaping health care
- Understand the social, political, and economic forces affecting health care
- Follow the government's involvement in health services

HISTORICAL EVOLUTION OF HEALTH SERVICES IN THE UNITED STATES

The modern American health care system has gone through three important phases in its development and has now entered a fourth (Table 1.1). The first phase began in the mid-nineteenth century (*circa* 1850) when the first large hospitals, such as Bellevue Hospital in New York City and Massachusetts General Hospital in Boston, were established. The development of hospitals symbolized the *institutionalization of health care* for the first time in this country. Before this time, health care in the United States was a loose collection of individual services functioning

Table 1.1. Major Issues in the Development of Health Care in the United States, 1850 to Present

Issues	1850–1900	1900 to World War II	World War II to 1980	1980 to Present
Predominant "targets" of the health system at the time	Epidemics of acute infections related to food, water, housing, and conditions of life	Acute events, trauma, or infections affecting individuals, not groups	Chronic diseases such as heart disease, cancer, and stroke	Chronic diseases, particularly emotional and behaviorally related conditions, as well as conditions related to work place, environment, and genetic inheritance
Technology to handle predominant health problems	Virtually none	Beginning and rapid growth of basic medical sciences and technology	Explosive growth of medical science; technology captures the health care system	Continued explosive growth and expansion of technology, with parallel rise in costs of health care
Social organization for health care	None; individuals left to their own resources or charity	Beginning societal and governmental efforts to care for those who could not care for themselves	Development of health insurance as the primary vehicle of social organization of health care in the United States	Increasing power of financial organizations to shape the health care system; increasing influence of governmental financial systems (e.g., Medicare and Medicaid)
Involvement of people in their health care	People actively involved in giving care to family; little factual knowledge	Beginning availability of medical knowledge to the general public	Increasing awareness of health care as a social and political issue by the public	Well-informed public, but increasing frustration with the complexity and expense of the system

independently and without much relationship to each other or to anything else. With the development of the first hospitals, health care personnel and technology began to cluster together around the most seriously ill patients, providing for the first time a centralizing, co-ordinating focus for what had been a dispersed and somewhat random collection of services. The arrival of the first hospitals in the United States brought a sense of order and concentration to health care in this country that had been lacking previously.

The second important phase of development began around the turn of the century (*circa* 1900) with the *introduction of the scientific method into medicine* in this country. Before this time, medicine was not an exact science but was instead a rather informal collection of unproven generalities and good intentions. After 1900, stimulated by the opening of the new medical school at Johns Hopkins University in Baltimore, medicine acquired a solid scientific base that eventually transformed it from a conscientious but poorly equipped art into a detailed and clearly defined science.

With the coming of World War II, the United States underwent a major social, political, and technological upheaval the effect of which was so marked that it ended the second phase of development of health care in this country and signaled the beginning of the third phase, the phase of *growing interest in the social and organizational structure of health care.* During this time, major attention was directed, for the first time, toward the financing of health care with the resulting growth of health insurance plans, such as Blue Cross and Blue Shield, in the nonprofit sector and numerous commercial insurance companies in the for-profit sector. This was also the time of rapidly increasing power in the federal government with regard to health care in the United States, as witnessed by the Hill-Burton Act (Hospital Survey and Construction Act), by the growth of huge research budgets of the National Institutes of Health (NIH), and, in 1965, by the passage and implementation of Medicare and Medicaid. Finally, during this time, largely as a result of the federal "War on Poverty," the principle of health care as a right, not a privilege, was widely discussed and widely accepted.

The Fourth Phase

Since the early 1980s, the health care system in this country has moved into a fourth phase of its development, an era of *limited resources, restriction of growth, and reorganization of the methods of financing and delivering care.* It has also been the era of the growth of the *influence of economic market forces* in the shaping of health care in America. Before this phase, it had been presumed that the health care system would always be encouraged to grow and expand, both in size and complexity, and that there would always be sufficient resources to support that expansion. Beginning in the 1980s, it seemed that the limits of our resources were being approached and that the health care system was being forced to consider options or alternatives to unrestricted growth and expansion.

Indeed, reimbursement policies introduced by Medicare and by health insurance plans in general have caused a decrease in the number of inpatient days provided by hospitals each year and an actual reduction in the operating size of most hospitals. The emphasis has been on doing less for patients rather than more. On all sides, there have been increasing pressures for smaller size, greater efficiency, and control of health care costs.

At the same time, the 1990s and early 2000s have witnessed the appearance of many new organizational pressures and models in health care, mostly as a result of forces generated by economic marketplace developments. Indeed, the use of the term *economic markets* with regard to health care would not have been widely accepted prior to the 1990s and not at all prior to the 1980s.

These new economic marketplace forces have spawned the growth of a wide variety of new organizational forms, both for-profit and nonprofit, that was previously unknown. The HMO that existed in relatively few sites in relatively small numbers throughout the country before the 1980s has given way to the broader "managed care plans" that are now present virtually throughout the country in great numbers and involve the majority of the population. (Indeed, "managed care" has become so important that a separate chapter of this book is devoted to that single subject.)

A variety of new enterprises have appeared to provide special services to patients and families at home, not only as a way of providing better services and answering to economic market forces for new products, but also as a way of reducing more expensive alternative services. Intermediary organizations have appeared to provide reviews of quality of patient care and appropriate utilization of services. The term *joint venture* has become an accepted part of our health care language, now used to describe new forms of partnership activities between previously separate components of the health care system: hospitals and physicians, insurance companies and pharmaceutical corporations, hospitals with other hospitals, and groups of physicians with other groups of physicians. Virtually no health care organizational model has been untouched by recent trends and changes in this latest phase of historical development in health care in the United States.

In order to fully understand the implications of this historical evolution of health care in the United States, this chapter will look at four separate topics across the time periods of the four phases of development. These topics are: (1) the predominant health problems that were the focus (targets) of the existing health system at the time; (2) the technology available to the health care system in each of the time periods; (3) the social organization of health care during these time periods; and (4) the involvement of the public in their health care and the system.

PREDOMINANT HEALTH PROBLEMS OF THE AMERICAN POPULATION

Since the dawn of recorded history, human beings have repeatedly suffered sudden and devastating epidemics of infectious disease. Plague, cholera, typhoid, smallpox, influenza, yellow fever, and a host of other diseases have raged almost at will, creating havoc wherever they struck.

During the period 1850–1900 in this country, these epidemics of acute infectious diseases were the health problem that drew the greatest attention from the then rather rudimentary health care system. Of particular importance were those diseases related to impure food, contaminated water supply, inadequate

sewage disposal, and the generally poor condition of urban housing. During this time, for example, a cholera epidemic occurred throughout the country, resulting in an official death toll of 5,071 in New York City alone and an unofficial toll several times higher. During this same period, yellow fever killed 9,000 in New Orleans in 1853, 2,500 in 1854 and 1855, and another 5,000 in 1858. Abraham Lincoln regularly sent his family away from the White House during the summer months in Washington, D.C. to escape the "fevers"—probably malaria—that swept through the city during those months. It can generally be said that the period 1850–1900 was a time in which the American health care system focused on epidemics of acute infectious diseases that were closely related to poor conditions of food, water, and housing.

By 1900, epidemics of acute infectious disease had generally been brought under control due to improved environmental conditions. In the latter years of the nineteenth century, cities had begun to develop systems for water purification, for sanitary disposal of sewage, for safeguarding the quality of milk and food, and for monitoring the quality of urban housing. Health departments had begun to grow in number and in strength and had begun to apply the methods of case finding and quarantine with satisfying results. Indeed, by 1990 those epidemics that had plagued humanity for centuries were eliminated as major causes of death in the United States.

After 1900, the predominant health problems that attracted the attention of the health care system were those acute events, either infectious or traumatic, that affected individuals one by one. The pendulum had swung away from epidemics of acute infection that affected large numbers of people in epidemics and toward conditions of a personal nature that required individualized treatment.

Relieved of the burden of epidemic illnesses, the newly developed medical sciences turned their attention to better surgical techniques, the discovery of new sera for the treatment of pneumonia, and the development of new tests for more accurate and rapid diagnoses. Hospitals began to grow rapidly, medical schools flourished, and there was a general air of excitement that suggested that the world was on the brink of significant advances in the treatment of individual illnesses.

Significant advances *were* being made. In Baltimore and Boston, the students of William Halsted, the pioneer surgeon at Johns Hopkins Hospital, began to operate on patients whose disease had previously been beyond the ability of surgeons. Advances in obstetrics now made it safer for women to have babies, and for the first time, women did not approach childbirth with a fear of dying in delivery. Research work by two physicians, Banting and Best, in the laboratories of the University of Toronto led to the discovery of insulin in 1922, and for the first time, diabetes could be effectively treated. Other research by Whipple, Minot, and Murphy on the causes of pernicious anemia led to successful medical treatments for that condition and further spurred the rush to find new treatments for other age-old conditions.

There were new discoveries on all fronts, each of which contributed some new advances in medical treatment. In 1928, however, in a cluttered laboratory at St. Mary's Hospital in London, a Scottish researcher, Alexander Fleming, produced the first of several discoveries that were to lead to the treatment of patients with penicillin for the first time in 1941. This discovery absolutely revolutionized medical care and totally changed the patterns of disease that threatened humanity. Within a few years after the treatment of the first patients with penicillin, antibiotics became readily available, and acute infections that had previously caused various illnesses and possible death now meant nothing more than the discomfort of an injection and a few days of disability. Many older people experienced the incredible effects of the antibiotic era; many of them had contracted pneumonia as children, and their families had admitted them to hospitals and prayed for their survival. Now, as older adults, they were told they had a "little pneumonia," given an injection of penicillin, and treated at home.

With the arrival of the antibiotic era in the 1940s and the subsequent conquest of acute infectious disease, the predominant problem for the American health care system became chronic illness. Because acute infections were no longer snuffing out the lives of children, people were living longer and beginning to manifest long-term chronic diseases such as heart disease, cancer, and stroke. As shown in Table 1.2, these three conditions alone now account for two-thirds of all deaths. A similar review of the causes of disability would show arthritis, blindness, arteriosclerosis, and other chronic diseases to be the predominant causes of morbidity and limitation of function.

The American health care system in the 1980s entered a new phase of organization that was accompanied by a sense of new predominant disease concerns. The rather sudden appearance of acquired immune deficiency syndrome (AIDS) in almost epidemic proportions in the early 1980s serves well to highlight the changing patterns of disease in this latest phase. AIDS is apparently initiated by a viral infection that triggers extensive damage to an individual's immune system, leading to susceptibility to other infections and to various forms of cancer. This combination of viral disease, immune system defects, and cancer as manifest in AIDS is probably only the first of many new combinations of disease causation we must face.

The Rising Importance of Chronic Illness

Chronic illness will certainly continue to be the predominant health problem of the American people in the future, but increasingly important will be chronic illness related to genetic makeup, personal lifestyles, and environmental hazards. Evidence is accumulating that would suggest that many important chronic illnesses are related to how we live our lives, what environmental hazards we subject ourselves to, and what genes we may have received from generations that preceded us.

Perhaps equally important are several kinds of chronic illnesses that have historically received very little attention and, in many instances, were not even considered "illnesses." The chronic mental illnesses, for example, are now only beginning to receive the attention that they deserve. These illnesses pose an enormous challenge for the health care system of the future. The rapid aging of the United States population makes it a certainty that a majority will live for at least eighty years, increasing the probability that they will need long-term care to help them handle the multiple physical and mental challenges of becoming

Table 1.2.   Death Rates for Leading Causes of Death in the United States, 1900 and 1996

1900		1996	
Causes of Death	**Crude Death Rate per 100,000 Population per Year**	**Causes of Death**	**Crude Death Rate per 100,000 Population per Year**
All causes	1,719.0	All causes	876.9
Pneumonia and influenza	202.2	Diseases of the heart	281.6
Tuberculosis	194.4	Malignant neoplasms	206.0
Diarrhea, enteritis, and		Cerebrovascular diseases	59.2
ulceration of the intestine	142.7	Chronic obstructive pulmonary	
Diseases of the heart	137.4	disease	39.1
Senility, ill-defined or unknown	117.5	Unintentional injuries	34.6
Intracranial lesions of vascular		Pneumonia and influenza	31.5
origin	109.6	Diabetes mellitus	21.2
Nephritis	88.6	Human immunodeficiency	
All accidents	72.3	virus infection	16.1
Cancer and other malignant tumors	64.0	Firearm injuries	15.2
Diphtheria	40.3	Suicide	12.4

SOURCES: *Vital Statistics of the United States, 1972,* Washington, D.C.: U.S. National Center for Health Statistics; *Health, United States 1996,* (Vol. II, Part A), Washington, D.C.: U.S. National Center for Health Statistics.

very old. These types of needs must now receive much more attention from the organized health care system.

Chronic illnesses have important characteristics that are different from acute illnesses and that will force a change in the way the American health care system deals with them. Chronic illnesses often begin early in life, long before overt symptoms appear and before medical attention is directed toward them. As a result, chronic illnesses have an opportunity to become firmly implanted before their actual symptoms call attention to their presence. For example, many studies of apparently healthy young people who were victims of automobile accidents or other sudden death have shown that large percentages have already begun to develop early signs of chronic illness detectable by pathological examination, but not yet by clinical tests. If the health care system is to be effective in preventing chronic illness, better methods for early detection need to be developed so that prevention and treatment can be initiated sooner.

The second major difference between chronic illness and acute illness is that once a chronic illness is present, it usually remains with the patient forever. Chronic illness is not cured by medical treatment, but rather its more prominent symptoms or external manifestations are treated. This means that an acute illness approach with its focus on "cure" over a period of short, intensive treatment no longer provides an appropriate paradigm for the treatment of chronic illness with its long-term and continuing presence. The acute illness treatment model is simply not suitable for many current chronic illnesses.

The Importance of Prevention

In the same fashion, our thinking with regard to prevention requires significant change to deal with chronic illnesses. Acute illnesses very conveniently have a clear-cut beginning, middle, and end; as a result, they are often amenable to one-shot solutions. If there is an epidemic caused by the contamination of the water supply, the construction of a sewage treatment facility will eliminate it completely. If there is a threat of polio infection, the use of polio vaccine once or twice will permanently protect a population.

With chronic illnesses, however, prevention cannot be a one-shot affair. Arteriosclerotic heart disease, for example, begins early in life and is probably affected by diet, cigarette smoking, stress, obesity, and several other factors that are directly related to personal habits and lifestyle. Prevention of these conditions cannot be accomplished by giving a person a single lecture on the evils of high cholesterol food or the dangers of heavy cigarette consumption. Rather, prevention must be long-term, continuous, and aimed at bringing about major changes in an individual's knowledge of disease, personal values, and behavioral patterns.

Optimal prevention and treatment for long-term, continuous illness will require a system of health care that is in itself long-term and continuous. Unfortunately, the organization of our health services is still modeled on the disease patterns that were predominant in the 1900–1945 period and concentrates on individual episodes of illness as if they were separate and distinct entities. As a result, the focus of the American health care system is primarily short-term and discontinuous in nature, and it treats chronic illness as if it were merely a series of separate and acute episodes. This trend is further reinforced by the current method of financing health care services, with its great emphasis on paying for and providing individual episodes of care, rendered as individual services, rather than on a long-term, continuous series of services coordinated around the needs of a long-term continuous illness.

It should be noted that the growth of managed care, with its emphasis on payment for services on a *per capita* basis rather than for individual services, may make it easier to develop programs of care that are longer term and continuous. Unfortunately, many of the new managed care insurance plans and their providers still have a short-term view of their beneficiaries who typically tend to change health plans frequently, thereby destroying any sense of long-term relationship. The increased emphasis on the use of managed care plans for the elderly under Medicare

may provide a stronger long-term focus within managed care and may allow managed care plans to develop strategies that are more appropriate to the chronic illness model.

A Challenging Future

It is entirely possible (and, indeed, probable) that the nation's predominant disease patterns will be changing again in the future, creating an entirely different set of conditions that may require an entirely different array of services and interventions. It will be important for future generations of health professionals to watch for changes in the major disease patterns to ensure a health care system that is genuinely appropriate and responsive to the problems of the day.

TECHNOLOGY AVAILABLE TO THE AMERICAN PEOPLE

During the various developmental periods of the American health care system, technology was available in different degrees to handle the diseases that affected the American people.

In the period 1850–1900, only a rudimentary technology was available for the treatment of disease. The scientific base of medicine was still very narrow, and the number of effective medical treatments was very limited. Indeed, a great deal of energy and effort was expended on treatment, but whether a patient recovered from an illness usually depended more on the patient and the disease than on the treatment.

Physicians during this period were poorly trained. They usually developed their skills by serving apprenticeships with physicians already in practice and then taking short courses at unsophisticated medical colleges. What physicians had to offer was usually contained in the black bags they took with them wherever they went. They spent a good deal of time in patients' homes and almost no time at all in the hospitals. In general, their practice was little different from that of their predecessors for centuries before them.

Nurses during the period 1850–1900 were not much better trained. Generally they were members of religious groups who volunteered to work in the few hospitals that existed, or they were poor, desperate, discarded women who frequented these institutions anyway and were pressed into service. Their work was nonscientific in the extreme and consisted simply of assisting patients with their usual bodily functions in any way possible. Not until the first training program for nurses was organized at Bellevue Hospital in the 1860s was there any formal preparation anywhere in the country for this important role.

Hospitals themselves were merely places of shelter and repose for the sick poor who could not be cared for at home. Anyone who could stay at home usually did so, since hospitals had little to offer that could not be obtained at home if one had the money. Indeed, the hospitals of those days were often a direct threat to the lives of patients: they were dirty, crowded, and disease-ridden. Infectious diseases frequently spread rapidly among hospitalized patients; during the typhus epidemics of 1852 in New York City, for example, the highest mortality for the disease was among the patients and staff of the hospitals themselves.

After 1900, conditions began to change, spurred on by new discoveries that were emerging from the research laboratories in this country and in Europe. In 1912, for example, a Polish chemist, Casimir Funk, published a paper, "The Etiology of Deficiency Diseases," in which he described "vitamines" and opened a whole new field of disease conditions to treatment. In 1908, James MacKenzie, in London, published his famous book, *Diseases of the Heart*, and patients throughout the world were the beneficiaries. In countless medical schools and hospitals throughout this country and Europe, major scientific advances were achieved, each of which contributed to easier and safer diagnosis and treatment of acutely ill patients.

The medical schools led the way in many of these advances as a result of some basic reforms that took place in the early 1900s. Before this time, a large number of small, poorly staffed, free-standing medical colleges existed throughout the country—fourteen in Chicago alone in 1910, and ten each in Missouri and Tennessee. In 1910, Abraham Flexner undertook a study of medical education for the Carnegie Foundation for the Advancement of Teaching and, in his report, *Medical Education in the United States and Canada*, recommended that medical education in this country

undergo radical reform. In particular, he strongly urged that the training of physicians be made a university function and that it be based on a firm scientific foundation. On the basis of Flexner's recommendations and the support of the Rockefeller Foundation, many of the small, unaffiliated schools began to close and many of the remaining ones became part of universities, with the important result that physicians began to be trained as scientists as well as practitioners.

Gradually, physicians began to have more effective tools with which to work, and the range of their capabilities expanded rapidly. They still continued to spend the majority of their time in their offices or their patients' homes, but they now also began to look to the hospital for the care of their more severely ill patients. The growth of radiology diagnosis during this period is a classic example of the new technology that physicians had available to them; it also emphasizes the new and growing importance of the hospital as the place where this new technology was available.

Hospitals and Technology

Hospitals in the 1900s began to play an increasingly important role in health care. As more technology developed, it tended to be concentrated in hospitals, with the result that patients and physicians began going to hospitals for the technology to be found there. St Luke's Hospital in New York City, for example, was fifty years old in 1906 when it opened its first private patient pavilion. Before that time, there had been no reason for private patients to go to a hospital because they could usually get the same type of care in their homes. Now, however, hospitals began to offer services and skills that were not available anywhere else.

Although the period 1900–1940 was one of rapid growth in scientific technology, it was nothing compared to what happened with the advent of World War II. With the start of the war, this country mounted a massive effort to organize the best talents available for the care of the wounded and for the solution of health care problems generated by the war. For the first time, relatively large efforts in research were begun under the direction of the federal government, and the results were impressive. The development of antibiotics accelerated rapidly, new surgical techniques for the treatment of trauma and burns were discovered, and new approaches to the transportation of the sick and wounded were developed.

The range and breadth of problems that were subjected to organized investigation were remarkable, opening the way for an even more greatly expanded research effort after the war ended. In 1950, the size of the research commitment begun during World War II rose to $73 million per year, $35 million of which was distributed through the National Institutes of Health (NIH). By 1974, only twenty-four years later, this expenditure had risen to an annual research budget of $2.5 billion, with $1.6 billion coming from a now greatly expanded NIH.

After World War II, hospitals were no longer the same. Previously, they had been places for the care of patients, with great emphasis being placed on the caring function. Now they became extensions of research laboratories, places where medical science was practiced and where curing was the order of the day. New procedures, new equipment, and new techniques all flourished to such a degree that the hospitals were now captured by their technology. The technology itself became the motivating force for hospitals, and most major decisions were based on that technology and its use.

The operation of these newly complex institutions called for waves of new workers, each more specialized and more highly skilled than the last. Before the war, there had been approximately twenty major categories of health care workers; by the 1970s, there were hundreds. With the increasing specialization of services and skills, there was also an increasing interdependence of health care workers on each other and an increasing reliance on the health care system to integrate the work of so many separate groups.

Technology, Physicians, and Medical Care

Physicians were seriously affected by these trends. With the explosive growth of scientific knowledge after World War II, it was impossible for one physician to know everything, and so the trend toward specialization in a particular subarea of medicine had a strong impetus. Before the war, approximately eighty percent of physicians had been general practitioners and twenty percent specialists. In the years after the war, these percentages were reversed. In their training and practice, physicians increasingly focused on the scientific aspects of diagnosis and treatment and, as a result, spent more time in hospitals and less time in patients' homes. The hospital became the emotional center of the physician's life because it was there that the most important, the most challenging, and most rewarding aspects of training and treatment occurred.

These trends affected nursing and the other health care professions as well. The training of nurses and other health care professionals became increasingly more scientific, more specialized, and more lengthy during the years after World War II. The desire to be recognized as competent in a particular area led to the proliferation of professional groups and to formal accreditation on the basis of scientific training and ability. It also led to university training programs in all of the health care professions.

In the latest period of evolution of the American health care system, the technology available to the American people has advanced to an incredible degree. Organ transplantation, gene therapies for various conditions, laser beams, and fiber optic surgical techniques are all accepted as merely the expected developments of the technological age. The merging of technologies from fields other than medicine, such as the development of computerized axial tomographic systems and magnetic resonance imaging systems, has further added to the immense range of technology available to the health care system. This explosion of technology in recent years, however, has not been without its problems. Indeed, the technology itself has *caused* a rather serious set of problems with which present and future generations of health care professionals must grapple.

Complex Issues Involving Technology

One important problem with medical technology is its impact on the form and configuration of the health care system and on the values, patterns, and practice of the professionals in the system. In many ways, the American health services system has been captured by its technology and has been subtly and seductively shaped by its demands. Decisions regarding the design of programs and institutions, the training of personnel, and the distribution of services have been governed by technological considerations that loom larger every year.

A still more profound effect of technology is its ability to insinuate itself into the values of not just the system but also of the people who work in the system. The student entering a health profession rapidly learns that academic success and, later, professional success comes from mastery of the scientific technology. Increasingly, the student is taught to view excellence as being reached through technical achievements and, as a result, inadvertently taught to give decreasing importance to the more personal, nontechnical aspects of disease. By the time the student becomes a fully accepted member of the profession, a value system may have been established that views illness as a series of technical problems to be solved by the application of specific technical solutions. This value system is then reinforced in practice by the expectations of the public and by the requirements of the regulators, both of whom have come to view quality in terms of technical excellence. The result frequently is professional performance that is excellent in technical terms and occasionally rather poor in human terms.

A quite different problem of technology arises not from its excessiveness but rather from its inequitable distribution to society. There is more technology available than can be provided equitably to all people due to limits on funding. Large portions of society do not benefit as much as they should from technological advances. Marked differences exist, for example, in mortality and morbidity measures for white versus nonwhite segments of society, possibly indicating an unequal access to modern health care technology. The answer obviously is to improve the health services system to ensure adequate distribution of available resources. But there has been relatively little movement in that direction, and the gap in equality of access to modern technology has probably widened rather than narrowed in recent years.

Indeed, the costs of the new technology have been one of the most important and difficult problems for the American health care system to face in this latest phase of its historical development. Expenditures for health care in the United States at the beginning of the twenty-first century have exceed fourteen percent of the country's gross domestic product (GDP). A large part of the increase in health care expenditures has been attributed to technology. As attempts are made to control the rising expenditures on health care, attention has naturally turned toward controlling the use of modern technology. The theory here is that if the use of modern technology, which had previously been widely available, could be reduced, the total expenditures for health care would in similar fashion be reduced (or at least would not increase as rapidly). According to this theory, modern technology is seen as extremely expensive, and its usage should be reduced or at least controlled more closely.

One interesting outcome of the attempts to use technology more carefully has been a growing interest in the evaluation of various new discoveries and techniques. In the past, many new technologies were adopted without appropriate evaluation of how effective they really were or, even more important, how much *more* effective they would be than already existing technology. Only limited examination of the cost implications of new technology was attempted. Now, the evaluation of new technology and its costs, and the comparison of the benefits of a new technology with the costs attendant to its use, have become much more common. In this latest period of health care evolution, with marketplace forces attempting to reduce (or at least rationalize) the use of services, it is increasingly common to read articles in leading scientific journals on the cost-benefit and cost-effectiveness analyses of new scientific or technical developments.

In summary, virtually no technology was available to treat disease before the 1900s. New technology began to appear and grow rapidly after the turn of the century. World War II fostered an incredible surge of research endeavors that were assisted after the war by major financial support for research provided by the National Institutes of Health. By the year 2001, technology has become such a major driving force in the American health care system, and such a major contributor to rising expenditures for health care, that its use is being challenged, primarily to reduce the use of technology or at least to control its growth. In this latest period of historical development of the American health care system, the emphasis on technology is no longer on unhindered growth and expansion, but rather on careful evaluation and controlled use and availability. At the same time that the use of technology is a subject for control and possible reduction, the number of people in the American population with limited access to technology has continued to grow.

SOCIAL ORGANIZATION OF HEALTH CARE IN THE UNITED STATES

In the four periods of historical evolution of health care in the United States, how has our society organized to use the health resources available to it? What has been the predominant ideology of social organization that has controlled the shaping and the functioning of the health care system? How has that social ideology changed over the various periods of evolution?

During the period 1850–1900, the social organization of health care in the United States was quite loose and simple. Public services were rudimentary and were concentrated on a very narrow range of problems. There were hospitals in a few areas, but they were generally started by religious or charitable groups for the care of those who were obviously and publicly impoverished. The predominant ethic of the time was that people should care for themselves and be self-sufficient. If they were to become dependent, they should take advantage of and be grateful for the various charities established for these purposes. Society did not believe that it had an obligation either to provide health services to the population or to ensure that the population received the services that it needed.

This philosophy of rugged individualism and relative lack of large-scale social organization for health care began to change somewhat in the early 1900s with the development of local efforts to provide care for people through city and county hospitals. Although there was virtually nothing of a national effort to effect the availability and distribution of health services and very little done by individual state governments, city and county governments, particularly those in large cities with large numbers of poor people, realized that something had to be done to provide care for those who otherwise could not obtain it. These local efforts were almost the only social stirrings of policy in the health area until the Great Depression of the 1930s struck with full force.

The Changing Social Role of Government

Prior to the Great Depression, the prevailing social ideology held that health care (and many other matters of social survival) were a concern of individual citizens and that government should intervene as little as possible. When economic forces beyond the comprehension of most Americans struck down many people, destroying their lives and leaving them destitute, this thinking began to change. With the arrival of Franklin Roosevelt in the White House, the New Deal was launched and a wide array of social programs appeared, all aimed at repairing the damage of the Depression. The importance of the New Deal in terms of changing American social ideology cannot be underestimated. For the first time, American society created large-scale national programs to assist those who could not assist themselves.

In health care, federal governmental activity was still minimal and limited to a few specific areas of grant-in-aid programs to states to improve certain public health services such as infectious disease control and maternal and child health. Although the services were limited and aimed primarily at the poor, this small start did signify at least a partial assumption of responsibility by the national government for the health of the public, at least in certain specific areas. It is interesting to note that proposals were made to President Roosevelt to develop a universal health insurance system connected with the Social Security program that was actively being developed, but Roosevelt decided that the addition of universal health insurance coverage would arouse too much opposition and would endanger the passage of the entire Social Security effort.

The arrival of World War II brought with it a major change in social organization, and social thinking in general, in the United States and also planted the seeds for some significant changes in social thinking about health care. As part of the mobilization effort for the war, millions of men and women entered the military service and, as a result, received a wide variety of health services simply by virtue of joining the military. The significance was twofold: (1) for many people in the United States, it was the first time that they had easy accessibility to a wide range of modern health services, and they began to realize the value and the benefits of having such services available; and (2) the services were provided as a right of those in the military—they were clearly not charity for people who could no longer take care of themselves, but rather came as a condition of work or service in the military.

The Growth of Health Insurance

Not only did World War II accustom the country to large-scale health care programs provided by society to its members, it also encouraged the growth of the health insurance industry. During the war a freeze was imposed on wages and salaries so that very little collective bargaining for increases in salary could occur. Considerable activity did occur in the development of pensions, disability programs, and health insurance plans, however, with the result that the private health insurance industry began to flourish. This industry provided the American public with a new form of social organization: the health insurance company or organization. Before the development of private health insurance, the public had no form of social organization to protect it from a sudden onslaught of medical bills. With the arrival of this new phenomenon—health insurance—the American public began to gain experience in the voluntary cooperative effort of pooling many individual contributions for a common group objective: protection from financial disaster.

The period immediately after World War II witnessed the growth of health insurance plans of both the nonprofit and the for-profit nature. The early Blue Cross and Blue Shield plans were started by voluntary hospital groups (Blue Cross) and state medical societies (Blue Shield). With the success and growth of Blue Cross and Blue Shield, commercial insurance companies also entered the field, offering health insurance plans to employers and industries as part of

their life/health/retirement/disability packages. With the rapid advances made by Blue Cross/Blue Shield and the commercial insurance carriers, the percentage of Americans covered by some form of health insurance rose from less than twenty percent at the end of World War II to over seventy percent by the year 2001.

The Acceleration of Government in Health Care Funding

In the early 1960s, a major battle was fought and won by those advocating a greater societal role in the organization of health care services. The battle involved the creation of government-sponsored health insurance plans for people over the age of sixty-five and resulted in the passage of legislation that created Medicare. Although Medicare itself was directed primarily to the needs of the country's elderly, its impact was soon felt throughout the entire health care system. The creation of the Medicare program had two immediate major social implications. First, Medicare provided financing for health care for all persons over the age of sixty-five simply on the basis of age; need was not a factor. American society, in effect, determined that there were certain things that society should do for all its members, regardless of individual needs, since society could ensure equity.

The second major effect of Medicare was the assumption by the federal government of the responsibility for planning, financing, and monitoring a significant portion of the health care services in this country. Society not only wanted social insurance programs for health care, but also wanted the federal government to assume a central role in operating these programs. In one legislative stroke, not only was a massive new program of health insurance coverage developed for an important segment of the American citizenry, but the federal government was given direct responsibility for that program and for the financial resources that were made available to it.

Either one of these developments would have been significant alone, but the two together (that is, the creation of a health insurance plan for the elderly in the United States and the assignment of the responsibility for that plan to the federal government) rather suddenly made the federal government a dominant force in shaping the organization and operation of health care in the United States after 1965.

A further significant change in the social organization of health care in this country involving the federal government came in the mid-1960s with the development of the Neighborhood Health Centers program of the United States Office of Economic Opportunity ("War on Poverty"). In this effort, a number of health programs were funded for underserved areas of the country by the federal government, each of which was required to have significant participation of consumers through governing boards and committees. This involvement of consumers of health care in the operation of the programs providing them with care was a substantial change from the thinking of the past, and soon became standard policy in new governmental programs, awakening people to the possibility of being directly involved in the operation and direction of health programs that had previously been considered the sole prerogative of health care professionals.

This philosophy was vigorously put forward in the National Health Planning and Resources Development Act of 1974, which required a majority of consumers on all local health planning boards. Although the health planning effort in this country has since been dismantled to a large degree, the involvement of consumer advocates in health policy matters was born and continues to be an increasingly important aspect of the United States health care system.

In short, the period from the end of the second world war to the early 1980s was marked by a rapid growth of national governmental involvement in the health care system as a result of the passage of Medicare. It put the federal government in charge of the single largest source of financing for health care in the United States and, almost overnight, completely reversed the lack of federal government involvement in the organization and delivery of health services. Indeed, during this period of historical evolution of health care in the United States, it was felt that there was a strong possibility that the United States might develop a national health insurance plan for all of its people, thereby giving the national government even greater control of the health care system and its functioning.

The Move to Limited Resources

In the early 1980s, the health care system of this country entered a fourth phase of its development, an era of resource limitation, restriction of growth, and reorganization of systems of financing for providing care. This was also a period in which general market forces began to play in health care throughout the country and to transform the system of financing and providing services in major ways.

In the early 1980s, with the federal Medicare program experiencing major increases in expenditure every year, interest began to shift toward a possible reduction of benefits, greater cost sharing by the elderly themselves, and a limitation on reimbursements to providers of service. Legislative observers of Medicare now began to fear for its long-term existence, with its present generous reimbursement and financing arrangements, and energy now became focused less on the development of new services or the expansion of coverage than on the control of costs through limitations and reductions. Changes in the manner in which Medicare reimbursed hospitals (by the use of prospective payment and "diagnosis-related groups") were designed to encourage hospitals and doctors to provide less in the way of services and to curtail or limit the number of services provided. This change of policy on the part of Medicare led to a reduction in admissions to hospitals and a great decrease in length of stay within hospitals, both of which led to a gradual shrinkage in the actual supply of operating hospital beds in the United States.

These developments were paralleled in the private sector by the realization of employers that their rapidly rising health care expenditures were a major threat to the long-term existence of their companies. With this understanding, private employers began to look for ways to curtail health benefits and to reduce the rise in their health insurance expenditures. Their efforts have included becoming much more aggressive in seeking lower cost insurance coverage when purchasing insurance as well as moving their employees into new forms of health insurance, such as managed care, that promise better cost and utilization control. In a very short period of time, the private sector in the United States has taken on a much more aggressive posture with regard to health care and health insurance, demanding lower prices and lower premiums in exchange for its continuing business.

In a remarkable and ironic development, the period since 1980 has seen the federal government and Congress talking about "health care reform" (with a possible objective of expanding benefits and coverage) while the private sector has aggressively carried out its own health care reforms that have rested largely on reduced coverage, reduced choices, and lower prices. The initial success of the private sector's efforts was demonstrated by national health care expenditures for private health care in 1995, which increased only 2.9 percent over the previous year, just about equivalent to the rate of inflation, while public sector (particularly Medicare and Medicaid) spending increased by 8.9 percent. It has become obvious that the private sector's cost containment efforts have worked for the private sector and have not worked for the public sector, at least until recent years.

In the period immediately following World War II, the federal government assumed a central role in health care financing, planning, policy, and regulation and seemed to be on its way to being the sole social organizing force for health care in the United States. The federal government controlled a significant portion of the financial support for health care (more than one-third of the total health care expenditures from all sources). By using these massive resources, the federal government set many of the rules by which health care, governmentally funded or not, was provided. It seemed that the health care system of this country, although by no means federally operated, was certainly going to be federally dominated or influenced.

In more recent years, the role of the private sector in reducing health care costs and controlling the use of services has become much more important, and in many states, such as California, is the predominant force shaping delivery of services. Although the role of the federal government and its programs remains massive, the more aggressive and effective shaping of the health care system in these states (and potentially throughout the country) may now have shifted the focus to the private sector, and particularly to employers who provide health insurance benefits and ac-

count for approximately one-third of the health care financing for this country.

In summary, with regard to social organization, the United States entered the twentieth century with a social philosophy that said that people should care for themselves or be satisfied with charity. After 1900, local governments became involved in providing some care for the indigent through local city and county hospitals, but federal and state governments played virtually no role at all. The limited federal role in health care is reflected in the absence of a federal cabinet level health department until 1953, when the Department of Health, Education, and Welfare was created.

With the passage and implementation of Medicare in 1965, it seemed as if the federal government would rapidly take on responsibility for the direction and control of health care in the United States in an almost unchallenged manner. But in the 1980s, private employers began to use their economic power and leverage to reduce health care utilization and costs in ways that the federal government had not imagined. The situation now suggests that the social organization and control of health care in the near future, if not necessarily in the distant future, will be shared between the federal government (operating primarily through its control of the Medicare and Medicaid programs) and the private sector (operating through its control of employer-provided health insurance).

INVOLVEMENT OF THE PEOPLE IN THEIR HEALTH AND HEALTH CARE

In the period from 1850 to 1900, a curious paradox seems to have occurred. People had almost no reliable information to guide them in their health care and, at the same time, they were probably more involved in health care than at any time since then. The reasons for this seeming paradox are simple to understand.

In the period of 1850 to 1900, the general level of education of the public was quite low. A high school education (let alone a college or university education) was somewhat rare. When it came to matters of health, even professionals had little factual scientific information on which to base their treatments. It should be no surprise that the general public had even less knowledge and insight than health care practitioners.

On the other hand, family members were the primary caregivers to the sick and were intimately involved in health matters, perhaps more intimately involved than they have been ever since. There were no hospitals or clinics to which sick patients could be taken (and left), medical practitioners were poorly trained and unreliable, and pharmaceuticals available at the time were mostly herbal remedies of little proven scientific value. Faced with these circumstances, the public was directly involved in health care and was as poorly prepared for this role as health service providers themselves.

By 1900, several important parts of this equation began to change. First of all, the general level of education of the public began to improve. Second, as the years went by, more information about health and illness began to be available to the public through the rapidly expanding media (at first, newspapers and magazines; later on, books and radio).

Probably most important, however, was the rapidly improving quality of, and access to, hospitals and better-trained physicians. The period after 1900 saw rapid improvements in the supply and quality of hospitals, as well as the appearance of a "new" medical science that rapidly caught the attention of the public. The last of these developments seems to have been the most important, with the apparent result that the public turned away from their own efforts to provide care to their sick family members and began to depend more and more on physicians and hospitals to do the job for them. One important implication here is that while the public seemed to have more information at its disposal, it was awed by scientific developments and less independent in its thinking.

World War II was very important to the development of an involved and informed American public for a number of reasons. For the first time, many Americans had access to regular health care and could appreciate its value. Prior to their induction into military service, many Americans had rarely (or never) seen a physician of their own and believed that health care was an unattainable luxury. Now they had

a chance to provide themselves with health services as a normal part of life.

There was a considerable attempt to educate both those entering the military and those remaining at home in the complexities of simple medical care and the ways in which the body actually worked. Military personnel received basic education and training in first aid and treatment of injuries and wounds, as well as the causes and cures of sexually transmitted diseases. Those at home who were living with a growing shortage of physicians and nurses received extensive educational training by the Red Cross in caring for their families and themselves. A small group of enlisted persons were given the chance to enter health care work as hospital corpsmen, beginning an active participation in the health care system which often lasted a lifetime.

The period immediately after the end of World War II saw a number of developments that increased the public's involvement in health care. First, the rapid development of television as a new medium of communication brought health and medical information directly into the homes of ordinary people all across the country. The explosive expansion of other media, such as magazines and inexpensive books, also expanded the knowledge base of the public. Parallel to this growing public knowledge about health care and its intricacies was a growing sense of health care as a social and political issue—an area in which the public could participate for the first time. With the movement toward Medicare as an issue of general political debate in the 1960s, the financing and organization of health care came within easy range of public interest and involvement. Slogans like "Health care is a right, not a privilege" and "Maximum feasible participation of the poor" (which came from the War on Poverty), as well as the requirement for direct public participation in the short-lived health planning system that developed in the 1970s, also reflected the public's taste for involvement.

In the 1980s and 1990s, the American public had become fully and directly concerned about, and involved in, health care issues. One factor in this involvement was enormous interest in physical fitness, jogging, and exercise in general, as well as an increased concern about diet and environmental issues. Although much of this activity may have been generated by a concern with personal appearance, the mental and physical health benefits were readily apparent and appreciated. Added to this was the revolutionary development of the Internet and other forms of digital media that bring a wealth of information and guidance to ordinary people in their own homes. Americans can now get more and better scientific information about health and health care than was available to medical practitioners themselves only a few years ago.

This rapid expansion of public knowledge and interest about health care has been accompanied by an increasing rigidity in the health care system that makes individual involvement more difficult. The rise of managed care and the increase in bureaucratic barriers to full public access to providers and treatments they think they deserve has caused a growing resentment among many toward the administrative complexity of the system itself. The public generally feels that it is more educated and more motivated to be active partners with the health care system at a time when that system has seemingly become less able to involve it directly. To its credit, the managed care industry has taken major steps to develop new information and communication systems to let people play a more active and involved role in their health care, but those efforts are still preliminary and the long-term results remain to be seen.

In summary, the involvement of the public in their own health and health care has come a long way since 1850. People are better educated and more motivated to participate, realize that they can participate, and are looking for ways to increase their participation. They understand that much of health care now is a major political issue that will be settled not in the doctor's office or hospital bed, but in elections and legislative actions. Finally, the public has a taste and appreciation for the best in health care but have little desire to pay more for it, as they are increasingly being asked to do. Because of these conflicts and energies, it is generally agreed that the public will play an increasingly important role in all aspects of health care in the years ahead.

A SUMMARY OF THE EVOLUTION OF HEALTH CARE IN THE UNITED STATES

An analysis of health care in the United States since 1850 makes it clear that our system has been continuously evolving for more than one hundred and fifty years. It has evolved in keeping with our scientific excellence, our social condition, our economic prosperity, and our political maturity. It will continue to evolve in the years ahead, with each level of development building on the previous one. Many of the underlying forces will remain the same, but many will be new and may impel our system in directions different from those we follow today.

One thing, however, is clear: To prepare for the future, it is imperative to understand the past. Where we have been as a system in the past will give us clues as to where we will go in the future.

CHAPTER
2

Overview of the Organization
of Health Services in the United States

Paul R. Torrens and Contributors*

Chapter Topics

- Ways of Looking at Health Care Organizations
- Health Services: A Summary of Perspectives
- Health Care Systems in Two Markets
- Assessing the Burden of Disease in Los Angeles County

*Portions of this chapter are reprinted with permission of the Center for Studying Health System Change, Washington DC, and adapted, with permission, from the Los Angeles County Department of Health Services and the UCLA Center for Health Policy Research, The Burden of Disease in Los Angeles County, January, 2000.

Learning Objectives

Upon completing this chapter, the reader should be able to:

- Apply three analytical models in examining health care systems in this country or abroad
- Describe a larger health care system in terms of the various subsystems that comprise it and serve different subsections of the population
- Describe a health care system in terms of its impact on the health status of the population being served
- Apply new measures of population health such as QALYs (quality adjusted life years) or DALYs (disability adjusted life years) as measures of a health system's effectiveness in improving health
- Describe a health system in terms of what is happening to the entire combination of patients, providers, and payors by looking at an entire market area as a single entity
- Explain how all parts of a health care system are related to each other and have a major impact on each other

The American health care system can be examined from three important perspectives. The first focuses on an understanding of its internal organization; the second, on an understanding of its impact on the health of the population it serves; and the third, on an understanding that all parts of the system within a market area are related to each other in important ways. The health care professional of the future will have to be capable of carrying out each of these types of analyses if internal efficiency and external effectiveness are to be maintained and improved.

In the previous chapter, the historical evolution of health care in the United States was reviewed in order to gain perspective about how the present structure and organization of our health care has come about. This chapter will present ways of looking at that organizational structure in order to gain a better idea of why the American health care system does some things very well and other things very poorly. Following this chapter, the remaining sections of this book will explore in more detail the individual component parts and how they relate to the overall system.

WAYS OF LOOKING AT HEALTH CARE ORGANIZATIONS

There are several ways of analyzing the organization of health care in this country or any country. This chapter will analyze our health care system from the point of view of different subgroups in our population and how they get their care. Not all Americans receive their health care in the same way or even from the same parts of the health care system, so it is useful to compare and contrast how different subgroups in our population are served. This is a method that can also be applied to other countries of the world; there are very few (if any) where a single health system provides all the care for all the people.

Development of Systems of Care

When visitors from abroad come to the United States, they frequently want to know about *the* American health care system and how it works, implying that there is a single system that describes all health care organization in this country. They are frequently puzzled when they learn that there is not a single American health care system, but rather a series of separate subsystems that serve different populations in different ways. Sometimes these subsystems overlap; sometimes they are entirely separate. Sometimes they are supported with private funds, sometimes with public funds, and sometimes with a mixture of both. Sometimes several different subsystems use the same facilities, but sometimes they use facilities and personnel that are entirely separate and distinct.

It should not be surprising that a multiplicity of health care systems (or subsystems) are present in the United States, given the historical development of health services in this country. In the earliest days, health care was entirely a private matter, and people were expected to take care of themselves by obtaining the services of private physicians and nurses when needed, purchasing medications from drugstores and chemist shops, and paying for all these services personally. For those persons who could not take care of themselves, charitable institutions were established as voluntary, nonprofit corporations to provide charity health care. These groups usually centered their efforts on hospitals and usually were located in larger towns and cities.

In the early twentieth century, a new element was added with the development of city/county hospitals. These hospitals were established by local governments to care for the poor in their area who could not get care either by their own efforts or from the voluntary nonprofit charity hospitals. These public facilities were generally large, acute care general hospitals, with busy clinics and emergency rooms and close connections to local government ambulance services, police departments, and other community services. At the same time, state governments were developing mental hospitals. Cities had previously been responsible for the care of lunatics and the insane, but after the turn of the century, state governments began to assume this burden. Every state soon had at least one mental hospital where the emotionally disturbed were offered what little care was available.

With the explosive growth in the size of the federal government and in the numbers of persons in the armed forces during World War II, separate systems of care developed for active-duty military personnel and their dependents, retired military personnel, and veterans. These were almost entirely self-contained systems, employing salaried physicians and nurses working entirely in military or veterans hospitals directly operated by the federal government.

As the cost of health care began to increase rapidly after World War II, the United States experienced a sudden and bewildering development of a wide variety of health insurance plans. The first to be operated were community-based, nonprofit Blue Cross and Blue Shield plans, developed by hospital and physician associations to spread the cost of health care more widely among the population. These were followed by labor union health and welfare trust funds, established as a consequence of benefit negotiations for union members. At the same time, the private, for-profit commercial insurance companies expanded their efforts on behalf of both individuals and large groups of employees. Finally, several large government-sponsored and publicly supervised health insurance plans evolved, such as Medicare and Medicaid, the latter to aid the medically indigent.

Private medical practitioners, voluntary non-profit hospitals, city and state government hospitals, military and veterans' hospitals, and health insurance plans with a variety of forms and origins all developed in the United States at the same time, separately and for specific purposes. The resulting picture has been described as having a rich diversity of opportunities and approaches for meeting the health care needs of a population that has in itself a rich diversity of people and situations. It has also been described as chaotic, uncoordinated, overlapping, unplanned, and wasteful of precious personal and financial resources. The reality probably lies somewhere in between.

If there is no single, easily described American health care system, at least some of the subsystems that compose the larger entity can be identified. Although an endless set of variations is possible, it seems appropriate to examine four models or subsystems of health care in the United States, each of which serves a different group. By looking at the components, the system as a whole may be better understood. These systems serve (1) regularly employed, middle-income families with a continuous program of health insurance coverage; (2) poor, unemployed (or underemployed) families without continuous health insurance coverage; (3) active-duty military personnel and their dependents; and (4) veterans of United States military service.

For each of these systems, the manner in which basic elements of health care are provided will be reviewed. These basic elements of a health care system are given in Table 2.1, and include all the services from health promotion/disease prevention services to ambulatory-patient services for simple and complex illness, inpatient services for simple and complex illness, long-term care, rehabilitation, mental health services, dental care, and pharmaceutical/supplies/medical equipment. For each of the subsystems mentioned, the pattern by which a patient/subgroup member obtains care will be described. As the description proceeds, the variation in the sources of care for the same element of care will become apparent.

Employed, Insured, Middle-Income America (Private Practice, Private Insurance)

It is appropriate for two reasons to consider the system of health care used by the typically employed, insured, middle-income individual or family. First, this system is frequently described as *the* American health

Table 2.1. Basic Service Components of a Health Care System

- Health promotion and disease prevention services
- Emergency medical services (including transportation)
- Ambulatory care for simple/limited conditions
- Ambulatory care for complex/continuing conditions
- Inpatient care for single/limited inpatient conditions
- Inpatient care for complex/multiple inpatient conditions
- Long-term care (either in-home or institutional services)
- Services for social/psychological conditions (both inpatient and ambulatory)
- Rehabilitation services (both inpatient and ambulatory)
- Dental services
- Pharmaceutical services

care system (all others, therefore, immediately becoming somehow secondary to it); second, this system is frequently said to include the best medical care available in the United States and perhaps the world.

The most striking feature of the employed, insured, middle-income system of care is the absence of any *formal* system. Each family puts together an *informal* set of services and facilities to meet its own needs. The system, therefore, has no formal structure or organization and is different for each individual or family. Indeed, each family's system may vary widely according to the particular situation in which it is used. The only constant feature of this system is the family itself; all other aspects are transient, changeable, and widely varied.

Two other characteristics are also noteworthy. First, the service aspects of the system focus on, and are coordinated by, physicians in private practice. Second, the system is financed by personal, nongovernmental funds, whether paid directly by consumers or through private health insurance plans, including managed care plans. As the system is described, it will become readily apparent that not only are these two features important descriptively, but they have been important in shaping the system in its present form.

Public health and preventive medicine services for the employed, insured, middle-income system are provided by two different sources. Those services designed to protect large numbers of people, such as water purification, sewage disposal, and air pollution control, are provided by local or state governmental agencies. Frequently these agencies are called *public health departments.* They usually provide their services to the entire population of a region, with no distinction between rich and poor, simple and sophisticated, interested and disinterested. Indeed, these mass public health services are common to all the systems of health care to be discussed. Those public health and preventive medicine services that are aimed at individuals, such as well-baby examinations, cervical cancer smears, vaccinations, and family planning, are provided by individual physicians in private practice. If a middle-income family desires a vaccination in preparation for a foreign trip or wants the blood cholesterol level of its members checked, the family

physician is consulted and provides the service. If it is time for the new baby to have its first series of vaccinations, the family pediatrician is usually the one who provides them.

Ambulatory patient services, both simple and complex, are also obtained from private physicians. Many families use a physician who specializes in family practice, while others use an array of specialist physicians such as pediatricians, internists, obstetrician/gynecologists, and psychiatrists who provide both primary care and specialty services. Increasingly, these physicians are employed by, or under contract to, a practice management corporation and sometimes a managed care plan. When special laboratory tests are ordered, X-ray films required, or drugs and medications prescribed, private commercial for-profit laboratories or community pharmacies are used. Many of these services, from individual preventive medicine services to complex specialist treatments, are financed by individuals through out-of-pocket payment; most health insurance plans do not provide complete coverage for their needs. When the middle-income family begins to use institutional services, such as hospital care, the source of payment shifts almost completely from the individual to third-party health insurance plans, including various forms of managed care.

Inpatient hospital services are typically provided to the employed, insured, middle-income family by a local community hospital that is usually voluntary and nonprofit or, increasingly, part of a for-profit system. The specific hospital to be used is determined by the institution in which the family physician has medical staff privileges or by the managed care plan. Generally, the smaller, less specialized, more local hospitals will be used for simple problems, whereas the larger, more specialized, perhaps more distant hospitals will be used for more complicated problems. Many of these larger hospitals have active physician training programs, conduct research, and may have significant charity or teaching wards.

The employed, insured, middle-income family obtains its long-term care from a variety of sources, depending on the service required. Some long-term care is provided in hospitals and, as such, is merely an extension of the complex inpatient care the patient has already received. This practice was more commonly in the past, but utilization review procedures have increased the pressure on hospitals to reduce the length of time people are hospitalized. More commonly, long-term care is obtained at home through the assistance of a visiting nurse or voluntary nonprofit or for-profit community-based nursing service. If institutional long-term care is needed, it is probably obtained in a nursing home or a skilled nursing facility, usually a small (50–100 patients) institution, operated privately, for profit, by a single proprietor or small group of investors. Recently, there has been a general increase in size (100+ patients per facility) and a trend toward absorption of individual facilities into larger multifacility proprietary chains. The employed, insured, middle-income family usually pays for its long-term care with its own funds; most health insurance plans provide relatively limited coverage for long-term care.

When employed, insured, middle-income families require care for emotional problems, they will again use a variety of mostly private services. As the illness becomes more serious, however, families may, for the first time, rely on government-sponsored service. When emotional problems first begin to appear in the employed, insured, middle-income family, the patient will probably turn to the family physician, who provides simple supportive services such as medication, informal counseling, and perhaps referral for psychological testing. The physician may even arrange for the patient to be hospitalized in a general hospital for some nonpsychiatric diagnosis. If the emotional problems become more severe, the family physician may refer the patient to a private psychiatrist, or to a community mental health center that most likely will be a voluntary nonprofit agency or under the sponsorship of one (such as a voluntary nonprofit hospital). If hospitalization is required, the psychiatrist or the community mental health center is likely to use the psychiatric section of the local voluntary nonprofit hospital if it seems that the stay in a hospital will be a short one. If the hospitalization promises to be a long one, the psychiatrist may use a psychiatric hospital, usually a private or for-profit, nongovernmental community

facility. Increasingly, both inpatient and ambulatory mental health care will be obtained in a contracted managed care environment.

In those cases in which extended institutional care is required for an emotional problem and the patient's financial resources are relatively limited, the middle-income family may require hospitalization in a state mental hospital. This event usually represents the first use of government health programs by the middle-income family, and as such, it frequently comes as a considerable shock to patient and family alike.

In summary, the employed, insured, middle-income family's system of health care has been an informal, unstructured collection of individual services put together by the patient and the private physician to meet the needs of the moment. The individual services themselves have had little formalized interrelationship, and the only thread of continuity is provided by the family's physician or by the family itself. In general, all of the services are provided by nongovernmental sources and are paid for by private funds, either directly out-of-pocket or by privately financed health insurance plans.

For all of its apparent looseness and lack of structure, the employed, insured, middle-income family's system of health care has allowed for a considerable amount of decision and control by the patient, more than that of the other systems to be discussed. The patient is free to choose the physician, the health insurance plan, and frequently even the hospital. If additional care is required, the patient can seek out and use (sometimes overuse) that care to the limit of the financial resources available. If the patient does not like the particular care being provided, dissatisfaction can be expressed in a more effective manner: the patient can seek care elsewhere from another provider.

On the other hand, the employed, insured, middle-income family's system of care has been a poorly coordinated, unplanned collection of services that frequently have little formal integration with one another. It can be very wasteful of resources, and without central control or monitoring, it is difficult to determine whether it is accomplishing what it should. Each individual service may be of very high quality, but provide little evidence of any "linking" taking place to ensure that each service complements the others as effectively as possible.

One special subset of the middle-income model now involves millions of patients in this country. When people reach age sixty-five, they are automatically eligible for Medicare, the federally sponsored and supervised health insurance plan for the elderly. A patient covered by Medicare benefits can utilize the same system of care as the middle-income family, including private practice physicians and voluntary nongovernment hospitals. The main difference now is that the bills are paid by a federal government health insurance plan, rather than the usual private plan in which the typical middle-income family is enrolled. The physicians are the same and the hospitals are the same; only the health insurance plan is different.

Alternatively, individuals can increasingly elect to enroll in a managed care program. As managed care has become more prevalent, an employed, middle-income, insured individual may no longer have an entirely open choice of physician and hospital; rather, the choice now may be limited to only the physicians and the hospitals with which the managed care plan contracts. Also, under managed care, access to specialists may not be as easy to achieve and may not be solely at the choice of the patient, since there may now be a primary care physician who must authorize referral to specialists, and that primary care physician may have incentives to reduce referrals. Because managed care is increasingly the plan of choice for employers and other purchasers of private health insurance, and because Medicare is now strongly advocating the use of managed care by its recipients, the more open, patient-initiated, and patient-controlled use of health care services may change very markedly and very rapidly in the near future.

Unemployed, Uninsured, Inner-City, Minority America (Local Government Health Care)

A second major system of health care in the United States serves those people who are not regularly employed, do not have continuous health insurance coverage, and often are minority group members living in the inner city. While the specific details may vary from city to city, the general outline is well known in all major cities of the country. If it is important to study the system of health care for the employed, insured, middle-income population because it represents the *best* health care possible in this country, it is equally important to study the care of the poor, unemployed, and uninsured because it frequently represents the *worst*.

The most striking feature of the health care system of the poor, inner-city resident is exactly the same as that historically characterizing the middle-income family system: there is no *formal* system. Instead, just as in the middle-income system, each individual or family must put together an *informal* set of services, from whatever source possible, to meet the health care needs of the moment. There is one significant difference, however: the poor do not have the resources to choose where and how they will obtain their health services. Instead, they must take what is offered to them and try to put together a system from whatever they are told they can have.

There are two important characteristics of the system. First, the great majority of services are provided by local government agencies such as the city or county hospital and the local health department. Second, patients have no real continuity of service with any single provider, such as an employed, insured, middle-income family might have with a family physician. The poor family is faced with an endless stream of health care professionals who treat one specific episode of an illness and then are replaced by someone else for the next episode. While the middle-income system of health care can establish at least some thread of continuity by the ongoing presence of a family physician, the poor family cannot.

The poor obtain their mass public health and preventive medicine services, including a pure water supply, sanitary sewage disposal, and protection of milk and food, from the same local government health departments and health agencies that serve the middle-income system. In contrast to the middle-income system, however, the poor also get their individual public health and preventive medicine services from the local health department. When a poor family's newborn baby needs its vaccinations, that family goes to the district health center of the health department, not to a private physician. When a low-income woman needs a Papanicolaou smear for cervical cancer testing, it is most likely that the local government health department will give the test.

To obtain ambulatory services, the poor family cannot rely on the constant presence of a family physician for advice and routine treatment. Instead, they must turn to neighbors, the local pharmacist, the health department's public health nurse, or the emergency room of the city or county hospital. It has often been said that the city or county hospital's emergency room is the family physician for the poor, and the facts generally support this contention: when the poor need ambulatory patient care, it is quite likely that the first place they will turn is the city or county hospital emergency room.

The emergency room also serves the poor as the point of entry to the rest of the health care system. The poor obtain many of their ambulatory services in the outpatient clinics of city and county hospitals. To gain admission to these clinics, they must frequently first go to the emergency room and be referred to the appropriate clinic. Once out of the emergency room, they may be cared for in two or three specialty clinics, each of which may handle one particular set of problems but none of which will take responsibility for co-ordinating all the care the patient is receiving.

When the poor need inpatient hospital services, whether simple or complicated, they again usually turn to the city or county hospital to obtain them. Admission to the inpatient services of these hospitals is usually obtained through the emergency room or the outpatient clinics, thereby forcing the poor family to use these ambulatory patient services if they wish later admission to the inpatient services. The poor may also turn to the emergency room, the outpatient clinics, and the inpatient ward or teaching services of the larger voluntary nonprofit community hospitals. Because these hospitals are frequently teaching hospitals for the training of physicians, they often maintain special free or lower-priced wards. It is to these wards that the poor are usually admitted. Because the care in teaching hospitals is generally as good as or better than any that might be obtained at local city or county hospitals, many poor are willing to become teaching cases in the voluntary nonprofit hospitals in exchange for better care in better surroundings. By and large, however, city and county hospitals carry the largest burden of inpatient care for the poor.

If the long-term care situation of middle-income people is generally inadequate, the long-term care of the poor can only be described as terrible. In contrast to the system of care for middle-income families, most of the long-term care of the poor is provided in the wards of city and county hospitals, although not by intent or plan. The poor simply remain in hospitals longer because their social and physical conditions are more complicated and because hospital staffs are reluctant to discharge them until they have some assurance that continuing care will be available after discharge. Because this status is often uncertain, poor patients are likely to be kept longer in the hospital so that they can complete as much of their convalescence as possible before discharge.

Most of the long-term care of the poor is provided in the same types of nursing homes or skilled nursing facilities that are used by middle-income people: either the smaller (50–100 patients) facilities, operated for profit by a single proprietor, or the larger (100+ patients) facilities operated by a proprietary chain. One major difference between the systems used by the poor and the middle-income population is the quality of the facility used. The middle-income generally have access to better-equipped and better-staffed nursing homes, while the poor are admitted to less expensive, less well-equipped facilities. Another important difference between the middle-income and the poor is that employed, insured, middle-income patients are more likely to pay for their own care in these institutions, while the poor have their care paid by welfare, Medicaid, or other public funds.

It is interesting to note that the system of health care for the employed, insured, middle-income utilizes entirely private, nongovernmental facilities until long-term care for mental illness is required; at that point, a governmental facility, the state mental hospital, is used. By contrast, the system of health care for the poor is composed almost entirely of public, government-sponsored services until long-term care is required. This care is usually provided in private, profit-making facilities, the first use of such private facilities by the poor.

The convergence of the poor and the middle-income systems of care in the private profit-making nursing homes is noteworthy because it represents an important feature of our multiple subsystems of health care. In many cases, several systems of health care that are otherwise separate and distinct merge in their common use of personnel, equipment, and facilities. The emergency rooms of city or county and voluntary nonprofit teaching hospitals, for example, serve as the source of emergency medical care for the middle-income family that cannot reach its own family physician. They also serve as the family physician for the poor family that has none of its own. The private, for-profit nursing home serves as the source of long-term care for the middle-income family and may provide the same function for the poor. The radiology department of the voluntary nonprofit teaching hospital provides X-rays for the middle-income patient whose care is supervised by the private family physician, as well as for the poor patient whose care is supervised by a hospital staff physician in training. This does not mean that there is any real, functional integration of the separate systems of care because of their use of the same facility or personnel. Rather, the model is more like that of a busy harbor in which a variety of ships berth side by side for a short period of time before going their separate ways for separate purposes.

In their use of services for emotional illnesses, the poor turn once again to an almost totally public, local government system. Initial signs of emotional difficulties are haphazardly treated in emergency rooms and outpatient clinics of the city or county hospital. From there, patients may be referred to the crowded inpatient psychiatric wards of these same hospitals, but they are just as likely to be referred to community mental health centers operated by local governmental or voluntary nonprofit community agencies. When long-term care in an institution is required, the poor are sent to the psychiatric wards of the city or county hospital, and from there to the large state governmental mental hospitals, frequently many miles away.

In the past, health services for the poor were usually free, at least to the patients. The local health department, the city or county hospital, or the state mental hospital generally did not charge for its services, regardless of the patient's ability to pay. In the last few years, both local health departments and city and county hospitals have been forced to initiate a system of charges for services that were previously free. They have done this to recapture third-party payments to which the poor patient might be eligible, and patients who are unable to pay are still ordinarily provided the services they need. The imposition of these charges for previously free health services has probably changed the perception of these programs by the poor, but it is still too early to determine the implications of these changes.

As with the employed, insured, middle-income system, there is a subset of the health care system for the poor that requires special comment. Certain persons who are poor enough by virtue of extremely low income or resources may qualify for Medicaid, the federal-state cooperative health insurance plan for the indigent. Under Medicaid, people whose income and resources are below a level established by individual states can use a state government-sponsored health insurance program to purchase health care in the private, middle-income marketplace. The purpose of this program is to move the poor out of their usual local government health care system and into the supposedly better private practice health care system of middle-income people. Unfortunately, the ability of Medicaid to move the poor into a better system of care has been limited by the reluctance of private physicians and private hospitals to assume responsibility for many Medicaid patients. This reluctance has been based on what has been seen as a low rate of reimbursement by Medicaid for services provided, an often cumbersome system of paperwork and prior authorizations in order to provide care, and a frequently irrational system of retroactive denials of payment for services already provided.

Just as the situation of the employed, middle-income, insured population is changing to the use of managed care, so too is the situation of the poor, uninsured, Medicaid recipient changing, with somewhat different directions and results.

In many states, some or all of the Medicaid population is being moved out of the standard Medicaid fee-for-service model into a managed care model. Although the models vary from state to state, the central idea is for Medicaid recipients to establish a more permanent relationship with a single primary care physician who will then coordinate (manage) that patient's use of specialist and hospital services. Just as it does for the employed, insured individual, the use of managed care for Medicaid recipients moves them into a more intentionally organized and monitored system of care, with rigorous standards of service and serious attempts to measure outcomes. Medicaid managed care will significantly change the organizational form for many poor, uninsured patients, probably for the better.

A second subset of the system of care for the poor and uninsured is that for poor people who turn sixty-five. Immediately upon reaching age sixty-five, they are eligible for Medicare and ostensibly should be able to take their new insurance coverage and move into the private, middle-income system of care. Unfortunately, this movement from public to private provider systems by poor people who become sixty-five years of age is limited by the deductible and coinsurance features of Medicare. Under Medicare, everyone (poor included) is expected to spend several hundred dollars for health care first, before Medicare begins to pay bills. Even when this deductible requirement is met, the elderly person is also required to pay a substantial amount for any hospitalization. The level of available cash to pay these deductibles and coinsurance limits the ability of many poor people to take full advantage of the benefits of Medicare when they become eligible at age sixty-five.

In summary, the system of health care for the poor is as unstructured and informal as that for the employed, insured, middle-income, but the poor have to depend upon whatever services the local government offers them. The services are usually provided free of charge or at low cost, but the patient has relatively little opportunity to express a choice and exercise options. Poor patients often cannot move to another set of services if they dislike the one first offered; those first offered are usually the only services available.

Like the system of health care for the middle-income, the system for the poor is poorly coordinated internally and almost completely unplanned and unmonitored. It is certainly as wasteful of resources as the middle-income system, but because it is a low-cost, poorly fi-

nanced system, the exact amount of waste is difficult to document. At the same time, the great virtue of the health care system for the poor—its openness and accessibility to all people at all times for all conditions (albeit with considerable delays)—is difficult to evaluate adequately as well, and the introduction of managed care is now seeking to provide some rationalization, as is the case for the middle class.

Military Medical Care System

A person joining one of the uniformed branches of the American military sacrifices many aspects of civilian life that nonmilitary personnel take for granted. At the same time, however, this person receives a variety of fringe benefits that those outside the military do not enjoy. One of the most important of these fringe benefits is a well-organized system of high-quality health care provided at no direct cost to the recipient. Certain features of this military medical care system (the general term used to include the separate systems of the United States Army, Navy, and Air Force) deserve comment. First, the system is all-inclusive and omnipresent. The military medical system has the responsibility of protecting the health of all active-duty military personnel everywhere and of providing them with all the services they may eventually need for any service-connected problem. The military medical system goes where active-duty military personnel go and assumes a responsibility for total care that is unique among American health care systems.

The second important characteristic of the military medical care system is that it goes into effect immediately whether the active-duty soldier or sailor wants it or not. No initiative or action is required by the individual to start the system; indeed, the system frequently provides certain types of health services, such as routine vaccinations or shots, that the soldier or sailor would really rather not have. The individual has little choice regarding who will provide the treatment or where, but at the same time, the services are always there if needed, without the need to search them out. If a physician's services are needed, they are obtained; if hospitalization is required, it is arranged; if emergency transportation is necessary, it is carried out. There is little that the individual can do to influence how medical care is provided, but at the same time, there is never any worry about its availability.

The third important characteristic of the military health care system is its great emphasis on keeping personnel well, preventing illness or injury, and finding health problems early while they are still amenable to treatment. Great stress is placed on preventive measures such as vaccination, regular physical examinations and testing, and educational efforts toward prevention of accidents and contagious diseases. In an approach that is unique among the health care systems of this country, the military medical system provides health care, and not just sickness care.

In the military medical system, the same mass public health and preventive medicine services that are provided to a locality or a community by a local government health department or health agency may also be provided to active-duty military personnel. Whenever personnel are actually within the boundaries of a military reservation or post, however, an additional set of mass public health and preventive medicine services may be provided by the military itself. Sanitary disposal of sewage, protection of food and milk, purification of the water supply, and prevention of vehicular or job-related accidents may be provided for by a local government agency, but each military installation usually has a second, separate system of its own, staffed by its own public health and safety officers. Individual public health and preventive medicine services are also provided by the military medical system according to a well-organized, regularly scheduled routine of yearly examinations, surveys of patient records, vaccinations, and other measures. The persons providing the specific preventive service (for example, a routine tetanus shot) are usually medical corpspersons or other nonphysician personnel; however, their work is carried out according to carefully developed guidelines and is monitored by well-trained supervisory medical personnel.

Routine ambulatory care is usually provided to most active-duty military personnel by the same medics who provide the individual preventive services. These services are usually provided at the dispensary, sick bay, first-aid station, or similar unit that is very close to the military personnel's actual place of work. These ambulatory services may also be provided by physicians or nurses at the same locations, but this is less likely. More complicated ambulatory patient care services are usually provided by physicians, frequently specialists, working at the same dispensary or medical station as the medics or, more likely, in a clinic or outpatient department of a larger facility such as a military hospital. Patients are usually referred by medics or physicians who have first cared for the patients for simpler problems; laboratory tests, X-ray examinations, and medications are obtained at the same military facility to which the patient is referred.

The simplest hospital services are provided using short-stay beds at base dispensaries, in sick bays aboard ship, or at small base hospitals on various military installations around the world. Usually the range of services that can be offered at these installations is limited, and referral to larger institutions is routinely carried out if a more complex problem is suspected. More complicated hospital services are provided to active-duty military personnel in regional hospitals that possess a wide variety of specialized services and facilities. Frequently, these hospitals also have large teaching and training programs, where the atmosphere and the quality of care are similar to what might be expected at a university hospital or a large community teaching hospital.

The military medical system does not pretend to offer the same extensive range of long-term care services that it provides for more acute short-term problems. The military medical system does provide care for potentially long-range problems in military hospitals, as long as there is some reasonable expectation that the patient will someday be able to return to full active duty. Whenever it is determined, however, that the problem is genuinely long-term in nature and that a complete return to active duty is not possible, the patient is given a medical discharge from the service and long-term care is provided through the Veterans Administration (VA) facilities.

If military personnel develop emotional difficulties, care is most likely to be provided initially by the medical corpsperson, and then by a physician assigned to that military unit. These personnel provide short-term nonpsychiatric support and counseling, and possibly prescribe certain medications such as tranquilizers. For more severe problems, patients are referred to the psychiatric services of larger military hospitals where the severity of the problem is determined. If the problem is short-term and is not believed to seriously affect the patient's work, an attempt may be made to provide the short-term treatment at the military hospital itself, first on an inpatient and later on an outpatient basis. If there is a significant psychiatric diagnosis, the patient is most likely to be given a medical discharge, with follow-up care to be provided through the psychiatric services of the VA hospitals.

The military medical system is a closely organized, highly integrated, rational, and regionalized approach. A single patient record is used, and the complete record moves from one health care service to another with the patient. Once the need for health care is identified, the system itself arranges for the patient to receive required care and usually even provides transportation to the services. The patient does not have to search out the necessary service or determine how to use it. This service is provided at no cost to the patient, requires little effort by the patient to initiate it, and generally involves a relatively high-quality product. The system is centrally planned, uses nonmedical and nonnursing personnel to the utmost, and is entirely self-sufficient and self-contained. The services are provided by salaried employees in facilities that are wholly owned and operated by the system itself. The system is not generally available to persons who are not active-duty military personnel or their dependents, although in cases of emergency or pressing local need, it can be. Generally, the patient has little choice regarding the manner in which services will be delivered, but this drawback is counterbalanced by the assurance that high-quality services will be available when needed.

Dependents and families of active-duty military personnel are served by a special subsystem of military medicine that combines the services of the middle-class, middle-income system and the active-duty military system. Active-duty personnel, dependents, and families are covered by health insurance plans: the Civilian Health and Medical Program of the Uniformed Services (CHAMPUS), and a managed care plan, TRICARE, provided by the military. These health insurance plans allow active-duty personnel and their families to obtain medical care from private practitioners, from health maintenance organizations, and from local community nonmilitary hospitals when similar services cannot be provided at a military installation within a reasonable distance. The dependents and families of active-duty military personnel can also use the same military services that the active-duty personnel use, provided space and resources are available and military authorities determine that this procedure is appropriate. The resulting subsystem of care for military dependents and families generally allows them to participate to some degree in two separate systems of care: the middle-class, middle-income private practice system and the military medical system. Their participation in either is generally not as clearly focused or as active as it would be for someone firmly planted in either system exclusively, but it still provides them with two viable options for obtaining care.

Veterans Administration Health Care System

Parallel to the system of care for active duty military personnel is another system operated within the continental United States for retired, disabled, and otherwise deserving veterans of previous United States military service. Although the VA system is in many respects larger than the system of care for active-duty military personnel, it is not nearly as complete, well-integrated, or extensive. At the present time, the VA system focuses largely on hospital care, mental health services, and long-term care. It operates 171 hospitals throughout the country that provide most of the VA care. In recent years, the VA has increasingly provided outpatient services and now maintains more than 200 outpatient clinics. In very recent years, the VA has announced plans to become a much more comprehensive and complete system of care, with major emphasis to be placed on primary care.

A second important characteristic of the VA system is the great preponderance of male patients with multiple-system problems. By and large, the patients using the VA health care system are older, inactive men in whom the occurrence of multiple and chronic physical and emotional illnesses is much higher than in the general population.

A third important feature of the VA system is its existence as only one part of a much larger system of social services and benefits for veterans. Many of the people eligible to use the VA health care system are also receiving other kinds of financial benefits; indeed, access to the VA health care system is sometimes directly dependent on eligibility for financial benefits of various types, including educational assistance grants and disability compensation. Because health care is only one of many VA programs, a great variety of social services interact with and compete for available resources.

A further feature of the VA health care system is its unique relationship with organized consumer groups. Because the VA is organized to provide care exclusively for veterans, and because many of those veterans are members of local and national veterans' clubs and associations, the VA health care system is constantly in direct communication with groups representing the interests of veterans. In a manner that is unparalleled in any other health care system in this country, the interests of veterans are constantly conveyed to individual VA hospitals, to the VA administrative body in Washington DC, and to the United States Congress. In no other health care system in this country does organized consumer interest play such a constant, important, and influential role.

Because the VA system is primarily a hospital system, there are few attempts to provide general public health services or routine ambulatory care services. Veterans usually obtain these services from some other system of care—either the middle-income system or the local government system that serves the urban poor. The VA does provide the more complicated ambulatory services, usually through its hospital outpatient clinics. This care is in preparation for possible hospital admission or as a follow-up after hospitalization. Many veterans who require these services obtain them from other systems of care and come to the VA system only after a condition is apparent and hospitalization is required. Admission to VA hospitals can be gained through the ambulatory

patient care services operated by the VA itself, by direct referrals from physicians in private practice, or by referrals from hospitals in the community. The services in VA hospitals are provided by salaried, full-time medical and nursing personnel; as in the military medical system, most of the VA hospitals are self-contained, relatively self-sufficient units that require little outside support or staff.

The VA health care system provides a tremendous quantity of long-term care for both physical and emotional illnesses. Indeed, the VA is probably the largest single provider of long-term care in the country, if not the world. In addition to providing considerable long-term care in the acute, short-term care hospitals, the VA also operates a number of domiciliaries and nursing homes and pays for care in local community nursing homes and skilled nursing facilities.

The VA system of care is difficult to describe fully for two important reasons. First, it is a system that does not attempt to provide a complete range of services, but instead concentrates on acute hospital services and on long-term care for physical and emotional problems. Second, eligibility for entry into the system is somewhat unclear and sometimes open to variable local interpretation. The system is designed to serve veterans with service-connected disabilities, but offers services to other veterans if they cannot obtain adequate care elsewhere and if adequate VA resources are available. In practice, the actual eligibility requirements and patient mix may vary substantially from one VA hospital to the next.

If the system of health care for active-duty military personnel focuses on preventive, ambulatory, and acute inpatient care, the VA system of care stresses long-term, chronic inpatient care for both physical and emotional problems. Whereas the military medical system offers a complete, well-integrated, well-coordinated package of health care services, the services that the VA offers are primarily hospital-related. In contrast to the military medical system, which actively seeks out and offers services to patients as part of their work environment, the VA provides its services to patients only when they come forward to seek them. Despite these reservations about the VA as a complete system of health care, it should be stressed that the VA serves as the primary source of inpatient hospital care for hundreds of thousands of veterans each year and is a potential source of inpatient care for millions more. As such, it is one of the largest single providers of health care services in this country and must be considered an integral, important component of the American health care scene, both now and in the future.

HEALTH SERVICES: A SUMMARY OF PERSPECTIVES

In reviewing each of these major systems of health care for Americans—the system for employed, insured, middle-income families who use the private sector services; the local government system for the urban poor; the military medical system for active-duty military personnel and their dependents; and the VA system for veterans—it becomes apparent that there are a number of additional systems that could be included as well. Other systems of health care include the one used by rural farming families and the Indian Health Service operated for Native Americans by the federal government. There are also many possible variations within the four systems discussed here. The purpose, however, is not to be exhaustive in describing the systems themselves but rather to point out that there are multiple systems providing services to different populations with different needs. No one system predominates in terms of persons served or benefits provided. Indeed, the purpose here is to point out that there is no one single American health care system but rather a mosaic of subsystems, each with its own characteristics and moving in its own direction.

Is it bad to have so many separate subsystems? Why is it even worth pointing out the obvious fact that many such subsystems exist? There are several pressing reasons for reviewing this country's compartmentalized organization of health care. The first and most important reason is quite simple: in order to improve health service to everyone in the country, an understanding of the component parts of the present health care structure is essential. Without a fundamental understanding of the separate component parts, it is impossible to understand the whole structure. Without an understanding of the interaction among the component parts, one cannot design appropriate and effective interventions and changes.

The second reason for considering the various separate systems of health care in this country is the vigorous competition for scarce resources of money, people, and facilities. Although the four systems described are separate from one another, they all compete for the same resources because they are all dependent on the same economy and the same supplies of health personnel and skills.

Whenever there is vigorous competition for resources, two things frequently happen. First, the stronger, more vigorous, more aggressive, or better connected competitors obtain the larger portion of the resources, whether or not this outcome is justified by their needs. In practice, this has meant that the middle-income/private practice system, the military medical system, and the VA system have all done relatively well, while the local government health care system for the poor has always been severely underfinanced and understaffed, a situation that seems to be getting progressively worse.

Second, intense competition for resources frequently results in wasteful duplication and ineffective use of resources. For example, in the same region, a city or county hospital, a private teaching hospital, a military hospital, and a VA hospital may all be operating exactly the same kind of expensive service, although only one facility might be needed, and undoubtedly one large integrated service would provide more efficient use of resources than four smaller ones. Because each institution is part of a separate system, serves a different population, and approaches the resource pool through a different channel, no really purposeful planning or controlled allocation of resources is possible. In the past, this situation might have been acceptable because the resources seemed endless, but in these days of very limited resources, this is no longer acceptable.

In addition to this economic inefficiency, there are other reasons for looking with a critical eye at multiple systems of care, reasons that are related to the quality and accessibility of services. Unfortunately, not all of these subsystems of care serve people in the same way with the same results. There is great inequality among the various systems of health care, with the result that different people receive different levels of care simply by accident of birth or membership in a special group.

Because all the separate systems of health care in this country ultimately depend on public funds for their continued existence, it is imperative that the inequalities among them be removed as rapidly as possible. This does not necessarily mean eliminating the various separate subsystems of care, but rather requires that all the systems rise to a common high level and equitably share responsibilities and resources.

In the past, there have been various approaches to the question of multiple subsystems of care serving different portions of the American population. All of these approaches have used specific mechanisms of financing, planning, or regulation with the shared purpose of developing a more integrated, more effective, and less costly health care system for the country. Although these proposals have often been limited in nature, their overall purpose generally has been to move the various pieces of the American health care system into a better relationship with each other. These approaches are interesting not only in themselves but also because they tell us more about ourselves and about the possibilities of health care in the United States.

One approach to rationalizing the health care system has been to develop a system of universal health insurance coverage for all people in the United States. Under this type of approach (sometimes referred to as either "national health insurance" or "universal coverage"), the differences in financing disappear and all people are able to approach the delivery system with equal resources and access. Once the differences in health insurance status are removed, it is argued, the system for providing health care will function in a much more rational fashion, with populations approaching individual providers because they chose to do so, not because they must because of their membership in one group or another. Unfortunately, national health insurance and universal coverage have not been easy to develop, and there is little indication that things will be any different in the near future.

Another proposal that has been considered and actually tried for a short while has been the voluntary (or semivoluntary) health planning approach. With the passage of the original Comprehensive Health Planning legislation and, more important, with the passage of the National Health Planning and Resources Development Act of 1974, it had been thought that providers, consumers, and public officials might come together and develop plans for all states and localities that would then become blueprints for a more rationally organized system of care. This hope did not turn into reality, primarily because of conflicts concerning power and control, and with the demise of the health planning system, this approach toward more rational coordination of health care services has been virtually abandoned. It is doubtful that there will be a return to anything resembling a government-sponsored health planning system again; it is also doubtful that planning without control of subsequent financing of health services (sometimes called "planning without teeth") has any chance of success.

A somewhat different approach to rationalizing the American health care system focuses on the use of financing mechanisms to encourage efficiencies or to force increased coordination of effort throughout the system. The proponents of this line of thought suggest that the power to withhold financial reimbursement to providers who do not comply with efforts to improve the system would be so strong as to be irresistible. Although the argument is used more visibly by many of the proponents of a national health insurance plan, it has also become a major lever by which the Health Care Financing Administration (HCFA) uses Medicare and Medicaid funds to encourage compliance with its long range objectives. It is also evident in the actions of private employers who espouse a return to a more free-market approach to health care; in this approach, purchasers use the power of their economic leverage to force the system to become more efficient and deliver a better product at a lower price. Indeed, it would have to be said that, whatever the specific source, the greatest forces shaping the health care system at present are financial and the greatest power to effect change in the system in the future is in the hands of the large third-party payers for health care: employers, Medicare, and Medicaid.

In the end, it should be realized that the American health care system is not a single, coordinated, well-integrated organization that provides care to all parts of our population in the same fashion, with the same standards, and achieving the same outcomes. There are many subsystems of health care in the United

States that are determined by characteristics having nothing to do with health status or the need for health care; they are determined by membership (or lack of membership) in one population subgroup or another. This reality is neither fair nor equitable in a country founded upon the values of fairness and equality. Neither is it efficient or effective. It is important that all health care professionals understand the deficiencies in our current health care subsystems so that in the future all Americans can be guaranteed the same level of health services regardless of the subsystem from which they obtain their care.

HEALTH CARE SYSTEMS IN TWO MARKETS

To illustrate the principles and practices of health care systems and their organization, this section of the chapter presents descriptions and analyses of the health care delivery systems of two major markets. The first of these is Boston, Massachusetts and the second is Orange County, California. The markets were selected for presentation due to the complexity of the issues and changes faced by providers and consumers in both locations, and their relevance to the concepts presented in the first section of this chapter.

Community Report for Boston, Massachusetts

After a series of health plan and hospital mergers before 1996, Boston's health care market entered a period of greater organizational stability. Five nationally renowned not-for-profit organizations still dominate: two large care systems based in academic medical centers, Partners and CareGroup, and three large health plans, Harvard Pilgrim Health Care, Tufts Associated Health Plan, and Blue Cross and Blue Shield of Massachusetts (BCBSM). While there have been some shifts in the competitive position of these entities, no single organization or sector controls the market.

Alongside this continuity there have been important changes in the market:

- Health plans have assumed a defensive posture as they encounter increased anti-managed-care sentiment.
- The focus of large care systems has shifted from finding partners to managing large networks and risk contracts.

- Medicaid enrollment has increased, but consolidation, market exits, and state contracting changes have left fewer plans serving this population.

Boston Retains Distinctive Market Features

The Boston health care market—with a forty-six percent HMO penetration rate—has several features that make it different from other high managed-care communities. It is dominated by three well-regarded not-for-profit health plans and is influenced by an activist government with a strong consumer orientation. A large proportion of families report being satisfied with their health care—more than in other HSC study sites with high managed-care penetration. There are more hospital beds and physicians per capita, and health costs are significantly higher than the national average. These costs are viewed by purchasers, plans, and providers as a reasonable trade-off for access to Boston's academic medical centers, key contributors to the local economy. Indeed, desire to maintain teaching and research capabilities was the main justification for the merger of Massachusetts General Hospital and Brigham and Women's Hospital that created Partners in 1993.

While cost cutting has not been the major focus of attention, some organizations have tried to reduce operating costs in the last two years. BCBSM reports that it eliminated fifty percent of its staff in an effort to shed unprofitable business and streamline its operations. Boston Medical Center also made significant cuts, and Harvard Pilgrim recently announced plans to lay off at least 100 staff members.

At the same time, employers are accepting moderate increases on an already high premium base, although they are pushing plans to deliver added benefits and better customer service in return. Premiums in Boston rose by about 3 to 5 percent in 1998, on par with the national increase of 3.3 percent.

Government Continues to Act as a Shaping Force

State government has long played a major role in shaping the Boston health care market. Extensive protections and mandates are already in place in Massachusetts, and the state government continues to play an active, behind-the-scenes role in shaping the health care market. Health care organizations pay close attention to concerns voiced by legislators and government officials and often proactively change their strategies to address these issues. At the same time, health care organizations try to achieve their competitive goals through policy initiatives.

Although little new legislation was passed in the late 1990s, much debate has taken place on managed-care issues. Reforms that were proposed would have introduced more state oversight of managed-care plans, instituted a standardized appeals process, and increased state-mandated services by requiring coverage for reasonable emergency room visits. Similar laws are expected to be proposed in the next legislative session.

Managed-care proposals mobilized employers and health plans in opposition. The managed-care debate also brought physicians and consumer groups into an unprecedented alliance in support of increased state oversight. Recent legislative effort has had a lasting impact on the market. Plan respondents indicate that local HMOs that have long been highly regarded have suddenly become unpopular.

As Plans Retrench, Provider Systems Strengthen Market Position

Confronted by increasing anti-managed-care sentiment, plans are perceived to be assuming a lower profile. They seem to have limited their scope of activities, selling off owned provider capacity, reducing product lines, and transferring some responsibilities to providers. BCBSM sold its nine health clinics to MedPartners to support its goals of generating cash and returning to core functions. Harvard Pilgrim spun off its fourteen health centers, the centerpiece of the original Harvard Community Health Plan, into a physician-directed enterprise, Harvard Vanguard.

The major plans have pursued regional strategies by affiliating with, buying, or establishing plans in the other New England states to offer products to multistate employers. At the same time, there have been shifts in the market position of the three large plans. Harvard Pilgrim is still the largest plan in Massachusetts, but Tufts has moved into second place, due in large part to the strength of its Secure

Horizons Medicare managed-care product. BCBSM, once the largest insurer by far, is now in third place. While the Blues plan appears to be on the upswing, it has faced significant problems over the last few years with financial losses that prompted close oversight by the state's Department of Insurance and an enrollment freeze on its Medicare risk plan initiated by the federal Health Care Financing Administration.

Meanwhile, local provider systems appear to be operating from a position of relative strength, as they move from a period of finding partners to one of making existing partnerships work. They have expanded their range of activities in the last two years by implementing mergers, building networks, and establishing risk-management infrastructures. Respondents point out that large academic hospitals were notably silent during recent managed-care debates in the legislature. These organizations seem well served by having plans take the heat from consumers and advocates.

Other health care entities in Boston are trying to increase their market power by affiliating either with the five major organizations or with other entities. For example, Neighborhood Health Plan (NHP), a Medicaid HMO formed by the city's community health centers, was recently acquired by Harvard Pilgrim Health Care. New England Medical Center, one of the last unaffiliated academic medical centers, was recently acquired by Rhode Island-based Lifespan. And Lahey Clinic recently announced a new partnership with CareGroup, after Lahey's merger with the New Hampshire-based Hitchcock Medical Center fell apart. These changes highlight the continued importance for plans and providers of being part of large, regionally powerful organizations.

By 1996, three large care systems had formed from a series of mergers with the stated goals of gaining market power and reducing excess capacity. Different consolidation strategies were pursued, with some integrating more than others. Two years later, it appeared that the systems that did more to integrate and consolidate had not yet seen a payoff in market position.

Partners retained the autonomy of its two flagship hospitals, Massachusetts General and Brigham and Women's, and sought integration opportunities that promised immediate returns and little opposition, especially from influential department chairs. While most of the managed-care contracting and many administrative functions such as human resources and purchasing were centralized, Partners' two main hospitals have remained operationally and clinically autonomous. The degree of independence of the hospitals was demonstrated when Massachusetts General opened an obstetrics unit, even though Brigham and Women's is the preeminent maternity hospital in the area. Although a significant downsizing in Boston's academic hospital capacity has long been predicted, Partners' two academic institutions have opened previously closed beds during the past two years to accommodate increasing patient volume.

CareGroup devoted extensive effort and resources to combining Beth Israel Hospital and Deaconess Hospital into one entity. Significant progress has been made, including merging all departments and appointing single department chiefs. However, the process has been contentious and difficult. According to several reports, most of the chiefs selected for the merged departments were from Beth Israel, alienating many Deaconess physicians. While CareGroup reports that it has been successful in reducing costs as a result of the consolidation, some respondents note that its internal focus has damaged the system's competitive position. However, the partnership with Lahey Clinic may improve CareGroup's standing in the market.

The Boston Medical Center merger consolidated Boston City Hospital (BCH) and Boston University Medical Center (BUMC) into one entity. Benefits of the merger include complementary clinical expertise and substantial cost savings. However, Boston Medical Center is viewed by many as being financially and operationally vulnerable. The consolidation also brought out cultural conflicts. Boston City's physicians tended to be primary-care-oriented, while BUMC's physicians were more academic and subspecialty-focused. Physicians from BCH were concerned that the BUMC doctors would not support the public hospital's mission of community service and care for the poor. These concerns, however, appear to have subsided somewhat since the merger was implemented.

Overall, Partners appears to be in a better competitive position than the other two large care systems, CareGroup and Boston Medical Center, which both did more to integrate and consolidate. However, some have noted that Partners' success may hinge more on the reputation and access to capital of its two hospitals than on its integration strategy.

Large Care Systems Focus on Managing Risk Contracts

The number of lives covered under providers' risk-based contracts has increased substantially over the last two years, and the two large academic medical center-based systems—Partners and CareGroup—have turned greater attention to implementing these contracts and managing their provider networks. Although these agreements still represent a relatively small share of the academic hospitals' business and reportedly have not been profitable, they are seen to be important because the number of risk contracts is expected to grow and because the networks are significant referral sources for the hospitals. The two systems have apparently invested heavily in the information and staff infrastructure needed to support these contracts, and observers predict they will push for payment increases when their plan contracts are renegotiated.

Partners and CareGroup have established management service organization (MSO)-like structures to manage this business, and these entities are now considered the dominant physician contracting organizations in the Boston market. Partners Community HealthCare, Inc., has 915 primary care physicians in its network while CareGroup's Provider Services Network has about 500. Both organizations have reportedly slowed acquisitions of physician practices, favoring affiliations and joint ventures.

For most of these risk contracts, the MSO is slated to receive seventy to eighty percent of the premium for enrollees from plans. Population-based budgets are established, and providers are paid on a fee-for-service basis with year-end reconciliation. The large care systems pass some of the risk along to risk units, each consisting of a group of physicians, such as the Massachusetts General physician group, and its affiliated hospital. Risk is assigned to these units based on the enrollee's choice of primary care physician.

The increasing focus on risk contracts has highlighted the underlying tensions between academic medical centers and community hospitals about how to structure payments to the multiple-risk units within their networks. Physicians affiliated with the academic medical centers want to institute risk-adjustment methodologies to avoid penalties for attracting sicker patients who require more services.

Meanwhile, physicians based at community hospitals are concerned that the drive for better risk-adjustment methodologies is part of a larger academic medical center strategy to attract patients who had historically received care at community hospitals. This concern may ultimately drive community hospitals and their physicians to seek contracting vehicles that are less closely tied to the academic medical centers.

With the increase in risk contracts comes the critical issue of who controls referrals. Partners and Care-Group are directing patient referrals for at-risk business to their own affiliated physicians and hospitals. This raises concerns among health plans that patients will not have full access to the broad networks they are building and promoting in response to purchaser and consumer demands.

Plan reactions to provider referral management have varied. Harvard Pilgrim Health Care allows primary care providers who are at risk to make their own referral decisions, but also allows enrollees to switch primary care providers at any time. Tufts Associated Health Plan has told providers who accept risk that enrollees must have access to the full Tufts network. BCBSM is also concerned about referral restrictions, especially because its signature asset is the breadth of its network, but it has not taken any action to counter referral management by providers, in part because it believes that could generate negative publicity.

The large care systems also want to control more care-management functions to obtain a larger share of the capitated dollar. So far, plans have retained many care-management responsibilities, including functions such as tracking and developing care plans for enrollees with chronic diseases. Plans have resisted handing over more responsibility on the grounds that care systems have not demonstrated their ability to implement system-wide quality improvement initiatives.

Medicaid Enrollment Increases, But Fewer Plans Participate

Medicaid enrollment increased significantly as a result of program expansions in 1997 and 1998, when more than 100,000 children and adults gained coverage under the state's Medicaid program, MassHealth. With these expansions in place, some speculate that the state may reduce funding for the uncompensated care pool, which pays for health services for eligible uninsured.

The largest recipients of uncompensated care pool dollars, Boston Medical Center and Cambridge Hospital, have developed their own managed-care programs to attract MassHealth enrollees and the uninsured. These two hospital systems negotiated higher Medicaid payments and approval to develop shadow managed-care programs for the uninsured. Under these new programs, the hospitals use pool dollars to fund a comprehensive package of services for the uninsured. Rather than receiving treatment on an episodic basis, the uninsured enrollees will be linked with primary care providers and have access to preventive services.

While the number of Medicaid eligibles has grown, the number of HMOs serving the Medicaid market has declined. Two commercial plans in the market—BCBSM and Tufts Associated Health Plan—are no longer contracting with the state's Medicaid program. The two plans had a combined enrollment of more than 60,000 Medicaid recipients and very broad provider networks. BCBSM withdrew because it was losing money on Medicaid. Tufts, which was also reported to have lost money on Medicaid, indicated it could not comply with the state's increased reporting requirement along with the information technology demands presented by year 2000 computer problems.

With these two plans out, Harvard Pilgrim is the only remaining commercial plan serving the Boston Medicaid market. At the same time, the plan has stopped enrolling Medicaid beneficiaries in its large Pilgrim network, relying instead on the narrower networks of Harvard Vanguard and NHP providers. While beneficiaries still have access to a very broad network of providers under the state's primary care case-management (PCCM) program it maintains as an alternative to HMOs, there are concerns about the implications of these changes. According to market observers, changes in plans' participation in Medicaid indicate that HMOs with broad and more loosely managed networks have had trouble surviving with the current rates.

Summary for Boston

The large academic care systems have grown stronger, and tensions have increased between these organizations and the three leading health plans. At the same time, Boston's health care system has retained many of its unique attributes: high managed-care penetration, high costs, renowned plans and academic hospitals, and an activist government.

Community Report for Orange County, California

Orange County's health care market has undergone dramatic upheaval over the past few years as cost pressures mounted. Area health plans have long delegated risk and medical management to physicians, leading to the emergence of large physician organizations that play a critical role in the delivery system.

Market Defined by Managed Care and Consolidation

Situated between Los Angeles and San Diego, the Orange County health care market is shaped, on the one hand, by being a part of southern California, where statewide purchasing pools and large regional employers influence the strategies of health plans and providers. On the other hand, the vast geographic scope of the region leaves Orange County a distinct local market for health care, shaped by a strong local economy, a politically conservative environment, and a rapidly growing population marked by ethnic diversity and economic disparity.

Orange County has extensive experience with arranged care, and today it is one of the defining features of the health care system. Even more notable, however, is the prevalence of capitation in the market. Orange County's health plans have delegated significant risk to physician organizations, typically paying

capitation for primary and specialty care as well as some ancillary services. Unlike many other markets, physician organizations in Orange County also typically share risk for hospital utilization and have responsibility for care management. While plans have broad networks and most providers contract with most plans, capitation has resulted in tightly managed gatekeeping systems with clearly defined subnetworks controlled by physician organizations. As a result, consumers' access to care is largely directed by their primary care physician and associated provider network.

Significant consolidation has taken place or is underway in all sectors of the market. Four of the major health plans in the county have consolidated, resulting in substantial concentration in the market. A series of mergers and acquisitions in the Orange County hospital market concentrated more than half of the hospital beds in three major systems. As a result of its national merger with OrNda, Tenet Healthcare Corp.'s eleven local hospitals alone control more than twenty-nine percent of the market's beds. In the physician sector, consolidation is underway, with the formation and growth of several large physician intermediary organizations led by PPMCs and local hospitals. All three sectors have shifted from planning the mergers to consolidating and leveraging the merged entities. Physician organizations have pursued these objectives while continuing to expand as well.

Physician Organizations Squeezed by Cost Increases

While Orange County's health care organizations grappled with how to consolidate, industry costs began to rise. In contrast to other markets where plans bear the brunt of these types of cost increases, the extensive use of capitation in Orange County meant that, in this market, physician organizations were financially at risk for delivering care under prepaid arrangements. Because physicians were often locked into long-term capitated contracts that did not account for rising costs, they had to tap into reserves or owner investments to fulfill this obligation.

In the late 1990s, physician organizations sought to expand the scope of their capitated services to increase their potential margin, driven partly by the belief that capitation rates for basic physician services were fairly bare-bones. Physicians continued to seek hospital risk-sharing arrangements, reasoning that good management of ambulatory care would result in lower hospital utilization and greater savings.

In addition, some of the more advanced physician organizations pursued capitation for pharmacy costs; others took it on, though reluctantly. Some physician organizations also sought global capitation—a consolidated payment to cover all medical services, including both physician- and hospital-provided care.

As physician capitation arrangements expanded in scope, local health care costs grew beyond expectations. Several federal and state policy changes led to cost increases that physicians needed to absorb under capitation. For example, a variety of mandated benefits guaranteeing coverage of certain services led to considerable cost increases. Costs also rose due to new requirements of physician-level encounter data for Medicare risk products and purchasers' quality and patient satisfaction measures.

More loosely managed HMO products—such as point-of-service (POS) products that cover enrollees for out-of-network care—were gaining in popularity among consumers, who felt constrained by tightly managed physician networks. In an effort to be more consumer-friendly, many health plans also instituted new grievance procedures, which resulted in increased retrospective approval of services.

Providers reported that these arrangements drove up costs, while in some cases decreasing physicians' capitated payment. For example, under POS products, plans typically reduced physician capitation to account for enrollees treated by out-of-network providers. However, enrollees reportedly would go out-of-network for referrals, then come back to in-network physicians for treatment. As a result, providers reported that in-network utilization was higher than expected under POS products, leaving physicians with insufficient payment to cover costs and diminished control over utilization.

And, keeping with national trends, local expenditures on pharmaceuticals and new medical technologies have grown rapidly. Locally, where many new contracts delegated risk for pharmacy, physician organizations had to absorb these costs.

While costs rose and revenues plateaued, physician organizations struggled to realize the expected benefits of consolidation. Integration efforts proved more difficult and time-consuming than expected, however, and the costs associated with consolidation exceeded the benefits achieved—at least in the short term—for three major reasons. First, physician organizations paid high prices for the practices they acquired. In competing for geographic depth and breadth, PPMCs and other buyers bid up the price for physician practices. Second, the cost of integrating practices and the difficulty of melding the practice styles of diverse physician organizations was greater than anticipated. For example, there was difficulty in translating care-management techniques across diverse practice arrangements. Third, the organizations needed to renegotiate plan contracts, rationalize physician payment arrangements, and establish common information systems. New and often costly and redundant layers of overhead were added to manage these larger, more complex organizations.

There were some gains for a few physician organizations, but overall, physician organizations did not realize quick returns on their investments, nor did they achieve one of their major promises: the advancement and broad-scale dissemination of sophisticated clinical information systems.

Physician Organizations Falter

As cost pressures outpaced the benefits of integration, physician organizations faced significant financial difficulty in the late 1990s. The 600-member Monarch IPA reported a fifteen percent drop in commercial revenue by 1998. And in 1998, the prominent Bristol Park Medical Group laid off staff and closed four clinics.

The most significant disruption was the downfall of the two major PPMCs, motivated largely by Wall Street investors, who, disappointed by poor initial returns, pulled out their capital. The demise of these organizations had profound implications for the market. They had purchased the assets of numerous physician practices and IPAs in Orange County and established intermediaries that assumed risk; their dissolution disrupted key arrangements for the delivery and financing of care.

The San Diego-based PPMC, FPA Medical Management, Inc., had grown rapidly in response to pressure from Wall Street investors. It acquired 600 physician members in Orange County through its March 1998 purchase of a large, local medical group and its affiliated IPA. Only weeks later, FPA was in trouble: it was saddled with debt from its various acquisitions, had disappointing earnings, and reportedly suffered from accounting and management problems. The company filed for bankruptcy in July, and by the end of 1998, it had sold all of its California practices and relocated its headquarters to Miami.

At roughly the same time, MedPartners was faltering. It experienced a failed merger with another national PPMC, PhyCor, in January 1998, and its stock value subsequently collapsed. By November 1998, the company announced its decision to get out of the physician-practice management business nationwide.

Shaken by its failure to foresee FPA's financial problems, the state Department of Corporations (DOC) acted quickly upon discovery of financial irregularities in MedPartners' California operations. DOC intervened in March 1999 to seize control of the assets of MedPartners' risk-bearing subsidiary, MedPartners Network (MPN), to make sure that health plans' payments to the intermediary were used to pay providers locally and not to help bail out the corporate parent in Birmingham, Alabama. DOC put MPN under a state conservator, who filed for bankruptcy on its behalf.

These developments raised serious concerns in the market about who is accountable under capitated arrangements for care that is paid for, but not yet delivered or reimbursed. Plans are holding physician intermediaries responsible, and providers who are owed money under FPA and MedPartners' global capitation arrangements—an estimated $60 million and $73 million, respectively—want plans to be held liable. The California Medical Association (CMA) has filed a petition with DOC to force plans to cover FPA debts to providers, but this issue remains unresolved.

The PPMC failures also disrupted physicians' contracts, raising concerns about patients' ability to maintain access to their regular providers. Health plans and purchasers moved rapidly to establish alternative arrangements with physicians to minimize the disruption and to protect consumers' access to their usual physicians. For example, one purchaser in Orange County intervened to ensure that its health plan would continue contracting with a physician group that had left the MedPartners network.

The state, however, has expressed concern that actions to protect plan and consumer interests could hurt efforts of physician organizations to stay afloat. Blue Cross of California attempted to transfer enrollees from MedPartners' network providers throughout California in March 1999, but DOC blocked this action, fearing it would only further undermine MedPartners' precarious financial position.

MedPartners and DOC reached a tentative settlement in April under which MedPartners agreed to pay its debts in California and to continue funding its California clinics and IPAs until they were all sold. In return, the state retreated from its aggressive oversight of MPN, allowing MedPartners to resume responsibility for day-to-day operations. Significantly, the deal extended DOC's oversight of MPN to include MedPartners' California clinics and IPAs, which strengthened the state's ability to ensure that patients maintain access to MedPartners' physicians, and that physicians and hospitals are paid.

California's increasingly vigorous oversight of health plans and risk-bearing entities is expected to continue. The 1998 election of the first Democratic governor in sixteen years has also raised expectations for increased market regulation. Meanwhile, health plans have increased their scrutiny of physician organizations and have expressed a greater willingness to initiate corrective action when signs of financial trouble develop. On the whole, however, plans appear reluctant to drop capitation, and instead have focused on ways to improve delegated risk contracting.

Ultimately, physicians will feel the greatest effect from the failure of these organizations. Not only do they face potential financial liability for these entities' unpaid claims, but now they are confronted with the decision of whether to stay with the organization when it is sold, join another group or IPA, or go solo. This decision is particularly difficult for physicians who sold all the assets of their practices to the PPMC.

This turmoil contributes to a general sense of uneasiness among physicians in the market. Overall, physicians in Orange County are concerned about declines in income. Anecdotal reports indicate that some are retiring early, leaving the area, or targeting lucrative niches in the nonmanaged-care market. Several respondents suggested that physicians were more cautious now of physician intermediary organizations; for example, avoiding exclusive affiliations and refusing to share data with them and health plans. Moreover, physician organizations are re-evaluating their risk exposure, which could lead some to push for new contracts to reduce their risk for pharmacy costs and Medicare business.

Finally, there is concern about the implications of these developments for care-management efforts. Struggling with organizational growth and mounting cost pressures, physician organizations in Orange County found it more difficult than expected to focus on advancing and further disseminating techniques for managing clinical care delivery. As physician organizations evolve in this market, it remains to be seen whether they will have the incentives and capital to adequately invest in these activities.

Soaring Enrollment Leads to Financial Losses for Kaiser

Kaiser Foundation Health Plan, the local leader in market share, experienced its first losses on its business nationally, driven largely by problems in the California market. As a group-model HMO, Kaiser cushioned its physicians from the cost increases that other plans had passed on through contractual arrangements with independent physician organizations.

Perhaps of greater consequence, however, Kaiser also had continued its aggressive efforts to build market share by limiting premium increases. With premiums five to twenty percent lower than most other plans, Kaiser enrollment soared to almost 300,000 members in Orange County, an increase of nearly thirty percent since 1996.

This burgeoning enrollment severely strained the capacity of Kaiser's physicians and its hospitals. Kaiser has an exclusive relationship with its owned physician group and hospitals and referral relationships with a few contracted providers. In Orange County, Kaiser owns one hospital and leases wards at

two other hospitals, but each of these was filled to capacity, so Kaiser had to pay high daily rates to place patients at other facilities. Moreover, the physician group absorbed the increased enrollment at a time when it was improving enrollees' access to primary care physicians, further straining provider capacity.

To reverse its financial losses, Kaiser abandoned its strategy of holding down premiums and sought double-digit increases. The state public employee purchasing pool, for example agreed to an increase of almost eleven percent in 1999. The plan also increased its hospital capacity statewide to reduce referrals to outside providers, and it postponed opening two physician clinics in Orange County to reduce operating costs.

Hospitals Benefit from Consolidation

Against the backdrop of market turbulence, hospitals gained strength. Like physicians and health plans, Orange County hospitals had consolidated in the previous years. They have sought to integrate to achieve operations efficiencies and to bolster their leverage in the market.

St. Joseph's Health System, for example, pursued physician integration through a strategy of purchasing the assets of physician practices and IPAs and pressing for increased exclusivity under these arrangements. This allowed St. Joseph's to consolidate contracting so that it could enter into "single-signature contracts" with plans that encompass all the services provided by the hospital system and its affiliated physicians. By bringing together several large hospitals and numerous physicians under an arrangement with increased exclusivity, St. Joseph's was reportedly able to gain better rates from multiple health plans.

Tenet took a different approach—contracting with physicians and providing financial support for administration, rather than seeking ownership of groups. For example, Tenet was negotiating a ten-year capitated contract with MedPartners, although MedPartners' financial troubles ultimately resulted in a more modest preferred provider arrangement. Tenet also merged contracting functions across its eleven Orange County hospitals, a move that helped some of its hospitals obtain new plan contracts but did not bring the expected gains in payment rates. At the same time, individual Tenet hospitals sought their own arrangements with physicians, in keeping with the system's more arms-length approach.

In spite of initial gains from administrative integration, Orange County hospital systems have pursued little clinical integration to date. St. Joseph's has had discussions about developing a common electronic medical record across the system, but these efforts are still in the planning state. Tenet, likewise, has done little to integrate clinical functions, although it has achieved significant economies of scale through integration of some back-office functions and purchasing.

As Wall Street exited the local physician-practice management market, hospitals could increasingly become a source of capital. Hospitals are in a strong position to benefit from the instability in the physician market, particularly as PPMCs sell off practices at much lower prices than they had previously. St. Joseph's, for example, reportedly bought FPA's large physician group and affiliated IPA for a fraction of what FPA had paid just months earlier. Despite the added leverage that these physician organizations may bring, it is unclear whether hospitals will pursue this business aggressively, given its demonstrated risks.

Medicaid Managed Care Proceeds Smoothly, but the Safety Net is Strained

Orange County initiated major reform of its health insurance programs for low-income and uninsured people several years ago, and by all accounts, implementation of these efforts is proceeding smoothly. In 1993, Orange County created CalOPTIMA, a semi-autonomous entity charged with developing and overseeing a mandatory Medicaid managed-care program that relied on capitated contracting. CalOPTIMA became operational in 1995 and enrolled all recipients eligible through their receipt of cash assistance, as well as those eligible under programs for the aged and disabled. CalOPTIMA has won praise for expanding access to providers; currently, eighty-five percent of the county's physicians see Medi-Cal enrollees.

Through new contracts executed in the late 1990s, the program is increasing its attention to clinical care management and quality improvement. CalOPTIMA purchases services for its Medi-Cal members via capitated contracts with health plans or physician-hospital consortia (PHCs) created specially for the program. New contracts changed the payment split between hospitals and physicians in favor of physicians, and altered physician-hospital risk-sharing arrangements begun in 1995 to reduce hospitalizations and increase coordination between physicians and hospitals.

CalOPTIMA is also raising the minimum number of enrollees for PHCs and health plans from 2,500 to 5,000 in an effort to reduce the administrative burden to the participating plans and the program overall. This is intended to allow for a greater focus on quality improvement and to help plans manage enrollment declines due to welfare reform and improvements in the local economy.

From its inception, CalOPTIMA took steps to ensure the participation of traditional safety net providers, but began contracting with plans and PHCs that included other hospitals and physicians as well. There is no public hospital in the county, and two hospitals—the University of California at Irvine Medical Center (UCIMC) and Children's Hospital of Orange County (CHOC)—serve as the county's major safety net hospitals. CalOPTIMA has attempted to support these and other safety net providers by favoring PHCs that include them in the assignment of members who do not select a plan voluntarily.

While UCIMC's PHC has shown signs of enrollment growth recently, both safety net hospitals are now under significant financial pressure because many Medi-Cal beneficiaries enroll in other plans and PHCs that have broader geographic networks. UCIMC is seeking to increase its commercial patients to offset its declining Medi-Cal patient base, although commercial payments are also under pressure.

Complicating matters for CHOC, local hospitals began charging lower prices for advanced pediatric care. As a result, commercial plans were lured away from CHOC and the hospital's occupancy rate dropped to thirty percent. It subsequently reduced staffing considerably, consolidated admissions and some administrative functions with neighboring St. Joseph's, and closed a clinic. Meanwhile, UCIMC has also cut back staffing, even though emergency room visits by indigent persons have increased and UCIMC-affiliated specialists at three community clinics are reportedly experiencing great increases in demand. UCIMC is one of a few places in the county that provides free follow-up care with specialists for the indigent population.

Responsibility for care of the medically indigent remains the subject of much debate in Orange County. From the beginning, CalOPTIMA was slated to take over the county's program for the medically indigent, Medical Services for the Indigent (MSI). Under California law, counties are responsible for providing care to the medically indigent; they use a mix of state revenues and their own funds to support this care. Despite small increases to specialists, annual funding is fixed, and the program reportedly reimburses providers for less than one-fifth of the cost of providers' billed charges. While MSI has contributed to the cost of care for 20,000 indigent patients with medical need, this constitutes only a fraction of the estimated 335,000 uninsured adults in the county.

CalOPTIMA has been hesitant to take over MSI, wary of the overall financial implications of this responsibility and the lack of information about the size of this population and its health needs. CalOPTIMA and the county are now working on a pilot managed-care program to develop data on cost and clinical care requirements as a way to consider these issues more carefully. The county also recently stepped up eligibility verification standards to better ensure that the program focuses on its intended population, a move that is expected to limit MSI enrollment.

Advocates for the poor remain concerned about the ability of the safety net to provide care to Orange County's uninsured immigrant population, which continues to grow, particularly among Hispanics and Southeast Asians. Initiatives are underway to better serve this population, including a new community health center (CHC) serving Vietnamese immigrants and additional federal and grand funding for local CHCs.

However, many people in the county who need health care remain outside the mainstream of services, including immigrants, who may fear that using the public system could result in their deportation. This fear, as well as other cultural and socioeconomic barriers to care, has fueled reliance on so-called "back-office clinics," where unlicensed individuals provide health care and distribute pharmaceuticals illegally. County officials are exploring how to adapt the existing safety net to better serve the diverse populations in need of health care services.

Summary for Orange County

Many of the features of this mature, managed-care market appear to be fraying under financial pressures and consumer demands for more loosely managed insurance products. Integration efforts have been slow and costly for hospitals and physicians, and the high-profile failure of several large physician organizations and difficulties of others present serious challenges to a delivery system built on capitation and tight networks. Regulatory bodies are stepping up their scrutiny of risk relationships, and state policy changes appear likely.

The cost pressures that physicians have faced over the past years remain and may intensify. Additional benefit mandates and managed care regulations and decreasing Medicare payments may further constrain revenue for plans and providers. Health plans are raising premiums now. It remains to be seen whether premium increases will result in large enough payments to physician organizations to offset the severe financial pressures that confronted them over the past few years.

ASSESSING THE BURDEN OF DISEASE IN LOS ANGELES COUNTY

The final section of this chapter ties together the organizational issues of health systems with the underlying causes of illness and disease that are presented in the chapters that follow. An analysis of the impact of disease for Los Angeles County is presented using a new method that illustrates the impact of disease on populations and health systems. Thinking about the organization and operation of health care systems must be integrally and analytically tied into an understanding of the underlying needs of a population for health care. All of these issues must be combined with the policy issues associated with setting priorities and establishing public health and health care delivery goals and objectives. This section serves to illustrate this point and set the stage for the detailed analysis of the chapters that follow.

Monitoring the health status of the population is one of the core functions of local health departments and other public health agencies. Developing a clear understanding of the sources of morbidity and mortality in the population is critically important for establishing health priorities, allocating resources, and planning services. In Los Angeles County, assuring the availability of health services and developing a public health infrastructure that meets the needs of all residents and maximizes the health of the total population is an enormous challenge. The county is home to over 9.6 million residents, and is one of the most ethnically diverse jurisdictions in the United States. In addition, many county residents live in circumstances that make them especially vulnerable. For example, one-third of all children in the county live in households with incomes below the federal poverty level. In addition, an estimated one-third of adults and one-fourth of children have no health insurance and, therefore, have reduced access to health care services.

A new method—the Global Burden of Disease— used to assess the total burden of disease among county residents is described in this section. This method combines premature mortality and morbidity into a single measure known as Disability Adjusted Life Years (DALYs). Sources of disease burden are viewed broadly to include communicable diseases, chronic non-communicable diseases (such as coronary heart disease, cancer, and diabetes), mental illness, and injuries. The goal here is to provide perspectives on how to assess the burden of disease and injury and to advance discussion about how and where to allocate health resources to most effectively address health needs.

DALYs combine the impact of mortality and morbidity into a single measure of disease burden. Mortality rates are useful in identifying conditions with the worst health outcomes. However, conditions with low or moderate mortality rates may have a high burden of disease because of premature mortality or morbidity, or both. For example, intentional and unintentional injuries (e.g., injuries resulting from violence or motor vehicle crashes) most often involve younger individuals and thus have a higher burden of disease when premature death and equivalent years of life lost due to disability are taken into account. Chronic conditions such as arthritis and depression may have minimal impact on mortality, but be a major source of chronic disability and, therefore, exact a great toll on the quality of life and economic productivity. DALYs provide a common measure of disease burden that combines both the rate of mortality and the degree of morbidity. This combined measure can then be used to compare total disease burden across conditions to better plan health resource allocation and related program and policy efforts.

Methods of Analysis

DALYs are a composite measure of the number of years of life lost due to premature mortality plus the number of years lived with disability, appropriately adjusted for level of disability. It is, therefore, a measure of disease burden that combines the contributions of both premature death and disability associated with individual health conditions. DALYs associated with individual conditions can then be summed across all conditions to produce a comprehensive estimate of disease burden in a given population.

DALYs are the sum of two components. The first, Years of Life Lost (YLLs), measures the number of years lost when a person dies prematurely. Thus, the younger the age at which death occurs, the greater the number of YLLs due to premature mortality. The second component, Years Lived with Disability (YLDs), measures the number of years of healthy life lost due to temporary or permanent disability. The more severe or the longer the duration of disability associated with a given health condition, the greater the number of YLDs.

When a person dies, the number of YLLs attributable to that death is the decedent's remaining life expectancy; that is, the remaining number of years the person would have been expected to live. For example, a female infant who dies shortly after birth would lose all 82.5 years of life she would have been expected to live. A woman who dies at age seventy-five years would lose only twelve years of expected life, because her life expectancy at age seventy-five is eighty-seven years. Data on life expectancy at every age are contained in life tables. These tables are calculated separately for males and females because females live longer on average. For economically disadvantaged groups, such as African Americans, life expectancies are further reduced.

The burden of disease method does not calculate YLLs individually for each death. Instead, each death is assigned to one of nineteen age groupings and the midpoint of the age group is taken as the average age at death for every person in that group. Deaths (and the resulting YLLs) are combined into 140 broad categories of disease and injury (e.g., coronary heart disease, alcohol dependence, homicide/violence) based on the underlying cause of death. These disease categories are then used to characterize disease burden in the county population.

Many conditions, such as cerebrovascular disease (stroke), cause significant disability as well as death. Other conditions, such as depression and other mental illness, are seldom listed as causes of death, but may cause severe and prolonged disability. The calculation of YLDs takes into account the severity of disability due to a given disease as well as the average length of time the disability persists. For example, Alzheimer's disease often causes severe disability, but typically occurs late in life and is, therefore, of relatively short duration. In contrast, asthma frequently causes less severe disability, but may begin in childhood and persist for a lifetime. The YLD measure counts the number of years of reduced health caused by living with a disabling condition, adjusted by the percentage of disability. For example, two years lived with fifty percent disability contribute one YLD to the overall burden of disease, as do four years lived with twenty-five percent disability. According to this definition of morbidity, one YLD is *equivalent* to one YLL; so two years lived with fifty percent disability are the same as one year of life lost due to premature death. The degree of disability due to a given condition is expressed as a disability weight, ranging from 0.0 for no

disability to 1.0 for death. The complete calculation of YLDs is complex. YLDs for a given disabling illness and for a given age group are the product of the disability weight, the expected duration of the disability, and the incidence of the disability (that is, the rate at which persons develop the disability during the year of analysis). The YLD calculation can be simplified by using YLD-to-YLL ratios. This ratio method produces *estimates* of the amount of YLDs in a population based on *actual* rates of YLLs.

The total number of DALYs associated with each disease category is the sum of the YLLs and YLDs for that disease. Two additional adjustments are applied to each measure: an age weighting factor and a discounting factor. The age weighting factor quantifies the widely held perception that a year of life is valued more heavily at some ages than at others. The value of the weighting factor rises rapidly from zero at birth, peaks at age twenty-two years, and declines gradually thereafter. The discounting factor quantifies the perception most people hold that a year of life is more valuable the closer it is to the present. This is analogous to the application of financial discount rates that value a current dollar more than a future dollar. The discounting factor applied is three percent per year.

Results of the Analysis

A total of 59,786 deaths were included in the analysis, accounting for 99.5 percent of all deaths reported among Los Angeles County residents (1997). Heart disease accounted for the greatest number of deaths, followed by stroke, lung and other respiratory tract cancers, pneumonia, and emphysema. For the twenty conditions accounting for the greatest number of deaths, their respective ranks based on YLLs and DALYs are shown in Table 2.2. Considerable variation is apparent in the ranking of conditions based on the number of deaths (crude mortality) versus YLLs and DALYs. For example, although pneumonia was the fourth leading cause of death based on crude mortality, it was only the twelfth leading cause of premature death based on YLLs and only the twenty-first leading cause of premature death and disability based on DALYs.

Heart disease was also the leading cause of YLLs, followed by homicide and violence, lung and other

Table 2.2. Leading Twenty Causes of Death in Los Angeles County, 1997 (YLL and DALY ranks are shown for comparison)

Rank	Cause	No. of Deaths	YLL Rank	DALY Rank
1	Coronary heart disease	14,378	1	1
2	Stroke	4,168	4	7
3	Trachea/bronchus/ lung cancer	3,772	3	8
4	Pneumonia	3,364	12	21
5	Emphysema	2,671	11	9
6	Diabetes mellitus	1,747	10	5
7	Colon cancer	1,483	15	23
8	Homicide/violence	1,247	2	3
9	Breast cancer	1,242	9	19
10	Hypertension	1,241	17	30
11	Cirrhosis	1,045	8	14
12	Alzheimer's/other dementia	1,000	30	12
13	Inflammatory heart disease	927	13	20
14	Motor vehicle crashes	888	5	10
15	Prostate cancer	841	27	36
16	Lymphoma	804	16	29
17	Pancreatic cancer	795	19	37
18	Suicide/other self-inflicted injury	785	6	16
19	HIV/AIDS	680	7	13
20	Leukemia	620	18	32

Table 2.3. Leading Twenty Causes of Premature Death in Los Angeles County Based on Years of Life Lost (YLL), 1997 (Crude mortality and DALY ranks are shown for comparison)

Rank	Cause	YLL (Years)	Crude Mortality Rank	DALY Rank
1	Coronary heart disease	66,494	1	1
2	Homicide/violence	35,572	8	3
3	Trachea/bronchus/ lung cancer	27,414	3	8
4	Stroke	21,601	2	7
5	Motor vehicle crashes	19,908	14	10
6	Suicide/other self-inflicted injury	15,339	18	16
7	HIV/AIDS	14,939	19	13
8	Cirrhosis	14,123	11	14
9	Breast cancer	13,288	9	19
10	Diabetes mellitus	13,262	6	5
11	Emphysema	13,017	5	9
12	Pneumonia	12,977	4	21
13	Inflammatory heart disease	10,635	13	20
14	Drug overdose/ other intoxication	10,631	23	11
15	Colon cancer	10,154	7	23
16	Lymphoma	8,029	16	29
17	Hypertension	7,122	10	30
18	Leukemia	6,479	20	32
19	Pancreatic cancer	5,483	17	37
20	Endocrine/ metabolic diseases	5,070	24	15

respiratory tract cancers, stroke, and motor vehicle crashes (Table 2.3). Considerable variation in the rankings is again apparent. For example, because YLLs account for the impact of premature mortality, motor vehicle crashes moved up in ranking from fourteenth based on crude mortality to fifth based on YLLs. Likewise, HIV/AIDS moved from nineteenth based on crude mortality to seventh based on YLLs.

The leading twenty causes of disease burden based on DALYs are shown in Table 2.4. Heart disease was the leading cause of DALYs, followed by alcohol dependence, homicide and violence, depression, and diabetes. As indicated in the table, many of the leading causes of disease burden on the DALYs list are ranked considerably lower based on crude mortality

and YLLs. For example, osteoarthritis is ranked sixth based on DALYs, but only seventieth based on crude mortality, and eightieth based on YYLs. These disparities highlight the importance of these conditions as sources of disability and their relatively minimal impacts on mortality.

The relative burden (as measured in DALYs) of communicable diseases, non-communicable diseases, and injuries for the total county population varies by disease category, gender, age, and race. Overall,

Table 2.4.   Leading Twenty Causes of Premature Death and Disability in Los Angeles County Based on Disability-Adjusted Life Years (DALY), 1997 (Crude mortality and YLL ranks are shown for comparison)

Rank	Cause	DALYs (Years)	Crude Mortality Rank	YLL Rank
1	Coronary heart disease	72,886	1	1
2	Alcohol dependence	60,872	39	29
3	Homicide/violence	45,548	8	2
4	Depression	43,449	91	91
5	Diabetes mellitus	42,456	6	10
6	Osteoarthritis	39,811	70	80
7	Stroke	33,351	2	4
8	Trachea/bronchus/lung cancer	29,785	3	3
9	Emphysema	29,333	5	11
10	Motor vehicle crashes	29,040	14	5
11	Drug overdose/other intoxication	28,508	23	14
12	Alzheimer's/other dementia	27,626	12	30
13	HIV/AIDS	20,649	19	7
14	Cirrhosis	18,263	11	8
15	Endocrine/metabolic diseases	17,541	24	20
16	Suicide/other self-inflicted injury	16,568	18	6
17	Drug dependence	16,415	50	40
18	Asthma	16,326	44	42
19	Breast cancer	15,379	9	9
20	Inflammatory heart disease	14,666	13	13

eighty percent of disease burden was associated with non-communicable diseases (e.g., coronary heart disease, cancer, and diabetes), eleven percent with injuries, and nine percent with communicable diseases. The DALY rates were higher in men than women. Most of this difference is attributable to a fifty percent higher rate of YLLs among men than women. The DALY rates also varied by race and ethnicity. African Americans had the highest rate, followed by American Indians/Alaska Natives, Whites, Latinos, and Asians/Pacific Islanders. The rates of YLLs and YLDs were also highest in African Americans.

Summary for Los Angeles County

Chronic illnesses, drug and alcohol dependence, violence, and unintentional injuries produce a substantial burden of disease. The most important finding here is that DALYs produce a substantially different ranking of disease burden than do mortality rates

alone. Several conditions, including alcohol dependence, depression, drug dependence, and osteoarthritis, have a significant burden of disease not adequately captured by mortality rates because of the large number of years of disability associated with these conditions. Other conditions, including injuries from motor vehicle crashes, HIV/AIDS, and suicide, have a greater burden of illness and injury than is measured solely by crude mortality rates due in large part to the considerable premature mortality associated with these conditions.

Many of the twenty highest ranked conditions in Los Angeles County based on DALYs can be effectively addressed through public health efforts. Alcohol and other substance abuse, injuries from motor vehicle crashes, and HIV/AIDS are examples of conditions where mortality and disability can be reduced through education, health promotion activities, treatment services, and healthful policies. The disease burden of chronic conditions, such as depression, heart disease, diabetes, and arthritis, can also be effectively reduced through public health programs and improved access to medical care services and disease management.

For Los Angeles County, this better depiction of disease burden will be used to help allocate funding for public health services and programs. The DALYs analysis provides a broader picture of community health needs than traditional measures of mortality and morbidity. Further, this study shows substantial differences within the county by racial/ethnic group and by geographic area. Ultimately, the test of the incremental value of this method will be whether this information leads to a more rapid closing of the serious disparities in health among different ethnic and racial groups.

CHAPTER

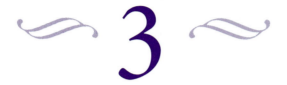

3

Medicine and Technology*

Institute for the Future
Menlo Park, CA

Chapter Topics

- Rational Drug Design
- Advances in Imaging
- Minimally Invasive Surgery
- Genetic Mapping and Testing
- Gene Therapy
- Vaccines
- Artificial Blood
- Xenotransplantation

Learning Objectives

Upon completing this chapter, the reader should be able to:

- Appreciate the complexity of today's technology
- Anticipate the nature of developing and new technologies
- Assess the impact of a selection of cutting-edge technologies
- Have a framework for understanding and assessing technology

New medical technologies are among the key driving forces in health care. In the years since its unscientific roots in the nineteenth century, medicine has made great strides in verifying the germ theory, creating aseptic surgical techniques, discovering antibiotics, developing anesthesia, and imaging the inside of the body. The impact has been huge in improving public health, extending our life span, saving lives, and heightening quality of life. The related cost impact has been equally large, especially in the United States, where new medical technologies are enthusiastically embraced as they become available.

This chapter examines eight medical technologies that will affect patient care over the next decade. Each is described, and then the magnitude and areas of impact as well as the barriers to change of the technology are discussed.

These technologies illustrate the dramatic turn of events in medicine today and help set the stage for the other chapters of the book. Technological change is the impetus for changes in how services are provided and paid for, and for the evaluation of clinical care itself. The technologies discussed here, while obviously not inclusive of the medical landscape, aptly illustrate the opportunities and challenges of the future.

Even after a medical technology or technique has been discovered, developed, approved, and commercialized, it may take years for it to be disseminated widely. Similarly, in many clinical areas, state-of-the-art knowledge is slowly adopted in community practice. Therefore, it is often difficult to know when each technology will be widely used in clinical practice or its full impact, especially on disease status, access to care, and costs. Other important technologies that will impact health care but are not discussed here are listed in Table 3.1.

Table 3.1. Additional Medical Technologies

• Ablative techniques	• Joint replacement
• Artificial livers	• Pain control
• Cloning	• Regional perfusion
• DNA sequencing/ diagnostics	• Tissue sealants
• Functional neural stimulation	• Treatments for drug-resistant disease strains
	• Virtual reality systems

RATIONAL DRUG DESIGN

Most drugs on the market today have been discovered in random screens of naturally occurring products or from analog development programs—once a time-consuming manual process. Today's robotic systems can screen millions of compounds in a year's time. This method of random trial and error is inefficient: of 10,000 agents tested, 1,000 typically show bioactivity, 100 are worth investigating, ten go to clinical trials, and only one reaches patients on the market. Most current pharmaceuticals were chanced upon after years of this research by trial and error; occasionally, researchers came across something that was not only safe for human use, but also beneficial. The chemicals identified from these experiments were discovered as they existed in nature. Happily, we are no longer just searching randomly in nature to find therapeutic chemicals. Now scientists are *designing* thousands every day.

Rational drug design is the development of new chemical or molecular entities by looking at the physical structure and chemical composition of a target—a molecular receptor or enzyme—and designing drugs that bind to those molecules, turning them on or off. Drug designers use physical chemistry to identify qualities of the specific agent that initiates a pathology; once a known chain of events is identified, designers attempt to intervene at a particular point with a specific method. Designers use several strategies and methods:

- *Structure-based design.* The central assumption of structure-based design is that good inhibitors must be complementary to their target receptor. The two-step process begins by determining the structure of receptors and then solving the 3-D jigsaw puzzle of matching molecular structures by using specially developed computer programs.
- *Molecular modeling.* This technique looks at the physical structure of a receptor and creates the model of a compatible chemical entity by using computer imaging. This can be done with incredible precision down to the level of DNA coding. With the help of computed chemical algorithms, designers can build—first virtually on the computer,

then "wet" in the lab—the molecule of perfect chemical fit.

- *Virtual reality modeling.* This is a form of computer-enhanced molecular modeling. It includes features such as a force feedback handle that permits tactile manipulation of a 3-D image of the candidate molecule model's orientation.

- *Combinatorial chemistry.* This technique allows drug researchers to quickly produce as many as several million structurally related compounds, which they then screen to find those that are bioactive and possibly have therapeutic value. The chemical attributes of those molecules are known, and the chemists working with them expect certain biological activity. With the development of more reliable and rapid screening tests, thousands of related chemicals can be tested in parallel processes for reactivity with a complement of human antibodies on a mass scale.

Rational drug design will shorten the drug discovery process. New chemical and molecular entities will get to clinical trials faster as the random and unpredictable time for discovering a compound by chance is replaced by these more predictable design processes based on the structure and complexity of the pathogen.

Because rational drug design may result in too many promising new chemical entities and not enough resources to test them all, prioritization and stratification of candidate products will be an important area of concern.

Magnitude and Areas of Impact

Rational drug design will have an impact in a number of therapeutic areas. Chief candidates include the following:

- *Neurologic and mental disease.* Drugs are being created that fit the receptors for various neurotransmitters, potentially to modify nerve activity and influence the function of the nervous system in different areas where neurological and mental pathology are manifested.

- *Antiviral therapies.* Protease inhibitors designed to combat viral disease will be an important area of development. Every virus uses proteases to chop proteins into amino acids, which the virus then uses as building blocks. Targeting and inhibiting these enzymes could lead to the creation of the first truly effective antivirals. In the next ten years, rational drug design will create antiviral therapies to combat diseases like human immunodeficiency virus (HIV), encephalitis, measles, and influenza.

Key Barriers

One of the key driving forces behind rational drug design has been the increasing power of computers. The techniques and processes involved in rational drug design are highly information intensive and well suited to computer processing. The pace of drug design advances is regulated in part by the availability of research teams that combine knowledge of biochemistry with that of computer technology.

As researchers seek to combat more complex pathogens, they need to develop drugs that interact with their targets in more specific ways. With increased specificity and complexity will come increased costs in developing the proper new chemical entity.

Because drug design can create an embarrassment of riches in terms of screened candidate compounds, much progress will need to be made in evaluating and prioritizing the candidates.

ADVANCES IN IMAGING

Imaging technologies present an enhanced visual display of tissues, organ systems, and their functions. They reveal the structural and functional aspects of organs, allowing clinicians to localize specific functions or conditions noninvasively.

Imaging has four elements: aiming energy at the area of interest; detecting or receiving that reflected or refracted energy; analyzing the data with computers, and displaying those data with technology that allows the clinician to view and interpret the information. Advances are taking place in each of these areas that will open up new functions for imaging technologies.

- *Energy sources* currently used for imaging include X-rays, ultrasound, electron beams, positrons, magnets, and radio frequencies. There is a constant trade-off in the energy sources used: on one hand, the more powerful the energy source, the more deeply it can penetrate and the more detail it can reveal in the image; on the other hand, powerful beams can injure tissues and organ systems. The same ultrasound energy that reveals "baby's first picture" to expectant parents can also, at a higher level, smash kidney stones in an electrolithotropter. Energy source technology is advancing as scientists find ways to more narrowly focus an energy beam to avoid damage to adjacent tissue. Research is also being conducted on alternate energy sources such as thermal differences in order to minimize residual damage.

- *Detector technology* is advancing along two dimensions. First, digital detectors benefit from the trends in microelectronics toward smaller and smaller features on devices. The resolution of those detectors is improving constantly. The first commercially available "megapixel" detector (able to detect an image that comprises a grid of 1,000 by 1,000 pixels, discrete elements of the image) became available more than a decade ago. By 2005, detectors that can resolve 6,000 by 6,000 pixels will become available. Second, there are advances in contrast media. These are chemicals that, when introduced into the body, enhance the contrast between light and dark regions of an image in specific ways; for example, by highlighting areas of malignant tissues or tissue abnormalities with more blood flow. Work is proceeding on contrast media that have organ, tissue, and cellular specificities.

- *Analysis of the image* is the next function in which there are rapid advances. Computer analysis of the masses of data from high-resolution detectors gets faster and better with increases in raw computing power. Breakthroughs in algorithms and techniques such as neural networks will speed the conversion from 2-D to 3-D images, improve pattern recognition through better detection of edges and other features of images, and ease the manipulation and enhancement of digital images.

- *Display technologies* are getting bigger, faster, and cheaper. There is spillover to medical imaging from a range of applications that require high-quality images. Improvements include larger displays, higher resolution, richer and more meaningful contrasts, and deeper color.

Magnitude and Areas of Impact

Advances in imaging are combining in several areas. *Electron-beam CT scanning*—in contrast to conventional CT scanning that uses X-ray beams—offers substantial improvements over old technologies. It allows for rapid acquisition of an image, reducing the discomfort patients experience from remaining immobile for the duration of a conventional CT scan. While this technology can detect calcium in the wall of the coronary artery, showing atherosclerosis, it does not show whether there is narrowing of the blood vessel. With the development of new contrast agents, electron-beam CT will be able to show visuals of the arteries themselves, making this technology competitive with MRI, although MRI has the additional value of showing blood flow.

- *Harmonic imaging* will overcome a number of barriers in ultrasonography. About one-third of all patients are "difficult to image," which means that a patient's body wall anatomy, for a variety of reasons, is difficult to "see" through. Specifically, someone who is obese or extremely muscular or someone with narrow rib spacing is often difficult to image. Smokers and people who have had radiation therapy can also fall into this category for cardiac imaging, and for OB/GYN a variety of impediments of the abdomen can cause difficulty. Harmonic imaging improves the quality of images in these patients. Ultrasound generally works as follows: sound waves are transmitted into the body at a relatively low frequency and are detected by a receiver that is tuned to the same frequency. In harmonic imaging, the receiver is turned to a higher frequency than the transmitter so that the clinician detects the harmonics, or the frequency-multiples of the echoes, that are produced inside the body itself. Higher frequency waves produce images with better resolution. Applications of harmonic imaging include better prediction of heart attacks by allowing the clinician to visualize blood flow through the myocardium.

- *Functional imaging*, which provides information about how a tissue or organ system is operating, will go far beyond the capabilities of conventional MRI, CT, and ultrasonography, which now provides only *structural* information about tissues and organ systems. PET has long been capable of metabolic imaging—detecting patterns of energy use in the body. High-resolution PET will offer pinpoint accuracy in these images, which will render many invasive diagnostic procedures such as surgical biopsy obsolete. Functional MRI is used to determine the location of neurological functions such as memory and reasoning in the brain, giving us the first look at how the brain works. Future applications of functional MRI will be in the study of disease and the body's response to treatment—for example, changes in the pattern of neural activity in the brain of schizophrenic patients being treated with new drugs.

Because developments in computing power have increased image display speed and improved the quality and content of digital images, *image-guided surgery* is becoming a mainstream procedure. Image-guided surgery is a new kind of minimally invasive surgical intervention. It improves on endoscopic and endovascular surgical methods by allowing the clinician to see a computed functional image superimposed on the surgical instrument's location and other relevant information. The current combination of nearly real-time imaging and functional mapping will result in real-time, high-contrast, and high-spatial-resolution images.

Overall, imaging technologies will improve the diagnostic process immensely. Clinicians will use these technologies to look at the form and function of organs that were once examined only by surgery, reducing the need for invasive diagnostic procedures.

Key Barriers

There are few barriers to the development of new imaging technologies, which benefit from the continual progress of computing power. Simple economics will limit the application of some technologies. Historically, imaging technologies have been additive—new technologies do not replace old ones, but rather sup-

plement their use. In a cost-constrained health system, more restraint will be exercised in the use of new imaging systems. Comprehensive analyses of cost-effectiveness, including the full life-cycle cost of the equipment, will become commonplace.

MINIMALLY INVASIVE SURGERY

Also called *minimal* or *limited-access surgery*, minimally invasive surgery was made possible by the introduction of fiberoptic technology, miniaturization of improved instruments and devices, image digitization, navigational systems for vascular catheters, and a sudden awareness that image-guided surgery was the wave of the future. Early examples of minimally invasive surgery were arthroscopic meniscectomy, endovascular obliteration of intracranial aneurysms, and laparoscopic cholecystectomy. More recent innovations are image-guided brain surgery, minimal access major cardiac operations, and the endovascular placement of grafts for abdominal aneurysms. Over the same period of time, open surgery biopsy has been replaced by fine-needle aspiration of many tumors, which is gaining general acceptance for use on tumors of the breast and thyroid gland.

The movement toward minimally invasive surgery has promoted the proliferation of ambulatory surgicenters. The consequent major reduction in the volume of surgical procedures performed in hospital facilities has achieved a remarkable reduction in the length of stay, as patients having procedures previously requiring hospitalization enjoy more rapid recovery and return to full activity because of the lowered morbidity of the less invasive operations. In areas where minimally invasive procedures have replaced their more disruptive antecedents, short-term as well as long-term outcomes have been the same or, in most examples, better, with a high level of acceptance and satisfaction by patients. In the case of invasive procedures, less *is* better.

Magnitude and Areas of Impact

To begin at the top, brain surgery has been a major beneficiary of image-guided technology. Operations requiring access to nonsurface areas of the brain beneath the surface are conducted by using navigational systems and image guidance through small openings in the skull. Even more dramatic has been the impact of endovascular surgery, the creation of a group of innovative interventional radiologists. Using current technology—digitized image guidance, catheter navigational systems, and an array of implantable materials—endovascular surgeons can treat almost all intercranial aneurysms and many arteriovenous fistulas. Moreover, subsequent open surgical procedures can be facilitated by preoperative reduction of blood flow to the tumor or congenital arteriovenous malformation.

Endovascular surgery has advanced and matured rapidly in the past decade. The practitioners of the art fall into three broad categories with a slight degree of overlap. The first, interventional neuroradiologists, deal with vascular pathology of the brain and spinal cord. In addition to the procedures described earlier, these neurointerventionalists can lyse blood clots in cerebral arteries and veins, dilate intracranial arteries narrowed by pathologic vasospasm, and open partially or completely occluded arteriosclerotic arteries that restrict blood flow to the brain.

The second and largest group of endovascular interventionalists are cardiologists whose major procedure is coronary angioplasty. With advances in intravascular stent technology and the introduction of pharmaceuticals that inhibit the principal cause of restenosis—postangioplasty proliferation of subendothelial smooth muscle in the arterial wall—percutaneous angioplasty will further reduce the indications for open operations for coronary artery bypass grafting. Cardiac interventionalists can also correct cardiac arrhythmias, treat selected cardiac valve disorders, and, by using improved technology, close congenital septal defects.

The third group of endovascular surgeons operate in sites other than the central nervous system and the heart; for example, they place endovascular prosthetic devices for the treatment of abdominal aortic aneurysms, create therapeutic vascular shunts, and perform angioplasty of narrowed arteries in the trunk and extremities.

Laparoscopy has truly revolutionized the practice of abdominal surgery for procedures on the gastrointestinal tract and female organs. The most recent addition to the laparoscopic surgeon's growing list of operations is bilateral adrenalectomy. Further advances will incorporate telepresence technology, which permits a surgeon to operate remotely, robotics, and 3-D imaging. Technological advances are proceeding with unprecedented speed, placing pressures on practicing general and gynecologic surgeons either to seek additional training or to drift into obsolescence with out-of-date skills.

Future refinements in minimally invasive surgery will expand the present scope and range of procedures. New arthroscopic procedures, wider use of image guidance in operations on the head and neck, and innovations in limited-access procedures for spinal and thoracic diseases are evolving; within the next five years they will be accepted practice. These advances will be aided by interventional MRI, currently used for liver and kidney biopsy, with its shortened acquisition time and 3-D capability.

For patients with acute stroke, interventional MRI will be a major addition to the surgical process. Pharmacologic brain protection will extend the viability of ischemic brain, and prompt transfer to a dedicated MRI facility will permit immediate assessment of the brain's viability and blood flow. When appropriate, occluded vessels can be opened by endovascular intervention under the guidance of MRI. By the year 2010, large population centers will have "vascular institutes" that are serviced by emergency transportation networks. Vascular institutes will facilitate rapid movement of heart attack, stroke, and other acute vascular accident victims to an institute staffed around the clock by endovascular surgeons who can prevent the death and disability that current technologies cannot. Current gaps in ancillary pharmaceuticals will be closed by products emerging from the biotech industry. The development of stent grafts that can be used in cervical vessels and at branchings will extend their application at sites currently beyond the reach of endovascular technology.

Key Barriers

• The American public wants big automobiles, RVs, and minimally—or even better, noninvasive—surgery. The appeal and marketability of minimally invasive operations have the effect of pulling these technologies into the health care system in advance of adequate technology assessment, including evaluation of cost-effectiveness. Adverse outcomes can and do result from prematurely applied minimally invasive procedures. One consequence could be restrictive legislation that would have the effect of creating major barriers to innovative clinical trials of promising technology.

• Insurers restrict or deny payment for new, minimally invasive procedures by declaring them experimental and therefore not a covered benefit.

• Currently, mechanisms for transfer of procedural technologies into the practicing medical community are barely adequate, bordering on inadequate. As computer-enabled procedural technologies evolve at an ever-increasing pace, their successful penetration into the delivery system will be restricted unless better models for teaching practicing physicians to use these technologies are designed and implemented.

GENETIC MAPPING AND TESTING

Until recently, most genetic tests have been used to detect rare and singular conditions. Many of these single-gene disorders become clinically apparent during infancy and childhood whereas others, such as Huntington's disease and polycystic kidney disease, are of adult onset. Genetic tests are used to detect carrier states and for prenatal counseling.

The special field of clinical genetics has evolved from observations of familial occurrences of inherited disorders to the use of the tools of human molecular genetics. Genetic tests have become available for more common and more complex diseases, many with onset in adult life. With the identification of cancer-susceptible genes and of genes leading to neurogenetic disorders including Alzheimer's disease, the Human Genome Project provided the engine that propelled the rapid identification of a wide range of genes that can cause complex diseases such as diabetes, cancer, and heart disease. These gene discoveries provided the basis for genetic susceptibility testing—recognition of a predisposition to disease—and with it unprecedented opportunities to inter-

vene with strategies for prevention, avoidance, or modification of the predisposed condition. Abruptly, clinical genetics assumed a role whose importance was only imagined a decade ago.

No scientific discipline is as fast-paced today as medical genetics. It seems that each week, disease-associated genes are identified and added to the genomic database to fuel a parallel growth of diagnostic and screening tests. To date, clinical tests have been developed for almost 500 human genetic disorders, a number that will continue to grow in the flurry of activity to complete mapping of the human genome.

The National Cancer Institute has established three primary goals with regard to genetic testing: (1) identification of every major human gene that predisposes individuals to cancer; (2) clinical application of these discoveries to people at risk; and (3) identification and remedial attention to psychosocial, ethical, and legal issues associated with inherited susceptibility. A secondary goal is developing an informatics system to collect, store, analyze, and integrate cancer-related molecular data with epidemiologic and clinical data.

Magnitude and Areas of Impact

Genetic susceptibility testing for cancer of the breast, colon, and prostate is moving into clinical reality, and in each instance, the hereditary pattern of disease provided the initial search for the identification of the critical gene or genes.

More complex genetic disorders, such as childhood asthma and late-onset Alzheimer's disease, suggest either a polygenic inheritance, in which more than one gene is responsible for the disease in a particular individual, or genetic heterogeneity, in which different combinations of genes produce the same condition in different individuals. Of even greater complexity are the conditions currently being studied in the emerging field of neurogenetics, where genes that increase susceptibility to schizophrenia, manic-depressive illness, and depression are studied to find out how they interact with nongenetic (e.g., environmental) factors to trigger the onset of the recognized disease state. In these psychiatric disorders, identification of the specific genes may give clues for designing pharmacologic interventions. The discovery of genetic susceptibility provides the basis for initiating preventive measures, whether through pharmacologic means or counseling. The new term *genometrics* has been applied to the discovery of a gene or genes responsible for a trait and to defining precisely the trait controlled by each gene involved in complex multifactoral illnesses.

Within a few years, our present methods of genetic analysis, sophisticated though they are, will be viewed as time-consuming, labor intensive, expensive, and myopic in scope and application. New technology will use microchips designed to interrogate DNA or RNA samples for sequence or expression information. The chemicals for these microchips can be synthesized cheaply, rapidly, and efficiently by using the synthetic methods borrowed from the semiconductor industry. With fluorescent methods for the detection of DNA and RNA targets, hybridization will occur in a special chamber, and the resulting signals will be detected by scanning microscopy in a matter of minutes. Current applications of this microchip technology will revolutionize the fields of diagnostics and genomics. Within the next decade, cancer tissue will be analyzed for differences in gene expression, and in another five years specific therapies can be assigned to individuals with identified cancer genotypes. Tumors of a particular type will be classified by genotypic profile, and once they are classified, even individualized treatment will be quite specifically administered. Applied to genetic testing, microchip technology will have predictive power for disease and disease predisposition that until now was almost unimaginable.

Key Barriers

Practicing clinicians—generalists and specialists alike—lack the knowledge base to practice genomic medicine. Genetic testing, particularly the predisposition genetic testing for late-onset disorders in adults, requires a multidisciplinary approach. People seeking such testing need appropriate pretest education and genetic counseling and post-test follow-up care. Before testing is done, the person must be informed that other factors, genetic and nongenetic, may influence onset and severity of the condition, and that, in many situations, testing is probabilistic rather than deterministic. Potential consequences must be understood, as must the clinician's inability to guarantee confidentiality despite all safeguards and legislative protections.

Genetic testing has a predictable future based on technological potential. This potential could be constrained, delayed, or lost entirely through several possible developments: the desire in prenatal testing to enhance specific attributes of offspring; technology's advancing too rapidly for rational assimilation and application because of an understaffed clinical genetics workforce; premature availability of self-administered testing kits as a consequence of unregulated commercial interests; and ethical roadblocks imposed because of misuse of genetic information contrary to public policy (e.g., sterilization of people afflicted with a serious heritable disease to prevent genetic transmission to offspring).

With proper safeguards, genetic testing will revolutionize prevention and treatment of many conditions and diseases, but without these safeguards, the possibilities for mass confusion, misapplication, discrimination, and lawful or unlawful commercial exploitation are sobering.

GENE THERAPY

A few years ago, a blue-ribbon panel of experts sharply criticized the rush to initiate clinical trials of gene therapy before an adequate scientific base was established. The consequence was a slowdown in clinical applications and a return to basic research in several critical areas: better vectors or delivery vehicles to ferry corrective genes into target cells; more precise targeting of genes to specific sites and tissues; and enhancement of gene expression following entry into the target cell.

Nevertheless, revolutionary advances in gene therapy are preparing medicine for an epochal shift to an era in which genes will be delivered routinely to cure or alleviate an array of inherited and acquired diseases. Gene therapy can be defined as "a therapeutic technique in which a functioning gene is inserted into targeted cells of a patient to correct an inborn error or to provide the cell with a new function." The successful delivery and insertion of a functioning gene leads to the expression of a therapeutic protein of some kind that will supplement or replace a defective gene or treat the effects of acquired diseases like cancer. Somatic gene therapy, discussed here, only affects somatic cells—the kinds that are neither sperm nor egg (Ronchi, 1996).

Current methods for gene therapy use directly harvested cells, cultured cell lines, genetically modified cell lines, and viral vectors, such as modified retroviruses or adenoviruses. In the *ex vivo* approach, cells from specific tissues are removed, cultured, and exposed to viral or nonviral vectors or DNA containing the gene of interest. After insertion of the genes into these cells, the cells are returned to the patient. In the *in vivo* approach, viral or nonviral vectors—or simply "naked DNA"—are directly administered to patients by various routes. A third approach involves the encapsulation of gene-modified cells and the reversible introduction of an encapsulated cell structure into the human body.

A challenge for genetic researchers is to develop methods that discriminately deliver enough genetic material to the right cells. Most gene vectors in current use are disabled mouse retroviruses. Retroviral vectors offer the most promising prospect for the transfer of useful gene sequences into defective tumor cells because they target only dividing cells and have the potential of long-term expression. They are considered safe and effective gene delivery vehicles and are attractive because they are designed specifically to enter cells and express their genes there. Retroviruses splice copies of their genes into the chromosomes of the cells they invade, and the integrated gene is then passed on to future generations of cells. Because cell entry by a retrovirus occurs only when cells are actively dividing, this feature is exploited in rapidly dividing cells such as bone marrow, but is not suitable for other tissues, such as muscle and lung. Unfortunately, retroviruses are somewhat indiscriminate and have been known to deposit their genes into the chromosomes of a variety of cell types, prompting research into viral envelope alteration in the hope of increasing target specificity. The specificity of the envelope—how the vector is "packaged"—ensures the appropriate receptors are triggered.

Other viral vectors are also being explored. These include adenoviruses and adenoassociated viruses, herpes viruses, alpha viruses, vaccina virus, and poxviruses. Each virus has a potential therapeutic niche established by its attributes and behavior. The next most commonly used vector after retrovirus is the adenovirus, a DNA virus that, although capable of entering a dividing as well as a nondividing cell, has produced disappointing results. Adenoassociated viruses appeal because they cause no known diseases in humans and they integrate their genes into human chromosomes. But because they are small, they may not be able to accommodate large genes. Herpes viruses do not integrate their genes into the host's DNA, but they are attracted to neurons and may be useful in neurological therapies.

Liposomes are yet another potential vector under examination. The synthetic liquid bubbles can be designed to harbor plasmids—stable loops of DNA that multiply naturally within bacteria—in which original genes have been replaced by those intended to be therapeutic. A synthetic, liposome-like vector, the lipoplex, can bind firmly to cell surfaces and insert its DNA package into cells at a significant rate. Mixing lipoplexes with DNA has become a standard technique for inserting genes into cultured cells.

Although currently undeveloped for clinical use, two new viral-based vector systems hold out the possibility of advancing toward the ideal delivery system for directly supplying cells with healthy copies of missing or defective genes. Both systems have the capacity to alter quiescent cells, such as the mature stem cells that generate the immune system. These viral vectors, HIV and simian virus 40 (SV40), share the preceding characteristics. Although HIV is a human pathogen whose use will be restricted at least initially to advanced cancers, origin from a human source may confer an advantage. SV40, an adenovirus, can be rendered harmless, is capable of infecting several resting and dividing cell types, is easy to manipulate, and is stable and nonimmunogenic, causing one to wonder why it has been ignored. Clearly this vector is not ready yet for clinical trials, and some safety concerns are unresolved. Still, SV40 appears to be as benign as any available viral vector and has the added attribute of being directly injectable into target tissues. Some investigators foresee the development of hybrid vectors that build on the best features of viral and nonviral vectors.

Magnitude and Areas of Impact

Scientists are currently debating whether gene therapy has definitively improved the health of the more than 2,000 patients in clinical trials worldwide. Current clinical trials are investigating the genetic treatment of several cancers and genetic diseases, such as cystic fibrosis. Gene therapy has succeeded in treating the symptoms of patients with hypercholesterolemia, and several children with severe combined immunodeficiency diseases are surviving as a direct result of treatment.

One of the most significant developments in this field is the application of this methodology to gene marking in the study of the biology of cancer. Close to 1.4 million Americans will be newly diagnosed with cancer this year alone, and the treatments currently available—surgery, radiation therapy, and chemotherapy—cannot cure fifty percent of those diagnosed. Although gene therapy was originally targeted toward single-gene deficiency diseases that are recessive and relatively rare, about seventy-five to eighty percent of the current clinical trials now focus on cancer.

For treating cancer, several approaches are being attempted. Some involve imparting cancer cells with genes that give rise to toxic molecules. When these genes are expressed, the resulting product then kills the cancer cells. Genetic marking of marrow cells used in similar *ex vivo* therapies permits physicians to monitor the effects of different cancer-purging methods. Another research focus is on the correction of compensation for acquired genetic mutations, particularly of the oft-mutated tumor suppressor gene p53.

Yet another field of cancer research is immunotherapy. Immunotherapeutic research concentrates on how tumors evade detection and attack via the immune system, how they spread away from their sites of origin, how they gain a new blood supply, and how they evolve and spread.

A different form of genetic marking is used in immunotherapy, also called *vaccine therapy*. Immunotherapeutic vaccinations tag cancer cells with certain genes that make them more visible to the immune system. One method being widely tested involves modifying a patient's cancer cells with genes encoding cytokines—the communication proteins of the immune system's B and T cells—to draw an attack from the immune system. Unfortunately, this method will benefit only patients with robust immune systems and not those with advanced cancer.

Key Barriers

Despite encouraging results, the field awaits answers to many unresolved questions. An area where enormous progress has been made, but where much more is needed, is developing gene-delivery vectors. Virus-based vectors have been the most efficient for inserting genes into cells in the laboratory, but in clinical applications, the results have sometimes been short lived, and there have been unwanted side effects.

In addition, the field needs to develop animal models to test the biological and clinical efficacy of the new vectors and procedures. As a result, gene therapy may take longer to reach patients than originally predicted. The progress of gene therapy also depends on adequate technical, financial, and training resources, and demands close interaction between academics, clinicians, and private-sector companies.

Private companies are playing a critical role in promoting the development of innovative medical technology. They have millions of dollars at risk: they have to choose technologies, knowing that the ultimately successful approaches are likely to require complex assemblies of new chemical tools and procedures. For industry, a necessary incentive is the award of exclusive protection of innovative breakthroughs. Limited access to enabling technologies for gene therapy—such as vectors—because of time consuming and expensive licensing processes could lead to prohibitive commercial burdens that would delay progress in the field.

By the end of the 1990s, there were 313 clinical studies involving gene transfer, of which 277 protocols involved new therapeutic applications with most (193) intended for patients with cancer. The same advisory group that in 1995 accused the scientific community of overselling the present benefits of gene therapy stressed the extraordinary potential of gene therapy for the long-term treatment of human disease. The lack of more efficient gene vectors was singled out as the major barrier to attaining better clinical results (Jenks, 1997).

With the intense, ongoing activity in vector development, it is likely that within ten years a number of efficient gene delivery systems will be in clinical use. Vectors that have both site- and cell-type specificities will deliver genes to treat a wide range of conditions in most, if not all, organs. The potential of using genes and gene products in novel strategies is an incredibly powerful incentive to pursue gene therapy as the equal of the future's most effective therapeutic modalities.

VACCINES

Since Jenner conferred smallpox immunity with inoculations of cowpox in the early nineteenth century, vaccines have been administered globally as preventive measures for acute diseases such as diphtheria, smallpox, and whooping cough, and have been used to avoid acute infection by creating a low-level immune response that remains as an acquired immunity. In the history of public health, vaccines have proved to be among the most effective disease prevention tools. Some diseases, such as smallpox, polio, and measles, have been eradicated or brought under control through mass vaccination programs.

The current use of vaccines includes any preparation intended for active immunization of the recipient. Until recently, vaccines were prophylactic—their sole objective was preventing a specific infectious disease. They were, therefore, directed against the causative infectious agent. Lately, vaccines have been used against noninfectious diseases. Patients with certain cancers have been vaccinated—either prophylactically, to prevent the emergence of micrometastatic tumors, or therapeutically, to boost the immunologic cytotoxic response to the tumor.

Vaccines can have preventive and therapeutic uses. Preventive vaccines permit the vaccinated individual to develop immunologic responses that prevent or modulate subsequent infection or disease. Recently

developed therapeutic vaccines use new recombinant DNA technology to provide genetic therapy to patients who already have a disease. The key to using this technology is specificity for tumor cells.

The application of molecular biology to the identification of virulent genes has led to a fundamental understanding of the pathogenesis of virulent microbes. With the molecular tools of the new genetics, the genes responsible for the organism's virulence can be identified and isolated. The molecular genetic definition of virulence has exciting and highly promising implications for vaccines. Given the side effects of antibiotics, including the emergence of resistant bacteria, novel strategies for controlling infectious diseases are evolving. One of the most promising strategies, that of using molecular microbiology and whole-gene sequencing to develop candidate vaccines, will be the wider use of gene-specific vaccines (Moxon, 1997).

Recent therapeutic vaccines are designed to attack certain chronic infections. Early cancer vaccines had few successes, but with the new knowledge and technology ushered in by molecular biology and recombinant DNA technology, anticancer vaccines are gaining increasing attention. This resurgence of interest in therapeutic vaccines reflects a new and broadened understanding of the immune system and its elements.

Vaccines have been effective in treating melanomas and renal cell carcinomas, two cancers that are unique in their responsiveness to the immune system. Vaccine therapies for cancer that stimulate the immune system and don't involve surgery, radiation, or cytotoxicity could become the least traumatic mode of treatment for particular cancer patients. A vaccine can activate the immune system by delivering a tumor antigen or by eliciting a nonspecific immune system response. A nonspecific response would simply boost the activity of the immune system, resulting in greater overall immune activity.

Magnitude and Areas of Impact

Prophylactic vaccination to prevent cancers caused by viruses would prevent an estimated 850,000 cases of cancer each year, roughly eleven percent of the global cancer burden. Examples of such viruses and their secondary cancers are Epstein-Barr virus and nasopharyngeal cancer, human papilloma virus (HPV) and cancer of the cervix, and hepatitis B virus and primary liver cancer. Because cervical cancer is diagnosed in 16,000 women in the United States each year, the impact of a vaccine for HPV will be substantial. In addition, a live, attenuated HIV vaccine may be a realistic projection by 2005, or even sooner.

A novel new vaccine against rotavirus, a major cause of childhood diarrheal disease mortality in developing countries that causes an estimated 600,000 deaths worldwide each year, is a live oral rotavirus vaccine. Incorporation of this vaccine into routine immunization could reduce severe rotavirus gastroenteritis by ninety percent.

Could some diseases currently believed to have a noninfectious cause be the direct consequence of an infection by an unidentified or unrecognized agent? If the recent connection of *H. pylori* infection to gastric carcinoma and lymphoma and the putative role of infectious prions with Alzheimer's disease are a prelude to the future, the answer is a resounding "yes." Among immediate candidates for such an etiologic connection are other cancers and rheumatoid arthritis. By the year 2010, prophylactic and therapeutic vaccines will compete with rational drug design for airtime.

Key Barriers

Advances in vaccine development are contingent on overcoming the same obstacles that must be overcome in gene therapy: delivering enough of the immune system trigger to the right cells. Vector development to increase the efficacy of delivery is what vaccine departments at most major pharmaceutical companies are working on now.

Clinical trials of HIV vaccines will undoubtedly be controversial and politically charged. Traditional approaches to vaccine development, such as "whole killed" or attenuated virus methods, raise special safety concerns with HIV because a faulty vaccine that actually infects a recipient would have lethal consequences. HIV vaccine research goals may focus on a product that can inhibit progression to disease or lower viral load in infected persons instead of preventing actual infection.

ARTIFICIAL BLOOD

Blood transfusions are given for two reasons: (1) to increase oxygen-carrying capacity, and (2) to restore intravascular volume. Intravascular volume can be restored by other fluids, such as crystalloids and colloids, which are free from the risks of transmitting an infectious agent. Thus, increasing oxygen-carrying capacity is rapidly become the *sole* indication for blood transfusion which, in most cases, is done by administering packed red blood cells. The only major risk of blood transfusion, assuming the absence of human error in the pretransfusion process, is transmission of an infectious agent that has eluded detection by the battery of screening tests currently performed before a unit of blood is cleared for use. The principal concerns are the HIV and hepatitis viruses, capable of producing fatal or crippling diseases for which no effective treatment currently exists. Availability of donated blood in the United States does not pose a problem; infrequent, temporary shortages are geographically restricted and short-lived.

Historically, the armed services have tried to develop artificial blood for military use under wartime conditions and in natural disasters. The features of an ideal blood substitute would be ready availability, safety, long shelf life, efficacy, and compatibility across all blood types. Interest in artificial blood peaked in the 1980s because of the seriousness of transfusion transmission of HIV and hepatitis infections.

Magnitude and Areas of Impact

Hemoglobin-free fluids carrying dissolved oxygen have been approved for clinical use, but because of their inability to achieve desired oxygenation of tissues these products have not been used much in practice.

Hemoglobin-containing products have been produced by using outdated human blood or bovine blood. A serious drawback of these hemoglobin products has been kidney damage caused by the splitting of hemoglobin into agents that were shown to damage the kidneys. Human hemoglobin can be chemically stabilized to avoid this splitting, and refined blood substitutes based on human hemoglobin are now in advanced clinical trials. The obvious problems are the supply of outdated blood and the risk, although reduced, of disease transmission.

One company, Somatogen, has produced a recombinant hemoglobin using *E. coli*. The recombinant hemoglobin acts like human hemoglobin, and the synthetic process can be programmed to produce a product with an ideal oxygen-release curve. The recombinant hemoglobin, like stabilized human hemoglobin, has a half-life of twenty-four hours. Refinements of synthetic hemoglobin molecules will lead to a near-ideal substitute for blood by 2010. This fluid will have a shelf life of one year or longer, obviate the need for cross-match (i.e., be a universal source of blood), and carry no risk of infection. Such a product will be used routinely for cardiac bypass procedures and renal dialysis as well as for transfusion.

Key Barriers

- The public may be reluctant to accept an artificial product that is perceived to be less valuable.
- An entrenched blood bank industry may be resistant to the use of artificial blood.
- Artificial blood may be extremely expensive due to a manufacturers' need to have an early return on its investment in product development.

XENOTRANSPLANTATION

Xenotransplantation—the transplantation of cells, tissues, and whole organs from one species to another—had its modern beginning in the early 1960s with the transplantation of kidneys from chimpanzees to six human patients. But these xenotransplants—and later other grafts of solid organs across species—resulted in immune rejection after brief periods of normal function in the new host. In contrast, allotransplantation—transplantation within species—of bone marrow and solid organs from related and unrelated human donors has become highly successful because of satisfactory, although less-than-ideal, means of avoiding

immune rejection, principally by using immunosuppressive drugs and avoiding major histoincompatibilities to the maximum extent possible.

Magnitude and Areas of Impact

The number of patients meeting strict criteria for receiving transplants of kidneys, lungs, livers, and hearts currently exceeds the supply of suitable donor organs. In the past ten years, the number of solid-organ allotransplants has increased slightly more than fifty percent, with the greatest increase being in lung transplants. Over the same span of time, the number of names on the waiting list for all organs reached 66,000 by the end of the 1990s, with about 5,000 persons dying annually while awaiting a suitable donor organ. Median waiting times at the end of the 1990s were 1.3 years for livers, more than 1.5 years for lungs, and more than 2.5 years for kidneys. Availability of a suitable donor organ poses a particular problem for infants and children because of organ size, and for ethnic minorities because of a lack of suitably matched donors.

As indications for organ transplantations have broadened, waiting lists have grown, and as waiting times for suitable human organs lengthened, research on xenotransplantation has accelerated by using new knowledge and methods of molecular genetics, transplantation biology, genetic engineering, and transgenic technology. Current xenotransplantation research focuses on the pig because of its size and favorable biologic factors.

The basic strategies fall in two areas: combined transplantation of bone marrow and the solid organ, and modification of the animal serving as the source of the organ. Both strategies are designed to avoid acute rejection. Combined transplantation, considered a high-risk but equally high-reward strategy, depends on first successfully grafting the foreign bone marrow into the patient, thus permitting later successful transplantation of the solid organ. The strategy more likely to be successful is genetic modification of the pig using transgenic technology.

Introduction of a new gene requires fourteen months, but this time will be shortened in the future.

The short-term goal will be to use organs from modified pig donors to bridge a human recipient for a matter of months while awaiting a suitable human organ. The use of pig organs as bridges will teach critical lessons essential to the creation of transgenic pigs whose organs can be transplanted for permanent replacement, an ideal that should be attained within ten years. Humans are presently living with xenotransplants of nervous tissue mechanically transplanted to the brain for the treatment of Parkinson's disease, so the feasibility of organ xenotransplantation is not far-fetched.

Transplantation of organs has been one of the great medical advances of the century and the one modality that treats a chronic disease successfully by replacing the diseased organ. The present limitation of solid-organ transplantation is the availability of donor organs, and for both social and economic reasons, current wait lists do not reflect the true need for organ transplants in our population. The applications of xenotransplantation go beyond eliminating the waiting lists for solid organs as they are now used. Chronic conditions, such as diabetes and Parkinson's disease, can be successfully treated with xenotransplants, and xenotransplants of cells and tissues can be used to transfer genes and their gene products for the treatment of genetic diseases, such as hemophilia, and acquired conditions, such as cancer. Pediatric organ transplants could be used in the treatment of congenital heart disease and as a prophylactic measure in the patient with Wilm's disease. The potential is incredible.

Key Barriers and Indicators

The principal scientific concern relates to disease transmission between animals and humans. The pig is known to harbor a retrovirus, but there is no known transmission of any infection or disease from pigs to humans. In theory, any infectious agent could be bred out of the donor animal, but the threat of disease cannot be dismissed entirely, nor can the successful treatment of a transmitted infection be assured. Preliminary vaccination of the organ recipient is a feasible option that could confer additional protection. Another concern is excessive inbreeding, and one goal of creating herds of pig donors is to use as little inbreeding as possible.

Two issues will need to be addressed: the economic consequences of applying a new technology on a scale that, today, would seem to be vast, but which is not precisely predictable, and the ethical and public policy implications of resource allocation and equity.

References

Jenks, S. J. (1997). Gene Therapy: Mastering the basics, defining details. *Journal of the National Cancer Institute, 89,* 1182–1184.

Moxon, E. R. (1997). Applications of molecular microbiology to vaccinology. *Lancet, 350,* 1240–1244.

Ronchi, E. (1996). Biotechnology and the new revolution in health care and pharmaceuticals. Special Issue on Biotechnology. *Science Technology Industry Review, 19,* 19–44.

CHAPTER
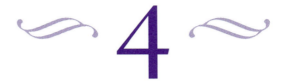

Patterns of Illness and Disease and Access to Health Care

Stephen J. Williams

Chapter Topics

- The Underlying Demographic Determinants of Health Services Utilization
- Fertility Trends in the United States
- Mortality Trends in the United States
- Specific Causes of Death for the United States Population
- Incidence of Infectious Diseases
- Lifestyle Patterns and Disease
- Health, Lifestyle, and Social Structure
- Access to Health Care Services

Learning Objectives

Upon completing this chapter, the reader should be able to:

- Trace twentieth-century United States demographic trends including births and deaths
- Understand correlates of mortality, especially with regard to the impact of population trends
- Understand disease patterns in the United States
- Relate lifestyle, behavior, and social patterns to health
- Appreciate cancer survival trends
- Understand issues of access to care

Disease patterns throughout history and the underlying social and demographic characteristics of our population provide empirical evidence from which to view the need and demand for health care services in the United States. The principal purposes of this chapter include the review of fundamental demographic, social, and economic trends in our nation, principally throughout the twentieth century, and patterns of morbidity, mortality, and other aspects of the measurement of the incidence and prevalence of disease. Analytical, epidemiologic measurement of these patterns illuminate the underlying factors that define the nature of health care services required for our nation.

An additional purpose of this chapter is to review population, disease, and illness trends and to relate these trends to issues of access to health care services. Access to care is a core theme throughout this book and a key health policy issue facing our nation. This chapter associates the various social, demographic, and disease patterns experienced by our nation with measures of access to health care and interpretation of these measures as a contributor to the national health policy debate.

The analysis presented here first focuses on the underlying demographic trends in our society during the twentieth century. Social and economic trends that define the character of our society and relate to the need and demand for health care services are also discussed. Finally, issues of access to health care are addressed.

The next section of the chapter focuses on disease patterns experienced in the twentieth century. Differential mortality and morbidity are presented to emphasize the importance of such variables as age, race, and sex in defining population groups at particular risk for various diseases. Ultimately, identification of risk factors and their association with various personal, sociodemographic, and physiological characteristics, and genetic markers will greatly heighten our ability to target health services to individuals in the greatest need for each category of care.

All aspects of this chapter are integrally related to virtually every other section of this book. The nature of the delivery system itself, including the settings in which services are provided, the nature of services, the technology of our system, and even the financing of care are all directly related to the underlying disease patterns that we experience.

This chapter sets the stage and forms part of the foundation of knowledge necessary for critically assessing how the health care system is structured. Our ability to measure performance within the system itself, including access to and outcomes of care, is related to these fundamental trends as well. Ultimately, the success of the system should be measured against criteria that recognize the true needs of the population with regard to the physiological and psychological manifestations of injury, illness, and disease, and their ability to obtain needed care.

Need, Demand, and Utilization

In discussions of disease patterns and their relation to the utilization of health care services, it is important to differentiate between the concepts of need, demand, and use of health care services. *Need* for health care services is defined as an interpretation of an individual's evaluated requirements for obtaining professional care through the health services system. *Demand* for health services is a function of an individual's actually seeking out, but not necessarily obtaining, health ser-vices. Demand may be a reflection of professional assessment of an individual's need for services or self-initiated desires for professional services, perhaps triggered by an individual's perceptions of potential illness. Finally, *utilization* is a measure of actual use of services, as discussed later in this chapter.

The extent to which there is a correlation between need, demand, and utilization is the central issue in addressing concerns of appropriateness of care, perceptions of when services should be obtained, and evaluation of access to health care services in our society. Many other issues related to these concepts are addressed throughout this book.

Data Sources and Quality

Morbidity, mortality, and other health status–related data are obtained from a variety of sources (National Center for Health Statistics, 2000). Information presented throughout this chapter and elsewhere in this book is based on such sources as national vital statistics data (National Center for Health Statistics, 1993). National vital statistics data are collected from birth, death, and marriage certificates. Mandatory data collection requirements in the United States provide the most consistent and generally highest-quality data available for determining the health status of our nation's population.

But even mandated vital statistics data collection produces information of inconsistent quality. All data should be viewed with a skeptical eye, recognizing the imperfections of the data collection effort. For primary demographic variables such as age, race, and sex, the quality of data recorded on the primary data source—the vital event certificate—is generally good. However, for more subjective data elements such as cause of death, the consistency and quality of data reported can vary appreciably, especially in past years, depending on the judgment of the individual, usually a physician, completing the certificate. Vital statistics data collected at the local level are compiled by the states and the federal government, and efforts are directed toward improving quality at each level.

Data on health services utilization, status, attitudes, and other variables are often collected through national probability surveys conducted by the federal government and some private organizations. The National Health Interview Survey collects data from a random probability sample of all Americans, asking questions regarding prior health services utilization, perceived health status, mobility, and other, often somewhat subjective, self-reported variables. Recall ability, response judgments, and other complex factors affect the quality of these types of data.

A third category of data collection for health services use involves the compilation of data from other sources. An example of this is the National Hospital Discharge Survey conducted by the federal government, which compiles the data from a sampling of hospital discharges in the country (Popovic and Kozak, 2000). Another example is the National Ambulatory Medical Care Survey, also conducted by the federal government, which is based on a sample of physicians who report on the characteristics, diagnoses, and use of services for all patients seen during a two-week interval of time (Woodwell, 1999).

Private data collection includes surveys of health services use, attitudes, and costs. National organizations such as the American Medical Association and the Medical Group Management Association conduct surveys on medical groups, physician practices, and hospital services. Various insurance companies, health care systems, and individual facilities also conduct surveys on patient satisfaction and other issues. Finally, data are collected by national voluntary accrediting agencies, health services researchers, and other organizations.

It is important to recognize the sources, quality, and contingencies associated with the data that are analyzed and presented throughout this book. The book's analytical perspective on health services is dependent on the assessment of population-based data, and the best available information is utilized for discussion purposes. Even the relatively solid data available in the United States, however, are subject to numerous limitations. Needless to say, data from many other countries in the world often lag far behind our own in this regard.

THE UNDERLYING DEMOGRAPHIC DETERMINANTS OF HEALTH SERVICES UTILIZATION

The dynamics of population are the most fundamental determinants of the need, demand, and use of health care services. The size and age composition of a population have a tremendous impact on total health services use as well as on the distribution of the use of specific services. Therefore, trends in population dynamics, including population size and demographic characteristics as well as births and deaths, are a basic starting point for assessing the need for health services in a population.

Population Size and Composition

Population size, as reflected in the total number of people in a population, as well as the distribution of population by age group, defined as the population pyramid, is the appropriate starting point. Table 4.1 presents the age-specific distribution of the United States resident population from 1950. These data, obtained from the federal government, are based on

Table 4.1. Resident Population: United States, Selected Years

Year	Total Resident Population (Population in Thousands)	Age Group (Population in Thousands)										
		Under 1 Year	1–4 Years	5–14 Years	15–24 Years	25–34 Years	35–44 Years	45–54 Years	55–64 Years	65–74 Years	75–84 Years	85 Years and Over
1950	150,697	3,147	13,017	24,319	22,098	23,759	21,450	17,343	13,370	8,340	3,278	577
1960	179,323	4,112	16,209	35,465	24,020	22,818	24,081	20,485	15,572	10,997	4,633	929
1970	203,212	3,485	13,669	40,746	35,441	24,907	23,088	23,220	18,590	12,435	6,119	1,511
1980	226,546	3,534	12,815	34,942	42,487	37,082	25,635	22,800	21,703	15,581	7,729	2,240
1990	248,710	3,946	14,812	35,095	37,013	43,161	37,435	25,057	21,113	18,045	10,012	3,021
1998	270,299	3,776	15,190	39,163	37,213	38,774	44,520	34,585	22,676	18,395	11,952	4,054

national census of population data. The federal government is required by the United States Constitution to conduct a census count of the population once every ten years to compile as complete a count as possible of all citizens (U.S. Bureau of the Census, 2000).

The United States Census of Population was most recently completed in 2000. Results of the 2000 census are currently available on a preliminary basis, and indicate an approximate United States population of 280 million individuals. Complete census results from the 2000 count are available in a variety of forms from the United States Bureau of the Census.

Population data between censuses and for future periods are determined through intracensual estimates and projections using prior data and adjusting for estimated population growth and migration. Intracensual data estimates are facilitated by using such available statistics as school enrollments, automobile registrations, and utility hookups. The original purpose of the census, of course, was to determine representation in the House of Representatives, although these data are now also used for an array of analytical, commercial, and social purposes.

The accuracy of the actual census count, of intracensual estimates, and of demographic projections into the future is a subject of considerable debate. The mobility of the population, the lack of tracking for internal migration, and illegal migration into the country complicate the picture. The cost of data collection, analysis, adjustment, and reporting has escalated greatly as the population has grown, as well.

The United States population has grown tremendously during the period presented in Table 4.1. This growth is a result of two principal factors. The first of these is the *rate of natural increase* attributable to the higher number of births as compared to deaths annually in the United States, leading to additions to the total population count. The second factor is the increase in population attributable to net in-migration, which historically has accounted for nearly all of the accumulated population of the country. The current United States population is over 275,000,000 people, nearly double the count in 1950. Further detailed data, not presented here, are readily available differentially by sex, ethnic group, and other sociodemographic variables. Depending on the nature of the analysis to be performed, use of the more detailed data can be quite revealing.

The age structure of the population is, as noted above, vitally important for health services purposes. The very young and the older population groups utilize considerably more health care services than other age groups. Table 4.1 also presents the age distribution, and hence the structure or pyramid of the population.

An important current trend is the aging of the population. On average, the typical American is getting older. This trend is the result of increased longevity and relatively lower fertility than was experienced

Table 4.2. Population Age Group Projections, Age 65 and Above

Age Group	Year (Population in Millions)			
	2000	**2025**	**2050**	**2075**
65 years and over	35.2	60.6	73.3	83.3
75 years and over	16.7	25.0	38.9	45.7
85 years and over	4.4	6.3	14.6	16.9

SOURCE: U.S. Social Security Administration Office of Programs: Office of the Actuary, 1993, Baltimore, MD.

earlier in the century. The consequences of this trend are reflected in Table 4.2. Projections for the older population groups over the next half century suggest substantial increases in health services utilization, assuming current technology, access to care, and patterns of use. The population aged sixty-five and above uses, on average, approximately twice the health care services as the younger population. This trend in the age structure for the United States is the underlying demographic reason for recent concerns over the future financial viability of the Social Security system and the Medicare program.

Parenthetically, many other countries in the world, especially in Europe, face an even more profound aging of their populations, so that future liabilities for social services, health care, and social security are even more serious than our own. Enhanced longevity as a result of biomedical advances is a two-edged sword leading to longer periods of economic and social dependency, while at the same time enhancing quality of life. As the population ages, the burdens on the younger working groups increase. This concept is reflected in the dependency ratio, which measures the proportion of a population that is working to those who are dependent.

FERTILITY TRENDS IN THE UNITED STATES

A key determinant of population that affects health services utilization is fertility. Fertility is a key determinant of the population pyramid, as well as of the use of services for mothers, infants, and children. Fer-

tility eventually influences total population size and has cohort effects in all age groups as a cohort ages.

Fertility behavior is also a socioeconomic characteristic of population. Developing nations, for example, are typically characterized by relatively high fertility rates, while developed, or postindustrial, societies usually experience low fertility rates.

Fertility is a measure of reproduction. Age-specific fertility rates are the primary indicator utilized in measuring this determinant of population. Age-specific fertility rates more accurately reflect differences in fertility patterns based on age groups of mothers than do birth rates, which are a cruder measure of reproduction. Birth rates are computed as the total number of births to total population. Age-specific fertility rates are computed as the number of births to women in a specific reproductive age group. The total fertility rate is the sum of all of the age-specific rates.

Table 4.3 presents age-specific fertility rates for the United States over the past half century. As for many of the other rates discussed in this chapter, age, race, sex, and other characteristics may be utilized to compute more specific rates than those presented.

Fertility, of course, differs greatly by age group, as reflected in Table 4.3. Fertility is highest for women in their twenties and generally declines thereafter as the age of the mother increases. Fertility rates drop off appreciably at the higher reproductive ages, with little fertility in the groups above forty-five years of age.

Recent technological advances have provided an occasional dramatic example of reproduction beyond the historical ranges. Historically, and in most societies, the reproductive ages begin with the physiological marker of menarche. A variety of sociological determinants of reproductive behavior, such as marriage, combine with physiology to produce actual behavior. The reproductive ages usually end with menopause. Other physiological factors, such as voluntary sterilization and infertility, and sociological patterns, such as family dissolution, also have a substantial impact on reproduction. The interaction of these dynamics can be quite complex.

Fertility has declined in most age groups over the past forty years, as reflected in Table 4.3. Reductions in fertility have been rather dramatic in the United States since peak fertility occurred in the mid-1950s.

Table 4.3. Live Births and Birth Rates by Age of Mother: United States, Selected Years

Year	Live Births	Age of Mother (Live Births per 1,000 Women)							
		10–14 Years	15–19 Years	20–24 Years	25–29 Years	30–34 Years	35–39 Years	40–44 Years	45–54 Years
1950	3,632,000	1.0	81.6	196.6	166.1	103.7	52.9	15.1	1.2
1960	4,257,850	0.8	89.1	258.1	197.4	112.7	56.2	15.5	0.9
1970	3,731,386	1.2	68.3	167.8	145.1	73.3	31.7	8.1	0.5
1980	3,612,258	1.1	53.0	115.1	112.9	61.9	19.8	3.9	0.2
1990	4,158,212	1.4	59.9	116.5	120.2	80.8	31.7	5.5	0.2
1993	4,000,240	1.4	59.6	112.6	115.5	80.8	32.9	6.1	0.3
1998	3,941,553	1.0	51.1	111.2	115.9	87.4	37.4	7.3	0.4

The dramatic decline in fertility that has occurred in the United States over the past forty years is primarily the result of increases in female labor force participation, marital dissolutions, and other economic and social forces in our society. In recent years, our nation has also witnessed a delayed average age of first marriage, reduced desired family size, delayed initiation of childbearing due to education and employment prospects, and a number of other important social and economic factors, all of which have further reinforced the primary underlying fertility trends.

Making predictions is a difficult business. Some demographers anticipated a resurgence of fertility to result from delayed childbearing associated with labor force participation by women and subsequent desires to "catch up." This has not occurred, although some slight increase in overall fertility has been experienced in recent years. A substantial change in the now well-established pattern of United States fertility is unlikely to occur in the foreseeable future.

Other societies have experienced many of the same general changes in fertility experienced by the United States in the twentieth century. The change from a high-fertility, high-mortality environment to a low-fertility, low-mortality environment is typical of most developing countries. This change is termed the *demographic transition*. Countries that achieve low fertility and low mortality combined with relatively affluent economic conditions typically experience substantial social and economic change that results in permanent reversals of the underlying social factors associated with high fertility.

Abortion Trends in the United States

Reproduction may be more appropriately measured in terms of conceptions rather than live births. Conceptions include spontaneous and induced abortions as well as live and dead births. However, the empirical data to accurately count conceptions is considerably weaker than that for live births.

National data are available on therapeutically induced abortions, as reflected in Table 4.4. The United States experiences an estimated 1.2 million abortions annually at the current time, and an unknown number of conceptions result in spontaneous abortions, primarily in the first month of gestation. Abortion practices vary considerably from society to society and over time, and the current acceptance of abortion services in the United States dates back nationally to the 1973 Supreme Court decision to restrict state barriers to such services.

Recent technological changes will likely substantially impact the provision of abortion services in the United States and throughout the world. Less invasive pharmacologically based approaches to termination of very early term pregnancies is beginning to shift the locus of abortion services to private physician offices and clinics without necessarily being associated with surgical procedures. Monitoring these

Table 4.4. Legal Abortions, According to Selected Characteristics: United States, Selected Years

Characteristic	Year	
	1973	1997
Total number of legal abortions (reported in thousands)		
	616	1,185
Period of gestation (percentage distribution)		
Under 9 weeks	36.1	55.5
9–10 weeks	29.4	21.9
11–12 weeks	17.9	10.7
13–15 weeks	6.9	6.2
16–20 weeks	8.0	4.3
21 weeks and over	1.7	1.4
Type of procedure (percentage distribution)		
Curettage	88.4	97.7
Intrauterine instillation	10.4	0.4
Other	0.6	1.9

services is extremely difficult. In addition, numerous political, economic, social, and psychological factors will continue to impact the provision of abortion services in the United States regardless of delivery mechanisms. However, it is likely that the database available for the analysis of these services will continue to deteriorate over time.

MORTALITY TRENDS IN THE UNITED STATES

Indicators of mortality are often used to measure a society's health status. Trends in mortality indicators over time also reflect a multitude of social, economic, health services, and other underlying trends in a society. Reasonably accurate mortality data are available for the United States population and for many other nations, although in some developing countries the quality of data may be limited.

Mortality data are collected at the time of death through the mechanics of the death certificate, a responsibility of local government. State and federal agencies compile data collected locally to produce the vital statistics for the entire country. Because various social and demographic variables are collected on the death certificate in addition to determinants of the cause of death, mortality data can be analyzed by selected characteristics of population.

Mortality Trends for the United States

This section of the chapter presents quantitative measures of mortality for the total United States population over time. Mortality data for infants and mothers and an analysis of specific causes of death are presented in later sections of this chapter as well. As for fertility, mortality data are generally age-adjusted to control for changes in the population age pyramid. Comparisons over time, in particular, require consideration of any substantial changes in the age structure of a population.

Life Expectancy

A common measure of mortality, particularly popular in the mass media, is life expectancy. Life expectancy is computed from mortality data and reflects a cohort effect for estimated years of life remaining.

Life expectancy can be computed for a population at any specific age, but it is most commonly presented at birth and at age sixty-five. Table 4.5 presents such data for selected countries in the world. Mortality and life expectancy data are typically presented on a sex-specific basis due to the consistent and substantial differences in mortality experienced comparing males and females.

International life expectancy comparisons reveal that, for both males and females, life expectancy at birth is greatest in Japan (United Nations, 2001). The United States falls somewhat short in these comparisons, which is a surprising finding for many people. However, the heterogeneity of our population and our complex social problems associated with violence, accidents, and infectious disease account for much of the cross-cultural deficiencies reflected in our mortality experience. Many Americans are surprised to see that mortality experience measured by life expectancy at birth is lower in the United States than in such countries

Table 4.5. Life Expectancy at Birth and at 65 Years of Age, According to Sex: Selected Countries, 1995

Country	Life Expectancy in Years		Country	Life Expectancy in Years	
	At Birth	**At 65 Years**		**At Birth**	**At 65 Years**
Male			*Female*		
Japan	76.4	16.5	Japan	82.9	20.9
Sweden	76.2	16.0	France	82.6	21.4
Israel	75.3	15.8	Switzerland	81.9	20.5
Canada	75.2	16.1	Sweden	81.6	19.8
Switzerland	75.1	16.1	Spain	81.5	19.9
Greece	75.1	16.2	Canada	81.2	20.1
Australia	75.0	15.6	Australia	80.9	19.5
Norway	74.9	15.2	Italy	80.8	19.4
Netherlands	74.6	14.7	Norway	80.7	19.3
Italy	74.4	15.5	Netherlands	80.4	19.1
England and Wales	74.3	14.7	Greece	80.3	18.5
France	74.2	16.6	Finland	80.3	18.7
Spain	74.2	16.0	Austria	80.1	18.8
Austria	73.5	15.2	Germany	79.8	18.6
Singapore	73.4	14.9	Belgium	79.8	18.9
Germany	73.3	14.7	England and Wales	79.6	18.5
New Zealand	73.3	15.0	Israel	79.3	17.8
Northern Ireland	73.1	14.1	Singapore	79.0	18.1
Belgium	73.0	14.5	United States	78.9	18.9
Cuba	73.0	15.7	New Zealand	78.9	18.6
Costa Rica	73.0	15.2	Puerto Rico	78.9	19.4
Finland	72.8	14.5	Portugal	78.6	17.7
Denmark	72.8	14.1	Northern Ireland	78.5	17.7
Ireland	72.5	13.4	Ireland	78.1	17.0
United States	72.2	15.6	Denmark	77.9	17.6
Scotland	72.2	13.8	Chile	77.9	17.9
Chile	71.6	14.6	Costa Rica	77.8	17.6
Portugal	71.2	14.3	Scotland	77.6	17.1

as Greece and France, perhaps owing a little to the value of red wine, paté, and olive oil!

Life expectancy at age sixty-five is also presented in Table 4.5 for selected countries. By age sixty-five, past the highest-risk periods for mortality attributable to nonphysiological causes, the differences between sexes are much less, as are the differences between countries. Sex mortality differentials drop by about half by age sixty-five, reflecting the higher risk

from violent accidents and lifestyle causes for individuals younger than sixty-five. The remaining differential is probably attributable to physiological factors such as hormones and genetics.

International differences are similarly moderated by age sixty-five, as many of these same causes of mortality in the younger ages have been factored out of the equation. Even at sixty-five, however, life expectancy is greatest in Japan, with females at age

Table 4.6.   Life Expectancy at Birth and at 65 Years of Age, According to Race and Sex: United States, Selected Years

Age Category and Year	White		Black	
	Male	Female	Male	Female
At birth				
1900	46.6	48.7	32.5	35.5
1950	66.5	72.2	58.9	62.7
1960	67.4	74.1	60.7	65.9
1970	68.0	75.6	60.0	68.3
1980	70.7	78.1	63.8	72.5
1990	72.7	79.4	64.5	73.6
1998	74.5	80.0	67.6	74.8
At 65 years				
1900	11.5	12.2	10.4	11.4
1950	12.8	15.1	12.9	14.9
1960	12.9	15.9	12.7	15.1
1970	13.1	17.1	12.5	15.7
1980	14.2	18.4	13.0	16.8
1990	15.2	19.1	13.2	17.2
1998	16.1	19.3	14.3	17.4

sixty-five expecting to live, on average, to about age eighty-six, a truly impressive result.

United States Life Expectancy Data

Table 4.6 presents life expectancy data for selected subgroups of the United States population. Again, mortality experience differs by sociodemographic characteristics such as sex and race. Dramatic differences appear in these data at birth for males as compared to females and for blacks as compared to whites. As noted previously, data are available for numerous subgroups of the population, and only selected illustrative data are presented here.

At birth, females have a substantially higher life expectancy than males, a difference of approximately six years of life. An equally dramatic differential is evident for whites as compared to blacks. These differences have been constant throughout modern United States history, as reflected in Table 4.6. At age sixty-

five, the differentials continue to exist, but as for the international comparisons, the differences are much more moderate, indicating that on a biological basis sex differences may be on the order of two to three years. Black/white differentials are also quite moderate at this point.

United States Mortality Rates

Table 4.7 presents age-specific mortality rates for the United States by selected demographic characteristics. These data conform to the life expectancy numbers presented earlier. As expected, mortality rates increase with age. The United States age-specific mortality rates are relatively moderate until the older ages, although notable differentials occur by sex and race. The higher mortality rate for younger black males compared to same-age-group white males is particularly startling; these data are discussed further later in this chapter in the discussion of specific causes of death.

Data on differential mortality help to identify problems in society with regard to causes of illness and disease and barriers to access to health care services. Trends over time reflect progress, or lack thereof, in achieving our goals for a greater quality and quantity of life.

Infant and Maternal Mortality

An oft-quoted set of data is mortality experience for infants and mothers. Table 4.8 presents international data on infant mortality. Infant mortality is measured as the number of infants who die in the first year of life per thousand live births. Related measures of mortality for infants include perinatal, postnatal, and other measures, all of which pertain to the time period before or after delivery in which the fetal or infant death occurs.

Once again, the United States falls short in international comparisons of infant mortality. Japan leads all nations in having the lowest infant mortality rate. The relatively poor performance of the United States population is again a function of population heterogeneity and such factors as lack of access to prenatal care,

Table 4.7. Death Rates for All Causes, According to Sex and Age: United States, Selected Years

Sex and Age	Year (Deaths per 100,000 Resident Population)					
	1950	**1960**	**1970**	**1980**	**1990**	**1998**
White male						
All ages, age adjusted	963.1	917.7	893.4	745.3	644.3	562.4
Under 1 year	3,400.5	2,694.1	2,113.2	1,230.3	896.1	673.8
1–4 years	135.5	104.9	83.6	66.1	45.9	32.5
5–14 years	67.2	52.7	48.0	35.0	26.4	21.2
15–24 years	152.4	143.7	170.8	167.0	131.3	107.6
25–34 years	185.3	163.2	176.6	171.3	176.1	133.9
35–44 years	380.9	332.6	343.5	257.4	268.2	232.7
45–54 years	984.5	932.2	882.9	698.9	548.7	489.6
55–64 years	2,304.4	2,225.2	2,202.6	1,728.5	1,467.2	1,215.5
65–74 years	4,864.9	4,848.4	4,810.1	4,035.7	3,397.7	3,082.3
75–84 years	10,526.3	10,299.6	10,098.8	8,829.8	7,844.9	6,988.5
85 years and over	22,116.3	21,750.0	18,551.7	19,097.3	18,268.3	17,048.3
Black male						
All ages, age adjusted	1,373.1	1,246.1	1,318.6	1,112.8	1,061.3	884.5
Under 1 year	—	5,306.8	4,298.9	2,586.7	2,112.4	1,717.8
1–4 years	—	208.5	150.5	110.5	85.8	69.2
5–14 years	95.1	75.1	67.1	47.4	41.2	35.6
15–24 years	289.7	212.0	320.6	209.1	252.2	194.6
25–34 years	503.5	402.5	559.5	407.3	430.8	282.0
35–44 years	878.1	762.0	956.6	689.8	699.6	483.1
45–54 years	1,905.0	1,624.8	1,777.5	1,479.9	1,261.0	1,082.6
55–64 years	3,773.2	3,316.4	3,256.9	2,873.0	2,618.4	2,269.3
65–74 years	5,310.3	5,798.7	5,803.2	5,131,1	4,946.1	4,186.0
75–84 years	—	8,605.1	9,454.9	9,231.6	9,129.5	8,311.4
85 years and over	—	14,844.8	12,222.3	16,098.8	16,954.9	15,540.9
White female						
All ages, age adjusted	645.0	555.0	501.7	411.1	369.9	355.2
Under 1 year	2,566.8	2,007.7	1,614.6	962.5	690.0	563.6
1–4 years	112.2	85.2	66.1	49.3	36.1	27.5
5–14 years	45.1	34.7	29.9	22.9	17.9	15.0
15–24 years	71.5	54.9	61.6	55.5	45.9	41.2
25–34 years	112.8	85.0	84.1	65.4	61.5	58.5
35–44 years	235.8	191.1	193.3	138.2	117.4	122.0
45–54 years	546.4	458.8	462.9	372.7	309.3	278.3
55–64 years	1,293.8	1,078.9	1,014.9	876.2	822.7	740.6
65–74 years	3,242.8	2,779.3	2,470.7	2,066.6	1,923.5	1,912.9
75–84 years	8,481.5	6,696.6	6,698.7	5,401.7	4,839.1	4,792.7
85 years and over	19,679.5	19,477.7	15,980.2	14,979.6	14,400.6	14,620.4

(continues)

70

Table 4.7. continued

Sex and Age	Year (Deaths per 100,000 Resident Population)					
	1950	1960	1970	1980	1990	1998
Black female						
All ages, age adjusted	1,106.7	916.9	814.4	631.1	581.6	540.9
Under 1 year	—	4,162.2	3,368.8	2,123.7	1,735.5	1,390.1
1–4 years	—	173.3	129.4	84.4	67.6	53.9
5–14 years	72.8	53.8	43.8	30.5	27.5	23.1
15–24 years	213.1	107.5	111.9	70.5	68.7	58.0
25–34 years	393.3	273.2	231.0	150.0	159.5	130.0
35–44 years	758.1	568.5	533.0	323.9	298.6	284.9
45–54 years	1,576.4	1,177.0	1,043.9	768.2	639.4	582.0
55–64 years	3,089.4	2,510.9	1,986.2	1,561.0	1,452.6	1,272.2
65–74 years	4,000.2	4,064.2	3,860.9	3,057.4	2,865.7	2,724.6
75–84 years	—	6,730.0	6,691.5	6,212.1	5,688.3	5,813.8
85 years and over	—	13,052.6	10,706.6	12,367.2	13,309.5	13,580.5

Table 4.8. Infant Mortality Rates and Rankings: Selected Countries, 1996

Country	Infant Deaths per 1,000 Live Births	International Rankings	Country	Infant Deaths per 1,000 Live Births	International Rankings
Australia	5.8	16	Italy	6.0	18
Belgium	5.6	13	Japan	3.8	1
Bulgaria	14.8	36	Kuwait	11.5	32
Canada	6.1	20	Netherlands	5.7	14
Chile	11.7	33	New Zealand	6.7	24
Costa Rica	11.8	34	Northern Ireland	5.8	16
Cuba	8.0	27	Norway	4.0	3
Denmark	5.7	14	Poland	12.2	35
England and Wales	6.1	20	Puerto Rico	10.4	30
Finland	4.0	3	Romania	22.3	38
France	4.9	9	Russia	18.2	37
Germany	5.0	10	Singapore	3.8	1
Greece	8.1	28	Spain	4.7	7
Hong Kong	4.1	6	Sweden	4.0	3
Hungary	10.9	31	Switzerland	4.7	7
Ireland	5.5	12	United States	7.3	26
Israel	6.3	23			

high fertility among high-risk young women, poor maternal nutrition, genetic risks, and other complex social, economic, and physiological factors. Differential infant mortality among United States population subgroups indicates that rates are substantially higher for blacks than for whites due to differences in access to health care, nutrition, social factors, and other variables that impact infant viability. These differences reflect underlying social and economic concerns faced by our society. Poor gestational outcomes may result in huge social and economic costs. Implications of inadequate prenatal care, nutrition, and related factors also extend to serious concerns of child intellectual development, social adaptation, and physical maintenance.

Maternal mortality, reflected in Table 4.9, has declined dramatically in the United States since 1950. In addition to the overall decline in these rates, the reduction in maternal mortality for the higher age groups is quite notable.

Again, a very significant differential exists by race. Black women have experienced a significant decline in maternal mortality since 1950, but they still have rates that are much higher than those of white women. The reductions in infant and maternal mortality discussed in this chapter represent a real success in our national efforts to improve the quality and quantity of life. But much remains to be done to achieve optimal results for all Americans and to fully invest in the future of our children.

SPECIFIC CAUSES OF DEATH FOR THE UNITED STATES POPULATION

Age-adjusted death rates for selected causes of death for the United States population from 1950 to the present are presented in Table 4.10. Heart disease, cancer, and stroke are, of course, the three leading causes of death in the United States and have been for quite some time. Interestingly, examination of equiv-

Table 4.9. Maternal Mortality Rates for Complications of Pregnancy, Childbirth, and the Puerperium, According to Race and Age: United States, Selected Years

Race and Age	Year (Deaths per 100,000 Live Births)					
	1950	1960	1970	1980	1990	1998
White						
All ages, age adjusted	53.1	22.4	14.4	6.7	5.1	4.2
Under 20 years	44.9	14.8	13.8	5.8	N/A	N/A
20–24 years	35.7	15.3	8.4	4.2	3.9	3.1
25–29 years	45.0	20.3	11.1	5.4	4.8	4.9
30–34 years	75.9	34.3	18.7	9.3	5.0	4.9
35 years and over	174.1	73.9	59.3	25.5	12.6	11.0
Black						
All ages, age adjusted	—	92.0	65.5	24.9	21.7	16.1
Under 20 years	—	54.8	32.3	13.1	N/A	N/A
20–24 years	—	56.9	41.9	13.9	14.7	12.7
25–29 years	—	92.8	65.2	22.4	14.9	17.2
30–34 years	—	150.6	117.8	44.0	44.2	27.7
35 years and over	—	299.5	207.5	100.6	79.7	37.2

Table 4.10 Age-adjusted Death Rates for Selected Causes of Death: United States, Selected Years

Causes of Death	Year (Deaths per 100,000 Resident Population)					
	1950	1960	1970	1980	1990	1998
All causes	840.5	760.9	714.3	585.8	520.2	471.7
Natural causes	766.6	695.2	636.9	519.7	465.1	422.6
Diseases of heart	307.2	286.2	253.6	202.0	152.0	126.6
Ischemic heart disease	—	—	—	149.8	102.6	79.5
Cerebrovascular diseases	88.6	79.7	66.3	40.8	27.7	25.1
Malignant neoplasms	125.3	125.8	129.8	132.8	135.0	123.6
Respiratory system	12.8	19.2	28.4	36.4	41.4	37.0
Colorectal	19.0	17.7	16.8	15.5	13.6	11.8
Prostate	13.4	13.1	13.3	14.4	16.7	13.2
Breast	22.2	22.3	23.1	22.7	23.1	18.8
Chronic obstructive pulmonary diseases	4.4	8.2	13.2	15.9	19.7	21.3
Pneumonia and influenza	26.2	28.0	22.1	12.9	14.0	13.2
Chronic liver disease and cirrhosis	8.5	10.5	14.7	12.2	8.6	7.2
Diabetes mellitus	14.3	13.6	14.1	10.1	11.7	13.6
Human immunodeficiency virus infection	—	—	—	—	9.8	4.6
External causes	73.9	65.7	77.4	66.1	55.1	49.1
Unintentional injuries	57.5	49.9	53.7	42.3	32.5	30.1
Motor vehicle crashes	23.3	22.5	27.4	22.9	18.5	15.6
Suicide	11.0	10.6	11.8	11.4	11.5	10.4
Homicide and legal intervention	5.4	5.2	9.1	10.8	10.2	7.3

alent data at the turn of the twentieth century would reveal a much greater prevalence of infectious as opposed to chronic diseases for the leading causes of death. Mortality attributable to such causes as nephritis and tuberculosis, which accounted for many deaths at the turn of the century, is far less common today. Influenza and pneumonia were also very important causes of death in the early 1900s. A dramatic outbreak of influenza occurred in 1918, causing considerable mortality.

Figure 4.1 illustrates the predominance of infectious diseases early in the twentieth century and the rise of chronic disease since midcentury. Chronic diseases, of course, are more prevalent because people are living longer and not dying early from infectious diseases. The control of many infectious diseases has been one of the most important successes in public health during the twentieth century. It is notable that the dramatic decline in infectious disease mortality had already occurred prior to the introduction of modern medical technologies such as antibiotic therapy.

Although the predominant challenges for mortality are now focused on chronic diseases, our nation must remain vigilant against outbreaks of infectious disease. Morbidity and mortality associated with the epidemic of human immunodeficiency virus illustrate the constant threat of infectious disease that we face even today. In many developing countries, infectious disease remains a principal cause of mortality, particularly among the very young and the very old. Such diseases as the Ebola virus and other startlingly virulent infectious diseases could become a threat to developed nations' populations at any time. Increased international mobility provides vectors of transmission for infectious disease that were not common years ago.

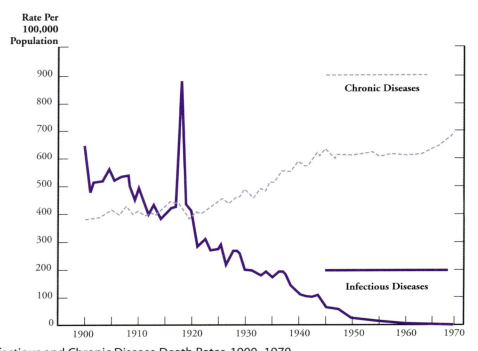

Figure 4.1. Infectious and Chronic Disease Death Rates, 1900–1970

SOURCE: Reprinted by permission of Appleton-Lange from *Dynamics of Health and Disease,* by C. L. Marshall and D. Pearson, 1972, Appleton-Century Crofts, Inc.

Number of Deaths for Specific Causes

Table 4.11 presents actual numbers of deaths for selected subgroups and causes for the United States population. The leading causes of death for each subgroup are listed. Although much more extensive analysis is available, these data sets dramatically demonstrate the tragic involvement of economic, social, and lifestyle factors in causing mortality in the United States. The high ranking for such causes as injuries and violence is quite striking in the younger age groups. Data for the older ages present a picture more common to our typical characterization of mortality causes in the United States.

Mortality attributable to selected causes is presented in the next few tables. Again, only limited data sets can be presented here; much more extensive sta-

tistical information is available from a variety of official governmental sources. Table 4.12 presents data for cardiovascular mortality in the United States. The data illustrate the dramatic and generally consistent decline in mortality from this cause over time and across age groups. Data for various population subgroups based on age, sex, race, and certain other variables would reflect similar patterns. As is typical in illness and mortality data, declines have occurred for many population subgroups, but the results lead to numbers for blacks, American Indians, and some other population groups that are not nearly as low as for whites. The reduction in cardiovascular mortality is attributable to improvements in living conditions, diet, and health care services, particularly interventions for such events as myocardial infarction and coronary occlusion.

Table 4.11. Leading Causes of Death and Number of Deaths, Selected Ages: United States, 1998

Age and Rank Order	Number of Deaths	Cause of Death	Deaths
Under 1 year	45,526	All causes	28,371
1	9,220	Congenital anomalies	6,212
2	5,510	Disorders relating to short gestation and unspecified low birthweight	4,101
3	4,989	Sudden infant death syndrome	2,822
4	3,648	Newborn affected by maternal complications of pregnancy	1,343
5	1,572	Respiratory distress syndrome	1,295
6	1,486	Newborn affected by complications of placenta, cord, and membranes	961
7	1,166	Infections specific to the perinatal period	815
8	1,058	Unintentional injuries	754
9	1,012	Intrauterine hypoxia and birth asphyxia	461
10	985	Pneumonia and influenza	441
1–4 years	8,187	All causes	5,251
1	3,313	Unintentional injuries	1,935
2	1,026	Congenital anomalies	564
3	573	Homicide and legal intervention	399
4	338	Malignant neoplasms	365
5	319	Diseases of heart	214
6	267	Pneumonia and influenza	146
7	223	Septicemia	89
8	110	Certain conditions originating in the perinatal period	75
9	84	Cerebrovascular diseases	57
10	71	Benign neoplasms	53
5–14 years	10,689	All causes	7,791
1	5,224	Unintentional injuries	3,254
2	1,497	Malignant neoplasms	1,013
3	561	Homicide and legal intervention	460
4	415	Congenital anomalies	371
5	330	Diseases of heart	326
6	194	Suicide	324
7	142	Chronic obstructive pulmonary diseases	152
8	104	Pneumonia and influenza	121
9	95	Benign neoplasms	84
10	85	Cerebrovascular diseases	82
15–24 years	49,027	All causes	30,627
1	26,206	Unintentional injuries	13,349
2	6,647	Homicide and legal intervention	5,506
3	5,239	Suicide	4,135
4	2,683	Malignant neoplasms	1,699

(continues)

Table 4.11. continued

Age and Rank Order	Number of Deaths	Cause of Death	Deaths
15–24 years (continued)			
5	1,223	Diseases of heart	1,057
6	600	Congenital anomalies	450
7	418	Chronic obstructive pulmonary diseases	239
8	348	Pneumonia and influenza	215
9	141	Human immunodeficiency virus infection	194
10	133	Cerebrovascular diseases	178
25–44 years	108,658	All causes	131,382
1	26,722	Unintentional injuries	27,172
2	17,551	Malignant neoplasms	21,407
3	14,513	Diseases of heart	16,800
4	11,136	Suicide	12,202
5	9,855	Human immunodeficiency virus infection	8,658
6	4,782	Homicide and legal intervention	8,132
7	3,154	Chronic liver disease and cirrhosis	3,876
8	1,472	Cerebrovascular diseases	3,320
9	1,467	Diabetes mellitus	2,521
10	817	Pneumonia and influenza	1,931
45–64 years	425,338	All causes	380,203
1	148,322	Malignant neoplasms	132,771
2	135,675	Diseases of heart	100,124
3	19,909	Unintentional injuries	18,286
4	18,140	Cerebrovascular diseases	15,362
5	16,089	Diabetes mellitus	13,091
6	11,514	Chronic obstructive pulmonary diseases	12,990
7	7,977	Chronic liver disease and cirrhosis	11,023
8	7,079	Suicide	8,094
9	5,804	Pneumonia and influenza	6,023
10	4,057	Human immunodeficiency virus infection	4,099
65 years and over	1,341,848	All causes	1,753,220
1	595,406	Diseases of heart	605,673
2	258,389	Malignant neoplasms	384,186
3	146,417	Cerebrovascular diseases	139,144
4	45,512	Chronic obstructive pulmonary diseases	97,896
5	43,587	Pneumonia and influenza	82,989
6	28,081	Diabetes mellitus	48,974
7	25,216	Unintentional injuries	32,975
8	24,844	Nephritis, nephritic syndrome, and neophrosis	22,640
9	12,968	Alzheimer's disease	22,416
10	9,519	Septicemia	19,012

Table 4.12. Death Rates for Diseases of Heart, According to Sex and Age: United States, Selected Years

Sex and Age Group	Year (Deaths per 100,000 Resident Population)			
	1950	1970	1990	1998
Male				
All ages, age adjusted	383.8	348.5	206.7	166.9
Under 1 year	4.0	15.1	21.9	16.2
1–4 years	1.4	1.9	1.9	1.5
5–14 years	2.0	0.9	0.9	1.0
15–24 years	6.8	3.7	3.1	3.5
25–34 years	22.9	15.2	10.3	10.8
35–44 years	118.4	103.2	48.1	44.0
45–54 years	440.5	376.4	183.0	152.2
55–64 years	1,104.5	987.2	537.3	411.1
65–74 years	2,292.3	2,170.3	1,250.0	997.3
75–84 years	4,825.0	4,534.8	2,968.2	2,377.2
85 years and over	9,659.8	8,426.2	7,418.4	6,330.6
Female				
All ages, age adjusted	233.9	175.2	108.9	93.3
Under 1 year	2.9	10.9	18.3	16.1
1–4 years	1.2	1.6	1.9	1.3
5–14 years	2.2	0.8	0.8	0.7
15–24 years	6.7	2.3	1.8	2.1
25–34 years	16.2	7.7	5.0	5.8
35–44 years	55.1	32.2	15.1	17.3
45–54 years	177.2	109.9	61.0	52.8
55–64 years	510.0	351.6	215.7	173.9
65–74 years	1,419.3	1,082.7	616.8	522.6
75–84 years	3,872.0	3,120.8	1,893.8	1,579.5
85 years and over	8,796.1	7,591.8	6,478.1	5,876.6

Table 4.13. Death Rates for Cerebrovascular Diseases, According to Age: United States, Selected Years

Age Group	Year (Deaths per 100,000 Resident Population)			
	1950	1970	1990	1998
All ages, age adjusted	88.6	66.3	27.7	25.8
Under 1 year	5.1	5.0	3.8	7.0
1–4 years	0.9	1.0	0.3	0.4
5–14 years	0.5	0.7	0.2	0.2
15–24 years	1.6	1.6	0.6	0.5
25–34 years	4.2	4.5	2.2	1.7
35–44 years	18.7	15.6	6.5	6.2
45–54 years	70.4	41.6	18.7	17.1
55–64 years	195.3	115.8	48.0	44.0
65–74 years	549.7	384.1	144.4	133.5
75–84 years	1,499.6	1,254.2	499.3	464.6
85 years and over	2,990.1	3,014.3	1,633.9	1,564.3

Cancer Mortality in the United States

Among those disease categories where our morbidity and mortality experience has been especially disappointing over the course of the last fifty years are various types of cancer. Mortality attributable to various cancers has remained fairly constant, in contrast to the dramatic declines experienced for cardiovascular and cerebrovascular disease. Furthermore, cancer survival rates after diagnosis generally have not improved very dramatically thus far.

Table 4.14 presents cancer mortality experience for the United States since 1950 by age group. As is evident from the data in this table, cancer mortality has actually increased over time. Increasing cancer mortality may be partially attributable to greater overall longevity, to genetic and environmental factors, to increased case-finding, to declines in other causes of death (leaving people more susceptible to cancer mortality), and to lifestyle issues.

Data for cerebrovascular disease-related mortality are presented in Table 4.13 and reflect a consistent decline over time and across age groups. Racial- and sex-specific data show similar declines as for cardiovascular mortality. Rates for whites are at lower levels at all points in time as compared to blacks.

Table 4.14. Death Rates for Malignant Neoplasms, According to Age: United States, Selected Years

Sex and Age	Year (Deaths per 100,000 Resident Population)				Sex and Age	Year (Deaths per 100,000 Resident Population)			
	1950	1970	1990	1998		1950	1970	1990	1998
Male					*Female*				
All ages, age adjusted	130.8	157.4	166.3	147.7	All ages, age adjusted	120.8	108.8	112.7	105.5
All ages, crude	142.9	182.1	221.3	213.6	All ages, crude	136.8	144.4	186.0	187.7
Under 1 year	9.7	4.4	2.4	2.2	Under 1 year	7.6	5.0	2.2	1.9
1–4 years	12.5	8.3	3.7	2.4	1–4 years	10.8	6.7	3.2	2.4
5–14 years	7.4	6.7	3.5	2.9	5–14 years	6.0	5.2	2.8	2.3
15–24 years	9.7	10.4	5.7	5.4	15–24 years	7.6	6.2	4.1	3.7
25–34 years	17.7	16.3	12.6	10.9	25–34 years	22.2	16.7	12.6	11.7
35–44 years	45.6	53.0	38.5	34.4	35–44 years	79.3	65.6	48.1	42.1
45–54 years	156.2	183.5	162.5	136.5	45–54 years	194.0	181.5	155.5	128.2
55–64 years	413.1	511.8	532.9	441.1	55–64 years	368.2	343.2	375.2	331.6
65–74 years	791.5	1,006.8	1,122.2	1,045.5	65–74 years	612.3	557.9	677.4	675.2
75–84 years	1,332.6	1,588.3	1,914.4	1,745.6	75–84 years	1,000.7	891.9	1,010.3	1,048.6
85 years and over	1,668.3	1,720.8	2,739.9	2,562.6	85 years and over	1,299.7	1,096.7	1,372.1	1,412.5

Tables 4.15 and 4.16 present cancer mortality for two major categories of malignant neoplasms: breast cancer in women and lung cancer. The dramatic increases in mortality attributable to lung cancer are, of course, primarily a function of exposure to tobacco products. Breast cancer mortality trends are more difficult to explain, particularly in light of current controversy regarding the etiology of this cancer.

Cancer Survival Rates

Cancer survival rates, presented in Table 4.17, are disturbing in that, for some categories of cancer, survival rates have not improved appreciably in recent years. Cancer survival is highly dependent on early detection and effective therapeutic intervention. Mass screening for various types of cancer, such as breast, cervical, testicular, and colorectal, can be beneficial for high-risk population subgroups. Population screening has complex cost-benefit trade-offs and other considerations regarding test accuracy, identification of

Table 4.15. Death Rates for Malignant Neoplasm of Breast for Females, According to Age: United States, Selected Years

Age Group	Year (Deaths per 100,000 Resident Population)			
	1950	1970	1990	1998
All ages, age adjusted	22.2	23.1	23.1	19.5
Under 25 Years	*	*	*	*
25–34 years	3.8	3.9	2.9	2.6
35–44 years	20.8	20.4	17.8	13.4
45–54 years	46.9	52.6	45.4	35.8
55–64 years	70.4	77.6	78.6	62.2
65–74 years	94.0	93.8	111.7	93.3
75–84 years	139.8	127.4	146.3	131.4
85 years and over	195.5	157.1	196.8	194.7

*Not large enough numbers.

Table 4.16.   Death Rates for Malignant Neoplasms of Respiratory System, According to Sex and Age: United States, Selected Years

Sex and Age	Year (Deaths per 100,000 Resident Population)				Sex and Age	Year (Deaths per 100,000 Resident Population)			
	1950	1970	1990	1998		1950	1970	1990	1998
Male					*Female*				
All ages, age adjusted	21.3	50.6	61.0	50.6	All ages, age adjusted	4.6	10.1	26.2	26.9
Under 25 years	0.2	0.1	0.1	0.0	Under 25 years	0.1	0.1	0.0	0.0
25–34 years	1.3	1.5	1.0	0.6	25–34 years	0.6	0.6	0.6	0.6
35–44 years	8.1	17.0	9.1	7.1	35–44 years	2.3	6.5	5.4	5.3
45–54 years	39.3	72.1	63.0	43.1	45–54 years	6.7	22.2	35.3	27.0
55–64 years	94.2	202.3	232.6	174.4	55–64 years	15.4	38.9	107.6	98.7
65–74 years	116.3	340.7	447.3	405.0	65–74 years	26.7	45.6	181.7	208.1
75–84 years	105.1	354.2	594.4	541.5	75–84 years	38.8	56.5	194.5	252.7
85 years and over	95.4	215.3	538.0	525.4	85 years and over	42.0	56.5	142.8	194.1

population subgroups appropriate for screening, and other concerns.

Although cancer morbidity, mortality, and survival rate experience has thus far been somewhat disappointing, particularly in comparison with certain other disease categories such as coronary artery and cerebrovascular diseases, prospects for the future appear much brighter. Current biomedical research is successfully elucidating the underlying molecular and biological factors associated with the causes, development, and proliferation of various cancers. Many new pharmaceutical products are in clinical trials or have, in some instances, been brought to market. An extensive commitment of our national research activity toward the development of additional interventions to address cancer in human populations is likely to lead to even greater successes in the coming years.

Because there is a substantial lag time in the collection, evaluation, and dissemination of morbidity and mortality data, particularly for cancer, it will take considerable time before the quantitative results of current biomedical research and clinical interventions become evident in the types of data presented here. Progress for certain types of cancers is already re-

flected in the results presented in these tables. However, most of these success stories focus on early detection and, in some cases, surgical intervention. A far greater impact from pharmaceutical progress and improvement in addressing more fundamental approaches to treating cancer based on an understanding of the biological causes of the disease is likely in the coming years. And, of course, as we conquer cancer as a cause of morbidity and mortality, we will see changes in the distribution of morbidity and mortality for other diseases.

Cancer Incidence Rates

Table 4.18 presents cancer incidence rates for selected sites for white males and white females in the United States over the latter part of the twentieth century. For many categories of cancer, particularly lung, prostate, and breast, incidence rates have increased, in some cases sharply. The extent to which increases in cancer incidence are the result of increased case-finding and greater patient awareness is difficult to elucidate. There is also controversy regarding the fundamental causes of cancer and the extent to which genetic, environmental, behavioral, and dietary factors trigger

Table 4.17. Five-year Relative Cancer Survival Rates for Selected Sites, According to Race and Sex: Selected Geographic Areas, 1974–1976 and 1989–1995

| Sex and Site | Percent of Patients Surviving More than Five Years | | | |
| | White | | Black | |
	1974–1976	1989–1995	1974–1976	1989–1995
Male				
All sites	41.9	59.2	31.3	46.5
Oral cavity and pharynx	54.3	51.7	31.2	28.4
Esophagus	4.3	13.2	2.1	8.0
Stomach	13.2	16.7	15.5	20.6
Colon	49.8	63.0	44.1	51.5
Rectum	47.8	60.0	34.1	52.0
Pancreas	3.1	3.8	1.4	3.2
Lung, bronchus	11.0	12.7	11.0	9.9
Prostate gland	67.7	93.0	58.0	83.6
Urinary bladder	74.5	83.9	54.1	66.6
Non-Hodgkin's lymphoma	47.7	47.7	43.1	37.6
Leukemia	33.5	45.5	32.6	29.7
Female				
All sites	57.4	62.6	46.8	49.1
Colon	50.8	61.9	46.6	52.1
Rectum	49.7	60.6	49.3	50.3
Pancreas	2.1	4.4	3.1	3.9
Lung, bronchus	15.8	16.4	13.1	14.0
Melanoma of skin	84.8	91.0	–	75.2
Breast	74.9	86.0	62.9	71.0
Cervix uteri	69.2	71.4	63.5	58.8
Corpus uteri	88.6	85.4	60.4	56.1
Ovary	36.3	49.9	40.1	47.1
Non-Hodgkin's lymphoma	47.3	57.3	54.1	47.5

its development. Further clarification of the causation and biological mechanisms of various cancers will be a product of ongoing epidemiologic and biomedical research.

Cancer remains one of the most challenging categories of disease with respect to detection and successful therapeutic intervention. Biomedical researchers are successfully elucidating the causes and mechanisms of various cancers, although the challenges from this complex category of disease remain great. Future therapeutic interventions hold great promise. The biomedical research pipeline is producing discoveries daily. However, cancer incidence rates continue to climb, and survival rates remain little improved from earlier years, based on available historical data.

Human Immunodeficiency Virus Mortality

The epidemic of AIDS can be traced back to the late 1970s with rapid progression throughout the 1980s (Centers for Disease Control and Prevention, n.d.). Mortality attributable to AIDS is reflected in Table 4.19. High-risk groups include male intravenous drug users and gays.

Table 4.18. Age-adjusted Cancer Incidence Rates for Selected Cancer Sites, White Males and White Females, Selected Geographic Areas and Years

Race, Sex, and Site	Year (Number of New Cases per 100,000 Population)	
	1973	1996
White male		
All sites	364.3	445.8
Oral cavity and pharynx	17.6	14.0
Esophagus	4.8	6.2
Stomach	14.0	8.4
Colon and rectum	54.3	50.7
Colon	34.8	34.9
Rectum	19.5	15.8
Pancreas	12.8	9.5
Lung and bronchus	72.4	68.4
Prostate gland	62.6	127.8
Urinary bladder	27.3	29.9
Non-Hodgkin's lymphoma	10.3	19.7
Leukemia	14.3	12.4
White female		
All sites	295.0	347.1
Colon and rectum	41.7	35.5
Colon	30.3	25.9
Rectum	11.5	9.6
Pancreas	7.5	7.1
Lung and bronchus	17.8	43.7
Melanoma of skin	5.9	13.2
Breast	84.4	113.3
Cervix uteri	12.8	7.0
Corpus uteri	29.5	21.8
Ovary	14.7	15.3
Non-Hodgkin's lymphoma	7.5	12.7

Table 4.19. Death Rates for Human Immunodeficiency Virus (HIV) Infection, According to Age: United States, Selected Years

Age Group	Year (Deaths per 100,000 Resident Population)		
	1987	1995	1998
All ages, age adjusted	5.5	15.6	4.6
Under 1 year	2.3	1.5	*
1–4 years	0.7	1.3	0.2
5–14 years	0.1	0.5	0.1
15–24 years	1.3	1.7	0.5
25–34 years	11.7	29.1	7.5
35–44 years	14.0	44.4	12.9
45–54 years	8.0	26.3	9.0
55–64 years	3.5	11.0	4.3
65–74 years	1.3	3.6	1.6
75–84 years	0.8	0.7	0.5

*Too small numbers to compute.

Recent biomedical research has produced tremendous progress in treating individuals with this disease. Earlier and more aggressive intervention, primarily utilizing new drug therapies, has led to a tremendous reduction in mortality. Individuals diagnosed with this disease were, in the earlier stages of the epidemic, condemned to a shortened life expectancy. Today, many of the affected individuals can expect to live longer, although the epidemic still exacts a substantial toll from the nation. The cost and complexity of treatment combined with uncertainty regarding the long-term prospects for patients suggest that this is one of the more challenging health concerns our nation must face.

However, to put this disease in perspective, more people die annually from many other causes, including accidents and violence. Parenthetically, it should be kept in mind that AIDS is an international epidemic with over 40,000,000 infected individuals worldwide and is virtually endemic in certain areas and population groups.

Other Causes of Mortality

Perhaps one of the most tragic causes of mortality and morbidity in our society is vehicular-related accidents. An estimated 40,000 people are killed and approximately 2,000,000 people are injured annually in vehicle-related accidents, resulting in a national tragedy. Safer

Table 4.20. Death Rates for Motor Vehicle Crashes by Age: United States, Selected Years

Age Group	Year (Deaths per 100,000 Resident Population)		
	1950	1970	1998
All ages, age adjusted	23.3	27.4	15.6
Under 1 year	8.4	9.8	4.3
1–4 years	11.5	11.5	5.0
5–14 years	8.8	10.2	4.8
15–24 years	34.4	47.2	26.9
25–34 years	24.6	30.9	18.4
35–44 years	20.3	24.9	15.6
45–54 years	22.2	25.5	14.3
55–64 years	29.2	27.9	15.3
65–74 years	38.8	32.8	18.5
75–84 years	52.7	43.5	28.9
85 years and over	45.1	34.2	31.5

Table 4.21. Death Rates for Firearm-related Injuries, According to Selected Sex, Race, and Age: United States, 1998

Sex, Race, and Age	(Deaths per 100,000 Resident Population)	
	White Male	Black Male
All ages, age adjusted	16.2	41.6
1–14 years	1.3	2.4
15–24 years	23.1	101.8
25–34 years	21.2	75.3
35–44 years	19.5	35.9
45–64 years	18.5	22.1
65 years and over	30.3	14.2

Table 4.22. Death Rates for Homicide and Legal Intervention, According to Selected Sex, Race, and Age: United States, 1998

Sex, Race, and Age	(Deaths per 100,000 Resident Population)	
	White Male	Black Male
All ages, age adjusted	6.4	43.1
Under 1 year	6.7	21.8
1–14 years	1.1	4.9
15–24 years	12.2	96.5
25–34 years	10.2	75.0
35–44 years	7.5	43.4
45–64 years	4.7	25.8
65 years and over	2.8	11.9

roads and vehicles and a lower driving speed have led to reductions in vehicular mortality over the past twenty years. The tragic toll of motor vehicle accidents is reflected in Table 4.20. Those at highest risk are young adult male drivers and the oldest age groups.

Mortality attributable to firearms is another inexcusable national tragedy. Table 4.21 reflects mortality rates by age group due to firearms-related accidents and violence. This includes mortality associated with suicide, homicide, police intervention, and accidents. Approximately 20,000 Americans are killed annually in firearms-related situations, with numerous others sustaining various injuries.

The violent nature of our society is also reflected in Table 4.22, which presents selected data on mortality attributable to homicide and legal intervention. These data partially overlap with firearms mortality when firearms are involved in the homicide or legal intervention.

As we seek to improve the quality and quantity of life in this country, we have to constantly appreciate the considerable morbidity and mortality attributable to social, economic, lifestyle, and other nonphysio-logical causes. Finding answers to problems of unhealthy diets and personal practices, consumption of alcohol, cigarettes, drugs, and other unhealthy substances, and the prevalence of social problems leading to violence in our society must be a high priority as we also seek biomedical solutions to our physiological problems. At the same time, we also face a wide range of psychological and mental health problems that cause tremendous disruption in our lives and our society; these, too, must be addressed from both biomedical and social perspectives.

INCIDENCE OF INFECTIOUS DISEASES

Our nation is now largely spared the tragedies of many of the infectious diseases that are still prevalent throughout the world. However, not all infectious disease has been eradicated in this nation, and new challenges continue to surface.

Table 4.23 presents the incidence of infectious disease over the latter half of the twentieth century for the United States (Centers for Disease Control and Prevention, 2000). The decline of many infectious diseases that are now avoidable through immunization and vaccination is evident in this table. At the same time, the table illustrates the continuing challenge of many infectious diseases that remain, especially those associated with sexual activity.

Likely further declines in reportable infectious diseases will occur with the use of immunizations for such diseases as chicken pox. For other diseases, such as gonorrhea, the challenge continues, particularly with physiologic resistance to many current drug treatments. And, of course, the AIDS epidemic dramatically illustrates the potential threat from new infectious diseases. Other particularly gruesome infectious diseases, such as the Ebola virus, have come to the forefront in recent years, clearly demonstrating how we can be challenged by disease even with the advancing state of our knowledge.

Table 4.23.   Selected Notifiable Disease Cases: United States, Selected Years

Disease	Year (Number of Cases)	
	1950	1998
Diphtheria	5,796	1
Hepatitis A	—	23,229
Hepatitis B	—	10,258
Mumps	—	666
Pertussis (whooping cough)	120,718	7,405
Poliomyelitis, total	33,300	1
Rubella (German measles)	—	364
Rubeola (measles)	319,124	100
Tuberculosis	121,742	18,361
Syphilis	217,558	37,977
Gonorrhea	286,746	355,642

LIFESTYLE PATTERNS AND DISEASE

Numerous behaviors and lifestyle patterns affect our health. Examples discussed previously in this chapter include exposure to violence, vehicular accidents, alcohol, drugs, and infectious agents.

An excellent example of the association between disease and behavior is the consumption of tobacco products. Cigarette consumption has been associated with numerous illnesses, including cardiovascular disease, lung cancer, and oral cancer. Reduction in cigarette and other tobacco product consumption has been a national goal for thirty years.

Government policy has been directed toward reducing morbidity and mortality by intervening in people's destructive behavior. Interventions include the use of taxation, public education, and restrictions on product production and distribution.

A reduction in cigarette consumption in the United States has occurred during the period of aggressive intervention, as reflected in Table 4.24. Many current smokers may be consuming greater

Table 4.24.   Current Cigarette Smoking by Persons 18 Years of Age and Over, According to Sex and Age: United States, 1965 and 1998

Sex and Age	Percent of Persons 18 Years of Age and Over	
	1965	1998
Males		
18 years and over, age adjusted	51.6	25.9
18–24 years	54.1	31.3
25–34 years	60.7	28.6
35–44 years	58.2	30.2
45–64 years	51.9	27.7
65 years and over	28.5	10.4
Females		
18 years and over, age adjusted	34.0	22.1
18–24 years	38.1	24.5
25–34 years	43.7	24.6
35–44 years	43.7	26.4
45–64 years	32.0	22.5
65 years and over	9.6	11.1

quantities of tobacco products than the typical smoker did in past years. Many of those giving up tobacco products were casual users.

The net effect on morbidity and mortality from tobacco product consumption is difficult to estimate. However, any reduction in use of these products is positive for the nation's health overall, probably substantially so.

HEALTH, LIFESTYLE, AND SOCIAL STRUCTURE

The relationship between lifestyle and health is well established with regard to practices such as tobacco products consumption, as discussed previously. Numerous other lifestyle issues also significantly impact health. Alcohol consumption and illicit drug use are examples of personal decision making and patterns of behavior that have tremendous adverse effects on health and on the nation's economy.

Alcohol consumption, beyond a very moderate level, is associated with numerous physiological complications including cirrhosis of the liver, various cancers, intestinal disorders, and brain function deterioration. Equally severe psychological and social complications ranging from divorce to poor job performance are also common. Alcohol abuse results in illness and injury to others, including—but certainly not limited to—vehicular accidents, job-place injuries, poor fetal outcomes associated with fetal alcohol syndrome, and spousal and child abuse.

Like alcohol abuse, illicit drug use results in a spectrum of adverse consequences for our society. In addition to many of the adverse consequences already mentioned for alcohol abuse, illicit drug use leads to high levels of violent crime, general social dysfunction, and many other untoward consequences.

The implications of tobacco, alcohol, and drug abuse alone are wide-ranging and contribute to the destruction of the fabric of our society and of individuals' lives. And these three areas constitute only a portion of dysfunctional behavior that impinges on health, with consequent increased morbidity and mortality.

The range of other behaviors that adversely affect health is tremendous. Enhanced morbidity and mortality have been associated with various complications of dietary behaviors such as elevated consumption of fat, sodium, and sugar. Sexual behaviors are associated with the spread of communicable diseases such as AIDS, gonorrhea, syphilis, and other sexually transmitted diseases, leading to increased levels of infertility, cancer, and other complications. Societal stress is associated with deterioration of the immune system and consequent morbidity and mortality, workplace violence, marital difficulties, spousal abuse, and other problems.

Thus, the etiology of much of our morbidity and mortality can be traced to behavior, social interaction, lifestyle, and other nonphysiological determinants. Solving the primary physiological causes of illness and disease may be easier than adequately addressing these social and behavioral ones. The challenges to modify behavior are great, and the complications introduced by our modern society make the task ever more difficult. As we move through the new century, the failure of our society in the twentieth century to adequately address the social, behavioral, and economic causes of disease and illness will continue to haunt us.

ACCESS TO HEALTH CARE SERVICES

As mentioned previously, various aspects of the measurement and assessment of access to health care services are extremely important in assessing the health care system's response to disease and illness and to the development of the national health policy. Assessing access to health care services can facilitate the determination of the degree to which the system responds to both consumer and professional assessments of need and demand for health care. Differentials in the measurement of access between population groups can reflect issues of equitable access to care and failures of the health care system to respond to perceived or actual needs on the part of consumers. Access trends over time, likewise, can reflect changes in the functioning of the health care system and its effectiveness in addressing the needs of the population (Andersen et al., 1996).

The concluding section of this chapter addresses issues of access to care, a core theme of this book, particularly as reflected in utilization of care in response to perceived needs by individuals with various diseases and illnesses. Trends in access to care, like trends in disease and illness patterns, are key assessment variables in our monitoring and evaluation of the health care system over time.

Models of Access

Numerous quantitative models of health services access have been developed over the years. These models typically emanate from analytical assessments based on psychological, sociological, financial and economic, or psychological perspectives and assessments of individual's access to health care services. Some researchers have attempted to provide more comprehensive and integrated models of access by combining a variety of perspectives as well.

As might be expected, discipline-oriented models of access to care reflect the variables typically assessed by such a disciplinary researcher. For example, sociological models of access to health care typically examine sociological variables such as population characteristics and interpersonal relationships and influences. Psychological models of access would focus more typically on perceptions by patients of severity of illness, health beliefs, attitudes and values, and health knowledge. Economic models of utilization and access typically address such factors as insurance coverage and income, health systems organization, and financing arrangements. Table 4.25 lists illustra-

Table 4.25 Discipline Oriented Models of Access to Care

Discipline	Variables
Demographic	Age, sex, marital status, family size, residence
Social structural	Social class, ethnicity, education, occupation
Social psychological	Health beliefs, values, attitudes, norms, culture
Economic	Family income, insurance coverage, prices of services, provider/population ratios
Organizational	Organization of physicians' practices, referral patterns, use of ancillaries, regular source of care
Systems	All or most of the above

tive variables typically measured by each discipline's approach to assessing health system access.

In most instances, for the variables listed in Table 4.25, extensive and relatively expensive survey questionnaires are required to collect and process the information necessary for the conduct of the analysis. In reality, and from a practical perspective, demographic, financial, and patient variables are those that are most typically utilized in assessing access to health care on an ongoing basis. These utilization variables are usually obtained from enrolled client populations in health services plans or from large-scale national surveys conducted by the federal government or by other organizations.

The predictive power of many models of utilization and their ability to influence national health policy are somewhat limited. And the often high costs associated with collecting and analyzing the data limit their actual application. Newer practice information systems are facilitating data collection and analysis. These models are valuable in providing a mechanism or forum through which to analyze issues of access and national health policy. The conceptualization of access to care and, even in a limited analysis, the use of some discreet readily available measures of utilization do provide valuable insight into access concerns that our nation faces.

As noted above, many complex models of access to health care have been developed, primarily by academic researchers, over the years. These include behavioral and sociological models that focus on the health behaviors of various population groups modified by their environments. These environmental factors include such measures as economic well-being and perceptions of health status. Measuring many of these variables is difficult and potentially expensive on an ongoing basis. But, as noted previously, these models hold great value in helping us understand how the health care system responds to consumer needs.

Many models, particularly those using sociological and economic concepts, focus on the resources available in the health care system and their organizational and financial arrangements. Characteristics of the population under scrutiny are also included in many models of utilization and access. Personal characteristics include such factors as health practices and prior utilization as well as demographic variables. Social structure and an individual's response to his or her environment may also be measured in the context of his or her ability to cope with health problems. Interaction with other individuals, other social influences, and social and cultural backgrounds may be considered as well. Health beliefs, attitudes, and knowledge have a significant effect on how an individual responds to health care needs and to signs and symptoms.

Many access models include a careful examination of the availability of community and personal resources. These variables include supply measures such as the availability of physicians and hospitals. They also include individuals' financial access to care as measured by income, health insurance, the availability of regular sources of care, and other practical considerations. Managed-care arrangements and other characteristics of the health care system are also considered in the development of these models.

Analysis of access to care frequently addresses professional assessments by physicians, nurses, and other health care practitioners of a patient's signs and symptoms of illness. Some models seek to incorporate patients' own perceptions of their health care needs, separate from professional evaluations. Professional assessments include quantitative assessments as a result of a physical exam or the conduct of laboratory tests. Numerous other aspects of professional assessment may also be included in more sophisticated modeling. Of course, professional assessment of individual needs may differ from the patient's own perceptions of what kind of care he or she needs.

Actual Measures of Access to Care

More common measures of access to health care services are used in this section to illustrate access and to examine trends over time. Selected measures of access are presented for the usual sources of care among children, use of mammography, and dental visits for selected United States populations.

Table 4.26 illustrates the increased availability, as measured by having a usual source of care, of health

Table 4.26. No Usual Source of Health Care Among Children, Selected Characteristics: United States, Average Annual 1997–98

Characteristic	Under 18 Years of Age	Under 6 Years of Age
	Percent Without Usual Source	
All children	6.7	4.5
Race		
White	5.8	4.1
Black	8.9	5.6
American Indian or Alaska Native	10.8	*
Asian or Pacific Islander	10.7	*
Race and Hispanic origin		
White, non-Hispanic	4.5	3.4
Black, non-Hispanic	8.8	5.4
Hispanic	13.2	7.6
Poverty status		
Poor	12.4	8.2
Nonpoor	3.5	2.0
Black, non-Hispanic		
Poor	9.1	5.4
Nonpoor	6.4	4.0
Hispanic		
Poor	16.9	8.4
Nonpoor	5.7	3.1
Health insurance status		
Insured	3.8	3.0
Private	3.3	2.4
Medicaid	5.1	4.0
Uninsured	27.6	17.3

*Too small sample

care services for white as compared to minority children. Lower income individuals also have less access to care as measured by this indicator.

Table 4.27 measures access to mammography services over time in the United States. Access has clearly improved over time by the indicators used in this

Table 4.27. Use of Mammography According to Selected Characteristics: United States, 1987 and 1998

Characteristic	1987	1998
Age		
40 years and over	28.7	66.9
65 years and over	22.8	63.8
Age, race, and Hispanic origin		
40 years and over:		
White, non-Hispanic	30.3	68.0
Black, non-Hispanic	23.8	66.0
Hispanic	18.3	60.2
65 years and over		
White, non-Hispanic	24.0	64.3
Black, non-Hispanic	14.1	60.7
Hispanic	13.7	59.0
Age and poverty status		
40 years and over		
Below poverty	15.0	50.5
At or above poverty	31.0	69.3
65 years and over		
Below poverty	13.4	52.2
At or above poverty	25.0	66.2
Age and education		
40 years of age and over:		
No high school diploma or GED	17.8	54.5
High school diploma or GED	31.3	66.7
Some college or more	37.7	72.8
65 years of age and over:		
No high school diploma or GED	16.5	54.7
High school diploma or GED	25.9	66.8
Some college or more	32.3	71.3

table. Access is still lower for poorer women and those with less education.

Finally, Table 4.28 measures access to dental services. Again, poorer people have lower access as measured by visits in the prior year. While this data does not adjust for dental health need, it is likely that lower income individuals do have poorer dental health.

Extensive data is available from various surveys, especially those conducted by the federal government, for tracking changes in access to care for various population groups. This information is extremely valuable for national policy-making and to contribute to the overall debate about the design of the health care system. Examples of current access-related issues reflected in these data would include lack of access to dental care for individuals without financial resources (a considerable percentage of the population, which is currently increasing) having no insurance coverage (or who are underinsured for health care services) and lack of adequate access to health care in the areas of long-term care and mental health services.

Access Issues for the Future

Access is a key issue that has challenged our nation's health care system throughout history. As a nation, we have long struggled with issues of who has the right to access which health care services and under what conditions. Assuring adequate access to care is an issue that permeates all aspects of health-care policy and delivery.

Managed-care organizations constantly struggle with the trade-offs involved in controlling access to care versus assuming increased costs. Social programs have long addressed issues of access. Medicare and Medicaid, as social programs, had their origins in the realization that access to health care for some population groups did not meet national social goals.

The formulation and measurement of indicators of access to care is a challenging area for health services researchers, but one that contributes substantially to improving the operation of the health care system. Addressing the challenges of access provides a key focal point for constant analysis of the nature of the health care system and our national goals for that system. Ultimately, it is the issues of access and cost that we must successfully address to assure that all citizens receive a level of health care services adequate for their most fundamental needs. It is also important to recognize that issues of access are intimately connected to factors associated with the quality of care, with satisfaction on the part of providers and consumers, and with national, political, economic, and social goals.

Table 4.28.   Dental Visits in the Past Year According to Patient Characteristics: United States, 1998

Characteristic	2 Years of Age and Over	2-17 Years of Age	18-64 Years of Age	65 Years of Age and Over
Total	66.2	73.5	65.6	56.4
Sex				
Male	63.6	72.0	61.7	57.8
Female	68.8	75.1	69.2	55.4
Race				
White	67.8	74.9	67.2	58.2
Black	58.0	69.8	58.3	36.9
American Indian or Alaska Native	56.1	72.6	53.7	41.1
Asian or Pacific Islander	65.5	67.8	63.4	67.4
Race and Hispanic origin				
White, non-Hispanic	69.5	77.1	68.9	58.7
Black, non-Hispanic	58.0	69.8	58.1	37.3
Hispanic	54.1	62.4	52.2	46.8
Poverty status				
Poor	48.3	63.5	47.1	32.6
Nonpoor	73.2	80.4	72.0	66.8
Race and Hispanic origin and poverty status				
White, non-Hispanic				
Poor	51.8	64.1	51.8	34.0
Nonpoor	74.4	81.5	73.3	67.7
Black, non-Hispanic				
Poor	47.1	67.7	46.6	22.5
Nonpoor	65.4	76.1	65.5	48.4
Hispanic				
Poor	41.7	58.7	37.4	36.3
Nonpoor	67.2	75.5	65.4	59.4
Geographic region				
Northeast	70.4	80.5	69.6	56.3
Midwest	69.4	76.9	69.2	56.2
South	62.2	69.1	61.2	53.9
West	65.6	70.1	64.7	61.2

SUMMARY

This chapter has traced many of the primary patterns of population dynamics and illness in our society during the twentieth century. A fundamental understanding of these trends is essential in interpreting the optimal structure of health services delivery systems as discussed in the remainder of this book. Understanding the relationships between these epidemiological trends and the physiological and psychological nature of the human body and of the determinants of health services utilization is important in defining the overall nature of a population's use of health care and, in turn, forms the basis for the organization and financing, and eventually evaluation, of that system.

References

Andersen, R. M., Rice, T. H., & Komnski, G. F. (Eds.). (1996). *Changing the U. S. health care system.* San Francisco: Jossey-Bass.

Centers for Disease Control and Prevention. (n.d.). *HIV/AIDS surveillance report* (published quarterly). Surveillance and Evaluation Branch, AIDS Program, National Center for Infectious Diseases. Atlanta, GA: Author.

Centers for Disease Control and Prevention. (2000). Summary of notifiable diseases. *U.S. Morbidity and Mortality Weekly Report,* Atlanta, GA: Public Health Service, DHHS.

National Center for Health Statistics. (1993). *Vital statistics of the United States, 1989* (Vol. I, Natality, DHHS Pub. No. (PHS) 93-1100 and Vol. II, Mortality, Pt. A, DHHS Pub. No. (PHS) 93-1101). Washington, DC: Public Health Service, U.S. Government Printing Office.

National Center for Health Statistics. (2000). *Health, United States, 2000 with adolescent health chartbook.* US Department of Health and Human Services. Hyattsville, MD.

Popovic, J. R., & Kozak, L. J. (2000). *National hospital discharge survey: Annual summary, 1998.* National Center for Health Statistics. *Vital and Health Statistics, 13* (148). Hyattsville, MD.

United Nations. (2001). *Demographic yearbook* (United Nations Pub. No. UNIS/PI/225). New York: Author.

U.S. Bureau of the Census. (2000). *2000 census of the population, general population characteristics* (Series 2000). Washington, DC: Author.

Woodwell, D. A. (1999). *National ambulatory medical care survey: 1997 summary.* (Advance data from *Vital and health statistics;* No. 305.) Hyattsville, Maryland: National Center for Health Statistics.

PART

2

Financing and Structuring
Health Care

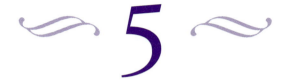

CHAPTER
5

Financing Health Services

Alma L. Koch

Chapter Topics

- Health Expenditures
- Health Insurance
- Medicare
- Medicaid
- Physician Reimbursement
- Initiatives in Health Care Finance
- Health Care Reform

Learning Objectives

Upon completing this chapter, the reader should be able to:

- Differentiate among types of health insurance: voluntary, social, and welfare

- Distinguish among various health financing schemes for provision of care and postulate future changes in these systems

- Understand provider incentives and disincentives stemming from the financing system for health care

- Intelligently discuss major health care financing issues of the day

- Compare the U.S. health financing system with that of other advanced nations

- Describe the principles of insurance and to apply them in evaluating health insurance plans

The system for financing health services in the United States reflects the fragmentation of health care as a whole. It is a patchwork of loosely connected financing mechanisms varying by sponsorship and provider type. It also reflects the age, health, and economic status of the specific patient groups that are being served. In view of the growing number of Americans who are uninsured for health care, one may say that it is a disappointing financing system. However, these observations do provide a touch point for studying the financing apparatus as it now exists. If one looks at the "system" in light of the role of tradition and the values of the American people, as well as the political philosophy of the times, the organization of health finance in the United States comes into better focus.

This chapter will examine the size and scope of the health care financing system in the United States. Where possible, comparisons will be drawn between the United States and other countries. Special attention will be paid to differences and similarities in the public and private financing components of the system, reimbursement of various provider categories, and trends that we may expect to see in the future. The role of health insurance as a financial conduit will be explored and monetary business objectives will be contrasted with the altruistic goals of health care as a human service.

HEALTH EXPENDITURES

Size of the U.S. Health Care Industry

The health care industry is by far the largest service industry in the country. In dollar volume, the health care industry ranks second after total durable goods manufacturing (U.S. Bureau of the Census, 2000). In 1998, Americans spent $1,149 trillion on health care, comprising 13.5 percent of the gross domestic product (GDP) and amounting to $4,094 per capita (USDHHS, 2000b). The United States spends far more on health care than other industrialized countries. For example, in 1997, the United Kingdom and Japan fell at the lower end of the spectrum, spending 6.8 and 7.2 percent of their respective GDPs on health care. Canada, France, Germany, and Switzerland came closer to U.S. figures, with 9.2, 9.6, 10.7, and 10.0 percent of

their respective GDPs spent on health, with most other industrialized nations falling in the established range (U.S. Bureau of the Census, 2000).

Growth in Health Expenditures

Since 1940, national health expenditures have grown at a rate substantially outpacing the GDP. Table 5.1 shows that, prior to World War II, only 4.0 percent of the GDP was devoted to health care, both public and private. By 1998, the proportion of the GDP expended for health care increased by almost ten percentage points. Since the onset of Medicare and Medicaid in mid-1966, national health expenditures have grown particularly rapidly, from about 6.3 percent of the GDP to the present figure. Most of this growth is quantitatively explained by nationwide inflation, excess medical inflation, and increased intensity in the provision of health care services, in that order. Only a small fraction of growth in health care can be attributed to the growth in the U.S. population. However, from 1993 to 1998, health care spending exhibited no change, stabilizing at around 13.5 percent of the GDP. This stability was precipitated both by a slowdown in the rate of growth of health care spending and to an upswing in overall economic growth.

A variety of qualitative factors is believed to have contributed to the disproportionate growth in health

Table 5.1. Aggregate and Per Capita National Health Expenditures, United States, Selected Years

Year	Total (Billions)	Per Capita	GDP (Billions)	Percent of GDP
1940	$ 4.0	$ 30	$ 100	4.0
1950	12.7	82	287	4.4
1960	26.9	141	527	5.1
1970	73.2	341	1,036	7.1
1980	247.2	1,052	2,784	8.9
1990	699.4	2,689	5,744	12.2
1998	1,149.1	4,094	8,511	13.5

SOURCE: Adapted from Health Spending in 1998: Signals of Change, K. Levit et al., Jan/Feb 2000, *Health Affairs, 19*(1), p. 125; and National Health Expenditures, 1995, K.R. Levit, et al., Fall 1996, *Health Care Financing Review, 18*(1), pp. 175–214.

care spending relative to the growth in GDP. These include (1) rapid development and dissemination of medical technology, which expanded the treatment of disease; (2) rising expectations about the value of health care services; (3) government financing of health care services; (4) the nature of third party reimbursement; (5) the growth in the proportion of elderly; (6) the lack of competitive forces in the health care system to increase efficiency and productivity in the delivery of services; and (7) the maldistribution of physicians and other providers of health services.

Monetary Flow

Payment Sources

Figure 5.1 contrasts the monetary inflow (i.e., "Where it came from") and outflow (i.e., "Where it went") in the United States for total health spending in 1999. Private health insurance finances less than one-third of all health expenditures; direct patient payment finances about fifteen percent. These payment sources, together with other private sources (mostly philanthropic), account for the fifty-four percent of all health expenditures that are privately financed in the United States. The other forty-six percent is financed publicly either by federal, state, or local governments. The largest single public program is Medicare (the federal social security health insurance plan for the elderly, the disabled, and other groups), followed by Medicaid (the federal/state welfare program for health care), and other government programs.

Spending for Medicare and Medicaid has been increasing even more rapidly than total national health expenditures. In 1999, Medicare and Medicaid together comprised thirty-four percent of the total health care bill; in 1967, the two programs represented only fifteen percent of the total health care bill. Out of approximately 270 million people in the United States in 1998, over one-quarter (74 million people) were enrolled in either or both programs. Medicare's role was clearly most substantial for hospital care; Medicaid's role was most prominent for nursing home care, and the growth in these two services has indubitably been spurred on by the two public programs (USDHHS, 2000a).

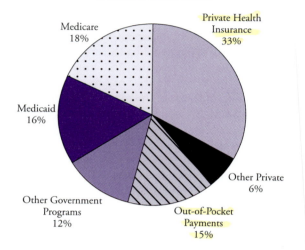

Where It Came From

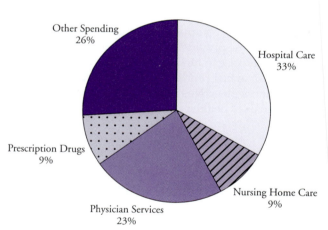

Where It Went

Figure 5.1. The Nation's Health Dollar, 1999

SOURCE: *National Health Expenditures, 1999.* Health Care Financing Administration, April 25, 2001, http://www.hcfa.gov/stat/nhe-oact/tables/chart.htm.

Outlays

In terms of outlays, forty-two percent of the money spent for health in 1999 was used to purchase hospital and nursing home services, although hospital expenditures, which totaled $383 billion, have dropped substantially as a proportion of health care expenditures in the past twenty years. Another forty-nine percent was divided among physicians' services and other personal care items (i.e., dental services, other professional services, vision services, home health care, drugs, eyeglasses and appliances, and other miscellaneous health care services and products). While physician services have increased slightly over the years, "other" health care costs have burgeoned. Prescription drugs accounted for the remaining nine percent of the health care dollar for 1999 (USDHHS, 2000a).

Personal Health Care

Figure 5.2 shows financing trends since 1950 for personal health care expenditures (PHCE), which include total health expenditures minus program ad-

ministration. public health activities, research, and construction. Government plus private insurance have grown enormously in the post-war era, funding just short of three-quarters of all PHCE. Direct payments by patients have dropped commensurately to just over fifteen percent of PHCE (USDHHS, 2000a).

For 1999, sources of funding for major providers of PHCE are depicted in Figure 5.3. Government funding dominates hospital reimbursement, with sixty percent financed by Medicare, Medicaid, and other government programs, in that order. Another thirty-one percent of the national hospital bill is footed by private health insurance. Physician outlays are clearly dominated by the private sector. Private insurance, direct patient payments, and other private sources account

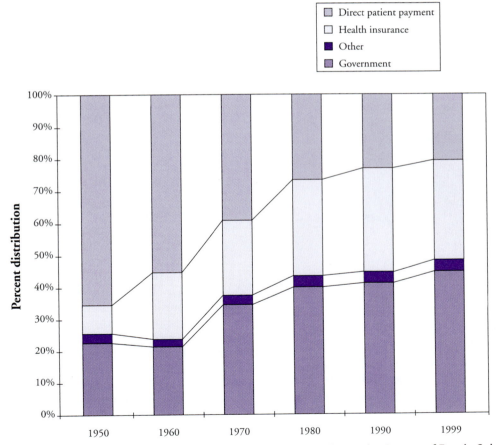

Figure 5.2.   Percentage Distribution of U.S. Personal Health Care Expenditures by Source of Funds, Selected Years

SOURCE: *Health Care Expenditures, 1999*. Health Care Financing Administration, April 25, 2001, http://www.hcfa.gov/stats/nhe-oact/tables/t4.htm.

Hospitals = $390.9 Billion

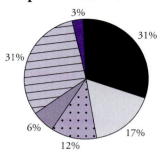

Physicians = $269.4 Billion

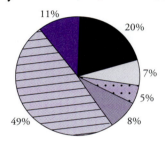

Nursing Homes = $90.0 Billion

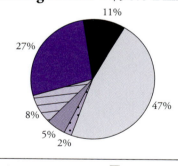

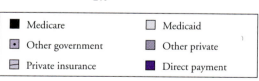

■ Medicare	□ Medicaid
▨ Other government	▨ Other private
▨ Private insurance	■ Direct payment

Figure 5.3. Personal Health Care Expenditures for Total U.S. Population by Type of Service and Source of Funds

SOURCE: *National Health Expenditures, 1999.* Health Care Financing Administration, April 25, 2001, http://www.hcfa.gov/stats/nhe-oact/tables/t5.htm.

for more than sixty-eight percent of physician funding; Medicare, which in recent years has diminished as a financier of physicians' services, picks up another twenty percent. Nursing home funding reflects the "rich man, poor man" dichotomy of the long-term care industry, wherein patients must "spend down" their assets in order to qualify for government assistance. About three-quarters of nursing home revenues are funded by direct patient payment and Medicaid. However, Medicare's share of funding for short-term nursing homes has risen almost six-fold since 1990. Private long-term care insurance, which was practically nonexistent ten years ago, has skyrocketed to eight percent of nursing home funding.

HEALTH INSURANCE

Origins of Health Insurance

Health insurance originated in Europe in the early 1800s, when mutual-benefit societies arose to lighten the financial burden for those stricken with illness. The focus was on low-skilled, low-income workers who were industrially employed. (Providers in Europe wanted to keep high-skilled employees in the private medical market.) The first government health insurance program arose in Germany in 1840, mandating workers below a certain income level to belong to a "sickness fund." The concept of health insurance as linked to employment in the industrial sector persists internationally to this day. The health insurance networks of many nations grew out of this linkage and still reflect an emphasis on nonagricultural employment and coverage of the worker, irrespective of dependents (Roemer, 1977; Roemer, 1978).

Today in the United States, the framework of health insurance stems clearly from its European antecedents and breaks down into three categories that, in some sense, reflect employment status. *Voluntary health insurance* (VHI) is private insurance usually denoting current industrial employment; *social health insurance* (SHI) reflects participation in a government entitlement program linked to previous (or current) employment; *public welfare* health care programs connote lack of employment, low-income employment, or the inability to gain employment stemming from a disabling condition.

Distributing Risk

Insurance is a way of pooling or distributing risk. Risk is the probability of incurring a loss. Risk stems from two kinds of occurrences: (1) unanticipated events such as fires, car accidents, or airplane crashes, and (2) anticipated events such as death, old age, and sickness. Health or, more correctly, illness is an anticipated event associated with old age and death. Thus, we know that illness is a likely event, but we do not know when it will strike, to whom it will happen, or how severe it will be. Therefore, health is uncertain for the individual but not for a group. Groups are actuarially (i.e., statistically) predictable.

Moral Hazard

In the theory of insurance, it is assumed that risks are independent of each other: (1) what befalls one person does not affect another, and (2) that for a single individual, risks are independent. Neither assumption is true in health insurance because one person's sickness may spread contagiously and illness in one part of the body may weaken another part. These phenomena, together with the *moral hazard* inherent in medical care, make health insurance and health costs, in general, extremely volatile. Moral hazard means that, to the extent that the event insured against can be controlled, there exists a temptation to use the insurance. (The classic example of moral hazard is setting fire to a failing business in order to collect the insurance.) Health insurance usage is highly discretionary; doctors and patients can conspire (intentionally or not) to use the insurance. An example is where a private patient with a traditional type of policy is kept in the hospital an extra day because it would be difficult or inconvenient for the family to receive the patient back home on the earliest possible discharge day. In this example, the insured extra day in the hospital, at a cost of $700 or more to the carrier, saves a loss in earnings for the family, and the expense is borne by purchasers of the policy, as reflected in the price of the premium.

Benefit Structure

Because of moral hazard, health insurance usually pays less than the total loss incurred by levying out-of-pocket or direct costs on the patient. In fee-for-service provider reimbursement, these take the form of deductibles and copayments. A *deductible* is a sum of money that *must* be paid, typically every year, before the insurance policy becomes active. Deductibles have long been criticized in health insurance for posing an impediment to first-contact care, discouraging the patient from seeking care until the condition becomes severe. Because higher costs may be incurred for more severe illness, deductibles have been postulated to contribute to health cost inflation, rather than stimulating parsimonious consumer utilization. A *copayment* is paid as the beneficiary uses the insurance. For example, in a policy with a traditional *indemnity benefit*, a fixed cash amount is paid to the beneficiary per procedure or per day in the hospital (e.g., $800 for a one-night stay in the hospital following a hernia repair). If the hospital charges $1,100, then the patient must pay a copayment of $300. Thus, the patient is liable for any amount in excess of the indemnity payment. An insurance plan with a *service benefit* reimburses on a percentage basis and the patient pays *coinsurance*. Using the example above, the insurance plan would pay eighty percent, or $880, of the surgeon's charges, leaving only $220 in coinsurance to be paid by the patient. Thus, if the percentage rate is high, the reimbursement structure of service benefits usually works to the patient's advantage compared to indemnity benefits.

Pure types of indemnity or service benefits are becoming increasingly rare. Nowadays, to control health cost inflation, there is a growing trend toward hybrid benefit structures, combining both service and indemnity features. A plan may, for example, pay a percentage of charges up to a specified limit, beyond which point the patient becomes responsible for the balance. Preferred provider organizations (PPOs) utilize this technique, often in concert with low price ceilings, to reimburse non-participating providers. Using the example above, the PPO might pay eighty percent up to an $800 limit on charges for a non-participating hospital. The plan would pay $640 and the patient would thus incur a $460 copayment. However, if the patient utilizes a hospital participating in the PPO, the plan might pay ninety percent of the discounted fee of $1,000 (i.e., a contractually determined "allowed amount" of $900), resulting in a copayment of only $100 for the patient.

Premium Determination

Due to the financial implications of choosing one type of health insurance plan over another and because the possibility of moral hazard is a real one in health care utilization, health insurance plans are particularly vulnerable to the phenomenon of *adverse selection*. Adverse selection may be at work when an insurance policy experiences a higher number of claims due to sickness than would be probable on a random basis. If an employee is offered an alternate choice of plans, for example, a "sicker" person or a potentially higher utilizer of health care services is likely to elect the plan with more generous provisions (i.e., lower deductible, copayments, and limitations or fewer exclusions), even if the employee's share of the premium is higher. Therefore, more liberal fee-for-service plans may experience an adverse selection of sicker enrollees compared to a more restrictive managed-care plan, such as a PPO, or a health maintenance organization (HMO). This may result in ever-spiraling claims for the liberal plan as costlier people join and as healthier individuals defect to the lower-cost alternative plans.

Because of adverse selection, most health insurance plans today are *experience rated;* the premiums are based upon the demographic characteristics, such as age and sexual composition, of the employer group or upon the actual experience of the group in that plan in prior years. *Community rating,* originated by Blue Cross and Blue Shield, bases premiums upon the wider utilization of the defined geographic area (e.g., census tracts, city, county, etc.). Today, most fee-for-service plans are experience rated, even the Blues, which must contend with stiff price competition from commercial carriers. HMOs use community ratings more widely for their enrolled groups than commercial carriers, but even this is fading as HMOs face stiff price competition in the for-profit arena.

Voluntary Health Insurance

Voluntary or private health insurance in the United States can be subdivided into three distinct categories: (1) Blue Cross and Blue Shield, (2) private or commercial insurance companies, and (3) health maintenance organizations. The respective sponsorships of these types of VHI may be providers, third parties or middlemen, and patients or independent carriers. Nowadays, it is common for the Blues and commercials to own and operate HMOs and other managed care plans.

Growth and Development

The year 1929 was a landmark year for VHI. In spite of active opposition from the American Medical Association (AMA) to any type of health insurance from 1920 onward, both Blue Cross and the HMO movement got their start in this last pre-Depression year. Blue Cross was initiated by Baylor teachers in Dallas, Texas, who organized to provide hospital care for three cents a day. Michigan and New Jersey were next in the movement for hospital insurance. In 1934, the depths of the revenue depression for hospitals, the American Hospital Association (AHA) united these plans into the Blue Cross network. Today, Blue Cross has broken away from its original AHA sponsorship, but the hospital-sponsored underpinnings remain strong in many locales (Roemer, 1977; Roemer, 1978).

In Oklahoma also in 1929, the Farmer's Union started their Cooperative Health Association, the first HMO. Independently, in the same year in Los Angeles, two Canadian physicians founded the Ross-Loos group practice and sold the first doctor-sponsored health insurance plan with prepayment to the Department of Water and Power and Los Angeles City workers.

As these and other plans grew during the 1930s, the AMA reversed its opposition to VHI in response to dwindling physician and hospital incomes and, in 1939, the California Medical Society developed and sponsored a plan known as Blue Shield to pay doctor's bills in a hospitalized environment (Roemer, 1977; Roemer 1978).

By 1946, private health insurance plans were experiencing astronomical growth as wage and price restrictions in the post-World War II period spurred the growth of fringe benefits, especially in unionized industries. Insurance companies, already having the inside track in sales and actuarial information in life insurance, went headlong into the health insurance business in competition with Blue Cross and Blue Shield.

Population Coverage

About eighty-four percent of the entire U.S. population in 1998 were covered by some type of health insurance, including private health insurance and public programs. In 1998, about seventy-one percent of the U.S. population under sixty-five had some form of VHI, over ninety-two percent of whom had their health insurance linked to group health policies (usually linked to employment) (U.S. Bureau of the Census, 2000). Firms that do not offer any health benefits at all tend to be small and non-unionized, hire seasonal workers, and employ relatively large numbers of low-wage employees with no college education. About seventy-five percent of the elderly, who with few exceptions are covered by Medicare, hold private insurance coverage (known as "Medigap" insurance) to supplement their Medicare benefits.

An unfortunate effect of employment-linked private health insurance is that people who are least able to pay for health care have the least insurance due to lack of employment (or full-time employment). The alternatives for these people are to purchase a nongroup or individual plan, usually a less generous and more expensive option in terms of out-of-pocket premiums, or to accept the risk of doing without any health insurance. Estimates vary, but according to the U.S. Census Bureau, about 16.3 percent of the total U.S. population in 1998 (44 million people) had no health insurance coverage at all, either public or private (U.S. Bureau of the Census, 2000).

Benefits

Private health insurance coverage varies widely in terms of benefits provided, the extent of reimbursement for covered services, and exclusions or limitations. General health insurance plans are designed to provide limited protection for the most expensive services and usually cover inpatient hospital and physician services, and outpatient hospital services, including laboratory procedures. Limits may apply to a group of related services such as those provided during the course of a hospitalization. The most commonly covered services for the privately insured are linked to inpatient hospitalization: room and board, surgeons' and other physicians' fees, and outpatient diagnostic services.

Most comprehensive health insurance policies extend basic benefits to such services as physician office visits, outpatient mental health care, prescribed medicines, durable equipment and supplies, ambulance services, and the like. Thus, they are designed to protect against large medical bills as well as many expenses associated with routine types of medical care. For a traditional indemnity claim, the insurer typically pays a specified share of total covered expenses (e.g., eighty to ninety percent) in excess of a deductible (e.g., $200 per year for an individual), with a high maximum allowance. The beneficiary pays the deductible and coinsurance, which comprise the share of the incremental expenses not covered by the plan, subject to a limited amount known as the "out-of-pocket limit" or "stop-loss provision." A limit of this kind may range from $1,500 to $3,000. Many major medical plans limit deductibles for family members to a specified amount (typically $300 to $600 per family), or waive the deductible for the rest of the family once two or three members have met their deductibles. The deductible and other provisions apply to expenses for all covered services. In contrast, "Medigap" plans are designed to reimburse only the deductibles and coinsurance associated with Medicare-covered services.

Hospital indemnity plans are another type of private insurance coverage that are noteworthy. Hospital indemnity plans offer specified cash payments (e.g., $200 per day) for each day of inpatient hospitalization, regardless of the expenses actually incurred. Thus, they are a type of disability insurance wherein the payment is not linked to the amount or type of medical services provided, but rather to length of the hospital stay, and the payment is not generous in relation to the actual hospital expenses.

Prepaid Plans

HMOs and other similar plans provide fairly comprehensive coverage in return for a prepaid fee, usually without deductibles and coinsurance for most services, and therefore offer coverage against the risk of large health care financial losses. Prepaid health plans are the most rapidly growing segments of the private health insurance market. In 1998, there were about 643 HMOs in the United States, covering about 81 million people, or thirty percent of the population (USDHHS, 2000b). This compares to about fifty HMOs in 1973, prior to the passage of the HMO Act, which required employers with over twenty-five employees to offer a dual choice of health plans including one HMO, if one was available locally.

It was anticipated that the HMO concept would foster incentives toward prevention and cost-consciousness on the part of physicians who would be encouraged to be frugal in the use of secondary services, particularly hospitalization. However, because the prepayment of premium does not necessarily translate into capitated provider reimbursement and tight prospective budgeting, cost-containment experience is mixed due to legislative and economic incentives that are sometimes perverse (Hillman, Welch, & Pauly, 1992).

Social Health Insurance

The U.S. government sponsors two major mandatory social health insurance programs: (1) workers' compensation for the costs and pain of suffering job-related accidents, and (2) Medicare for the elderly, disabled, and other special groups. Several states sponsor social insurance programs in the areas of temporary disability (California) or health insurance (Hawaii).

Workers' Compensation

Workers' Compensation is offered in all fifty states to some extent. It is usually the first type of social insurance enacted in a nation, and the vast majority of nations worldwide have some form of industrial accident insurance. The first workers' compensation law in the United States was passed by New York State in 1914 in response to the tragic Triangle Shirt factory fire in which 146 women lost their lives. In 1950, Mississippi became the last state to enact workers' compensation. In recent years, over eighty percent of the U.S. workforce is covered to some extent by workers' compensation, leaving the remaining workers, many of whom are agricultural, casual, and domestic workers, without coverage. Unfortunately, it is often these same people who are not covered by any type of health insurance (Roemer, 1978).

Workers' compensation provides two basic benefits: (1) cash replacement of a portion of wages lost due to disability, and (2) payment for all or part of the medical care necessary. Workers' compensation may be underwritten by a private insurance company, a state government insurance fund, or a corporate contingency fund. Premiums are usually determined by experience rating.

Medicare

In 1935, national health insurance almost became a reality as part of the Social Security Act. Due to strong opposition from the AMA and conservative members of Congress, national health insurance was scrapped from the Act by President Roosevelt, who did not want to risk passage by Congress. In 1939, and every two years for several Congresses thereafter, the Wagner, Murray, Dingell National Health Insurance Bill was proposed in Congress. The timing of this bill coincided with the growth curve of private health insurance enrollment, which precluded a pressing interest in national health insurance. However, private health insurance was largely sponsored by employers and thus did not serve the nonworking population, particularly the aged. Nonetheless, about fifty percent of the elderly enrolled in voluntary health insurance programs during the 1957–64 pre-Medicare period (Roemer, 1978).

In 1957, Representative Forand of Rhode Island introduced the bill that was the precursor of Medicare (Title XVIII of the Social Security Act). On July 30, 1965, Medicare became the first entry of the federal government into the provision of social health insurance rather than medical assistance (public welfare medicine) such as offered by the Kerr-Mills Act of 1960—"Medical Assistance for the Aged."

Strictly speaking, only Medicare Part A—Hospital Insurance (HI)—is social health insurance (see Figure 5.4). Part B—Supplementary Medical Insurance (SMI)—is neither compulsory nor funded by a trust fund. More than three-quarters of the funds for SMI come from the general treasury; the other quarter percent comes from Medicare Part A recipients who elect that Part B premiums be deducted from their monthly Social Security check (USDHHS, 2000a).

Medicare utilizes an *indirect pattern* of finance and delivery, wherein the Health Care Financing Administration (HCFA), recently renamed the Centers for Medicare and Medicaid Services (CMS), a branch of the U.S. Department of Health and Human Services, contracts with independent providers. Medicare recipients also access providers independently. HCFA sees to it that the provider is paid, but the providers are neither owned nor hired by the government, as in SHI systems utilizing the *direct pattern* of delivery. Generally speaking, if the private medical market is strong at the time when SHI is enacted, an indirect pattern of delivery emerges. If the market is weak, a direct financing route emerges.

Welfare Medicine

Public assistance, or *welfare medicine,* is sponsored by a plethora of federal, state, and local government programs, but the most far-reaching program is Medicaid (Title XIX of the Social Security Act). Administered at the federal level by HCFA, Medicaid is financed by an average federal contribution from the general treasury of fifty-seven percent and from state treasuries at an average contribution of forty-three percent (see Figure 5.4). Federal matching varies from fifty to seventy-five percent, depending on the income of the individual state (USDHHS, 1998; USDHHS, 2000a). General treasury funds are generated from personal income tax, corporate income tax, and various excise taxes and, to the extent that these taxes are borne by higher income individuals and organizations, Medicaid represents a type of transfer payment to the poor.

The distinction between welfare medicine and social health insurance, both of which are public programs, is an important one and rests on the philosophical difference between a transfer payment and entitlement. Medicaid is a *transfer payment* "in kind," meaning that medical services are provided as a

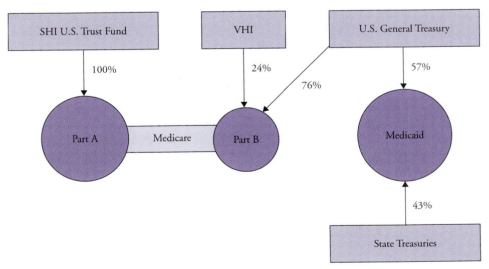

Figure 5.4. Flow of Federal and State Financing for Medicare and Medicaid, 1999 (Each circle reflects the relative size of the program)

welfare benefit in lieu of cash. Welfare recipients also receive cash subsidies to pay for their living expenses, but medical benefits are paid directly to the provider so that the recipients will not be tempted to spend the money on expense items other than health care. (Food stamps are another "in kind" benefit, providing vouchers solely for the purpose of purchasing food and groceries.) Thus, the transfer payment is a type of "relief" that government bestows upon the poor; it is a form of charity.

Social health insurance is an *entitlement program*, not charity. It is a right earned by individuals in the course of their employment. The funds for SHI programs are contributed by a payroll tax (for 2001, 2.9 percent of total wages—a stable percentage for many years), which, in the case of Social Security, is divided equally between the worker and the employer. In addition, Worker's Compensation is financed, at least in part, by worker contributions. When the worker retires or suffers a temporary or sustaining injury related to employment, SHI becomes active for the worker and dependents. The fundamental aim of a compulsory, government-provided or supervised SHI program is social adequacy: to provide members of society with protection against hazards so widespread as to be considered risks that individuals cannot afford to deal with themselves. Eligibility in SHI is derived from contributions having been made to the program, and benefits are a statutory right not based on need. Recipients are thus entitled to the benefits of SHI. About half the countries in the world have a SHI system for financing health care (Roemer, 1978).

In reference to Figure 5.4, it is interesting to note that the federal share of funding (coming from the U.S. General Treasury) for Medicare Part B has diminished in recent years.

MEDICARE

Medicare, the principal SHI program in the United States, provides a variety of hospital, physician, and other medical services for (1) persons sixty-five and over, (2) disabled individuals who are entitled to Social Security benefits, and (3) end-stage renal disease victims. In 1999, Medicare financed $206 billion in health services, comprising fifty-two percent of all

publicly financed health expenditures and 19.5 percent of PHCE. Medicare reimbursed thirty-one percent of all hospital expenditures, and twenty percent of all physician expenditures in 1999 (HCFA, 2001).

Hospital Insurance

Ninety-nine percent of the aged population of the United States is enrolled in Part A of Medicare, Hospital Insurance (HI). Part A finances four basic benefits for the covered population:

1. Ninety days of inpatient care in a "benefit period" (a spell of illness beginning with hospitalization and ending when a beneficiary has not been an inpatient in a hospital or skilled nursing facility for sixty continuous days). There is no limit to the number of benefit periods a beneficiary can use.
2. A lifetime reserve of sixty days of inpatient care, once the ninety days are exhausted
3. One hundred days of post-hospitalization care in a skilled nursing facility
4. Home health agency visits

Since the inception of the Medicare program, hospital insurance has required the beneficiary to participate in cost sharing. The patient is required to pay an inpatient hospital deductible in each benefit period, which approximates the cost of one day of hospital care ($792 in 2001). Coinsurance based on the inpatient hospital deductible is required for the sixty-first to the ninetieth day of inpatient hospitalization and is always equal to one-fourth of the deductible ($198 in 2001). For the twenty-first to 100th day of skilled nursing facility (SNF) care, the coinsurance equals one-eighth of the deductible ($99), and for the sixty lifetime reserve days, the patient pays one-half of the deductible ($396) for each day of inpatient hospitalization. As previously mentioned, about seventy-five percent of Medicare enrollees have private "Medigap" policies, which primarily cover some or all of the deductibles and coinsurance under Medicare. About six million of the aged and disabled have both Medicare and Medicaid coverage in combination (a group known as "crossovers" or "Medi-Medi"), and Medicaid usually assumes responsibility for the cost-sharing arrangements under Medicare (USDHHS, 2001).

While hospital expenditures have grown at a rapid rate since the inception of Medicare in 1966, skilled nursing facility, home health agency, and outpatient benefits have all shifted significantly as a percent of total Medicare benefit payments. Skilled nursing facility payments have dropped from 6.5 percent of payments in 1967 to 4.7 percent in 1999. Once the fastest growing component of Medicare—home health agency payments—fell to 7.0 percent from 8.4 percent of Medicare outlays in 1995. Outpatient outlays fell from 8.2 to 7.1 percent during the same period of time (USDHHS, 1996; USDHHS, 2000a; HCFA, 2001).

Catastrophic Coverage

In 1988, amendments to Medicare were enacted to shield Medicare beneficiaries from catastrophic hospital and doctors' bills related to acute illnesses. While the bill provided no new benefits for long-term care, it did provide for the first broad coverage of outpatient prescription drugs. Due to pressure from organized groups of elderly who objected to the additional income taxes and substantial premium increases targeted at them, Congress repealed the bill in 1989. Only a few minor provisions in the amendment were subsequently incorporated into the regular Medicare benefit structure.

Supplementary Medical Insurance

Ninety-five percent of Part A beneficiaries are enrolled in Part B—Supplementary Medical Insurance (SMI). SMI was designed to complement the HI program. It provides payments for physicians, physician-ordered supplies and services, outpatient hospital services, rural health clinic visits, and home health visits for persons without Part A. SMI requires the beneficiary to meet a deductible (currently $100) each year, in addition to paying a monthly premium ($50.00 in 2001). Under "buy-in" agreements, most state Medicaid programs pay the premiums for Medicaid enrollees who qualify to participate in SMI (USDHHS, 2000a).

Among items not covered by any part of traditional fee-for-service Medicare are prescription drugs on an outpatient basis, dental care, routine eye examinations and eyeglasses, preventive services, and long-term care services. However, hospice benefits became available for persons who are terminally ill in 1983. Enrollees in Medicare can elect the hospice benefit for two 90-day periods and one 30-day period, with a subsequent extension period during the individual's lifetime.

From 1967 to 1999, Part B of Medicare grew faster than Part A. Therefore, although Part B represented only thirty-eight percent of Medicare expenditures in 1999, Part B has increased as a proportion of Medicare expenditures since 1967, whereas Part A (focusing on hospitals) has shrunk commensurately (USDHHS, 1995; USDHHS, 1998; USDHHS, 2000a).

Provider Reimbursement

Hospitals

Until 1983, Medicare operated primarily on a fee-for-service basis for physicians' and related services, and on a cost-based retrospective basis for hospital services. Hospitals were reimbursed for any reasonable costs incurred in the provision of covered care to Medicare patients. Commencing in 1983, payment rates were prospectively determined on a per-case basis. The Medicare hospital Prospective Payment System (PPS), discussed in detail further on in this chapter, uses diagnosis-related groups (DRGs) to classify cases for payment. Except for four major classes of specialty hospitals (children's, psychiatric, rehabilitation, and long-term), all hospitals must participate in PPS to qualify for Medicare reimbursement, billing Medicare directly.

Physicians

To constrain SMI inflation, the Deficit Reduction Act of 1984 introduced the concept of "participating physicians," who are those who "accept assignments" for all services (i.e., claims) for all Medicare patients in that doctor's practice, with no exceptions. Several pecuniary and marketing incentives to participate were introduced and resulted in substantial increases in assignment. Nationally, the rate of participating physicians increased from fifty-one percent in 1983 to eighty-three percent in 1998, amounting to 96.5 percent of all Medicare Part B claims. A non-participating physician can continue to treat Medicare patients, accepting assignments or not on a claim-by-claim basis, but Medicare will reimburse only ninety-five percent of the amount given to participating physicians (USDHHS, 1995; USDHHS, 1998).

Under Medicare Part B, physicians may elect one of two reimbursement strategies. The first is to accept the Medicare Fee Schedule (MFS) as payment in full (i.e., participating physicians accepting the assignment), billing Medicare directly, and receiving eighty percent payment from the Medicare intermediary. The beneficiaries are liable for the remaining twenty percent coinsurance, also according to the MFS. On unassigned claims, the beneficiary is additionally liable for the difference between the physician's charge and the Medicare allowed charge.

Intermediaries or fiscal agents, such as Blue Cross or a commercial insurance company, which are contracted by the Medicare program to review and pay the bills, process claims. Enrollees can also join HMOs, and similar forms of prepaid health care and special reimbursement provisions apply to these organizations. The Tax Equity and Fiscal Responsibility Act of 1982 (TEFRA) included major revisions to the Medicare law to encourage growth in the number of HMOs and other comprehensive medical plans enrolling Medicare beneficiaries. By 1999, 393 prepaid plans, with 6.9 million members (nineteen percent of Medicare enrollees) held contracts with Medicare (USDHHS, 2000a). TEFRA also set limits on Medicare reimbursements for hospital costs at the per-case level—the harbinger of DRGs under PPS.

Utilization

The average Medicare enrollee spent over $5,772 in 1999. As in any insurance program, however, utilization is uneven. A study of 1992 data showed that one-third of the enrolled population had small claims of $500 or less, while another twenty-two percent had no claims at all. The highest 9.8 percent of users had reimbursements of $10,000 or more, and these enrollees consumed 68.4 percent of program payments (USDHHS, 1995). Other studies have demonstrated that high Medicare reimbursements are related to terminal illness. A seminal study by Lubitz and Prihoda (1984) found that reimbursements for decedents averaged $4,527 for the last year of life—620 percent of the average of $729 for a comparison group who survived the period under study. Fuchs (1984) showed that the greatest proportion of medical care costs is incurred in the year prior to death, regardless of the age of natural death. For Medicare enrollees, the average reimbursement for those in their last year of life was 6.6 times as large as for those who survived at least two years. Thus, one may surmise that the principal reason why health expenditures rise with age is that the proportion of persons near death increases with age. Other studies have found a great deal of consistency over time in the utilization of health expenditures by the highest users, with the top one percent accounting for twenty or more percent of health care dollars (Gornick, Greenberg, and Eggers, 1985).

MEDICAID

Program Structure

Medicaid was enacted into law on July 30, 1965, as Title XIX of the Social Security Act, and became part of the existing federal-state welfare structure to assist the poor. Until 1956, there had been no federal participation in health care for the poor. This public obligation was delegated to the states as part of their *police powers*. Prior to Medicaid, many doctors donated their services or used a sliding scale of fees in treating the poor and, as a rule, hospitals admitted charity cases. However, under the purview of the states, health care for the poor varied widely from state to state and manifested all the forms of discrimination tolerated in each locale. The Kerr-Mills Act of 1960—Medical Assistance for the Aged—was the forerunner of the Medicaid model and was later subsumed under Title XIX.

Eligibility

Supported by federal grants and administered by the states, Medicaid is limited to specific groups of low-income individuals and families. Medicaid is welfare medicine and thus has no strict entitlement features (although lately the word "entitlement" has been used indiscriminately, particularly by politicians and the media, in reference to Medicaid and other welfare programs). Recipients must prove their eligibility for Medicaid according to their income and, prior to 1976, states were even permitted to put a lien on a recipient's home or other personal property.

The program was designed to cover those groups who are eligible to receive cash payments under one of the two existing welfare programs established under Social Security: Aid to Families with Dependent Children (AFDC)—now known as TANF, Temporary

Assistance to Needy Families, and Supplemental Security Income (SSI). In most instances, receipt of a welfare payment under one of these programs means automatic eligibility for Medicaid. The mandatory eligibility groups covered by Medicaid include (1) families with children who receive AFDC, (2) pregnant and postpartum women with children under six years of age, whose incomes do not exceed 133 percent of the Federal Poverty Level (FPL), (3) aged, blind, and disabled individuals who receive SSI, and (4) certain other specifically defined groups.

Figure 5.5 compares the distribution of Medicaid recipients to that of expenditures by eligibility category. Needy families—adults and children—were the

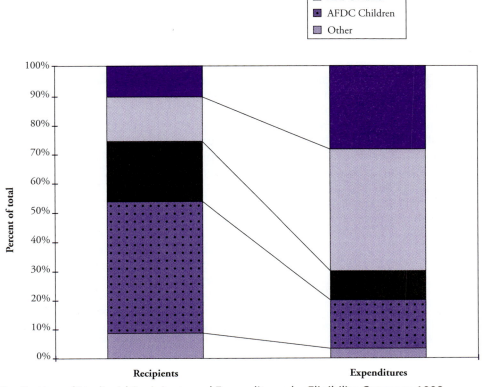

Figure 5.5. Distribution of Medicaid Recipients and Expenditures by Eligibility Category, 1998

SOURCE: U.S. Department of Health and Human Services (1998), Health Care Financing Administration, Office of Strategic Planning. 1998 data compendium. Baltimore.

largest group of recipients (66.2 percent) in 1998, but accounted for a relatively small part of the Medicaid budget (26.4 percent), which is a reflection of the relatively good health of most Medicaid children. Due largely to the high utilization of nursing home services, 28.5 percent of total Medicaid outlays was attributable to the aged, who comprise only 9.8 percent of the Medicaid population. Outlays for the blind and disabled totaled 42.4 percent of Medicaid expenditures, a disproportionately large amount as compared to the number of recipients (16.3 percent) (USDHHS, 1998). These facts serve to dispel the conventional wisdom that families on welfare incur the lion's share of Medicaid expense. The impoverished aged and the disabled (which includes the mentally retarded) have no alternative but to expend large per capita amounts in the Medicaid program.

States may choose to provide Medicaid to certain "optional eligibility" groups. Most of these optional groups share characteristics of the mandatory groups (parents and children, aged, blind, and disabled), but the income eligibility ceilings are higher (e.g., 1.33 to 1.85 times the federal poverty level of $13,003 for a family of three in 1998). "Medically needy" persons comprise another optional group—those who "spend down" their income and wealth, due to medical bills, to the medically needy standard. Under federal guidelines, states set income and asset levels for cash assistance and medical eligibility. Because there is considerable variation in the coverage of optional groups by the states and in income standards across Medicaid jurisdictions, the degree to which programs cover the poverty population varies considerably.

Benefits Provided

Services

Title XIX of the Social Security Act mandates that every state Medicaid program provide specific basic health services:

- hospital inpatient care
- hospital outpatient services
- certified nurse practitioner services
- laboratory and X-ray services
- nursing facility services for those aged twenty-one and older
- home health services for those eligible for nursing services
- physicians' services
- family planning services and supplies
- rural health clinic services
- early and periodic screening, diagnosis, and treatment for children under twenty-one years of age
- nurse midwife services
- certain federally qualified health center services
- medical and surgical services furnished by a dentist

States may determine the scope of services offered (e.g., limit the days of hospital care or the number of physician visits covered) and provide a number of other elective services. The most commonly covered optional services include the following:

- clinic services
- nursing services in a care facility for the aged and disabled
- intermediate care facility services for the mentally retarded
- inpatient psychiatric services
- optometrist services and eyeglasses
- prescribed drugs
- prosthetic devices
- dental care

Administration

Medicaid operates primarily as a vendor payment program. Payments are made directly to providers of service for care rendered to eligible individuals. With certain exceptions, a state must allow Medicaid recipients freedom of choice among participating providers of health care. Managed care plans, which are foremost among the exceptions, usually hold the ability to restrict freedom of choice to contracted providers.

Methods for reimbursing physicians and hospitals vary widely among the states, but providers must accept the Medicaid reimbursement level as payment in full. Payment rates must be sufficient to enlist enough providers so that comparable care and services are available to the Medicaid population as are available to the general population in the area. Notwithstanding, Medicaid physician reimbursement rates are usually less generous than those of Medicare.

In long-term care facilities, individuals are required to turn over income in excess of their personal needs and maintenance needs of their spouses (the monetary level being determined by the state) to help pay for their care. States may require cost-sharing by Medicaid recipients, but they may not require the mandatory amount eligible to share costs for mandatory services. As noted previously, most state Medicaid programs have buy-in agreements with Medicare in which Medicaid assumes the responsibility for the Medicare cost-sharing for persons covered under both programs. (Gornick, Greenberg, & Eggers, 1985; Waldo, 1990).

States participate in the Medicaid program at their option. All states except Arizona (which has a demonstration project of capitated health delivery that excludes long-term care services) currently have Medicaid programs. The District of Columbia, Puerto Rico, Guam, the Northern Marianas, and the Virgin Islands also provide Medicaid coverage.

The states administer their Medicaid programs within broad federal requirements and guidelines. These requirements allow states considerable discretion in determining not only eligibility, but covered benefits and provider payment mechanisms. Some states also include in the Medicaid program persons known as "state-only" enrollees, who do not meet federal requirements and hence do not qualify for federal matching funds. As a result of state options and policy decisions, the characteristics of Medicaid programs vary considerably from state to state. Medicaid expenditures also vary widely across the states, and states' benefit mix offerings change frequently.

Growth of Medicaid

From 1980 to 1999, growth in Medicaid expenditures (705 percent) exceeded that of Medicare, which grew by 567 percent over the same period. A disproportionately large share of this growth took place in the 1990 to 1995 period. During this time, Medicaid re-

cipients, as a percent of the total civilian population, rose from 10.2 percent to 13.8 percent, an increase of thirty-five percent, which was principally attributable to an expansion of those covered in the mandatory eligible groups and to the economic ravages of the early-1990s recession.

Providers

Hospital care (inpatient and outpatient) accounted for a much smaller proportion of 1998 Medicaid expenditures (19.4 percent) than Medicare hospital outlays (48 percent in 1998). Nursing home care, including skilled nursing, intermediate care, and intermediate care facilities for the mentally retarded (ICF/MR), commanded 29.4 percent of Medicaid budget for 1998 (USDHHS, 2000a).

Medicaid continues to be the largest payer of long-term care services, financing forty-seven percent of nursing home care in 1999. Although growth in spending for nursing facility care has slowed considerably in recent years, since the early 1970s, Medicaid has funded at least eighty percent of all public spending for nursing home care. Compared with other services that Medicaid provides, Medicaid payments for long-term care are also the most costly per user. HCFA statistics from 1999 showed that the average Medicaid payment for nursing facility services was $18,588, and for Institutions for the Mentally Retarded (i.e., ICF/MR), the payment averaged a whopping $68,250. In 1998, however, the highest growth rates were home services, prescription drugs, and other care (USDHHS, 1998).

State Spending

Since 1975, Medicaid has been the fastest growing component of aggregate state spending. In 1999, Medicaid spent $174.2 billion of combined federal and state funds for vendor payments for personal health care. Program spending for Medicaid recipients decelerated in the 1990s. Spending grew by 286 percent for the entire decade of the 1980s, whereas from 1990 to 1999, Medicaid spending grew by 250 percent. Nevertheless, Medicaid's share of personal health care expenditures grew from 11.3 percent in 1989 to 16.5 percent in

1999 (Levit et al., 2000; USDHHS, 1995; USDHHS, 2000a).

In order to curtail Medicaid growth, cost containment initiatives began in the early 1980s. During this time, important experiments were launched in prepaid managed health care, utilization review, case management, reimbursement via diagnosis-related group (DRGs), and new services for the elderly, disabled, and persons with AIDS. In 1990, Congress enacted careful and selective expansion of Medicaid coverage, particularly for low-income (and pregnant) women and children. Currently, the focus is on shifting Medicaid funding from the federal coffers to state budgets and encouraging states to model their systems using principles of managed care.

PHYSICIAN REIMBURSEMENT

Paying the doctor traditionally calls upon one of three reimbursement mechanisms: fee for service, prepayment, or salary. Health insurance plans, either public or private, may utilize any or all of the three reimbursement types. According to Reinhardt (1985), there is no optimal system for paying the doctor.

Fee for Service

Fee for service (FFS) is widely used throughout the world for paying the doctor and is typically the physician's preferred mode of payment. In FFS, the unit of remuneration is the medical act, either a service or a procedure. In the days before health insurance for physician reimbursement was widespread, most physicians had a sliding fee scale wherein the poor paid lower fees than wealthier patients. With the advent of health insurance in both the public and private sectors, physician payment became more regulated and physicians adopted one schedule of charges used for all payers, whether they were individuals or third parties. By the 1980s, however, fees schedules began to vary widely by the type of health plan or insurance organization, public or private.

One advantage of fee-for-service reimbursement is that remuneration adjusts automatically for case complexity, linking the providers' reward closely to the output of services. The billing system, in turn, provides a great deal of "transparency" of the physician's profile of practice. The ease with which patients may change physicians in a traditional fee-for-service system enables them to directly exercise considerable economic clout over practitioners (Reinhardt, 1985).

Indemnity

Insurance policies that reimburse on a fee-for-service basis offer payment either by indemnity or service benefits or by fixed fees. *Indemnity payment* stipulates a certain dollar value per procedure, usually according to a "Table of Allowances." These allowances may vary widely among insurance plans. In traditional indemnity, the provider can charge anything above the stipulated allowed amount and collect the remainder directly from the patient. Often, the Table of Allowances is based upon a "Relative Value Scale," in which each procedure is rated according to a point system—relative value units (RVUs)—which reflects the relative technical difficulty and time cost of the procedure, and each point is worth so many dollars. The dollar amount per RVU may also vary widely among insurance plans. This type of system is easy to administer and update for inflation and changing practice patterns, but no provision is made by the insurer to protect the patient from outlandish charges.

Service Benefits

Service benefits pay a percentage per procedure, usually eighty percent of "usual, customary, and reasonable" (UCR) fees. In this scheme, the UCR fee schedule protects the carrier from unlimited liability in the wake of high charges and also may give the patient information about reasonable fee norms. UCR means that the fee is "usual" in that doctor's practice, "customary" in that community, and "reasonable" in terms of the distribution of all physician charges for that service in the community. The latter is commonly expressed as a percentile (e.g., the policy will pay up to the seventy-fifth percentile). Up until 1992, Medicare Part B used a similar standard of "customary, prevailing, and reasonable fees."

Hybrid Fee-Based Systems

Hybrid systems came into vogue with the advent of PPOs, combining features of both indemnity and service reimbursement for cost containment. In a hybrid system, the intermediary contracts with the participating physician (or hospital) to accept a discounted version of the UCR table of allowances. The plan considers these "allowed amounts" to be the maximum covered expenses. For a participating provider, the PPO will typically pay ninety percent of the allowed amount for most procedures, with the remaining ten percent paid by the patient as coinsurance. This arrangement protects both the intermediary by effectively capping the reimbursement (as in an indemnity payment) and the patient by limiting the liability for the difference beyond ten percent of the allowed amount.

Fixed Fees

In some reimbursement plans, physicians can only charge, and will only be paid, according to fixed fees, usually with little cost sharing (e.g., $5.00 to $10.00 per physician office visit) or none at all on the part of the patient. If the provider accepts the plan, then the fee schedule must be accepted. This arrangement exists in Medicaid; many private plans also stipulate fixed fees in order to protect the patient and to contain costs. Many HMO plans also mandate fixed fees, especially for specialists contracted with the health plan.

Prepayment

In prepayment or capitation, the person served, rather than the medical act, is the unit of remuneration. The capitation payment takes care of reimbursement for a stipulated length of time, usually a year. Using capitation as a reimbursement methodology, HMOs have encouraged physicians to form networks linked to hospitals and have spurred the popularity of Independent Practice Associations (IPAs), in which the participating physicians actually sponsor and administer the HMO. Advantages to prepayment are that it is administratively simple, it facilitates advance

global budgeting, and it gives physicians incentive to control the cost of medical treatments. If patients are allowed to switch primary care physicians from time to time, they still retain some economic clout over physicians (Reinhardt, 1985).

Salary

Salary is payment to the doctor for time consumption, irrespective of the units of service or the number of patients. On a large scale, salaried practice almost always takes place in a highly organized network like the National Health Service in Great Britain. On a smaller scale in the United States, urban public hospitals, which serve indigent populations, often have large attending staffs that are salaried. Countries in which salaried practices are common rarely include specialists in this payment mechanism. Instead, general practitioners or primary care providers have a "panel" of patients in the community. Advantages to salaried reimbursement for physicians are that it is administratively simple, the medical treatments selected are not influenced by relative profitability, and it encourages cooperation among physicians. Furthermore, salaries facilitate budgeting for health expenditures *ex ante* (Reinhardt, 1985).

Monitoring

All payment mechanisms have faults and each must be monitored for abuses. In FFS, the incentives are for overwork by the physician and overutilization by the patients. FFS fosters unnecessary or duplicative service to the point where the high volume of services may actually affect the quality of care adversely. Unfortunately, in the United States, malpractice suits have encouraged defensive medicine, wherein overutilization and extra fees are simply passed on to the consumer in higher insurance rates. Also, if fees for all procedures do not stand in constant proportion to costs incurred, the choice of treatment may favor more profitable procedures. For these and other reasons that foster inflation, fee-for-service reimbursement is very difficult to budget in advance.

In prepayment, however, underutilization must be monitored because the incentives are to decrease costs and services provided vis-à-vis the capitation payment. In many prepayment schemes, any cost savings realized are distributed to the participating physicians, which may be an inducement to cut costs too much. In HMOs where only the primary care physicians are capitated, there also exists the incentive to excessively refer patients to specialists. Likewise, capitation gives physicians incentives for "dumping" patients with complex, costly conditions onto other providers. Finally, the administrative system for prepayment yields little insight as to the transparency physician's practice profile. Of late, many HMOs mandate that physicians submit monthly *encounter data* on patient visits and/or procedures delivered as a condition of participation in the health plan.

In salaried practice, incentives favor underwork or seeing too few patients. Doctors literally get paid by the hour, resulting in no inducement toward higher volume. According to Reinhardt (1985), unless the salary is linked to output and patient satisfaction, patients lose economic clout over the physician, who, in turn, may render care as an act of *noblesse oblige*. Like capitation, salaried practice gives little transparency as to the physician's practice profile.

INITIATIVES IN HEALTH CARE FINANCE

Factors in Health Care Inflation

The implementation of Medicare and Medicaid in 1966 heralded a twenty-five-year era of unprecedented health care cost inflation. Aaron (1993/94) attributes the continually rising costs of health care to three main factors:

1. Technology has transformed medical care, giving rise to new diagnostic techniques and new methods of treatment.
2. Consumers are demanding low-benefit care.
3. Budget limits on hospitals and fee controls on physicians are lacking.

He also notes that high administrative costs, compensation for medical malpractice, and bad health habits

of the populace are not important factors in the rising costs of care.

Cost Containment Measures

In the 1970s, the federal government experimented with a number of programs and reimbursement methods to contain health care costs. Major programs included (1) the establishment of reasonable cost limits for hospitals; (2) the initiation of state and local networks of health planning agencies along with the "certificate-of-need" procedure for augmenting capital plant and equipment; (3) the establishment of the Professional Standards Review Organization (PSRO) program to review care and to eliminate unnecessary hospital days for federally funded patients; and (4) the encouragement of the growth of HMOs to promote the use of preventive services and to decrease the utilization of hospital inpatient care. It can be safely said that the programs of the 1970s were unsuccessful in containing health care costs.

Early in the 1980s, during the Reagan Administration, legislative efforts to change the monetary incentive system in health care began in earnest. While the 1980s and 1990s have witnessed considerable flux in healthcare financing, along with inducements to reduce overutilization, cost containment efforts have shown mixed results (Rice, 1992). Furthermore, they have held painful consequences for many groups of people. The balance between reasonable costs and equitable access has not yet been struck, but what is clear is that the traditional health-care market has no apparatus to reflect social or economic rationing decisions regarding the provision of health care that might help to stem inflation. Managed care, particularly capitated prepaid care, holds better incentives for efficiency, productivity, and management coordination. Yet, even with more closely managed utilization, better quality management, and the continual expansion of government programs, universal access to health services remains elusive.

Pro-Competition

Early in the 1980s, Enthoven (1981) and other health economists exposited strategies of *pro-competition*, which were meant to restrain health care costs by creating competitive market conditions via direct incentives both for consumers and for employers who purchase group health insurance policies. Among these strategies were the imposition of a "tax cap" on employer income tax deductions for health insurance expenses, raising the threshold for individual income tax deductions, and offering multiple choices by employers in health insurance plans. While the threshold for personal income tax deductions for medical out-of-pocket expense was raised to 7.5 percent of gross income, the other strategies, while not formally enacted, had a profound effect on the thinking of health policymakers. The programs of the 1980s reflect this conservative philosophy and, in most cases, the scorecards for their success are mixed, at best.

TEFRA

The Tax Equity and Fiscal Responsibility Act (TEFRA), signed into law on September 30, 1982 and enacted the next day, set limits on Medicare reimbursements on a per-case basis for hospital costs and also placed a limit on the annual rate of increase for Medicare's reasonable costs per discharge. TEFRA was expected to reduce Medicare reimbursement by 4.5 percent in real dollars over the ensuing three years, during which time reimbursement increases, based on projected inflation rates, would be in effect. Due to the fast enactment of the Prospective Payment System one year later, it was difficult to evaluate the impact of the Act. However, TEFRA was the harbinger of prospective payment and a number of features of the latter program were borrowed from it. These features were part of the *Section 223 limits* on hospital costs. They included (1) grouping hospitals by bed size and size of locale, (2) wage adjustments by locality, and (3) an adjustment for case-mix index (Deloitte, Haskins, & Sells, 1982). Today, most hospitals which are excluded from the Medicare Prospective Payment System are reimbursed according to TEFRA regulations.

The Section 223 limits were calculated according to a complicated formula whereby the labor-related component for the hospital region, adjusted by a geographic wage index, was added to a regional non-labor component. The product was then multiplied by a case-mix index, specific to each hospital. These figures were all specified by HCFA and published in the *Federal Register*. The formula used to calculate the Section 223 limits was substantially retained for figuring reimbursement rates for the Prospective Payment System.

HCFA developed institutional-specific case-mix indices based on a diagnosis-related group (DRG) system designed at Yale University. The DRG classification system sorts patients into uniform, clinically compatible groups that have been categorized on the basis of traditional resource use by patients with similar diagnoses. The original Yale DRGs were modified to reflect variation solely in Medicare cases. For each hospital, HCFA used a twenty percent sample of the Medicare billing forms submitted for calendar year 1980. Using the 10,167 ICD-9-CM diagnosis codes from these claims and each hospital's Medicare cost report, HCFA developed the case-mix index. In essence, this case-mix index was intended to compare a particular hospital's case mix with that of all other hospitals in the nation. Table 5.2 shows how five hypothetical hospitals with five DRGs, each varying in volume by hospital, can calculate their case-mix indices, which reflect the relative severity of each hospital's caseload. Hospital D, with 62.5 percent of their cases in the high-weighted DRG 3, claims the highest case-mix index of 1.6031. This contrasts with Hospital A, which, with almost seventy percent of their cases in the low paying DRGs 2 and 4, holds a case-mix index of 0.8900. Extending this calculation to all cases in all hospitals participating in PPS, the national average case-mix index always equals 1.0000. The dollar amount ascribed to a DRG of 1.0000 is recalculated on a yearly basis.

Target Rates

Another ceiling established by HCFA, concurrent with the Section 223 limits, was the *target rate ceiling*. This target rate limited the allowable amount of growth in Medicare reimbursable inpatient operating costs limits. In essence, TEFRA reimbursement gave bonuses to hospitals whose inpatient operating costs per discharge were less than the target rate ceiling, providing that the target rate was below the Section 223 limit. Today, while the Section 223 limits

Table 5.2. Calculation of Medicare Case-Mix Index[a]

Hospital	DRG 1	DRG 2	DRG 3	DRG 4	DRG 5	Total (Percent)	DRG Weighted Expected Cost Per Case ($)[b]	Case-Mix Index[c]
A	2.5	27.3	10.5	41.5	18.2	100	1,660.40	0.8900
B	21.0	.9	30.1	2.0	46.0	100	2,401.30	1.2872
C	40.6	5.0	2.3	47.2	4.9	100	1,346.30	0.7227
D	5.1	18.4	62.5	10.0	4.0	100	2,990.70	1.6031
E	30.4	65.0	1.0	1.6	2.0	100	929.00	0.4980
Average Proportion for all hospitals	19.92	23.32	21.28	20.46	15.02	100	1,865.54	—
DRG cost weight	$1000	$ 800	$4100	$1500	$2000	—	—	—

[a] Adjusted to make these 5 DRGs hypothetically represent all 356 Medicare DRGs
[b] For hospital A, calculated as follows:
$0.025(1,000) + 0.273(800) + 0.105(4,100) + 0.415(1,500) + 0.182(2,000) = \$1660.40$
[c] For hospital A, calculated as $1,660.40 divided by $1,865.54 = 0.8900

SOURCE: *Tax Equity and Fiscal Responsibility Act of 1982: Management Strategies for Health Care Providers,* Deloitte, Haskins & Sells, 1982, New York: Author.

have been abandoned, the target rates have been retained for Medicare reimbursement for hospital categories exempt from PPS.

The Prospective Payment System

The Prospective Payment System (PPS) was enacted on October 1, 1983, two years ahead of schedule. The Social Security Amendments of 1983 initiated the new system and contained provisions to base payment for hospital inpatient services on predetermined rates per DRG. In 1998, out of a total of 6,190 hospitals in the United States, eighty-one percent participate in PPS. Of the remaining 1,158 hospitals in the United States, ninety-four percent still participate in Medicare under different reimbursement arrangements. (USDHHS, 1998). These "categorically exempt" hospitals are psychiatric facilities, rehabilitation hospitals, children's hospitals, long-term care hospitals, and other special medical facilities that have an approved waiver. Except for childrens' hospitals, which are still reimbursed according to costs, these facilities remain on TEFRA regulations.

PPS represents a major departure from the preceding reimbursement system—cost-based reimbursement—

in that payment bears no direct relationship to length of stay, services rendered, or costs of care. For a given discharge, a hospital with actual costs below the designated PPS rate for a given DRG is permitted to keep the difference in payment. If discharge costs exceed the payment level, the hospital is required to absorb the loss. Certain costs, such as capital depreciation and direct medical education costs, are exempt from PPS provisions and have their own payment formulas. Payment for hospital-based physician services (e.g., radiology, anesthesiology, pathology, etc.) that, previous to enactment of PPS were reimbursed on the basis of reasonable costs under Medicare Part A, are included in the hospital's PPS rate. As a result, many such physicians have defected to Part B of Medicare, billing patients directly for their services.

Standardized Payment Amount

PPS pays a standardized amount for each DRG. Standardized amounts are updated each year by HCFA according to the region of the country (e.g., New England, Middle Atlantic, etc.) and by urbanization of the area (large urban or other areas). This amount is further divided into two components: a labor-related amount and a nonlabor-related amount. To compute the payment amount for a DRG of 1.0000, the labor-related amount is multiplied by a wage index, specific to each locality, and the product is added to the nonlabor-related amount. For the 2001 fiscal year, for example, a hospital in San Diego is subject to a large urban labor-related amount of $2,864.19, times a wage index of 1.1955, plus a nonlabor-related amount of $1,164.21. Thus, the DRG payment for a hospital in San Diego is $4,588.35. This "final" figure is adjusted upward by an area-specific capital factor and other hospital-specific adjustments for indirect medical education and disproportionate share of low-income patients.

DRG Weights

The DRG weight classifications originally used in TEFRA were updated for use in PPS using a stratified sample of 400,000 medical records drawn from patient discharges in 332 hospitals during the last half of 1979. To date, over 500 DRGs have been developed, expanding on the original 468 principal diagnoses. A contracted fiscal intermediary, such as Blue Cross or a commercial insurer, assigns a DRG from a bill submitted by the hospital for each case. Using classifications and terminology consistent with the ICD-9-CM and the Uniform Hospital Discharge Data Set (USDHHS, 1995), the intermediary assigns the DRG using the Grouper Program (an automated classification algorithm), which compares information contained in the bill, with appropriate DRG criteria. Criteria include the patient's age, sex, principal and secondary diagnoses, procedures performed, and discharge status (American Medical Association, 1984). (Figure 5.6 presents a schematic diagram of the Grouper Program.) For all but a few DRGs that require clarification by the hospital before the payment amount is determined, the intermediary determines the payment amount and pays the hospital.

Outliers

Bills for "outliers," which result in extra payment for the hospital above the standard DRG rate, re-

quire special consideration. In the 2000 fiscal year (FY), 6.3 percent of the pool of total DRG payments was reserved for outliers. The hospital must identify cost outliers and request payment. (It is important to note that the classification of DRGs depends largely on the principal diagnosis, which may not be the diagnosis consuming the most resources, thus making the discharge an outlier.)

For a discharge to be considered as an outlier, the rules are very stringent. For FY 2001, HCFA set the outlier threshold to equal the prospective payment rate for the DRG (including adjustments for indirect medical education and "disproportionate share" hospitals) plus $17,550 (Deloitte & Touche, 2001).

Quality Indicators

A clear incentive in the PPS system is for hospitals to expand services still qualifying for cost-based Medicare reimbursement. Opportunities for marketing expansion include specific ambulatory programs, satellite clinics, health-related services such as family planning, chemical dependency treatment, and laboratory or other ancillary services used by physicians. Hospital-sponsored skilled nursing, rehabilitation, home health services, and other services that may facilitate earlier discharge of patients and provide additional sources of revenue for hospitals have experienced marked growth since the inception of PPS. Many of these programs may be accomplished by conversion of acute care beds, replacing services eliminated by PPS-induced financial considerations or making use of excess capacity.

The major deleterious incentives anticipated in the enactment of PPS included (1) multiple, unnecessary admissions of the same patient for a set of related procedures resulting in more discreet DRG payments, a practice known as *churning;* (2) *skimming* more profitable, less severely ill patients in each DRG, or *dumping* high-cost patients; and (3) reducing length of stay, tests, and procedures per admission to dangerously low levels, increasing mortality and morbidity.

Empirical findings as to the validity of these assertions have shown few ill effects of PPS or are inconclusive due to the rapidly changing nature of the health-care sector. Prior to PPS, hospital admissions

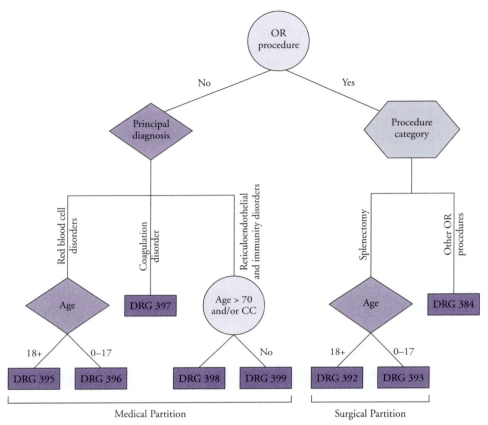

Figure 5.6. Flowchart of the Grouper Program for major diagnostic category 16: Disease and Disorders of the Blood and Blood-Forming Organs and Immunological Disorders (OR, operating room; CC, comorbidity and/or complication)

SOURCE: Reprinted with permission of American Medical Association. *Diagnosis-Related Groups (DRGs)*, 1984, Chicago: Author.

had been falling for all payers for a number of years. Once PPS was enacted, Medicare admissions went down as well. The figures for the fiscal year 1984 (the first full year of PPS) indicated an 11.3 percent decrease in admissions, resulting in a per-Medicare-enrollee decline of 15.9 percent, which was counter to the steady rise in Medicare admissions during the 1978–84 period. While anecdotal evidence of skimming and dumping did surface, widespread usage of these practices by hospitals had largely been documented for the uninsured and, in some states in particular, for Medicaid patients, rather than for Medicare patients. From 1990 to 1998, hospital discharges per

1,000 enrollees has remained fairly steady at about 315 (DesHarnais, Kobrinski, Chesney, Long, Ament, & Fleming, 1987; Guterman & Dobson, 1986; Guterman, Eggers, Riley, Greene, & Terrell, 1988; USDHHS, 2000a).

Length of stay has been falling for Medicare since the inception of the Act. Under the PPS system, an even steeper decline in average length of stay (down seventeen percent for the first three years of PPS), combined with reduced admissions, has resulted in declining patient volumes. This reduced length of stay has been achieved through shorter stays across the board, rather than efforts aimed specifically at patients who have the longest stays (i.e., the most severely ill). From 1990 to 1998, length of stay continued to decline from 9.0 days per admission to 6.2 days. These phenomena indicate that PPS has been effective in encouraging hospitals to become more efficient in the provision of inpatient care (USDHHS, 2000a).

The Medicare Case-Mix Index increased sharply and the percentage of hospital days spent in special care units increased after the implementation of PPS, possibly due to more judicious selections of candidates for inpatient hospitalization. Other studies of severity of illness at admission and discharge also show increases in the post-PPS period. The discharge of patients "quicker and sicker" has fostered rapid growth in the use of skilled nursing facilities and home health agency services by Medicare enrollees. Research indicates a tendency under PPS to increase the care provided to patients in other areas than inpatient settings. Under prospective payment, hospitals have encouraged physicians to reduce ancillary services, to shorten hospital stays, and to increase outpatient testing (Guterman & Dobson, 1986; Guterman, Eggers, Riley, Greene, & Terrell, 1988).

A number of criticisms have been levied against the incentives inherent in the DRG system. First, speculation exists that DRGs may not be "economically neutral" in that a hospital may be rewarded or penalized for performing an activity. To the extent that individual DRGs reflect procedures actually performed (e.g., types of surgery) as well as diagnosis, the choice of treatment may vary according to the "profitability" of that DRG and treatment decisions may not be made on purely clinical grounds. In a similar vein, physicians, in their clinical notes, and medical records administrators, in abstracting data for the DRG grouper program, might call upon *gaming* strategies to assure *DRG creep* to higher-level, revenue-enhancing diagnoses.

Financial Performance

Hospitals have generally fared well financially under PPS, but the distribution of results is uneven. The spate of hospital bankruptcies that were predicted at the inception of PPS has not taken place, but acquisi-

tions and mergers have been rampant in the health care industry in recent years.

PPS appears to have decelerated the rate of increase in Medicare inpatient hospital expenditures. Although outpatient payments, which are excluded from PPS, have mushroomed, total Medicare benefit payments are increasing at a slower rate due to the sharp decline in growth of Part A payments. Hospital inpatient expenditures comprise only forty-one percent of Medicare—only slightly more than total SMI payments in 1998 (USDHHS, 2000a).

It is interesting to note that prospective payment for hospitals based on DRGs has become an export item for the U.S. health care industry. As of 1992, nine other industrialized nations were already using or proposing to use DRGs, or a modification thereof, for hospital reimbursement. Nations in the process of phasing in DRGs include England, Australia, Belgium, Norway, Portugal, and Sweden (Wiley, 1992).

Medicare Physician Reimbursement

From 1975 to 1990, Medicare's total payments for physician services grew at a faster rate than payments for hospital services. By 1990, physician services reached a high of almost twenty-three percent of total Medicare spending. Over the same period, hospital care dropped drastically as a share of total Medicare expenditures. In 1998, physicians expenditures comprised only nineteen percent. The Reagan Administration plans to reform Medicare physician reimbursement were postponed due to pressures from opponents of government regulation in the private sector. Nonetheless, there was general agreement that physician payment under Medicare needed to be revised. In 1990, Congress directed the Administration to study physician payment reform when it established Medicare's DRG-based prospective payment system for hospital care.

Resource-Based Relative Values

On January 1, 1992, Medicare initiated a new system for reimbursing physicians using a resource-based relative-value (RBRV) scale. The new payment method divides resources needed to produce physician services into three components: physician work, practice expenses, and malpractice insurance costs. For each procedure, each of the three components is characterized by a numerical value representing its relative contribution to the expenses incurred in delivering the service (Table 5.3). In addition, as shown in Table 5.4, the relative values of the three components are each adjusted for geographic cost/price variations. The total units drive the fee, which is derived by multiplying the total units by a *conversion factor*. The conversion factor for 2001 is $38.26 for each unit of service. The final fee is thus a geographically weighted summation of the three components of the RBRVs times the conversion factor (American Medical Association, 2001; Hsiao, Braun, Dunn, Becker, DeNicola, & Ketcham, 1988a; Hsiao, Braun, Yntema, & Becker, 1988b).

For surgery, the RBRV payment schedule also establishes a uniform definition of "global surgery" to assure that identical payments are made for the same amount of work and resources expended in furnishing specific surgical services on a nationwide basis. The initial evaluation or consultation by a surgeon is paid separately from the global surgery package. The global fee includes all preoperative visits and all medical and surgical services related to a procedure, covering a ninety day postoperative period for all visits by the primary surgeon.

Simulations conducted by the Harvard University developers of the new reimbursement system (Hsiao et al., 1988a) showed that certain types of physicians would be financial winners and losers under RBRVs in comparison to what they would have earned under the old fee schedule. Pathologists, radiologists, thoracic surgeons, cardiovascular surgeons, and opthalmologists stood to lose from twenty-five to forty-five percent of their former Medicare fees. Physicians specializing in evaluation and management, such as internists, family practitioners, and immunologists, on the other hand, would be likely to gain from thirty-five to sixty-five percent over their previous Medicare earnings.

Hsiao, et al. (1992) later published an article criticizing HCFA for setting the monetary conversion factors at unreasonably low levels and pointed out that Medicare continued to reimburse invasive services with more units than research justified, according to the RBRVs actually assigned in the Medicare Fee Schedule. This practice by HCFA continues to this day, and now most types of physicians are feeling the pinch of restricted Medicare fees.

Selective Contracting

In 1982, the California legislature cleared the way for the state Medicaid program (Medi-Cal) and private

Table 5.3. Geographic Practice Cost Indices Used in the Medicare Fee Schedule: Selected Procedures, 2000

Description	Physician Work	Practice Expense	Malpractice Insurance	Total Units[*]
Appendectomy	8.70	5.06	0.86	14.62
Coronary artery bypass graft, four vein	31.95	30.60	4.11	66.66
Hysterectomy and vagina repair	15.00	9.60	1.15	25.75
Insertion of heart pacemaker	12.48	12.66	1.45	26.59
Knee arthroscopy/surgery	9.46	9.78	0.98	20.22
Magnetic Resonance Image, face/neck	1.48	12.00	0.56	14.04
Psychiatric treatment, 45–50 min	1.86	0.62	0.05	2.53
Repair detached retina	14.84	15.27	0.58	30.69
Repair inguinal hernia	5.84	4.54	0.56	10.94
Replacement of aortic valve	32.30	30.84	4.18	67.32

SOURCE: Adapted from Gallagher, P. E., & Smith, S. L. (2000). *Medicare RBRVs: The physician's guide.* Chicago: American Medical Association.

[*]Total units reflect the hypothetical number of RVUs existing in an area where all three GPCIs are 1.000.

insurers to enable payers to draw up contracts for the delivery of health services to their beneficiaries, selecting only hospitals and physicians that agreed to accept a negotiated price for their services. This practice of *selective contracting* was first embraced by the Medi-Cal program to contract hospitals at low per diem rates. The selection rule was uncomplicated: if the price was right and other specified conditions were met, a contract would be secured.

Not all hospitals competing for contracts, including large traditional Medi-Cal providers, gained them and, as a result of these shockwaves in the health care marketplace, the contracting process was enormously successful, with sixty-seven percent of California hospitals, accounting for seventy-two percent of the Medi-Cal patients, awarded contracts by the end of the first year of negotiations. Furthermore, for the first two years of selective contracting, there was no evidence of reduced access to health resources for Medi-Cal patients or any change in the quality of care they received. Savings to the state

were enormous for the first years of the program (Johns, Anderson, & Derzon, 1985; Johns, Derzon, & Anderson, 1985).

Cost cutting on an unprecedented scale was reported by hospitals receiving Medi-Cal contracts, demonstrating that competitive bidding shifts the burden of proof in hospital rate setting and encourages an active search for economies of operation. For contracted hospitals, total payments (in constant dollars) fell 9.6 percent in the first year of the program; average payments per day fell 18.4 percent and payments per admission fell 19.7 percent. Teaching hospitals, nonprofit hospitals, and investor-owned hospitals absorbed the largest reductions in average payment per day. Even though the per diem rates held incentives for increasing inpatient stays, length of stay fell 1.5 percent. Hospital financial analyses showed that contractors were, on the whole, not adversely impacted by selective contracting in the first two years. Anecdotal evidence, often citing the monies supplied by federal legislation for hospitals

Table 5.4.   Geographic Practice Cost Indices Used with Components of RBRVs: Selected Cities, 2000

Locality	Physician Work	Practice Expense	Malpractice Insurance
Arizona	0.995	0.971	1.189
Atlanta, GA	1.006	1.034	0.951
Birmingham, AL	0.978	0.872	0.876
Boston, MA	1.039	1.196	0.713
Chicago, IL	1.027	1.088	1.693
Colorado	0.987	0.970	0.795
Dallas, TX	1.010	1.016	0.930
Detroit, MI	1.042	1.022	3.069
Houston, TX	1.020	1.007	1.418
Iowa	0.958	0.882	0.648
Los Angeles, CA	1.055	1.199	0.846
Miami, FL	1.015	1.077	2.350
New Orleans, LA	0.998	0.950	1.153
New York, NY (Manhattan)	1.093	1.353	1.654
Puerto Rico	0.882	0.729	0.359
San Francisco, CA	1.067	1.299	0.667
Seattle, WA	1.005	1.080	0.742
St. Paul-Minneapolis, MN	0.989	0.967	0.507
Vermont	0.973	0.984	0.548
Washington DC, Area	1.050	1.161	1.032

SOURCE: Adapted from Gallagher, P.E., & Smith, S.L. (2000). *Medicare RBRVs: The physician's guide.* Chicago: American Medical Association.

serving a "disproportionate share" of Medicaid patients, supports the continued cost-saving effects of selective contracting by Medi-Cal. Zwonzinger & Melnick (1996) confirm that, in competitive managed-care markets in California, where selective contracting is the norm, hospitals showed far slower growth and lower relative costs since 1982.

Preferred Provider Organizations

The entry of private insurers and firms into selective contracting began in earnest in 1984 and quickly became known as "preferred provider organizations" (PPOs). PPOs have become a rapid growth area in health insurance. By 1993, enrollment in PPOs had increased to twenty-six percent of health plan participants.

A PPO is an arrangement or contract between a panel of health care providers, usually hospitals and physicians, and purchasers of health care services; the providers agree to supply services to a defined group of patients on a discounted fee-for-service basis. The exclusive provider organization (EPO) is the narrowest form of a PPO, wherein services provided by nonparticipating providers are not reimbursed at all (forcing the patient to pay the entire cost out of pocket unless care is rendered by an affiliated provider). Many PPO plans are sponsored by health insurance companies or self-insured employers.

PPOs generally have five key elements: (1) a limited number of physicians and hospitals; (2) negotiated fee schedules; (3) utilization review; (4) consumer choice of provider with lower out-of-pocket costs as an incentive to use participating providers; and (5) more expedient settlement of claims (de Lissovoy, Rice, Ermann, & Gabel, 1986).

Utilization review is the principal mechanism used by PPOs for controlling costs via reducing inappropriate use of services. Typical methods of utilization review include preadmission certification for hospital stays and certain types of high-cost outpatient procedures. Other mechanisms utilized by PPOs for cost control are contracting with low-cost providers and establishing a reimbursement system that realizes saving through discounted provider charges or incentives for reduced utilization. Discounts are generally in the range from ten to twenty percent below usual charges

and insurers are able to reduce premiums by a commensurate amount below standard indemnity plans.

HEALTH CARE REFORM

National Health Insurance

National health insurance (NHI) is a concept that has been espoused by many for over sixty years for containing health care costs and for providing universal access for the U.S. population. NHI came close to becoming part of the Social Security Act of 1935, and numerous bills, representing a spectrum of schemes, have been introduced and seriously debated by most Congressional sessions ever since then. In the mid-1970s, the issue of NHI became so heated that both political parties introduced some bills that were strikingly similar. NHI bills ran the gamut from expanding Medicare to new population groups (e.g., children under five years of age) to a national health service (NHS) concept like that of Sweden or Great Britain, where the government owns the hospitals and the doctors are paid on the basis of capitation or salary by the NHS.

When President Carter was elected in 1976, many in the health arena assumed that NHI would be an eventuality in a Democratic administration, but early on, it was evident that Carter took little interest in health issues. In the 1980s and early 1990s, the Reagan and Bush administrations were active in introducing cost containment measures, such as PPS and RBRVs for Medicare, but no serious consideration was given to sweeping reform of the entire system.

Strategies for Reform

American Medical Association

An unprecedented issue of the *Journal of the American Medical Association (JAMA)* appeared in May 1991. The entire issue was devoted to health system reform proposals, a subject traditionally anathema to organized medicine. Thirteen articles, by authors spanning a plethora of special interests, detailed a variety of strategies for achieving a new system.

Most proposals called for a revised system administered by private insurers with employer/employee premium sharing, supplemented by some form of government financing for nonworking individuals and families. With few exceptions, the proposals called for universal access to health care and for the provision of health insurance to all employees. Looking to the political left, it was interesting that no plan advocated a national health service model. On the right, only one of the plans called for increased privatization and freedom of choice.

In what can only be called a courageous editorial, Lundberg (1991), then the editor of the *JAMA*. summed up the findings:

> Although there may be consensus that our society must provide basic medical/health care for all of our people, we seem not to be close to a consensus on how to do it. Virtually all comprehensive health care proposals involve major legislation of some sort. Since consensus means "general agreement or unanimity; group solidarity in sentiment or belief," it is unlikely that, either as a society or as a profession, we will ever reach a true consensus on how to proceed, so we must not wait for one. To pass federal legislation requires only a simple majority in both houses of Congress plus presidential approval. (p. 2566)

Bush Proposal

In 1992, President George Bush unveiled his proposal for health care reform. Calling upon conservative principles, he advocated a type of voucher system whereby needy families would be allowed to take up to a $3,750 family tax credit, inversely related to income, for the purchase of private health insurance. With the goal of providing better access to the poor, states would be financially induced to capitate and expand Medicaid programs.

Critics of the Bush proposal noted that the tax credit voucher approach, linked to income taxes, might bypass many nonworking poor. Further, they held that it would take as much as $100 billion in additional government revenues to compensate for taxes lost to the credits, and the President gave no indication as to how such a shortfall in revenues would be avoided. Finally, the plan did not elucidate on how cost controls would be achieved in the market-based

approach. Needless to say, the Bush proposal was cast to oblivion.

The Clinton Health Security Plan

Health care reform then became one of the hottest domestic political issues of the early 1990s. Pressures for such reform have come from a wide variety of groups including providers, the elderly and disabled, labor unions, state and local governments, and insiders within the Washington establishment. Even health insurers and managed-care organizations have called for change. The two main targets of discontent are (1) the growing numbers and financial burden of uninsured and underinsured Americans, and (2) the high cost of health care, which eroded American competitiveness in the international marketplace.

In response to these pressures, President Clinton introduced *The President's Health Security Plan* (The White House Domestic Policy Council, 1993), which was largely the work of a task force headed by First Lady Hillary Rodham Clinton. The plan was subject to a great deal of criticism (and negative television advertising) from a large number of wealthy special interest groups, with the result that the plan died in Congress within a few months.

The essence of the plan was to create regional health alliances (i.e., health insurance purchasing cooperatives), wherein various competing insurance plans would be offered, at various premium supplements, to all participating employers and thus their employees. The model was based, in part, upon the California Public Employees Retirement Program (CalPERS) health insurance, which has been quite successful for more than a decade in containing costs, maintaining quality, and offering a wide range of comprehensive traditional and managed-care plans to its members. The Clintons' plan would also have created a separate risk pool for the uninsured.

Perhaps the ultimate reason that the Health Security Plan failed was that its implementation depended on global prospective budgeting for health care at a national level, the monies from which would be dispersed to state budgeting agencies and then on to the regional alliances. Many influential opinion makers maintained that the United States had no viable administrative apparatus whereby such complex prospective budgeting could take place. They predicted that a large and costly new government bureaucracy would emerge at a time when the electorate was seeking to curtail the size of government and its possible intrusion into peoples' personal lives.

The irony of the failed outcome of the Clinton Plan is that, in many regions of the country, such health alliances are emerging within the private sector, spurred by consolidation of health plans and providers into large health systems and managed-care plans. Government purchasers are also mimicking the CalPERS marketing formula.

President Clinton, in the face of his defeated plan, remained active in pushing health reform legislation incrementally, based upon the research conducted for the Health Security Act. Among areas of federal legislative reform enacted late in the Clinton Administration were (1) increasing the portability of health benefits from one employer to another, (2) encouraging growth for Medicare managed-care plans, (3) expansion of mental health benefits in health plans so that they would be comparable to physical health benefits, and (4) incentives to form Medical Savings Accounts (MSAs). MSAs, drawing the greatest amount of conservative political approval, are similar in concept to Individual Retirement Accounts, offering upscale "savings accounts" with comprehensive benefits subject to high yearly deductibles (e.g., $6,000 per year). However, MSAs attracted only a few thousand people during their first years as an option in Medicare.

Medicaid Reform

The Welfare Reform Act of 1996 placed new restrictions on eligibility for AFDC, SSI, and other federally funded welfare programs, including Medicaid. Furthermore, greater discretion was given to the states as to how to organize and enact welfare programs. Chief among the new provisions is that Medicaid will be delinked from cash assistance programs and states will be required to redetermine Medicaid eligibility for all welfare recipients. Another new provision is that states may deny Medicaid and cash assistance to current legal immigrants. Legal immigrants who ar-

rive after the bill is enacted are subject to a five-year waiting period before they become eligible for means-tested programs. (This provision holds great cost-cutting opportunities for states with high rates of immigration, like California and Texas, but may hold dire consequences for public health and communicable disease.) Finally, new criteria for SSI will result in about 50,000 children, most with behavioral disorders, losing Medicaid coverage.

SCHIP

In 1997, Congress enacted the State Children's Health Insurance Program (SCHIP), which provides states with $40 billion in federal funding over ten years to expand coverage for low-income children. Implementation of SCHIP is meant to reduce the number of low-income children lacking insurance coverage. Unlike previous expansions, which built upon existing Medicaid programs, states can set up separate programs to serve SCHIP enrollees. States that choose to participate have greater flexibility in designing benefit packages and may impose some cost sharing, resembling private insurance plans more than Medicaid. The majority of states are taking advantage of this opportunity.

Medicare Changes in the George W. Bush Administration

The addition of a presciption drug benefit to Medicare was an important issue in the 2000 presidential campaign. Although the Republican proposal was less generous than the Democratic plan, a new prescription drug benefit was nonetheless highly touted by President Bush.

Six months into the Bush Administration, no proposals for a Medicare drug benefit have been brought to Congress. Indeed, health care reform, in any incarnation, has not been addressed since Bush took office. However, vast changes in the federal political landscape (i.e., the May 2001 change in the Senate majority from Republican to Democrat) may serve to resurrect the Medicare prescription drug benefit as a pressing issue for Congress and the President.

The Uninsured

Health reform cannot be discussed without addressing the growing plight of the uninsured. In 1998, approximately 16.3 percent of the U.S. population, comprising about 44 million people, was not covered by health insurance, either public or private. This percentage is up from 1987, when about 12.9 percent of the population was uninsured for health care. Groups that predominate among the uninsured are Hispanics and, to a lesser extent, African Americans, those eighteen to twenty-four years old, and those with low household incomes. Males are more likely than females to be uninsured. The South and the West are also disproportionately represented among the uninsured, with the highest rates in Texas, Arizona, California, Nevada, New Mexico, and Mississippi (USDHHS, 2000a). Needless to say, the majority of the uninsured were poor or hovering close to the poverty level.

In addition to the growing ranks of the uninsured, anecdotal evidence attests to the transience of private insurance coverage for all Americans, linked as it is to employment status and subject to fluctuations in the economy. Constantly changing eligibility requirements for Medicaid and other public programs also add to the problem of frictional uninsurance for many of the nation's low-income population.

The problem of uninsurance impinges on the health care of all Americans for several reasons. First, it results in reduced access to care for the uninsured themselves, who are likely to postpone needed care to a time when their medical conditions have escalated in severity. Thus, the heightened intensity of caring for sicker people increases the cost of their care. Second, providers must recoup the costs of serving the uninsured from their paying customers—private insurers or the government. Insurance premiums go up commensurately and the taxpayer's burden enlarges. Third, this cost-shifting imposes yet another pressure on the efficient production of American goods and services, many of which stand to lose their competitive advantage in the world economy. Finally, in a spiral effect, uninsurance feeds on itself. With health insurance premiums constantly escalating, many businesses—especially small businesses—cannot afford to initiate or continue health insurance, thus adding to the problem.

International Comparisons

A great deal of interest in recent years has been focused on the health care systems of other industrialized nations, particularly Canada and Germany (Hurst, 1991; Iglehart, 1986a; Iglehart, 1986b; Neuschler, 1990; Reinhardt, 1990). While each system has its flaws, comparable countries have achieved universal access, ostensibly high quality, high-volume care, and significant cost controls. The Canadian system is financed equally by federal and provincial government general revenues in most provinces; Germany relies primarily on social health insurance linked to employment, supplemented by public general revenue funds. In both systems, global budgets are prospectively determined on an annual basis. In both systems, providers are predominantly private, independent contractors with the relevant health ministry acting as third party payer—the sole purchaser and reimburser of health services. Many assert that it is this monopsony purchasing power that fosters coalition building around issues of cost control, negotiated rate setting, and sustained quality of care. It is also argued that a universal reimbursement system promotes efficiencies that vastly reduce administrative costs.

In contrast to the Canadian and German national health insurance systems, the national health service model has been a growing movement in Europe (Abel-Smith, 1985). Among twelve nations in the European community, six now have a national health service model: the United Kingdom. Denmark, Spain, Italy, Greece, and Portugal. France, West Germany, Belgium, Luxembourg, Ireland, and the Netherlands remain without a NHS. Increasing regulation of health care is also notable in Western Europe.

SUMMARY

Financing health services in the United States involves a plethora of institutions and activities. The growth of employer-based private health insurance has stimulated unprecedented growth in health expenditures and biomedical advancement for the nation in the post-war era. The advent of Medicare and Medicaid in 1966 heralded a period of even more rapid growth, along with unbridled inflation, that persists to this day.

Inequities in access to health care, thought to be alleviated by Medicare and Medicaid, and the extensive provision of voluntary health insurance for employed groups, have not been resolved. Universal health coverage has not been realized, and a substantial and growing percent of the U.S. population go uninsured. State revenues have grown at rates slower than health care costs, inducing across-the-board reductions and more restrictive eligibility requirements for state Medicaid programs. Very recently, the Prospective Payment System, the new Medicare Fee Schedule for physicians, selective contracting, and managed-care plans have shown some success in ameliorating uncontrolled inflation in health care spending. However, effective means for identifying and monitoring the adequacy and appropriateness of health care, in an environment of either overutilization or underutiliztion, have not been developed.

The cry for health care reform resounds in all sectors of the U.S. economy. While most policy-makers agree upon universal access, they are far from agreement on how to finance the system, reimburse the providers, and impose cost controls. Whatever transpires in the future is likely to revolve around the fundamental politic of health finance: private versus public, entitlement versus social welfare, monopsony purchasing versus competitive concessions, fee-for-service versus prepayment.

This chapter has provided an historical and methodological framework for understanding and analyzing health care finance in the United States today. The principles that have been presented will apply to health finance, no matter how dynamic the future of the health care sector proves to be.

References

Aaron, H. J. (Winter 1993–94). Paying for health care. *Domestic Affairs*, 23–78.

Abel-Smith, B. (1985). Who is the odd man out? The experience of western Europe in containing the costs of health care. *Milbank Memorial Fund Quarterly, 63*, 1–7.

American Medical Association. (1984). *Diagnosis-related groups (DRGs) and the Prospective Payment System.* Chicago: American Medical Association.

American Medical Association. (2001). *2001 conversion factor and payment formula* [On-line]. Available: <http://www.amaassn.org/ama/pbu/printcat/3232.html>.

deLissovoy, G., Rice, T., Ermann, D., & Gabel, J. (1986). Preferred providers organizations: Today's models and tomorrow's prospects. *Inquiry, 23*, 7–15.

Deloitte, Haskins, & Sells. (1982). *Tax Equity and Fiscal Responsibility Act of 1982: Management strategies for health care providers.* New York: Deloitte & Touche.

Deloitte & Touche. (2001). Payment analysis of final FY 2001 PPS Rule. *Washington Commentary.* New York: Deloitte & Touche.

DesHarnais, S., Kobrinski, E. J., Chesney, J. D., Long, M. J., Ament, R. P., & Fleming. S. T. (1987). The early effects of the Prospective Payment System on inpatient utilization and the quality of care. *Inquiry, 24*, 7–16.

Enthoven, A. (1981). The competition strategy: Status and prospects. *New England Journal of Medicine, 304*, 109–112.

Fuchs, V. R. (1984) "Though much is taken": Reflections on aging, health, and medical care. *Milbank Memorial Fund Quarterly, 62*, 143–166.

Gornick, M., Greenberg, N. J., & Eggers, P. W. (1985). Twenty years of Medicare and Medicaid: Covered populations, use of benefits, and program expenditures. *Health Care Financing Review: Annual Supplement*, 13–59.

Guterman, S., & Dobson, A. (1986). Impact of the Medicare Prospective Payment System for hospitals. *Health Care Financing Review, 7*, 97–114.

Guterman, S., Eggers, P. W., Riley, G., Greene, T. F., & Terrell, S. A. (1988). The first three years of Medicare prospective payment: An overview. *Health Care Financing Review, 9*(3), 67–77.

Health Care Financing Administration. (1999). *National health expenditures, 1999* [On-line]. Available: <http://hcfa.gov.stats/nhe-oact/tables/chart.html>.

Hillman, A. L., Welch, W. P., & Pauly, M. V. (1992). Contractual arrangements between HMOs and primary care physicians: Three-tiered HMOs and risk pools. *Medical Care, 30*(2), 136–148.

Hsaio, W. C., Braun, P., Dunn, D. L., Becker, E. R., Yntema, D., Verrilli, D. K., Stamenovic, E., & Chen, S. P. (1992). Results and impacts of the resource-based relative value scale. *Medical Care, 30*(11), NS61–NS79.

Hsaio, W. C., Braun, P., Dunn, D., Becker, E. R., DeNicola, M., & Ketcham, T. R. (1988a). Results and policy implications of the resource-based relative-value study. *New England Journal of Medicine, 319*(13), 881–888.

Hsaio, W. C., Braun, P., Yntema, D., & Becker, E. R. (1988b). Estimating physicians' work for a resource-based relative-value scale. *New England Journal of Medicine, 319*(13), 835–841.

Hurst, J. W. (1991). Reform of health care in Germany. *Health Care Financing Review, 12*(3) 73–101.

Iglehart, J. K. (1986a). Canada's health care system: Part one. *New England Journal of Medicine, 315*(3), 202–208.

Iglehart, J. K. (1986b). Canada's health care system: Part two. *New England Journal of Medicine, 315*(12), 778–784.

Johns, L., Anderson, M. D., & Derzon, R. A. (1985). Selective contracting in California: Experience in the second year. *Inquiry, 22,* 335–347.

Johns, L., Derzon, R. A., & Anderson, M. D. (1985). Selective contracting in California: Early effects and policy implications. *Inquiry, 22,* 24–32.

Levit, K., Cowan, C., Lazenby, H. Sensenig, A., McDonnell, P., Stiller, J., & Martin, A. (2000). Health spending in 1998: Signals of change. *Health Affairs, 19*(1), 124–132.

Lubitz, J., & Prihoda, R. (1984). Use and costs of Medicare services in the last two years of life. *Health Care Financing Review, 5,* 117–131.

Lundberg, G. D. (1991). National health care reform: An aura of inevitability is upon us. *Journal of the American Medical Association, 265*(19), 2566–2567.

Neuschler, E. (1990). *Canadian health care: The implications of public health insurance.* Washington, DC: Health Insurance Association of America.

Reinhardt, U. E. (1985). The compensation of physicians: Approaches used in foreign countries. *Quality Review Bulletin, 11,* 366–377.

Reinhardt, U. E. (1990). West Germany's health-care and health-insurance system: Combining universal access with cost control. In the Pepper Commission, *A call for action: Final report of the U. S. bipartisan commission on comprehensive health care.* Washington, DC: U. S. Government Printing Office.

Rice, T. (1992). Containing health care costs in the United States. *Medical Care Review, 49*(1), 19–65.

Roemer, M. I. (1977). *Comparative national policies on health care.* New York: Marcel Dekker.

Roemer, M. I. (1978). *Social medicine: The advance of organized health services in America.* New York: Springer.

U. S. Bureau of the Census. (2000). *Statistical Abstract of the United States: 2000* (120th ed.). Washington, DC: U.S. Government Printing Office.

U. S. Department of Health and Human Services, Health Care Financing Administration, Office of Research and Demonstrations: Medicare and Medicaid Statistical Supplement. (1995). *Health Care Financing Review* (HCFA Publication No. 03348): U.S. Health Care Financing Administration, U.S. Department of Health & Human Services.

U. S. Department of Health and Human Services, Health Care Financing Administration, Bureau of Data Management and Strategy. (1996). *1996 HCFA Statistics* (HCFA Publication No. 033394).

U. S. Department of Health and Human Services, Health Care Financing Administration, Office of Strategic Planning. (1998). *Data compendium.* Baltimore: U.S. Health Care Financing Administration, U.S. Department of Health & Human Services.

U. S. Department of Health and Human Services, Health Care Financing Administration, Office of Strategic Planning. (2000a). *1999 HCFA statistics.* (HCFA Publication No. 03421): U.S. Health Care Financing Administration, U.S. Department of Health & Human Services.

U. S. Department of Health and Human Services, Centers for Disease Control and Prevention, National Center for Health Statistics. (2000b). *Health United States 2000.* Hyattsville, MD: U.S. Department of Health & Human Services.

U. S. Department of Health and Human Services, Health Care Financing Administration. (2001). *Medicare and You, 2001.* Baltimore: U.S. Health Care Financing Administration, U.S. Department of Health & Human Services.

Waldo, M. O. (1990). Addendum: A brief summary of the Medicaid program. *Health Care Financing Review: Annual Supplement,* 171–172.

White House Domestic Policy Council. (1993). *The President's health security plan.* New York: Times Books.

Wiley, M. M. (1992). Hospital financing reform and case-mix measurement: An international review. *Health Care Financing Review, 13*(4), 119–133.

Zwanzinger, J., & Melnick, G. A. (1996). Can managed care plans control health care costs? *Health Affairs, 15*(2), 185–199.

C H A P T E R

6

Managed Care:
Restructuring the System

Paul R. Torrens
Stephen J. Williams

Chapter Topics

- What Is Managed Care?
- The Components of Managed Care
- How Managed Care Works
- Key Concepts and Principles of Managed Care
- Issues for the Future of Managed Care
- Managed Care and the Future of Health Care

Learning Objectives

Upon completing this chapter, the reader should be able to:

- Understand the variety of arrangements included under the term *managed care*
- Appreciate the roles of all key players, especially the consumer, in managed care
- Understand the underlying mechanisms of managed care
- Appreciate the complex challenges involved in the future of managed care
- Analyze the appropriate role of managed care in the nation's health care system

Although the term *managed care* has become increasingly familiar to anyone involved with health care in the United States in the last few years, there are two major misunderstandings with regard to the term and its use. First, the term is sometimes used as though all forms of managed care are the same, or that managed care were a single organizational structure that functions like a tightly unified entity. Unfortunately, nothing could be further from the truth on both counts; managed care covers a wide variety of organizational forms, and in any one of the organizational forms, there are three or four separate subunits that make up the whole.

The second misunderstanding with regard to managed care often involves the impact of the arrival of managed care on the American health care system. Sometimes, managed care is discussed as if it were merely one more change in the way health insurance is organized and in the way that providers of health services are paid. Frequently, managed care is described as yet one more technical innovation in what has become an increasingly specialized field of insurance.

Unfortunately, viewing managed care as merely a new set of technical changes misses the point that managed care has brought about a major change in the way health care in the United States is delivered by providers and utilized by patients. It should be understood that although the technical changes included in managed care are very interesting, it is much more important to realize the structural and policy changes in American health care that are currently being wrought by the increasing presence of managed care.

This chapter examines both aspects of managed care: the technical and descriptive aspects of managed care itself, and the impact on the American health-care system. The implication for changing objectives and incentives is emphasized.

WHAT IS MANAGED CARE?

It is virtually impossible to provide a definition of managed care that satisfies all participants in all circumstances because the applications of the term are so wide and varied (Fox, 1997; Miller & Luft, 1994). One definition might be: "managed care is an organ-

Table 6.1. Objectives of Managed Care

- enhance cost containment
- implement some forms of rationing
- promote administrative and clinical efficiency
- reduce duplication of services
- enhance appropriateness of care
- promote comprehensive contracting mechanisms
- manage care processes by managing provider and consumer behavior

ized effort by health insurance plans and providers to use financial incentives and organizational arrangements to alter provider and patient behavior so that health care services are delivered and utilized in a more efficient and lower-cost manner." This definition includes the central principles of managed care: it is an organized effort that involves both insurers and providers of health care; it uses financial incentives and organizational structures in reaching its goal; and its purpose is to increase efficiency and reduce health care costs (Table 6.1) (Drake, 1997).

THE COMPONENT PARTS OF MANAGED CARE

Managed care includes at least four basic components (Figure 6.1). These parts are: the purchaser/ultimate payer for health care; the health insurance plans/intermediaries; the providers of care (that is, hospitals, physicians, and others involved in the direct delivery of personal health care); and the patients/public receiving care.

The *purchaser/payer* of managed care is generally one of three large groups: employers who purchase health insurance for their employees, the federal Medicare program, or state Medicaid programs. *Health insurance* plans are organizations licensed by their individual states to offer health insurance coverage that is bought by the purchasers/payers. Health insurance plans create the benefit packages, market the plans, enroll the beneficiaries, arrange for the provision of health care services to these beneficiaries, and monitor the results. The *providers of care* are licensed health care professionals, organizations, and institutions that actually deliver the needed health

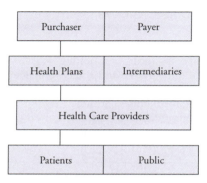

Figure 6.1. Components of Managed Care

care services to the individual beneficiaries under the terms of the health insurance plans' benefit packages. The *patients/public* are the individuals covered by health insurance plans who receive health care services from providers. In recent years, it has been suggested that a fifth important component part of the managed-care structure might be the health insurance *brokers*, as an increasingly high percentage of health insurance (particularly that provided by employers) is arranged through the technical and organizational assistance of brokers.

In many instances of managed care, these four (or five) components are separate organizational units, linked together by negotiated contracts. In some forms of managed care, such as the Kaiser-Permanente Health Plan, the insurance and provision of care functions are seemingly joined together in a single organ-

ization that appears to be both the insurer and the entity providing services. In most other managed-care arrangements in the United States today, this is not the case, and it is perhaps better to consider the insurance and the provision of services functions as separate organizational subunits that can be either more loosely or more tightly linked together.

HOW MANAGED CARE WORKS

The process of making the managed care system work begins with certain important decisions made by the purchaser/payer (Enthoven & Singer, 1996). With these decisions, the purchaser must decide how many and what type of health insurance plans are to be offered and how much the purchaser/payer will pay for each premium. In the past, purchasers frequently selected a wide range of plans and paid different amounts for each plan. More recently, purchasers are selecting fewer health insurance plans to offer and are paying the same amount of money for their health insurance premium, regardless of which plan the beneficiary chooses, with the employee paying any difference.

Specifically, purchasers/payers must decide whether they wish to give their beneficiaries a wide-open range of choices of providers or whether they wish to limit, in some fashion, the choices available to the beneficiaries. The more restrictive plans offer fewer choices of provider and greater restrictions on consumer behavior, but may yield lower costs (Figure 6.2). In the same fashion, the purchasers/payers must decide whether

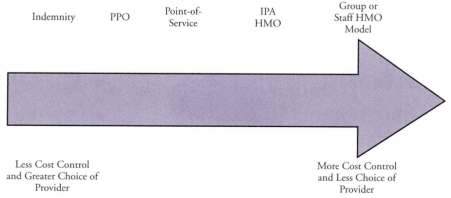

| Indemnity | PPO | Point-of-Service | IPA HMO | Group or Staff HMO Model |

Less Cost Control and Greater Choice of Provider

More Cost Control and Less Choice of Provider

Figure 6.2. Continuum of Cost Control in the U.S. Health Care System

they want to have their beneficiaries enrolled in health insurance plans that pay providers on a fee-for-service or capitation (that is, a fixed amount per person per month covered) basis. In this set of choices, the purchasers/payers usually find themselves choosing between a preferred provider organization (PPO) or a health maintenance organization (HMO). The PPO allows the recipient of health insurance a wider choice of providers and pays those providers on a modified fee-for-service basis; the HMO offers a more constrained range of choices among providers and usually pays the provider organization on a *per capita* (a fixed amount per person) basis.

A survey of employer-sponsored health insurance provided in the 1990s showed that eighty percent of the firms surveyed offered health insurance benefits of some kind. Of the health insurance benefits offered, seventy-three percent of the plans included some type of managed care; this was a significant increase from only a few years earlier. The types of managed care plans offered to employees were HMOs, PPOs, and "point-of-service" (POS) plans. Point-of-service plans combine elements of both HMOs and PPOs, allowing an enrollee to obtain care from providers outside the PPO network but with a substantially higher copayment, as discussed in more detail later (Jensen, et al., 1997).

Types of Managed-Care Plans

The two main representative types of managed-care health plans now offered to purchasers/payers by insurance organizations, preferred provider organizations (PPOs), and health maintenance organizations (HMOs) are both types of managed care. But these plans differ significantly in their major characteristics.

The PPO is essentially a fee-for-service type of health plan that allows a beneficiary to use a wide-open range of providers or select from a narrower list of providers who have agreed to give the health insurance plan a discount. If the beneficiary chooses to use a provider on the narrower list, the plan, the provider, and the beneficiary all benefit. The health plan generally has negotiated a discounted rate for the provider's services (sometimes a very significant discount), so the plan uses its purchasing power to get

a lower price. The providers agree to take a lower price but, in return, hope that the health insurance plan's members will choose them more frequently because they are now put on a special list of "preferred providers" that are made available to the health plan's members.

The health plan members benefit by choosing a preferred provider because, if they do, the member's share of the cost (as expressed by the plan's deductibles and coinsurance) is reduced, so the member may actually pay nothing at all to use the preferred provider. In other words, financial incentives are used to create a buyer/seller/user network that benefits all three parties.

For purchasers/payers, the PPO is a very attractive option, because it means that the purchaser/payer is not forcing the beneficiaries to limit their choices or change their behaviors if they do not want to. However, if they do wish to save some money and choose the preferred provider, they benefit, and the purchaser/payer has not coerced them to do something that they would rather not do.

The HMO type of managed-care plan, now quite prevalent (Table 6.2), has many significant differences when compared with the PPO type of managed care. Indeed, the differences in the two types are so major that it is confusing to describe them under the same general heading of managed care, as though both are closely related and are only minor variants of each other.

The HMO type of managed-care plan offered to purchasers/payers of health insurance plans has a number of important premises built into its framework. First, the HMO form of managed care depends upon the fact that the health plan has developed a contract with a group of physicians to take on total responsibility for a list of enrolled patients. The HMO form of managed care depends upon an individual's choosing to sign up with one particular group of physicians and then to receive virtually all medical care—both primary and specialty—through that group of physicians, either directly or by referral. That particular group of physicians, in return, is paid a fixed fee per patient (capitation rate) that the group agrees to take on for total responsibility. This *per capita* form of reimbursement to the medical provider and

Table 6.2. Health Maintenance Organization Enrollment: United States, Selected Years

Plans and Enrollment	1980	1999
Plans	*Number*	
All plans	235	643
Model type		
Individual practice association	97	309
Group	138	123
Mixed	N/A	208
Geographic region		
Northeast	55	110
Midwest	72	179
South	45	239
West	63	115
Enrollment	*Persons in millions*	
Total	9.1	81.3
Model type		
Individual practice association	6.4	32.8
Group	14.6	15.9
Mixed	N/A	32.6
Federal program		
Medicaid	0.6	10.4
Medicare	1.1	6.5
Geographic region	*Percent of population enrolled in HMOs*	
Northeast	3.1	36.7
Midwest	2.8	23.3
South	0.8	23.9
West	12.2	41.4

the continuing, comprehensive responsibility for total patient care of the enrolled population is what makes the HMO form of managed care significantly different from the PPO form of managed care.

In the HMO form of managed care, the linkages are tighter and more formal, and the payment is on a *per capita* basis rather than on a fee-for-service basis, modified or not. In this form of managed care, just as in the PPO form, the three participants (health plan, providers, and patients) form a network of mutual benefit, but it is much tighter and based on different

principles. The health plan benefits because it is able to limit its financial exposure by paying the provider group a fixed amount for taking care of the enrolled population. The plan knows that no matter how much care the provider is required to give patients to handle their medical problems, the health plan will not be asked for any additional financial payments. From the provider's point of view, these planned contractual arrangements provide a steady stream of revenue, whether individual patients seek care or not. The provider organizations are able to plan on a more stable and long-term basis than they could if they were in the situation of a company's fee-for-service plan, dependent as it is on individuals' choices; the providers' contracts with the plan guarantee financial stability, at least to some degree. The patient benefits as well, as there are usually few or no copayments, deductibles, or other payments in an HMO form of managed care. The patient knows, therefore, that once the premium is paid each month, there will be little or no additional financial claims directed at the patient for covered services.

Providers have a wide variety of ways in which they may relate to managed-care plans. Hospitals, for example, may agree to contract with PPOs and offer substantial discounts when PPO members are actually hospitalized at a contracting hospital. Hospitals also may contract with HMOs to provide hospital care for an enrolled population on a *per capita* basis, although this type of *per capita* contract with hospitals is less common. Hospitals may also agree to take part in joint contracting efforts involving physician groups/organizations/or independent practice associations (IPAs) that agree to take on an enrolled population for a *per capita* payment, with the *per capita* later being divided by mutual agreement between the physician group and the hospital.

For their part, physicians have a variety of ways to take part in managed-care health plans, either singly or in larger groups and organizations. With regard to PPOs, physicians working alone or in groups can simply agree to take members of PPOs on a fee-for-service basis, the fee usually being a decrease or discount from the physician's usual fee. This type of arrangement is organized around individual patients making individual visits to a doctor and implies no long-term commitment to a relationship between the physician and the health plan, or between the physician and an individual patient.

By contrast, when physicians are faced with HMOs, their decisions are more critical because they have much broader and much longer-term implications. In the IPA, the physician in practice voluntarily joins a collaborative group of physicians, all of whom are in independent practice and all of whom join the IPA in order to be able to take part in large contracts with HMOs. In the IPA, the physician remains in independent practice and agrees to care for those patients whom the IPA attracts and assigns to that physician. The physician in practice usually has many other patients that come from other sources, some of whom may be paid for on a fee-for-service basis and others for whom payment may be from other managed-care arrangements, including HMOs. The IPA allows individual physicians the benefits of independence, multiple sources of patients, and involvement in other contracting arrangements. The individual physician may also be an owner of the IPA, but that is not usually a necessary condition of the physician's involvement with the IPA as a provider of care.

When IPAs first began to appear, it was believed that they might merely be a transitional form of medical organization that might gradually give way to tighter forms of group practice and staff model HMOs, but that has not been the case. The IPA model of physician involvement has many advantages to physicians, as well as to health plans, and probably will be a permanent feature on the health-care scene. The longer they are in existence, the more tightly IPAs are organized and managed, but the fundamental model of physicians in independent private practice who voluntarily join a collaborative contracting group remains the same.

Physicians can also participate in HMO managed care by joining organized medical groups and having the medical groups contract with HMOs to provide care to an enrolled population. In this form of involvement in managed care, a physician chooses to become a formal member of an organized medical group that practices together, shares premises, and may share patients and revenues. The formal contract with the HMO is between the medical group and the

HMO, not necessarily with individual physicians. The HMOs may prefer this type of arrangement, as the internal discipline of an organized medical group is usually, though not necessarily, much tighter than the internal discipline of an IPA (made up as it is of large numbers of doctors who work in separate locations). The physician selection process here is that a physician first must decide to join an organized medical group and practice medicine actively together with other physicians. Then the physician is a member of an organized medical group that contracts with an HMO to care for patients enrolled in that HMO.

In relatively few circumstances, a physician may decide not to go into independent practice and not to join a medical group that is separate from an HMO, but may instead decide to join a "staff" model HMO that actually employs its own physicians. In this model, the doctor decides to become directly associated with the HMO itself, rather than to become a part of a contracting medical group that is separate from the HMO. In this type of organization, the physician is in effect becoming a salaried member of a larger corporation that may actually have its own hospitals and clinics in a number of locations and that markets its own HMO under its own name. In some instances, due to state medical practice laws, physicians may actually form a partnership that then exclusively contracts with the HMO.

There are other types of physician relationships with managed-care plans, but these three—the IPA model, the medical group, and the staff model—are the most common forms of physician-managed care collaboration.

In summary, it can be seen from this brief review that managed care is not a single monolithic organization, nor is it characterized by a single form of operation. Managed care involves a variety of choices in a variety of organizational relationships on the purchaser/payer level, on the health insurance plan level, and on the provider level. In considering any issues related to managed care, therefore, it is important for the health care professional to first identify which level of the managed-care structure is actually being discussed and which issue is under review.

Depending upon the level of the managed-care system or structure and depending upon the issue being discussed, the details and outcomes of such discussions may vary greatly. Managed care is not a single, all-encompassing, unified structure, but rather a series of separate subunits, linked together by a series of decisions, contracts, and administrative structures. The result is a wide variety of managed-care activities and operations.

KEY CONCEPTS AND PRINCIPLES OF MANAGED CARE

In the previous section, we stressed that managed care is more of a concept and a process than a specific, single entity; it is a series of organizational subunits that are linked together in different ways to achieve certain outcomes. A managed-care program serving any one particular person may be quite different in the details of its organization from a managed-care program serving another. In the same fashion, an individual physician or a hospital may participate in many different types of managed-care programs at the same time, each having some significant variation from the rest.

There are some important concepts and principles, however, that are common in a general sense to all types of managed-care programs. It is important to understand these key principles because they apply in a general way across the entire spectrum of managed care.

The Need for Education/Preparation of the Insured in Managed Care

One of the most important principles of managed care is the need for careful preparation and education of the insured about the way in which managed care works. If managed care is to succeed in its goals, it is important that the insured be told very specifically what managed care is and what it is not. Because the use of health care under a managed-care arrangement may be quite different from previous patterns of utilization and behavior, it is important that patients be instructed about what services are covered, how care can be obtained, and how care might be different from more conventional fee-for-service coverage.

Unfortunately, there is very little preparation carried out by the purchasers/payers when they make a decision to use managed-care plans for the provision of health insurance coverage to their beneficiaries. Often the purchasers/payers leave it to the health plans to inform the enrolled members that there are certain new procedures they must follow and new behaviors they must assume, as purchasers/payers may actually wish to stay away from passing on the bad news themselves.

Unfortunately, many health insurance plans do not do a very good job of instructing their members in detail about how the plans function. It is clear that if managed care is to succeed in the future and is to be accepted by patients/people, a better job of information exchange and education must be done by the purchasers/payers at the time of the decision to enroll beneficiaries in a managed-care plan.

The Importance of an Information System and the Insistence on Quality and Outcome Measures

One of the central characteristics of all forms of managed care is the absolutely central necessity of much more advanced information systems that will provide more accurate and timely data on the utilization of services and on the quality and outcomes of those services. In the past, under fee-for-service forms of health insurance, the key information that was collected came from claims data (that is, data from requests for payment for the provision of specific items of services). Under an HMO type of managed care, claims data are no longer gathered, as payment is based on a *per capita* rather than fee-for-service basis. In addition, the previous claims data usually revealed very little about the quality of the services provided or the effect/outcomes of those services on the health status of the insured.

The importance of these new information systems is further heightened by the requirement of the purchasers/payers of care to the health plans that they be able to report to the purchasers on the quality of services provided, often using standardized data sets such as the HEDIS (Health Plan Employer Data and Information Set) format. In the same manner, the plans themselves are requiring the provider groups and systems to gather and report more sophisticated utilization and quality/data outcomes to enable the plans to better evaluate the services of the providers and also to make it possible for the plans to report back to the purchasers/payers on the quality of services for which they are paying.

It is felt that only a small portion of the data being gathered at the present time is being utilized to its maximum potential. However, it is clear that this situation will change very quickly, given the increasing demands for better data and for better use of the data that is being generated.

Plan/Provider Control of Utilization

Control of costs, utilization, and, to an extent, consumer behavior depend heavily on influencing provider, and especially physician, behavior (Table 6.3). There are numerous considerations involved in influencing physicians, ranging from careful selection of efficient participating providers (economic credentialing) to overt utilization reviews and controls. Enhanced controls on both providers and consumers, sometimes using highly restrictive mechanisms, are a central hallmark of managed care.

Because one of the main objectives of managed care is to reduce the unnecessary use of services and to provide health care in a more efficient fashion, review and control of the utilization of health services are central to the idea of managed care. The control of the utilization of services begins with decisions that are made by the purchaser/payer with regard to what services should be included in the benefits package. Increasingly, the range of services to be included as a

Table 6.3. Influencing Physician Behavior in Managed-Care Practices

- feedback and comparisons to the norm using quantitative data
- physician recruitment and selective contracting policies
- socialization to group goals and philosophy
- positive rewards such as money, benefits, on-call preference, and leave time
- promotion of teamwork and quality management
- financing and reimbursement incentives
- efficiency and productivity enhancements

benefit of managed care is being narrowed by purchasers, who are ever more anxious to limit their financial exposure. Many times, health plans find themselves blamed for not paying for certain health care services when the actual decision to limit services has been made by the purchaser/payer in designing the benefit package.

Health plans themselves also have methods for reviewing the utilization of services and frequently require the provider to report on the use of expensive services such as inpatient care and high-technology diagnostic and treatment services. The basic contract between the insurance organization and the providers frequently stipulates the nature and extent to which providers must review their own utilization of services and provide summary data.

Most utilization review and control occur at the level of the provider organization itself, however, which is usually in the IPA or medical group providing medical services. Because these medical groups are increasingly being paid on a *per capita* basis and are, therefore, at risk for the financial consequences of any high utilization, it is logical that the most active and aggressive control of utilization occurs within the medical group or IPA itself (Kerr, 1996). Indeed, as IPAs and medical groups learn that their financial futures now depend upon the medical group providing fewer rather than more services, the utilization control processes used within the medical group or IPA can become increasingly stringent. In some instances recently, IPAs and medical groups have begun using hospital-based physicians to handle all of their admissions ("hospitalists"), thereby reducing variation on inpatient admissions and length-of-stay patterns.

At the heart of any utilization control system is the concept of the primary care physician (PCP) as a "gate-keeper." The gate-keeper concept rests on the idea that one physician, usually a PCP in family practice, internal medicine, pediatrics, or, less often, obstetrics/gynecology, is responsible for providing all of the primary care for the patient. The PCP also determines when referral to specialists is needed and then provides oversight and coordination for the use of the specialist on an ongoing basis. The gate-keeper concept is designed to control the patient's use of expensive resources, to reduce the self-initiated use of specialty physicians, and to ensure overall coordination of care.

Placing the primary care physician in the position of gate-keeper is increasingly being seen as a potential source of conflict of interest for physicians playing this role. If the primary care physician aggressively seeks to ensure that the patient has all possible diagnostic procedures and specialists' opinions, that PCP may also be draining the IPA or medical group's total financial pool under capitation. The PCP realizes very quickly that the more aggressively the patient's best interests are pursued, the less advantageous it may be to the physician personally. The subject is one of serious concern to physicians and medical organizations.

Capitation

Central to the HMO type of managed-care program is the concept of capitation, the payment of a fixed fee per person to physicians or hospitals in exchange for their willingness to assume responsibility to provide a complete range of services as needed. In contrast to the fee-for-service form of reimbursement for the provision of health services, capitation provides entirely different incentives to those providing care. Under fee-for-service, the more services that are provided, the more the provider is paid. Under capitation, the fewer services that are provided, the more funds there are left over for the provider. The incentives, therefore, are for the provider to be more careful and frugal in the use of health services resources and in the referral of specialists, as the provider is rewarded for doing less rather than more.

The use of *per capita* payments for coverage of services exists throughout the entire managed-care structure. The purchaser/payer pays the health plan on a *per capita* basis, providing a fixed amount in exchange for a guarantee of a range of services by the health insurance plan. The HMO type of managed care health insurance plans, in turn, generally use *per capita* payments to medical groups or combined hospital/medical group joint enterprises, also in exchange for a guarantee that the

providers will offer a wide range of services to those covered by the health insurance plan.

Within the IPAs or medical groups, capitation can also be used to reimburse individual physicians in different ways. For example, it is quite common for an IPA to reimburse primary care physicians on a *per capita* basis, but then reimburse specialists within the IPA or medical group on a modified fee-for-service basis. In recent years, various IPAs and medical groups have begun to experiment with the use of capitation in exactly the reverse fashion: Primary care physicians are now occasionally being paid on a fee-for-service basis and specialists are occasionally being paid on a *per capita* basis. The point remains that capitation is a powerful tool in managed care, is central to the concept of managed care, and can be used in different ways throughout the entire managed-care structure.

Risk Sharing

Of increasing importance and interest in managed care is the use of risk-sharing pools of various sorts. These vary widely, but in general, they involve the establishment of a pool of money from which certain services are paid for throughout the year. Funds remaining at year end are then divided, either between the providers and the health insurance plan or between the physicians and a hospital with whom those physicians have joined in a collaborative effort.

The general concept of the risk pools is to provide an incentive to reduce use, particularly with regard to hospitalization, specialty referrals, and high-technology diagnostic and treatment services. The extent to which risk pools are effective in reducing use and saving money is not clear. It is also not clear whether risk pools (and the previously mentioned use of capitation payments) result in underuse of needed services. The greatest fear in managed care, both on the part of patients and of providers, is that the incentives to control overuse of health services that have been so common in the past under fee-for-service forms of reimbursement will now lead to serious underuse and denial of needed services, with a resulting negative impact on the health status of the covered population. Indeed, of all of the questions involved in managed care, this is probably the most critical one to examine continuously over the next few years.

The Importance of Contracts in Managed Care

With the exception of staff model HMOs that employ their own physicians, managed care consists of a series of separate subunits that are linked together by legal contracts. Indeed, managed care can be seen as a series of separate entities whose only connection is through legally negotiated systems of contracts.

Unfortunately, many clinical professionals in health care are not used to the negotiating and contracting process and, as a result, pay less attention to it than they should. In effect, managed care consists of a series of legally binding contracts and documents that set the terms and boundaries for everything that happens within the managed-care structure. Therefore, the negotiation of proper contracts and the clear understanding of all the details in the contracts by all parties to those contracts is essential for the long-term success of managed care. At the present time, the negotiation and creation of contracts between the various parties in managed care are challenging and uncertain.

It should also be pointed out that the least informed and prepared party in the managed care structure is probably the person covered by the health insurance policy. If the health insurance policy is considered a contract between the health plan and the patient/person, it is very important that the patient/person understand better what is in that contract, even if he or she has no part in the actual negotiations. There is growing interest in and concern for methods of better education and preparation of patients/public in the interpretation of their health insurance contracts, as well as a growing interest in discovering ways in which patients/public can take a more active part in the actual negotiation of better contracts for themselves, either with the purchasers/payers or with the health plans. One of the most interesting and potentially important areas of future activity in managed care is the possible increase in the power of groups of patients/public as members of the managed-care structure.

ISSUES FOR THE FUTURE OF MANAGED CARE

In the future, several important issues must be considered with regard to the development of managed-care programs and their services to patients. Among the important issues are consolidation among health plans, the impact of managed care on the provider system, Medicare and Medicaid managed care, managed behavioral health care, conflicts of interest, and protection of the public.

Consolidation Among Health Insurance Plans

As managed care matures, one phenomenon that is developing rapidly is consolidation among health insurance plans. Every year sees more and more of the nation's health insurers merging with or acquiring other health insurers in what can only be described as a major change in the health care financing landscape. This consolidation of health insurance providers and plans is a concern for several reasons.

The first concern about consolidation of the health insurance industry is the tendency of plans to become so large that they have an unfair advantage in dealing both with purchasers/payers and providers. The larger a health insurance plan becomes, the more financial assets it has and the more enrolled lives it controls. This means that the leverage among the plans may become unduly strong and make it difficult to have an even balance among purchasers/payers, health plans, and providers. In their defense, health plans very frequently say that they must consolidate because purchasers/payers and providers are themselves consolidating into larger bargaining units; the plans must consolidate if they are not to be overwhelmed by the larger size and strength of their negotiating partners.

The second reason why consolidation among health plans may be a concern in the future is the potential reduction of variation among health plans and their products. At a time when everyone is still trying to learn about managed care and when there still seems to be considerable experimentation about the insurance products being offered, consolidation among health plans may reduce this variability significantly.

The opportunity to learn exactly what are the best forms of managed-care insurance products for our various subpopulations may be prematurely ended before we have had a chance to learn the lessons that should be learned.

Consolidation that leads to a reduction in the number of health plans also reduces the competitive nature of the marketplace, which in itself may be a bad outcome for purchasers/payers and the public. Healthy competition among providers of any service is critically important to the success of any market-oriented industry, and this is no less true when considering the managed-care health insurance industry. A purchaser/payer who goes into the marketplace seeking health insurance and is confronted with a limited choice of competing health insurance plans is less able to engage these plans in a marketplace dialogue on price and quality of services than that purchaser/payer would be if there were a wide variety of plans competing among themselves for the business.

There are obviously major antitrust and monopoly issues to be considered in regard to consolidation. The formal legal and regulatory mechanisms in this area move so slowly that significant reshaping of the managed-care health insurance industry may take place before the formal governmental protections are able to come into effect (Kuttner, 1997). Also, because there are very few legal or regulatory precedents in this area of the health care industry, those formal governmental protections may be even slower to come into effect than in a well-established industry.

Impact of Managed Care on the Provider System

It has been stressed in this chapter that managed care is really a series of subunits that are linked together by a series of legal, contractual, and organizational mechanisms. Therefore, a change in any one subunit tends to bring about changes in other subunits that are linked to it. This means that any change in the methods for financing health care through health insurance (such as the growth of *per capita* HMO insurance mechanisms) will cause changes in the provider system as well.

In practice, what has happened among provider systems has been a growth of new organizational forms and new operating principles with regard to the provision of care, in response to change on the financing side (Table 6.4). This has led to the growth of larger groups of physicians working together, groups of physicians entering into joint ventures of one kind or another with hospitals, a drive for increased efficiency of operation, and an overall rethinking about the most appropriate organizational structure for the delivery of personal health care services.

The rethinking may have both positive and negative effects. On the positive side, the reorganization of the provider system may lead to greater efficiency and better effectiveness of that system and, therefore, to better patient care with improved outcomes. This scenario suggests that the previous organizational structure of health care under a fee-for-service stimulus may not have been the most efficient or effective and that managed-care-driven changes in the delivery system are a distinct improvement.

On the negative side, the drive for increased efficiency of operation, the emphasis on providing fewer services rather than more, and the overwhelming concern about economic issues may all serve to dampen or reduce the humane and compassionate personal aspects of health care as it was previously delivered in the United States. Under this scenario, the provider system for health services in the United States may become more coldly efficient and effective in an organizational sense, but it may be less satisfying

Table 6.4. Provider Concerns Under Managed Care

- enter into contracts carefully
- know practice strengths and weaknesses
- use clinical protocols and other control guidelines
- establish performance goals and measures of success or failure
- ensure that management information systems are adequate
- continually monitor results and respond to information
- reduce inpatient utilization
- be cost conscientious
- emphasize primary care
- monitor and manage risk
- maintain provider relationships
- enhance consumer controls and satisfaction

in a personal and psychological sense to the people receiving services.

A point to remember here is that changes in the way in which health care providers are paid are not merely financial or economic in nature. They also drive organizational changes, and those organizational changes may be either for the better or the worse, depending upon how they are developed.

Medicare/Medicaid in Managed Care

Although much has been said about the impact of managed care in reducing health-care expenditures for employers and the private sector, the major impact of managed care may actually be felt on the two major public sector financing programs in health care, Medicare and Medicaid. The impact on each of these programs may be quite different, given the different nature of the constituencies they serve and the specifics of their financing. They have in common the fact that they will both be impacted in a major way by the use of managed care.

With regard to the Medicare program, the federal Health Care Financing Administration (HCFA) had wanted to have approximately half of all Medicare beneficiaries enrolled in managed-risk/managed-care programs by the year 2007. With Medicare program expenditures increasing at a rapid rate HCFA felt that managed care should play a major part in the long-term solution of Medicare's financial woes.

The implications for patients served under Medicare are potentially good and bad (Wagner, 1996). On the positive side, Medicare beneficiaries may actually receive more benefits and services (particularly a much wider range of pharmaceutical benefits than are now available to them) and may also have their patterns of care and the outcomes of that care more closely monitored and controlled. Medicare beneficiaries may actually get better services and may have more confidence in the care that they are receiving from their providers, as that care may be more closely observed and measured.

On the negative side for Medicare beneficiaries is the effect of consolidation among the provider health care systems mentioned earlier. Medicare beneficiaries who may previously have been treated personally,

warmly, and humanely by an individual solo-practice physician with whom they have had a very close personal relationship may find that solo-practice physicians are becoming a thing of the past, replaced by comparative supermarkets of physicians whose hallmarks are efficiency of a less personal kind. Moving into a Medicare-managed-risk/managed-care program may mean that elderly Medicare patients have less time to talk with their physicians, less personal connection, and less personal involvement than they had under the previous fee-for-service arrangement.

Over the past few years, a number of corporate providers of Medicare managed-care services (including, for example, Pacificare Health Systems through its Secure Horizons product) have determined that federal reimbursement is inadequate to provide Medicare managed-care services in certain of their markets. A subsequent reduction in availability of such products in certain areas of the country has occurred with realignment of the marketplace in these regions. Less-concentrated population centers and particularly rural areas have been hardest hit. The availability of adequate numbers of contracting providers and the capability to achieve a critical mass in marketplace enrollments combined with federal reimbursement levels will continue to be a critical factor determining the geographic reach of the Medicare managed-care program.

In the same fashion, Medicaid programs around the country are moving very rapidly to use managed care for their recipients' care, and it seems clear that the impact on Medicaid recipients will also be quite marked, if different from the impact on Medicare beneficiaries (See Table 6.2). In the case of Medicaid, changes from the increased use of managed care are more likely to be positive than negative.

In the past, Medicaid recipients generally received their care in a somewhat random and scattered fashion from local governmental hospitals, clinics, and emergency rooms, interested physicians, and a wide variety of free clinics and other community organizations. There usually was very little cohesion among the providers and very little coordination in the patterns of care being given.

Under a managed-care structure, Medicaid recipients will have a firm and formal connection with a medical group or medical provider and will be required to have a designated primary care physician as the coordinator of all of their services. There will be a formal set of required services that must be provided on a regular basis, and there will be an organized method for determining whether these services were actually provided to Medicaid recipients. This will mean that, perhaps for the first time, Medicaid recipients will develop longer-term relationships with a primary care physician, will be mandated to receive a predetermined package of services, and will have outcomes that are measured in a formal fashion. In a very real sense, managed care presents a great opportunity to improve the quality of care received by Medicaid recipients across the country.

Mental Health and Managed Care

One of the most interesting areas of application of managed care, and also one of the most rapidly expanding, is the implementation of managed care for mental and behavioral health services. If the use of managed care is increasing in general health services across the country, it can only be said that managed mental health services are increasing at an almost explosive rate.

The reasons for the increased use of managed-care mechanisms to organize mental health benefits are fairly obvious to any student of the provision of mental health services in the past. The general criticism has been made of mental health services over the years that they were relatively unstandardized, poorly supervised, and without any meaningful measures of results or outcomes. It was also generally believed that there was an excessive use of expensive inpatient mental health services, the utilization of which was governed by the availability of health insurance payments for inpatient services.

The shift to managed care in mental health services is causing significant concern among both patients and providers of mental health services and is also forcing patients and providers to learn a new set of procedures and policies in obtaining and in providing mental health services. Rather than a wide-open patient-initiated selection of mental health practitioners, the managed behavioral health plans require beneficiaries to first use a "triage" process, which attempts to determine the severity of the problem and the most appropriate form of treatment. The triage process usually also arranges the connection for the patient with what is believed to be the most appropriate form of treatment. This means that an individual may no longer be free to pick the psychiatrist of his or her choice, call and make an appointment, and begin therapy for what may be an indefinite period of time. Now all of those previous forms of behavior are organized and managed by the managed mental health organization itself. That organization then also attempts to monitor results of treatment and determine outcomes.

From the patient's point of view, this means that there will be much more formal and supervised systems of determining the severity of the initial problem and a much more standardized process for obtaining care; there also will be a very deliberate attempt on the part of the managed-care organization to determine the credentials of the mental health practitioners before they are accepted as providers by the plan. For their part, providers of mental health services may now find themselves dependent upon the managed-care plan for a flow of initial patients to their practices and may find their ability to provide care limited by the number of encounters that are authorized by some other seemingly artificial time constraints. Mental health practitioners see this as an imposition on their independence and their clinical judgment, and, for the most part, mental health professionals are not very positive or supportive in their views about managed mental health programs.

Conflict of Interest in Managed Care

One of the most important issues facing managed care in the future is the question of conflict of interest among the various participants in any type of managed-care system (Gray, 1997). The conflict is centered around the need to reduce the use of various health services, products, and procedures. The economic survival and prosperity of all of the major players in managed care depends upon the imposition of tight controls on the use of health services, with the implication that services have been overused in the past and that this overusage must be eliminated.

Although there is general agreement that many types of health services have been overused in the past and that unnecessary health services have been provided, it is not always clear exactly which of those services have been used in excess (and, therefore, need reduction) and which services have not. The application of across-the-board methods to reduce the use of health services in general will affect both those services that may have been overused and overprovided in the past as well as those services that may not have been overused and overprovided. The net result may be that *all* health services utilization may be reduced, both those services that needed reduction and those that did not. The end result may be that patients who need some services may not get them in the future.

For the most part, purchasers/payers and health insurance plans have been unwilling to concede or even discuss the possibility of a conflict of interest affecting their participation in managed care, but increasingly physicians have been more vocal about the difficult situation in which they find themselves. Indeed, because physicians are directly involved with their patients on a face-to-face basis, it is very likely that the issues of conflict of interest will be most apparent in this part of any managed-care system. It is also very obvious that the discussion of conflict of interest in managed care will most likely be led by physicians, as it is there that the stresses and strains are felt most acutely (Kerr, 1996). As ethical principles and economic pressures begin to impede on each other more actively around the provision of physician services, that is where the most active discussion of this important issue will start. It certainly will not end there, however, because there is a fundamental conflict of interest throughout the entire managed-health care structure.

Protection of the Public

A final issue of importance to the future of managed care is the development of better mechanisms for the protection of patients and the public interest. At the present time, it appears that individual patients and the public in general are somewhat at the mercy of a managed-care structure that is consolidating very rapidly, from purchasers/payers, through health insurance plans, to provider systems (Bodenheimer, 1996). The only part of the managed care structure that is not consolidating itself (and, therefore, is better able to exert itself in the new economic marketplace) is the area of individual patients and the public in general.

For most individual people/patients who must make their way through the managed-care structure in a relatively unaided fashion, the complexities of managed care leave them very vulnerable and relatively unprotected. From the time when purchasers/payers select a health insurance plan under which the employees will be covered (sometimes without choice or options and other times with options that are not clearly explained), the individual is at a significant disadvantage because of the relative lack of information, experience, and sophistication. Later, in dealing with individual health insurance plans and their consumer relations departments, which are established ostensibly for the purpose of service to plan enrollees, the individual person/patient is also at a disadvantage, as he or she is dealing with a health plan staff member who is much more experienced and knowledgeable about the details of the plan's operation. The plan employee may also have been given the specific direction to constrain or reduce the utilization of services and may have the best interest of the health plan uppermost in mind—not necessarily the best interest of the patient (as seen by the patient).

Finally, when an individual person/patient must deal with a physician or a medical group in an attempt to get additional services, the group's process for approving or denying services may not be clearly described and may be implemented in widely varying forms and with different effects, depending upon the patient and/or the physician involved. All of these circumstances tend to make many members of managed-care health plans suspicious and distrustful even when the plans and the physicians are actually doing as much as they can to provide appropriate service. The sense of vulnerability among individuals when they are confronted with the various aspects of the machinery of managed care may tend to make them feel that they have fewer options and less power than they may really have.

One response to this sense of isolation and vulnerability among members of managed-care plans has been the passage of a series of legislative and regulatory efforts by the Congress, state legislatures, and state departments of insurance/corporations/industry to "protect" the interests of the public. Legislation mandating the number of days that a woman may remain in the hospital after a normal delivery and legislation prohibiting the performance of outpatient surgery for a specific condition (for example, mastectomy for breast cancer) are certainly well-intentioned, but raise a serious question about their wisdom. Nevertheless, until patients/people organize to more strongly protect themselves from the apparent imbalance of power, and until purchasers/payers and managed-care health insurance plans do much more in the way of direct communication and assistance to patients and the public, the only channel of recourse available to the patients/public will be through laws or regulation. It is in the best interest of patients and the public to organize into aggressive consumer protection organizations, and it is equally in the best interest of purchasers/payers and health plans to better serve the members of managed-care health plans to prevent further legislative or legal overreaction. Until that time, one can expect to see much more in the way of legal, legislative, or regulatory solutions governing the organization and the conduct of managed care.

MANAGED CARE AND THE FUTURE OF HEALTH CARE

Managed care represents an array of arrangements and mechanisms designed in one form or another to organize health care services. New forms of managed care are still emerging, and the conflicting political, economic, and social currents in our society are constantly influencing our assessments of the nature and ramifications of managed care. These are dynamic, not static, currents, and the pendulum of change will always be in motion.

The critical assessment of our managed-care experience continues unabated. Recognizing that the evolution of managed care to this point has not yielded an ideal health care system only reinforces the need to further assess which managed-care mechanisms are

effective in improving access, cost and payment, and patient and provider satisfaction (Veeder & Peebles-Wilkins, 2001). The accumulation of empirical evidence and perspectives has increasingly allowed for the assessment of various managed-care mechanisms and their contribution to improving the operation of the health care system (Kongstvedt, 2000a; Kongstvedt, 2000b). In addition, an increasingly sophisticated consumer base combined with changes in medical technology (particularly information systems technology through the Internet) has greatly enhanced the role of the consumer in improving the function of the nation's health care system and of managed-care organizations and services (Coddington, Fischer, Moore, & Clarke 2000; Goldsmith, 2000). The increasing sophistication of consumers and the backlash on the part of providers to managed-care methodologies attempted thus far combined with increasing cost pressures and national policy concerns on the part of government mandate continual refinement of managed-care systems and organizations and places tremendous pressure on those managing the nation's health-care system to find more acceptable and successful approaches to organizing these services.

Some of the complex issues faced in assessing the role of managed care are listed in Table 6.5. These concerns include the most fundamental factors involved in designing health care systems: How do we influence, and limit, provider and consumer behavior? Where do we draw the lines in rationing services? How do we collect information to monitor and control behavior? How do we provide leadership in the

Table 6.5. Complex Issues in Managed Care

- controlling physician behavior
- controlling consumer behavior
- rationing/caps on care
- monitoring care and reacting
- information collection and use
- administrative and medical leadership
- encouraging competitive markets
- protecting against underutilization
- measuring costs and ensuring access
- enhancing provider, payor, and consumer satisfaction

system? How do we assess costs? How do we promote both provider and consumer satisfaction while controlling use and costs? These are complex questions that require us to address the most basic issues and moral concerns in providing health care.

The future of managed care will be different from the past. Experimentation is ongoing. Some paths may prove politically, socially, or economically unacceptable. The use of information technology, in particular, will radically change our ability to measure, monitor, control, compare, and influence the behavior of all participants in health care. Dramatic technological change will also radically affect the incentives, alternatives, and costs of nearly all aspects of health

care, and increasing recognition of the need for more prevention, combined with a greater ability to actually prevent illness, will challenge the focus on individuals versus populations.

The ultimate forms of managed care arrangements that are implemented and, perhaps, new alternative health care systems in the future remain to be determined. But there is little likelihood that the payers of health care will allow any return to the open-ended systems and plans of the past. The challenge for managed care is to find the balance between choices and control that promotes efficiency, contains costs, enhances satisfaction, and assures quality.

References

Bodenheimer, T. (1996). The HMO backlash . . . righteous or reactionary? *New England Journal of Medicine, 335,* 1601–1604.

Coddington, D. C., Fischer, E. A., Moore, K. D., & Clarke, R. L. (2000). *Beyond managed care: How consumers and technology are changing the future of health care.* San Francisco: Jossey-Bass.

Drake, D. (1997). Managed care: A product of market dynamics. *Journal of the American Medical Association, 277,* 311–314.

Enthoven, A., & Singer, S. (1996). Managed competition and California's health care economy. *Health Affairs, 15,* 40–57.

Fox, P. (1997). An overview of managed care. In P. Kongstvedt (Ed.), *Essentials of managed health care,* Aspen Publishers: Gaithersburg, MD.

Goldsmith, J. (2000). The Internet and managed care: A new wave of innovation. *Health Affairs, 19,* 42–56.

Gray, B. (1997). Trust and trustworthy care in the managed care era. *Health Affairs, 16,* 34–49.

Jensen, G., Morrisey, M., Gaffney, S., & Liston, D. (1997). The new dominance of managed care: Insurance trends in the 1990s. *Health Affairs, 16,* 125–136.

Kerr, E. (1996). Quality assurance in capitated physician groups. *Journal of the American Medical Association, 276,* 1236–1239.

Kongstvedt, P. R. (2000a). *Managed health care handbook* (4th ed.). Gaithersburg, MD: Aspen Publishers.

Kongstvedt, P. R. (2000b). *Essentials of managed health care* (4th ed.). Gaithersburg, MD: Aspen Publishers.

Kuttner, R. (1997). Physician-operated networks and the new anti-trust guidelines. *New England Journal of Medicine, 336,* 386–391.

Miller, R., & Luft, H. (1994). Managed care plans: Characteristics, growth, and premium performance. *Annual Review of Public Health, 15,* 437–459.

Veeder, N. W., & Peebles-Wilkins, W. C. (2001). Managed care services: Policy, programs, and research. New York: Oxford University Press.

Wagner, E. (1996). The promise and performance of HMOs in improving outcomes in older adults. *Journal of the American Geriatrics Society, 44,* 1251–1257.

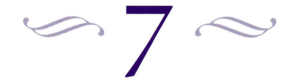

C H A P T E R

7

Private Health Insurance and Employee Benefits

Gary Whitted

Chapter Topics

- Insurance Concepts
- A Brief History of United States Health Insurance
- Alternate Health Insurance Taxonomies
- The Commercial Health Insurance Industry
- Blue Cross and Blue Shield Plans
- Health Maintenance Organizations
- Private Health Insurance as a Financing Mechanism
- Health-Related Insurance Programs
- Funding Alternative for Group Health-Related Insurance
- Core Medical Employee Benefits
- Changes Facing the Health Insurance Industry

Learning Objectives

Upon completing this chapter, the reader should be able to:

- Understand the history, structure, and role of health insurance
- Appreciate the commercial health insurance industry's size, objectives, products, and marketplace
- Identify the impact of managed care on private health insurance
- Differentiate various health insurance provisions, terms, conditions, and product types
- Understand related insurance products
- Appreciate the challenges facing this industry in the future

After Medicare, private health insurance is the most prevalent source of financing for the United States health care system. Few other industrialized countries maintain systems of private medical insurance programs that even approximate those established in the United States. Private health insurance coverage is by far the most comprehensive source of medical care financing for Americans, and it continues to play a pivotal role in influencing the direction and structure of the United States medical care system.

The term *health insurance* often is employed to mean a wide array of health care financing mechanisms: The social insurance of Medicare, the public assistance of Medicaid, the "self-insurance" techniques adopted by large employers, and the managed-care programs of health maintenance organizations (HMOs) and preferred provider organizations (PPOs). This chapter expands on the concepts in Chapter 5, focusing extensively on the private sector. Because health insurance and employee medical benefits are inextricably linked for most American families, this chapter will often look at these two concepts together, even though many medical benefits programs are not "insurance" in the technical or legal sense.

INSURANCE CONCEPTS

Central to any definition of *insurance* is the notion of risk. One standard insurance text defines *risk* as "the possibility of an adverse deviation from a desired outcome that is expected or hoped for," or more simply as a "possibility of loss" (Vaughn & Elliott, 1978). Insurance is a mechanism for managing or controlling the financial exposure to this risk through two basic principles: (1) transferring or shifting risk from an individual to a group, and (2) sharing losses on some equitable basis by all members of the group. Depending on individuals' or employers' preferences about how much risk they want to assume, as well as their various abilities to withstand the economic consequences of the losses, the amount and type of insurance required can vary substantially.

When health insurance began in the United States, it was conceptually similar to most other types of insurance—for example, auto insurance. In both cases,

insurance was purchased to protect an individual from an expensive loss: hospital care or a badly damaged automobile. As private health insurance evolved to cover more people and a wider variety of medical expenses, however, it began to assume characteristics very dissimilar from traditional forms of insurance by violating certain implied rules.

1. A *loss* is supposed to be something out of the ordinary, as well as something to be avoided. However, ill health is not a substantially abnormal event for most people, and in many cases, the loss being indemnified (for example, a physician office visit) is not necessarily an event to be dreaded.
2. Losses are intended to be fairly independent events. In contrast, the very nature of infectious illness (or, in the extreme, an epidemic) implies a great degree of dependency among insureds' losses.
3. The loss should be of such financial magnitude that it is realistically unbudgetable for most insureds. The growth of so-called "first-dollar" base/major medical health plans (prominent in the 1970s and early 1980s) directly violated this tenet. Even today, providing insurance coverage for items such as pharmaceuticals or vision care stretches the limits of the "insurance" principle.

Thus, it is not surprising that health insurance has become a fundamentally different product than most other forms of insurance. And many health care observers have noted that these unique characteristics of health insurance, when added to the economic structures of the medical care marketplace, have made health insurance a chief contributor to the continued rapid growth of health expenditures in the United States. Ironically, the presence and growth of health insurance in the 1950s and 1960s provided a financial foundation for much of the medical-industrial complex that now fuels medical expenses. And the presence of health insurance creates a catch-22 situation in which the existence of the insurance mechanism (often distorted to include first-dollar coverage of non-catastrophic expenses) stimulates demand and increases medical care prices, thereby raising the cost of health care and encouraging even greater insistence on more comprehensive coverage.

A BRIEF HISTORY OF UNITED STATES HEALTH INSURANCE

The history of medical expense insurance in the United States, discussed briefly in the previous chapter, goes back to the middle of the nineteenth century, when in 1850 the Franklin Health Insurance Company of Massachusetts offered coverage for bodily injuries that did not result in death (Health Insurance Association of America, 1991). Ten years later, the Travelers Insurance Companies first extended health coverage in a form similar to today's insurance. By 1866, sixty other insurance companies were writing forms of such coverage. At the end of the century, accident and life insurers were writing health insurance policies, primarily to indemnify against loss of income and for certain acute illnesses. The real beginning of modern private health insurance took place in 1929, however, when a group of teachers made a contract with Baylor Hospital in Dallas, Texas, to provide coverage against certain hospital expenses, thereby starting the first Blue Cross plan.

During the 1930s and until the wartime period of the 1940s, health insurance coverage grew rather slowly, in terms of both the insured population and the types of coverage offered. In 1940, insurers provided some form of medical expense protection to 12 million people, which was nine percent of the total United States population (Table 7.1). A series of legal and tax developments in the mid-1940s and early 1950s provided nontrivial inducements for both employers and employees to purchase comprehensive health insurance benefits (Congressional Budget Office, Congress of the United States, 1991; Feldstein & Friedman, 1977; Greenspan & Vogel, 1980). In 1942, only thirty-seven insurers wrote group health insurance coverage; by 1951, this number had climbed to 212 (Congressional Budget Office, Congress of the United States, 1991). By 1950, the number of people covered by the nation's health insurers had climbed to nearly 77 million, or fifty-three percent of the United States population. Fueled by the strong union gains of the 1950s and 1960s, collectively bargained employee benefits packages quickly became the norm throughout industrial America.

In 1960, 123 million Americans held some type of health insurance protection, generating about $5 billion in payments and accounting for nearly twenty-one percent of the financing for personal health care expenditures (see Tables 7.1 and 7.2). During the 1960s, health insurance coverage was expanded to an additional 36 million Americans, while health insur-

Table 7.1. Historical Distribution of Covered Persons, by Type of Private Health Insurance

Year	Net Number of Persons with Private Health Insurance (Millions)	Percentage Distribution		
		Commercial Insurance Companies	Blue Cross/ Blue Shield Plans	HMOs and Self-Funded Plans
1940	12.0	31%	50%	19%
1950	76.6	46%	48%	5%
1960	122.5	56%	47%	5%
1970	158.8	52%	43%	5%
1980	187.4	47%	38%	15%
1990	181.7	35%	30%	36%

Note: Percentages may not sum to 100%, as persons with duplicate coverages are counted multiple times.

SOURCE: *Source Book of Health Insurance Data, 1996* (p. 41), Health Insurance Association of America, 1997, Washington, DC: Author.

Table 7.2.   Private Health Insurance as a Health Care Financing Vehicle

Year	Private Health Insurance Expenditures (Billions)	Per Capital Health Insurance Expenditures	Private Health Insurance as a Percent of Total Personal Health Care Expenditures
1960	$ 5.0	$26	21%
1970	$ 14.8	$69	23%
1980	$ 62.0	$264	29%
1985	$113.8	$460	30%
1990	$201.8	$776	33%
1995	$276.8	$1,014	31%

SOURCE: "National Health Expenditures, 1995," by K. R. Levit, et al., 1996, *Health Care Financing Review, 18*(1), Table II, p. 205.

ance payments tripled to $15 billion, representing more than twenty-three percent of total United States personal health care expenditures. The inauguration of Medicare and Medicaid in 1965 greatly expanded Americans' protection against catastrophic medical expenses for our most vulnerable citizens, the elderly and indigent. But these two programs also gave substantial impetus to the notion that affordable access to the health care system was a right for Americans.

The decade of the 1970s witnessed another 29 million Americans added to the roster of the health-insured population, as the health insurance industry plateaued in terms of the depth of medical coverage, while introducing new forms of health insurance protection (principally dental and prescription drug insurance). By 1980, health insurance paid twenty-nine percent of the nation's personal health care bill, more than $62 billion. Although the 1980s saw proportionately slower growth in the number of Americans with private health insurance protection than did earlier decades, private health insurance expenditures more than tripled to $202 billion by 1990, even though neither the depth nor breadth of coverage increased nearly as dramatically as in previous eras. By 1995, private health insurance and employee benefit programs were responsible for financing nearly one-third of all personal medical care expenditures (see Table 7.2).

Despite an increase from 12 million people protected by private health insurance in 1940 to about two-thirds of the total United States population covered now, political concern has escalated about the number of individuals without any financial protection for health care expenses (Bilheimer and Colby, 2001).

The substantial number of Americans made vulnerable to the economic consequences of serious medical illness (or for low-income individuals, even relatively routine medical care) has become a potent political cause as the United States enters the twenty-first century. Lack of health insurance protection is greatest for the unemployed, minority, younger-age, and low-income/moderate-income segments of the United States population.

Yet even among the employed population under age sixty-five, many are without health insurance protection, due principally to lapses of coverage between jobs, the preexisting condition clauses of most employee benefits programs, and lack of benefits for employees in many small businesses and the self-employed (Table 7.3). Indeed, two-thirds of the uninsured population are in families of full-year, steadily employed workers, most of whom are employed full-time. Nearly half of the uninsured workers are self-employed or are employed in small companies with fewer than twenty-five employees (Health Insurance Association of America, 1997). Employees working in small establishments are particularly vulnerable to inadequate or nonexistent health insurance coverage.

Table 7.3 Health Care Coverage for Persons Under 65 Years of Age, According to Type of Coverage and Selected Characteristics: United States, Selected Years

Characteristic	Private Insurance Total		Private Insurance Obtained through Workplace		Medicaid		Not Covered	
	1984	1997	1984	1997	1984	1997	1984	1997
	Number in millions							
Total	157.5	165.8	141.8	152.5	14.0	22.9	29.8	41.0
	Percent of population							
Total, age adjusted	77.1	70.9	69.2	65.1	6.7	9.6	14.3	17.4
Age								
Under 18 years	72.6	66.1	66.5	61.4	11.9	18.4	13.9	14.0
18–44 years	76.5	69.4	69.6	64.4	5.1	6.6	17.1	22.4
45–64 years	83.3	79.0	71.8	70.8	3.4	4.6	9.6	12.4
Race								
White	80.1	74.3	72.0	68.0	4.6	7.5	13.4	16.3
Black	59.2	56.1	53.3	53.7	18.9	20.5	20.0	20.2
Asian or Pacific Islander	70.9	68.2	64.4	60.5	9.1	9.4	18.0	19.3
All Hispanic	57.1	47.9	52.9	44.5	12.2	16.0	29.1	34.3

ALTERNATE HEALTH INSURANCE TAXONOMIES

Most of what falls into the category "health insurance" is a combination of true insurance and employee benefits. One methodology for gaining an overview of health insurance is to subdivide the general area using different criteria. First, the principal insurance vehicles provide benefits associated with ill health: (1) basic employee benefits (primarily medical, dental, vision, and prescription drug coverage); (2) disability (short- and long-term insurance offered as part of many employee benefits programs, as well as compulsory temporary disability insurance mandated by five states); and (3) workers' compensation. Employers pay for some or all of each category of insurance, with the first type of insurance reimbursing most of the expenditures attributed to health insurance.

A second major categorization of health insurance is by the type of organization furnishing the coverage. First and foremost among such organizations are the approximately eight hundred insurance carriers that comprise the commercial health insurance industry. Second are Blue Cross and Blue Shield plans. While technically offering insurance, the Blues historically maintained a different tax status from that of the commercials. (The Tax Reform Act of 1986, PL 99514, removed the federal tax exemption for Blue Cross and Blue Shield organizations engaged in providing commercial-type insurance.) Third, health maintenance organizations (HMOs) offer a form of health insurance, although not in the same legal definition as either the Blues or the commercials. HMOs, in addition to retaining different tax and regulatory structures than those of either the Blues or commercials, differ from those two entities in one very fundamental sense: HMOs are not guaranteeing to *reimburse* the insured for medical expenses. Rather, their obligation to the insured is more direct: to actually provide medical services to them. A fourth major entity in furnishing health insurance is employers (primarily large corporations) that self-fund or partially self-fund employee benefits for workers and their families. Although declining in importance, unions are a fifth type of health insurance sponsor. Finally, corporations and unions sometimes jointly sponsor and administer Taft-Hartley health and welfare funds.

A third taxonomy of health insurance is by funding mechanism: (1) fully insured, (2) partially insured, and (3) self-funded or self-insured. The funding mechanisms of health insurance should not be confused with the three principal administrative intermediaries: (1) insurers, (2) third-party administrators (TPAs), and (3) self-administration. The market shares for these types of intermediaries have changed drastically in past time frames.

THE COMMERCIAL HEALTH INSURANCE INDUSTRY

There are several ways to describe the commercial health insurance industry. Perhaps the most fundamental distinction is between *mutual* and *stock* insurers. Mutual insurance companies (examples are Prudential and Metropolitan) essentially are owned by their policyholders, in contrast to stock insurance companies (for example, Aetna/U.S. Healthcare and United HealthCare), which are owned in the more traditional corporate fashion by stockholders. Within each type of insurer are so-called "multiline" carriers and "single-line" insurers. Multiline insurers offer life insurance and accident and health insurance, as well as property/casualty insurance (for example, auto, homeowners, workers' compensation, comprehensive general liability, and so on). Many multiline insurers also operate businesses that offer a range of financial products and services, particularly in the pension and investment areas. In contrast, single-line insurers usually offer the majority of their insurance products in the life insurance, property/casualty, or health insurance/employee benefits arena.

Despite the approximately 800 companies that participate in writing health insurance and/or providing employee benefit programs, the commercial health insurance industry is moderately concentrated. Because most of the major United States self-funded employee benefits programs are administered by the largest accident and health insurers, the concentration of the total generic health insurance/employee benefits industry is even more pronounced than indicated by accident and health insurance premium volume alone. Use of the word *premium* generally refers only to true insured products, not to partially insured or self-funded medical payments that flow through insurance companies via other administrative arrangements. These latter monies are often described as "premium-equivalents" and usually are several times the size of true premiums.

BLUE CROSS AND BLUE SHIELD PLANS

As noted earlier, Blue Cross plans initiated the modern era of private health insurance in 1929. Throughout the early portion of their history, Blue Cross plans focused attention on medical insurance for hospital costs, and Blue Cross itself was closely affiliated with the hospital industry. Approximately ten years after its establishment, Blue Shield began offering medical insurance protection for physicians' services. As with Blue Cross, Blue Shield was loosely affiliated with organized medicine because of its focus on insuring physician expenditures.

Since their inceptions, many Blue Cross and Blue Shield plans have merged their activities, becoming essentially a single insurance entity in a state. By the 1980s, however, a number of Blue Cross and Blue Shield plans reversed this posture and divorced themselves from each other, in a few cases becoming bitter rivals. In recent years, the national Blue Cross and Blue Shield Association, which heretofore had provided only a minimal amount of integration among its member constituents, has become more aggressive in attempting to marshal the resources of individual plans (for example, in the area of centralized claims processing). This cooperation has been necessary in order to compete effectively with large national commercial insurance companies for the business of employers operating in more than one state. The Blue Cross and Blue Shield Association also developed a national HMO network for the same reason.

Unlike commercial insurance companies, which are regulated in most states by a state insurance department, most Blue Cross and Blue Shield plans are subject to special enabling state legislation. In addition to the close affiliations of the Blues with hospital and physician providers, the Blues have differentiated themselves historically from commercial insurers by establishing premium levels using a community-rating methodology (in contrast to the experience rating most often used by commercial insurers) (Hall, 2001).

Another key area of differentiation historically between the Blues and commercial insurers is the former's adoption of service benefits (that is, reimbursement for the total costs of covered benefits), rather than the indemnity benefits (that is, payment of a fixed sum for a covered benefit) of commercial insurers. Today, however, particularly for group insurance, commercial insurers offer service benefits; major exceptions are some individual and supplementary policies, as well as specialty insurance (for example, cancer insurance).

One final point of distinction for the Blues is their traditional reluctance to underwrite quite as rigidly as commercial carriers, particularly with respect to refusing coverage for entire industry groups or for individuals. In some states, for some populations, the Blues are the only health insurer of any significant size. All of these historical differences between the Blues and commercial insurers, however, are rapidly disappearing.

The 1990s witnessed profound changes in the structure and organization of Blue Cross and Blue Shield plans. First, the number of Blues plans decreased steadily. This consolidation has occurred primarily due to mergers between Blue Cross and Blue Shield plans. Second, pseudoconsolidation is occurring on a marketing or administrative basis, as Blues plans collaborate formally (but without legal mergers), usually on a regional basis. Third, in an attempt to compete effectively for the business of multistate employers, Blues plans throughout the country are cooperating to market and administer their services jointly. Fourth, many Blues plans have converted, or are seriously planning to convert, to for-profit status. (In some cases, Blues plans are only creating separate for-profit subsidiaries.) The rationale for this conversion is primarily to gain access to capital markets for the extensive investments needed to pursue managed-care initiatives. Fifth, Blues plans will continue to emphasize managed care with greater zeal than historically has been the case.

HEALTH MAINTENANCE ORGANIZATIONS

Although coining of the term *health maintenance organizations (HMO)* was attributed to Dr. Paul Ellwood in the early 1970s, these insurance-like organizations have been in existence for over a half-century. In 1929, the Ross-Loos Clinic in Los Angeles was the first generally recognized HMO (or prepaid group practice) to use the pre-Ellwood term; however, one can argue that the true roots of prepaid group practice began at the Mayo Clinic in the late 1800s.

Beginning with Kaiser's coverage of the health needs associated with workers building the Grand Coulee Dam in the 1930s, HMOs grew relatively slowly until the Nixon administration sparked new interest in these providers of predominantly group medical benefits. Enrollment has been strongest since the mid-1980s (Table 7.4), fueled by employers' dissatisfaction with the escalating costs of their employee medical benefits programs and the concomitant published research demonstrating the cost-containment success of many HMOs. Growth of HMOs was also stimulated by the HMO Act of 1973 (PL 93-222) and its subsequent amendments. These statutes required employers with more than twenty-five employees to offer an HMO option if a local, federally qualified HMO so mandated. The legislation also required employers to contribute toward the HMO premium of its employees an amount equal to that contributed toward indemnity plan premiums—the so-called "equal contribution" rule.

Table 7.4. HMO Growth, 1970–1999

Year	Number of Plans	Enrollment (Millions)
1970	N/A	2.9
1975	N/A	5.7
1980	235	9.1
1985	391	18.8
1990	553	33.6
1999	643	81.3

Table 7.5. Private Health Insurance by Health Maintenance Organization (HMO) and Other Types of Coverage According to Selected Characteristics: United States, Selected Years

| | Private Health Insurance | | | |
| | Health Maintenance Organization | | Other | |
Characteristic	1989	1997	1989	1997
	Number of persons in millions			
Total	45.1	76.5	140.2	111.5
	Percent of population			
Total, age adjusted	18.4	29.1	58.0	41.2
Age				
Under 18 years	20.1	29.9	51.7	36.2
18–44 years	20.3	31.4	55.2	38.1
45–64 years	17.6	31.3	65.0	47.7
65 years or more	10.4	12.5	67.0	57.0
Race				
White	19.1	29.3	61.4	44.7
Black	19.7	27.9	37.2	25.8
Asian or Pacific Islander	24.1	35.2	45.0	30.5
All Hispanic	18.8	25.4	33.3	20.4
Geographic region				
Northeast	20.1	37.7	61.4	36.2
Midwest	20.2	25.6	61.6	51.5
South	11.7	23.6	60.3	43.2
West	25.7	34.9	46.6	29.8

In the 1990s, HMO growth slowed somewhat, due to several factors (Table 7.5). First, the emergence of competing alternative delivery systems, such as preferred provider organizations and, more recently, point-of-service managed-care options, has provided employers with cost-effective, middle-of-the-road medical benefit plan options. Principal among the attractions to employers of these non-HMO options is the enhanced employee freedom of choice regarding providers, particularly physicians. Second, the wave of enthusiasm for HMOs regarding their potential cost-containment prowess was tempered when many

HMOs' premium increases reached levels nearly as great as those of indemnity insurers and the Blues. In addition, research findings (aided by the gut feelings of many large employers) indicted HMOs for "cream skimming" the healthier risks toward the HMO, supposedly leaving the remaining indemnity medical plan options saddled with the "sicker" insured (Reschovsky, Kemper, & Tu, 2000). Finally, for reasons of administrative ease and fear of the financial and liability consequences of dealing with potentially insolvent HMOs, some employers have substantially trimmed the numbers of HMOs offered to employees, particularly beginning in 1995 when the dual-choice mandating provision of the 1973 HMO Act no longer applied to employers due to legislative amendments enacted in 1988. This same legislation also permitted greater employer flexibility in determining their required contributions to HMO premiums.

As discussed in detail in Chapter 6, HMOs generally are characterized by their form of organization according to principal structures: (1) group, (2) staff, (3) independent practice association (IPA), and (4) network. In group plans (Kaiser is the most prominent one), a physician medical group contracts with an entity that is financially responsible for covering enrollees. For example, the Kaiser Permanente Medical Care Program is actually a combination of three different groups: (1) The Permanente Medical Groups (providing professional services), (2) Kaiser Foundation Hospitals (providing hospital care), and (3) Kaiser Foundation Health Plans (providing administrative and financial services). In the network model, the HMO contracts with two or more dependent group practices. Staff model HMOs (such as Group Health Cooperative of Puget Sound) employ most primary care physicians and major specialty physicians on a full-time, salaried basis. Hospital services and the rarer physician specialties are arranged through separate contracts. IPA-model HMOs forge the same types of hospital arrangements as staff-model HMOs, but physicians' services are established with a relatively large number of generally small or medium-sized group practices, with physicians receiving some type of discounted fee-for-service payment from the HMO, rather than the salaried reimbursement of staff-model HMO physicians.

As stated earlier, HMOs fundamentally differ from the true insurers (that is, commercials and Blue Cross/Blue Shield) because HMOs are not offering reimbursement for health care outlays. Rather, HMOs actually guarantee the *provision* of covered health services. Like the historical record of Blue Cross and Blue Shield plans, HMOs generally have relied on community—not experience—ratings. (Indeed, the HMO Act of 1973 required federally qualified HMOs to price insurance in this manner.) Due to both competitive pressures and employers' increasing paranoia about perceived cream skimming by HMOs, however, HMOs are being pressured to engage in experience rating, which has been permitted since 1989 by subsequent amendments to the HMO Act of 1973. Another distinction between HMOs and their pure insurance colleagues is that HMOs often are regulated by an entirely different set of statutes and organizations than either commercial insurers or the Blues.

Not only can HMOs be freestanding organizations, but the Blues and commercial insurers also own and operate HMOs. Although the earliest large HMOs (such as Kaiser, Health Insurance Plan of New York and Group Health Cooperative of Puget Sound), as well as some of the newer, well-respected HMOs (such as the Harvard Community Health Plan in Boston), were organized as not-for-profit entities, many of the newer, rapidly expanding HMOs (such as United HealthCare) and most of the commercial insurance company-sponsored HMOs are for-profit organizations.

PRIVATE HEALTH INSURANCE AS A FINANCING MECHANISM

Private health insurance is made up of the three principal entities just described (commercial carriers, the Blues, and HMOs), plus self-funded plans. The importance of private health insurance as a source of financing for personal health care expenditures has increased slowly but steadily.

As noted earlier, private health insurance began with coverage principally for hospital and physicians' services. In 1960, virtually all of the total net private health insurance payments were devoted to these two types of health care (Figure 7.1). Private health insurance has funded a steady one-third of personal health care expenditures for hospital services since 1960. Private health insurance has grown in importance as a source of financing for physicians' services. The largest percentage impacts of health in-

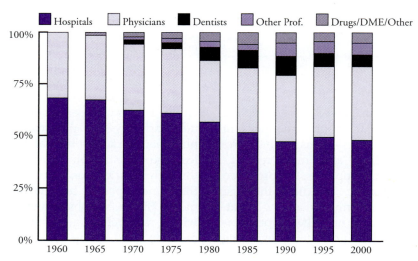

Figure 7.1. Recipients of Private Health Insurance Payments

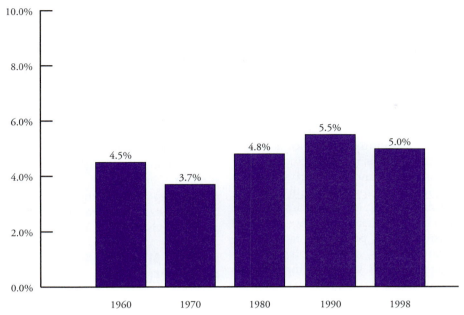

Figure 7.2.   Program Administration and Net Cost of Private Health Insurance as a Percent of Total National Health Expenditures

surance financing have occurred in the areas of dental services, nonphysician professional services, and pharmaceuticals. Private health insurance for these expenses was negligible until about 1970, and even at that time, reimbursements from private health insurance were less than seven percent of total payments in each of the three categories.

As political debates in the United States continue regarding health insurance, there has been considerable argument and criticism about the overhead generated by the private health insurance mechanism. (Woolhandler & Himmelstein, 1991). In 2000, the total administrative costs of public medical programs, philanthropic organizations, and the net cost of private health insurance amounted to about five percent of total national health expenditures (Figure 7.2). This estimate excludes the nontrivial administrative costs to providers regarding the filing of claims. Americans pay about fifteen percent in net cost of private health insurance. This cost includes insurers' administrative

costs, net additions to reserves, rate credits and policyholder dividends, premium taxes, and carriers' profits or losses.

Although there is no denying that some government health insurance programs such as Medicare deliver benefits at far less administrative cost per dollar of reimbursement than the private health insurance industry, health insurance *by itself* is not always a profitable business for insurers. This is particularly true at the high end of the market, where self-funded administrative-services-only customers generate relatively narrow profit margins for most group insurers. Indeed, the health insurance industry suffered a net underwriting loss (the difference between premiums and claims paid) in many years since 1976. Health insurance is beneficial for many insurers because it serves as a vehicle for selling other, more profitable products (such as life insurance) and because health insurance premiums generate revenues via investment income.

HEALTH-RELATED INSURANCE PROGRAMS

Individual Coverage

A number of insurance entities (including commercial carriers and the Blues) offer insurance coverage for individuals (Pauly & Percy, 2000). Some of the nation's largest commercial accident and health insurers sell few or no individual policies.

Much of the current individual insurance sold is supplementary in nature; that is, it picks up coverage for the many expenses that another plan such as Medicare does not cover, or covers only with significant cost sharing. Ordinary individual policies for basic medical (hospital and physician) coverage are extraordinarily expensive: Policy premiums can easily reach several thousand dollars, even for plans with extensive cost-sharing provisions. Underwriting guidelines for individual policies have become increasingly stringent, so many people who might wish to purchase coverage are not able to do so (Saver & Doescher, 2000). In some states, the only recourse for such individuals is through high-risk state insurance pools. Many states have enacted broad-based pools for uninsurable individuals to provide some protection (Rogal & Gauthier, 2000).

Demand for individual medical policies has diminished with the enactment of PL 99-272, the Consolidated Omnibus Budget Reconciliation Act of 1985 (COBRA). Under this statute, employers with twenty or more employees are required to extend group health care coverage to former employees after they leave their jobs (voluntarily or not) and for dependents of employees following events such as death or divorce. Employers can charge a premium of the average cost of group health insurance for that employer.

Group Coverage

In the United States, employment not only provides the financial means of support for families, but it is the principal source of insurance protection against medical expenses and income loss associated with both on- and off-the-job illness and injury. Through sponsorship by a number of different groups (principally employers, but also unions, employer/union Taft-Hartley plans, multiple-employer trusts [METs], and multiple-employer welfare arrangements [MEWAs]), Americans receive the preponderance of their health insurance protection. The United States is the only major industrialized country in which voluntary, employment-based health plans are the primary source of health insurance for its citizens.

The rapidly accelerating costs associated with medical care and the tax-exempt nature of employee medical benefits have stimulated the expansion of group health coverage. As noted earlier, small employers often provide meager health insurance benefits, if they provide them at all. But for workers of medium-size and large employers, medical insurance protection is nearly a universal benefit.

FUNDING ALTERNATIVE FOR GROUP HEALTH-RELATED INSURANCE

As mentioned earlier in this chapter, there are three principal options to funding health-related insurance: (1) fully insured, (2) partially insured, and (3) self-funding. At least for conventional health insurance (defined as non-HMO and non-PPO health plans), substantial differences exist in the use of funding alternatives among the Blues, commercial insurers, and self-administered/third-party administrator plans. For certain health-related benefits, such as accidental death and dismemberment (AD&D), travel accident, long-term care, and long-term disability, funding (even within large corporations) is usually on a fully insured basis. This funding mechanism is employed because premiums are relatively small and stable, and the frequency of loss is so small that the only sound actuarial basis for establishing a premium is to combine exposures from many different employers.

For medical and dental employee benefits, however, all three of the aforementioned funding alternatives are used (Park, 2000). Which one makes most sense to an employer is primarily a function of the size of its employee population and the employer's degree of risk aversion. Clearly, for employers with more than several thousand employees, pure self-funding is actuarially viable because medical expenses are relatively predictable. With 100% self-funding, employers basically choose some organization (an insurer or third-party administrator) to administer their medical benefits program and perform claim adjudication. Depending on the self-funding contract, additional services (for example, actuarial, employee communications, and so on) also may be performed for the employer. Thus, the employer basically pays two types of employee benefits expenses: (1) medical service claim expenses submitted to the administrator for reimbursement by employees, and (2) an administrative fee, usually called *retention.* This latter fee can be computed as a per capita charge, a percent of claim payments, or a transaction-related fee.

Self-funding of employee benefits is one of the principal trends in health insurance since the late 1970s. There are four principal advantages to self-funding. First, the employer avoids the risk charges paid to the insurer that are inherent whenever any entity purchases insurance. Second, employers may be able to avoid administrative fees for services that are bundled with a normal insurance premium, but which the employer may wish to purchase through alternate channels (for example, actuarial or loss-prevention services). Third, because self-funding is technically not insurance, employers can avoid the nontrivial premium taxes (usually amounting to several percentage points) assessed by states on insured group health products.

Finally, and perhaps the biggest enhancement of self-funding, the Supreme Court ruled in June 1985 that the 1974 federal Employee Retirement Income Security Act (ERISA) statute preempted states from regulating self-funded group medical programs (*Metropolitan Life Insurance Co. v. Massachusetts,* 1985; Rublee, 1985). The most important advantage of this preemption is the ability of employers to avoid the mandated benefit provisions of states, which require insured benefit plans to cover specific types of benefits. These state mandates originally served as a useful stimulus to encourage appropriate coverage for types of care or for conditions not previously covered by typical group health plans. (Alcoholism is a notable example.) In recent years, however, state legislatures have greatly expanded the scope and specificity of coverage to include personal preferences of powerful state legislators and for care where cost-effectiveness is unproven. Mandated benefits increase the costs of medical benefits, especially for small employers, thereby exacerbating the uninsured problem. In effect, large employers began to see that their multimillion-dollar employee benefits programs were being crafted by politicians who bore no responsibility for the financial impact of their decisions. Thus, self-funding not only provides financial savings for large employers but also permits the employers significantly greater flexibility in designing benefit plans and establishing employee cost-sharing responsibilities.

Many employers, particularly those with 500 to 5,000 employees, are reluctant to assume the financial risk of a fully self-funded arrangement. For these employers, there are several forms of partial self-funding, the most common of which is usually referred to as a "minimum premium plan." Generally, these financial options permit the employer to self-fund claim expenses up to a certain predefined maximum amount, after which an insured policy assumes financial liability. Another variant of self-funding involves the purchase of stop-loss (or specific and aggregate) insurance. Again, the employer pays directly for all medical claims, except for those that, either in the aggregate or individually, exceed a predetermined threshold.

Finally, there is the standard fully insured program, which remains the principal funding mechanism for the millions of small and medium-size businesses that form the foundation of employment for most Americans. For the small employer, premiums for this coverage are set prospectively (akin to auto insurance premiums, for example). For larger employers, a form of retrospective experience rating is often used, so that this year's premium is affected (either positively or negatively) by the previous year's claim expense history for each individual employer.

All three of these standard funding mechanisms are employed by both commercial carriers and the Blues. In contrast, most HMOs price their services prospectively, on a *per capita* basis. HMOs are then financially responsible for providing all necessary, covered medical services for this capitated premium. Historically, these capitation amounts were community-determined, unrelated to the claim experience of individual employers. As stated earlier, however, competitive pressures and amendments to the 1973 HMO Act are now stimulating funding approaches for HMO services that are more similar to the approaches used by the Blues and commercial insurers, particularly in the area of experience rating.

CORE MEDICAL EMPLOYEE BENEFITS

Today's core medical employee benefits consist primarily of medical and dental coverage. In addition, larger employers may offer separate plans for coverage of prescription drug and vision services (although coverage for these expenses can be combined under the general medical plan).

Medical Plans

This coverage is the oldest and most vital form of health insurance, as it protects against those financial expenses that can be truly catastrophic. Employer costs are reflected in Table 7.6. For most major types of providers (for example, hospitals, physicians, nonphysician providers, laboratory and radiology, and so on), there is somewhat uniform coverage under indemnity group policies, but with different cost-sharing responsibilities for employees. The most generous plans (but also the type of plan rapidly losing favor with employers) are called *base/major medical* plans. Under these arrangements, there is first-dollar coverage for a few key providers (for example, hospitals and sometimes physicians), then more limited cover-

Table 7.6. Employers' Cost Per Employee Hour Worked for Health Insurance, According to Selected Characteristics: United States, Selected Years

Characteristic	Health Insurance		Health Insurance as a Percent of Total Compensation	
	1991	1999	1991	1999
	Amount per employee-hour worked			
State and local government	$1.54	$2.12	6.9	7.6
Industry				
Goods producing	1.28	1.52	6.9	6.6
Service producing	0.79	0.88	5.5	4.9
Region				
Northeast	1.08	1.19	6.2	5.7
Midwest	0.95	1.07	6.3	5.8
South	0.76	0.89	5.5	5.2
West	0.92	1.00	5.8	4.8
Union status				
Union	1.63	2.02	8.2	8.2
Nonunion	0.78	0.89	5.4	4.9
Establishment employment size				
1–99 employees	0.68	0.77	5.1	4.7
100–499	0.90	1.01	6.3	5.6
500 or more	1.40	1.64	6.8	6.2

age (for example, with twenty percent employee coinsurance required) for all other services. Except for so-called "corridor" deductibles that may exist between the base and major medical expenses, these plans generally contain no up-front employee cost sharing. Perhaps the biggest disadvantage of base/major medical plans is that many do not place any upper limit on the expenses borne by the patient in a calendar year.

In contrast, the most prominent type of medical benefit plan today, the comprehensive design, retains little (if any) first-dollar coverage. A comprehensive plan design usually has a relatively small annual deductible (for example, $200) that pertains to all medical expenses; then it reimburses the patient a fixed percentage (most commonly eighty percent) of all medical claims that exceed the deductible, up to a maximum out-of-pocket patient expense (typically $1,000 to $2,000 per insured person). When the patient reaches this out-of-pocket maximum, 100% of all subsequent expenses are borne by the medical plan. Both base/major medical and comprehensive plans sometimes place lifetime maximums on the total amount of benefits that will be paid to any individual. Most medical plans today impose at least some managed-care requirements on plan participants, the most common programs being utilization review and case management.

The benefit structure of medical plans offered by HMOs is somewhat different from fee-for-service indemnity coverages. First, the scope of coverage often is broader in HMO plans than in indemnity programs (although there are notable exceptions, particularly regarding the coverage of psychiatric and substance abuse illnesses). Second, the more generous HMO plans usually have no deductibles. Third, instead of coinsurance, HMOs feature fixed-dollar copayments for selected services, most commonly physician office visits ($5 to $15 per visit) and medications ($5 to $10 per prescription). Finally, HMOs traditionally have displayed greater attentiveness to fostering health promotion than have indemnity insurers. Therefore, covered expenses in HMO benefit plans often include medical care not covered in indemnity plans, such as immunizations, well-child care, and physical examinations.

Dental Plans

Although Continental Casualty Company, in 1959, was the first commercial insurer to issue a comprehensive group dental insurance plan, insurance for dental expenses was not generally available until the 1970s. Plan designs for dental insurance generally follow a comprehensive rather than base/major medical structure. Usually there are three tiers of benefits. For preventive services (for example, semiannual prophylaxis and routine dental X-rays), coverage often is 100%, without a deductible. For the two remaining benefit tiers, there is a small annual deductible ($50 to $100 per insured person) the patient must satisfy before any benefits are paid. Restorative services (for example, amalgams), oral surgery, endodontics (for example, root canal), and periodontics are then paid with relatively standard coinsurance (usually eighty percent). Services such as crowns, inlays, and prosthetics are reimbursed only fifty percent by the dental plan. Cosmetic dentistry (for example, bonding) usually is covered at this lower level, or it may be excluded from coverage entirely. Orthodontic services usually receive a relatively limited lifetime benefit (for example, $1,000), unless special orthodontic coverage is elected. Plans of dental HMOs (DMOs) and Delta Dental plans are analogous to medical HMO coverages, with slightly broader coverage and fewer cost-sharing requirements for the employee when compared to indemnity dental plans. Unlike medical benefits, dental plans are more restrictive in terms of annual limits on reimbursement.

Vision Plans

Expense benefits for vision care were first introduced by private insurers in 1957. Many health care observers believe that vision care is a prime example of what should not be covered by an insurance program, as vision care is relatively inexpensive for most Americans. For those individuals covered for vision services, nearly all received coverage for examinations, while two-thirds were covered for eyeglasses and contact lenses. Usually there are limits regarding the frequency with which examinations and lenses are reimbursable. With the advent of managed care, vision care may be available as a "carve-out" benefit, sometimes with a separate deductible. These vision care programs are usually offered in conjunction with large, national chains of vision care products, offering employees substantial discounts on these products if they are purchased through the preferred providers.

Prescription Drug Plans

This benefit is another example of a specialized employee benefit that is increasingly carved out of the regular medical benefit program in order to take advantage of managed-care features. Generally, coverage assumes one of two forms. In the traditional fashion, prescription drugs simply are a covered expense under the medical benefit plan. There may be individual copayments per prescription, and sometimes these copayments are higher for branded drugs than for generics. (Traditional coinsurance, typically eighty percent, may be substituted for the copayment type of cost sharing.) Nearly all types of prescription drugs are eligible for reimbursement, with common exceptions being certain injectibles (except insulin), contraceptives, and experimental drugs. Prescription drugs for acute conditions (for example, antibiotics) may be covered in part by the regular medical plan, while "maintenance" drugs are available through mail order. Mail-order plans permit employers and employees to take advantage of steep discounts and some drug use review, while offering the convenience of home delivery. Mail-order programs have been particularly well received by older employees and retirees. The latest trend in pharmacy programs, however, is a full "carve-out" program for all prescription drugs, a feature that may or may not include a mail-order companion product.

Long-Term Care Coverage

The most recent option for a number of corporate employee benefits programs is long-term care insurance, which first became available for groups during the last half of the 1980s. Many of these benefits are paid by individual long-term care policies and group medical plans (although nursing home coverage usually is

quite limited for the latter programs). The group policies now available are largely 100% employee-funded, as employers are fearful of assuming any additional fiscal liability for insurance protection, even though the long-term actuarial value of this type of insurance is highly uncertain. Unlike the service benefits of most group medical and dental plans, long-term care insurance is largely an indemnity product, offering a fixed daily reimbursement payment for nursing home care and related services.

The purchase of long-term care insurance received a significant stimulus with the passage of the Health Insurance Portability and Accountability Act of 1996 (commonly known as Kennedy-Kassebaum), which modified the tax treatment of long-term care insurance. If a long-term care plan is provided by an employer, premiums are deductible by the employer and the benefits received by the beneficiary are tax-free to specified limits (Pincus, 2000).

Retiree Medical Coverage

The foregoing description of the principal forms of group health insurance applies to active employees. (Of course, a very small percentage of active employees or their family members may receive primary insurance coverage through Medicare, such as individuals with chronic renal failure who require dialysis.) For active employees between the ages of sixty-five and seventy, the Tax Equity and Fiscal Responsibility Act (TEFRA) of 1982 required employers' group health insurance plans to remain the primary payers, with Medicare retaining only secondary coverage. In 1984, the Omnibus Deficit Reduction Act (PL 98-369) extended Medicare as the secondary payer for aged spouses of workers under age sixty-five. These statutes are just two examples of how the federal government has shifted fiscal responsibility for the financing of some medical care from government to the private sector.

For retirees, there has been a profound reexamination by employers of providing continuing medical expense protection, particularly for early retirees who have not yet reached age sixty-five (and therefore are ineligible for Medicare). This rethinking of retiree medical coverage has occurred for several reasons.

First, the unrelenting growth in employers' medical benefit expenses acceleration, which is two or three times as rapid as the increase in other costs of doing business, has forced most employers to reassess whether they can afford to finance retiree medical expenses as generously as in the past.

Second, as one would expect, early retirees' average annual medical expenses easily can be double or triple those of the active population. For employers with significant numbers of retirees (such as long-standing manufacturing companies like auto and steel producers), early retiree medical costs can significantly raise an employer's overall average financial liability for medical benefits. Third, all employers (even relatively young firms) are faced with the undeniable aging of America, so the pressures on employers' total medical benefit expenditures will become more severe over the next several decades.

Finally, regulations promulgated by the Financial Accounting Standards Board (referred to as FASB 106) became effective at the beginning of 1993. Before 1990, virtually all employers used the pay-as-you-go approach to value the cost of retiree medical benefits on their financial statements. Now employers must accrue retiree health-care liabilities as an expense against earnings from the date an employee is hired until that employee becomes eligible for benefits. In addition, retiree health liabilities that have accumulated as of the date that employers adopt FASB 106 accounting rules must be recognized at once or be amortized (generally over twenty years).

Because incorporation of these amounts on corporate balance sheets results in only a minimal diminution of actual cash flow (as FASB 106 is merely an accounting acknowledgment of future liabilities), its direct effect on employers' day-to-day operations is minor. However, the enormous financial impact of FASB 106 has jolted senior corporate executives into explicitly acknowledging the increasingly onerous burden of all medical benefits (not just retiree obligations) on employers' overhead expenses, perhaps more than any other single legislative or regulatory rule enacted to date.

As a result of these combined forces, most employers are reexamining how (and even if) they want to provide medical coverage for retirees. Some employers have even attempted to rescind retiree health insurance coverage. The courts generally have ruled that employers retain the right to rescind or amend retiree medical benefit programs, as long as this option is clearly stated in the employers' benefit documentation (Geisel, 1989). For retirees under age sixty-five, benefit protection often is the same as that for active employees. For retirees over age sixty-five, employers' liability is diminished significantly because the group health insurance plan becomes secondary to Medicare coverage. For both groups, however, employers are reconsidering their funding options.

One approach is to eliminate retiree medical coverage entirely for all new hires, or to link coverage with length-of-service requirements, much as pension plans are linked with vesting periods. Another option is to require retirees to contribute much more generously than in the past to their medical coverage. Unfortunately, tax laws often impeded the ability of employers to establish tax-exempt trusts to fund retiree medical benefits.

But the most fundamental choice most employers must make these days is whether they will continue to offer medical benefits to retirees under a defined-benefit concept or whether (like pensions) retiree medical benefits should be switched to a defined-contribution program. This latter option generally limits employers' future liabilities by making them much more predictable (like pension benefits) and clearly places most of the concern over the ultimate magnitude of medical care cost escalation squarely on retirees. If defined-contribution programs for retiree medical benefits become the norm, retirees will need to be much more concerned about issues of plan design and cost containment than they have in the past. Active employees also will be required to assume significantly more responsibility for funding their retiree medical benefits far ahead of when they will be incurred, just as workers must plan now to ensure that they will retain enough retirement income via pension benefits and 401(k) plans.

Disability Insurance

Serious illness or injury not only creates economic hardship due to the high costs of medical care but also inhibits the ability of workers to maintain a wage stream to support the everyday costs of living. Thus, loss-of-income policies are one of the oldest forms of health-related insurance. In contrast to the disability programs available through Social Security for chronic loss of income via disability, private insurance vehicles have focused on the short to medium term. Unlike most health insurance, disability insurance pays indemnity benefits, not medical service benefits. Except for the compulsory temporary disability insurance programs mandated by some states such as Rhode Island (1942), California (1946), New Jersey (1948), New York (1949), and Hawaii (1969), which combine wage replacement with medical expense reimbursement for nonoccupational disabling illness or injury, short- and long-term disability programs do not reimburse for expenses associated with medical services.

Short-Term Programs

Coverage for loss of income due to illness can be available to workers through two avenues: (1) sick leave or salary continuation benefits, or (2) short-term disability insurance. While sick leave benefits usually replace all or most of an ill employee's wages, reimbursement often is limited to no more than a few weeks, at best. Eligibility for sick leave and the length of sick leave benefits are usually related to an employee's length of service.

Short-term disability insurance retains several important features, many of which differentiate disability insurance from health insurance. First, there is a short elimination period (usually one to seven days) between the onset of disability or illness and the date when benefits begin to be paid. In the most generous short-term income protection employee benefits, sick leave benefits dovetail with short-term disability insurance so that the ailing worker has no front-end gaps in coverage.

Second, as their name implies, short-term disability programs protect workers only for relatively brief periods. Many short-term disability insurance plan participants have a length-of-service requirement before they are eligible for coverage, usually three months or less. This period of time to become eligible for coverage is called a *waiting period*.

Long-Term Programs

Long-term disability insurance can be perceived in two different lights. In its most generous version, this coverage dovetails with an employer's short-term income maintenance program to create a seamless layer of wage protection for periods of several years. In its more primal role, long-term disability insurance is the disability equivalent to a catastrophic medical benefit plan: Benefits are paid only after the insured has retained a significant amount of loss.

Premiums are often entirely employer-financed. Like short-term coverage, long-term disability insurance maintains a waiting period before employees are eligible for coverage. Plan participants may have an elimination period (no coverage) of six months.

In order to induce workers to return to the job and because long-term disability payments can be exempt from both state and federal taxation, benefits are paid at rates usually in the range of fifty to sixty-seven percent of a worker's wages, although there are often maximums to these payments. Due to the existence of Social Security disability programs, most long-term disability policies include provisions that permit benefits to be reduced commensurate with the amount of Social Security disability benefits paid. This provision is analogous to the coordination-of-benefits feature common in most medical and dental insurance policies.

Workers' Compensation Insurance

Like Medicare, workers' compensation insurance is a social insurance program. Usually, employee benefits professionals do not consider workers' compensation a health insurance program. However, changes in the nature of workers' compensation benefits over the years, as well as the way in which these programs are now being affected by new managed-care techniques, argue that workers' compensation should be discussed as a vehicle providing nontrivial medical benefits.

Workers' compensation programs really were the first types of broad-coverage, health-related insurance in the United States. Beginning with a federal statute in 1908, workers' compensation–type insurance programs were enacted by nine states in 1911, and by 1920, all but six states had inaugurated such a program (Workers' Compensation, 1991). Today, there are fifty-five workers' compensation programs in operation, one in each of the fifty states as well as in Puerto Rico, the District of Columbia, and the Virgin Islands. There are also two special federal workers' compensation programs covering government employees, longshoremen, and harbor workers. In addition, there are unique occupational illness and injury programs for coal miners suffering from pneumoconiosis (black lung disease) and railroad workers.

Workers' compensation insurance is compulsory for most private employment, except in a very few states. This protection provides workers and their families with three types of benefits: (1) indemnity cash benefits to help replace lost wages, (2) medical expense reimbursement, and (3) survivors' death benefits. Despite generally broad-based coverage, many state workers' compensation programs do not cover domestics, agricultural workers, and casual laborers. Also, many programs cover public employees, as well as workers in nonprofit and charitable institutions, with varying degrees of comprehensiveness. Initially focusing on workplace injuries, workers' compensation programs increasingly are being pressured financially by the long-term effects of occupational illness.

There is a large difference between premiums and benefit payments reflecting the long payout time frame on workers' compensation claims, so premiums collected in one year must anticipate claims filed for many subsequent years. Employers provide funding for virtually all workers' compensation premiums. About twenty percent of premiums are contributed to state high-risk pools, which provide coverage for high-risk employers that cannot obtain workers' compensation insurance through commercial carriers. Each state establishes its own regulatory mechanisms, eligibility rules, benefit schedule, and funding alternatives.

In most states, employers may purchase workers' compensation insurance through private insurers, either property/casualty single-line carriers or multiline carriers. In some states, however, commercial insurance is not permitted. There is an exclusive state workers' compensation insurance fund, or employers can purchase workers' compensation coverage through the state program or they can self-fund.

One important development in workers' compensation programs over time has been the degree to which they provide reimbursement for medical benefits. This percentage has been increasing slowly but steadily since 1980. This trend is due both to states' restrictions on cash compensation benefit levels and to the higher growth rate for medical care when compared to wages. Nearly all standard employee benefit medical programs contain provisions that exclude coverage for medical care for work-related accidents, in order to avoid duplicate payments by both the medical plan and workers' compensation.

Many employers are observing that their workers' compensation expenses are accelerating like the costs of medical benefit programs. Thus, it is no surprise that many of the cost-management techniques (particularly managed care) that have been used to try to moderate medical benefit plan expenditures are now being modified for workers' compensation programs. These strategies are more workable in some states than in others, however, as states differ in the degree of provider freedom-of-choice that is afforded to the injured worker. It is not surprising that some of the most aggressive transference of managed-care techniques from the employee benefits arena to workers' compensation is occurring in those states that provide employers with unilateral physician selection powers.

CHANGES FACING THE HEALTH INSURANCE INDUSTRY

Profound changes have been sweeping through the private health insurance sector during the past decade:

1. *Increasing challenges to control employers' medical benefit costs.* The cost-control mania of corporate America during the 1990s has created an atmosphere of very aggressive cost-management expectations by group health purchasers.
2. *Increasing competition from nontraditional health insurance models.* Health insurers face a growing array of competitive threats to their control of the medical benefits arena. First, providers are showing increased

interest in direct contracting involvement with group purchasers and in creating managed-care entities of their own (for example, provider-sponsored organizations [PSOs] for Medicare risk contracting). With the emergence of these types of managed-care arrangements, the distinction is blurring between "providers" and "insurers." Second, private insurers are facing new competitors in the medical benefits administrative arena from human resources consultants and outsourcing firms. Third, the advent of technological developments such as the Internet permit many traditional health benefits activities (for example, enrollment) to be undertaken by firms that are primarily technology experts, not medical benefits experts.

3. *Continued consolidation of major health insurers.* Beginning with the purchase of Equicor's health insurance business by CIGNA in 1990, the private health insurance industry has undergone considerable and continued consolidation on two fronts. First, many smaller health insurers have elected to leave the health insurance arena entirely, and their business has been purchased by the remaining large firms (for example, the purchase of John Hancock's group health insurance operations by WellPoint Health Networks). Second, there have been mergers among the largest of the health insurers. Examples are the 1995 merger of United HealthCare and MetraHealth (MetraHealth itself was the merger of the health insurance operations of Travelers Insurance Company and Metropolitan Insurance Company just a year earlier); the purchase in 1996 by Aetna of HMO powerhouse U.S. HealthCare; and two major mergers during 1997 of California-based HMOs (Foundation Health Corporation/Health Systems International and FHP/Pacificare).

4. *Movement away from "bricks-and-mortar" managed-care structures.* Although staff model HMOs traditionally have been viewed as the ultimate form of managed care, the high fixed infrastructure costs are proving to be too onerous and inflexible in today's dynamic managed-care competitive environment. Even Kaiser Health Plans has been experimenting in different parts of the United States with operations that utilize non-owned hospitals and permit its HMO members to utilize non-Permanente physicians.

5. *Increasing growth of less restrictive forms of managed care.* The fastest-growing forms of managed care today are HMOs with opt-out provisions, and open-access HMO and POS plans, where members can seek care directly from any network physician without gaining authorization from a primary-care physician "gate-keeper." Continued attacks by managed-care critics are likely to force health insurers to decrease the "hassle factor" for both patients and providers.

6. *Escalating regulation and oversight of the managed care industry.* Critics of managed care, especially those groups whose vested self-interests are threatened by the increasing control of their activities by the managed-care industry, are becoming much more sophisticated and successful in placing the health insurance industry on the defensive regarding its more aggressive cost-management practices. Mandated benefits at the state level (affecting primarily *insured* medical benefit programs) will be supplemented by attempts to also control the structure and process of managed care (for example, "any-willing-provider" statutes, "prudent layperson" restrictions on denial of emergency room usage, and so on) (Jensen & Morrisey, 1999). Of concern to large employers is the movement away from state-based legislative initiatives to federal ones, which remove the ERISA preemption and thus subject even self-funded medical benefit plans to their consequences. (Examples are the federal Mental Health Parity Law and the so-called "drive-though-delivery" restrictions that mandate minimum lengths of stay for pregnancies.) Given the failure of broad-based health care restructuring initiatives such as the Clinton health plan in the early 1990s, more incremental legislative changes are being sought to address more narrowly focused issues. The Health Insurance Portability and Accountability Act of 1996, which (among other impacts) dramatically limits the use of preexisting conditions in group health plans, is an example of legislation that was

enacted relatively expeditiously and with considerable bipartisan support.

7. *Growing use of managed care in medical benefit programs, especially for retirees.* Given the level of provider discounts available from most major managed-care insurers, very few employers can afford any longer to offer pure indemnity medical benefit offerings. And those employers with less aggressive forms of managed care (for example, PPOs) increasingly are attempting to move their employees toward more aggressive managed-care alternatives, namely, POS and HMO plans. But, proportionately, the largest growth in managed-care enrollment likely will come in the *retiree* population segment (both retirees younger than sixty-five and Medicare-eligible retirees) for three reasons. First, the FASB 106 accounting standards have significantly raised the visibility of retiree medical expenses, so there is increased pressure to manage these costs as aggressively as is feasible. Second, corporate America's hard look at providing *any* retiree medical benefits will pressure employees to accept more stringent medical plan offerings. Fi-

nally, the enormous growth of interest by most major managed-care insurers in Medicare risk programs will offer employers powerful financial incentives to migrate Medicare-eligible retirees to such plans as quickly as possible.

8. *Increasing focus on measuring and monitoring quality.* As medical benefit trends have moderated, and as the stridency of managed-care criticism has escalated, both employers and health insurers have faced mounting pressure to define, measure, and monitor medical care quality. Iterations of the Health Plan Employer Data and Information Set (HEDIS) standards and growing demands for health plans to be formally accredited are the most visible signs of slow progress in this arena. Particularly as other avenues of cost-management opportunities continue to dwindle, progressive insurers and employers finally are beginning to realize that quality improvement and health-promotion strategies ultimately may be the biggest weapons of the future in continuing to moderate the cost escalation of employer-sponsored medical benefits programs.

References

Bilheimer, L. T., & Colby, D. C. (2001). Expanding coverage: Reflections on recent efforts. *Health Affairs, 20,* 83–95.

Congressional Budget Office, Congress of the United States. (1991). *Rising health care costs: Causes, implications, and strategies.* Washington, DC: U.S. Government Printing Office.

Feldstein, M., & Friedman, B. (1977). Tax subsidies, the rational demand for insurance, and the health care crisis. *Journal of Public Economics, 7*(2), 155–178.

Geisel, J. (1989). Court says firm can't alter retiree health plan benefits. *Business Insurance, 2*(7).

Greenspan, N. T., & Vogel, R. J. (1980). Taxation and its effects upon public and private health insurance and medical demand. *Health Care Financing Review, 1*(4), 39–46.

Hall, M. A. (2001). The structure and enforcement of health insurance rating reforms. *Inquiry, 37,* 376–388.

Health Insurance Association of America. (1991). *Source book of health insurance data, 1990.* Washington, DC: Author.

Health Insurance Association of America. (1997). *Source book of health insurance data, 1996.* Washington, DC: Author.

Jensen, G. A., & Morrisey, M. A. (1999). Employer-sponsored health insurance and mandated benefit laws. *Milbank Quarterly, 77,* 425–459.

Metropolitan Life Insurance Co. v. Massachusetts, 84–325 (S. C. 1985).

Park, C. H. (2000). Prevalence of employer self-insured health benefits: National and state variation. *Medical Care Research Review, 57,* 340–360.

Pauly, M. V., & Percy, A. M. (2000). Cost and performance: A comparison of the individual and group health insurance markets. *Journal of Health Politics Policy and Law, 25,* 9–26.

Pincus, J. (2000). Employer-sponsored long-term care insurance: Best practices for increasing sponsorship. *EBRI Issue Brief, 220,* 1–22.

Reschovsky, J. D., Kemper, P., & Tu, H. (2000). Does type of health insurance affect health care use and assessments of care among the privately insured? *Health Services Research, 35,* 219–237.

Rogal, D. L., & Gauthier, A. K. (2000). Introduction: The evolution of the individual insurance market. *Journal of Health Politics Policy and Law, 25,* 3–8.

Rublee, D. A. (1985). Self-funded health benefit plans. *Journal of the American Medical Association, 255*(6), 787–789.

Saver, B. G., & Doescher, M. P. (2000). To buy, or not to buy: Factors associated with the purchase of nongroup, private health insurance. *Medical Care, 38,* 141–151.

Vaughn, E. J., & Elliott, C. M. (1978). *Fundamentals of risk and insurance.* New York: Wiley.

Woolhandler, S., & Himmelstein, D. (1991). The deteriorating administrative efficiency of the U.S. health care system. *New England Journal of Medicine, 324*(18), 1253–1258.

Workers' compensation. (1991). *Social Security Bulletin, 54*(9), 28–36.

PART

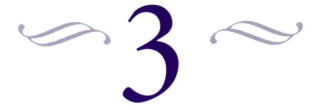

3

Providers of Health Services

CHAPTER
8

The Evolution of Public Health:
A Joint Public-Private Responsibility

Paul R. Torrens
Lester Breslow

Chapter Topics

- Levels of Prevention
- Historical Evolution of Health Promotion and Disease Prevention in the United States
- The Structure of Organized Public Health Efforts in the United States
- The Role of the Private Sector in Health Promotion and Disease Prevention
- Summary

Learning Objectives

Upon completing this chapter, the reader should be able to:

- Understand the role of public health services in protecting the health of populations
- Differentiate the various levels of prevention
- Appreciate the history of public health in the United States
- Understand the roles and duties of each level of government in providing public health services
- Appreciate the increasingly important role of the private sector in public health
- View public health services as a collective requirement of all participants of the health care system

In the past, if one were discussing the organization of health services in the United States, that discussion would most likely not include a great deal of detail with regard to health promotion or disease prevention. It would probably not cover in very great detail the organization of governmental public health services either. *Health services* in the past meant curative and treatment services for the most part, and health promotion or disease prevention services were considered only peripherally, if at all.

This is not to suggest that the providers of health care services in the past were uninterested in keeping their patients healthy over a long period of time. Rather, it is meant to suggest that the model of health care in the past was focused around acute treatment of short-term illnesses (with some notable exceptions). Public health was the job for governmental agencies and was seen as something quite distinct and very rarely overlapping with curative and treatment services.

In recent years, fortunately, a new paradigm for health promotion and disease prevention has emerged that is based on a public-private partnership to protect and preserve the health of the American public. This chapter will examine this new paradigm of health promotion and disease prevention and will provide the modern health care practitioner with a better framework for understanding and dealing with the major health problems of the public.

LEVELS OF PREVENTION

In order to understand the new framework for health promotion and disease prevention, it is important first to provide background information about the levels of prevention, as included in the terms *primary, secondary,* and *tertiary prevention* (Commission on Chronic Illness, 1957; Leavell & Clark, 1958). Without a clear understanding of the levels of prevention, it would be difficult to understand the relative roles of the public and the private sectors with regard to the enhancement of the health of the public.

Primary prevention means averting the occurrence of disease. It includes those measures that are applied or brought into effect *before* disease is present. These may include general attempts to promote better

health by efforts to educate the public, to establish standards of appropriate sanitation, to apply specific methods of protection such as immunizations, to remove occupational hazards, and to protect from known carcinogens. Primary prevention focuses on the promotion of healthy lifestyles and specific protections from known hazards.

Secondary prevention means halting the progression of disease from its early, unrecognized stage to a more severe one and preventing the complication or sequelae of disease. It focuses on early diagnosis and/or prompt treatment of a health problem that would otherwise have serious impacts on the health of individuals. This means identifying the presence of a problem before it breaks the clinical horizon and before it becomes symptomatic in most cases, although it also includes attempts to discover disease early while it is still effectively treatable. In the case of coronary artery disease, for example, secondary prevention would focus on identifying individuals at high risk for disease—people, for example, who have a strong family history of heart disease, a history of heavy smoking, a lack of exercise, or a blood lipid profile that is abnormal. These early screening efforts can lead to more specific and focused tests and examinations that might further establish the early diagnosis of potential disease while it can still be constructively handled.

Tertiary prevention involves the prevention (or at least, the limitation) of the effects of disease once it has been identified. This level of prevention operates on the premise that simply because disease is present does not mean that its course should be allowed to run unhindered. In the case of coronary artery disease, for example, tertiary prevention would include efforts at cardiac rehabilitation and exercise programs, control of stress, maintenance of optimum weight and diet, and possibly adherence to a medical regimen that might reduce the future risk of further worsening of the disease.

In the new paradigm of public/private partnership in health promotion and disease prevention, there is a role for both the public and the private sectors at each level of prevention. Sometimes the roles are quite different and separate; other times the roles are similar, and perhaps overlapping, requiring some collaboration and coordination. The important message, however, is that there are several different levels on which health promotion and disease prevention can focus and a wide variety of interventions that can be sponsored by both public and private sectors.

HISTORICAL EVOLUTION OF HEALTH PROMOTION AND DISEASE PREVENTION IN THE UNITED STATES

In order to understand the present circumstances in the United States with regard to health promotion and disease prevention, it is important to review the history of public health activities in the United States. Much of our tradition and organizational framework for public health activities in the United States today is the product of the thinking and actions of previous generations. Therefore, it is important to know these developments and to understand how they affect our current thinking.

In the eighteenth century in the United States, public health activities were, for the most part, limited to individual cities and were focused on protection of the public in those cities from diseases introduced by travelers arriving from elsewhere. Early public health efforts in the United States in the eighteenth century focused on inspection of ships arriving in harbors along the eastern sea coast and included laws for the isolation and quarantine of persons suspected to be carrying diseases that might be spread to the general population. In some of these cases, local governments established institutions (pest houses) to voluntarily (or involuntarily) contain suspected disease carriers until they either became noninfectious or, more likely, expired from their illness. During this period, the focus of public health activity in the United States was carried out by local governments and was limited to preventing the introduction of disease into the populations of port cities.

The nineteenth century marked a great advance in public health and was described by C.E.A. Winslow as "the great sanitary awakening" (Winslow, 1923). In this period, problems of sanitation were identified as a cause of disease, and public health efforts were focused on the improvement of social and environmental conditions. Housing, water supply, and sewage disposal were all the focus of organized public health

activities, with the intent of reducing the disease burden on the public by improving the physical environment. As in the eighteenth century, these activities in the nineteenth century were generally carried out by cities and local governments, with the thrust of organized public health services being carried out on a local level, not necessarily on a state or national one.

In Massachusetts, Lemuel Shattuck published a landmark report in 1850 (*Report of the Sanitary Commission of Massachusetts*) that, for the first time, collected vital statistics on the population of Massachusetts, pointing out the variable threats to health throughout the state as a result of variable sanitary conditions (Shattuck, 1850). His report recommended, among other things, new census schedules, regular surveys of local health conditions, supervision of water supplies and waste disposal, and special studies on specific diseases such as tuberculosis and alcoholism. Probably most important was the recommendation of the establishment of a State Board of Health to enforce sanitary regulations. Massachusetts did set up such a State Board of Health in 1869, becoming the first state in the United States to do so.

From the late nineteenth century to the early twentieth century, many of the sanitary threats to public health were brought under control, and emphasis shifted to the prevention of acute illnesses by use of increasingly available immunizations and vaccinations. This shift of emphasis from sanitary and environmental threats toward individual bacteriological threats to health signaled a major change in the role of health departments. In previous years, organized public health services focused more on problems that were sanitary and environmental in nature and did not necessarily involve individual people; the efforts were more engineering in nature than they were directly clinical. After the turn of the century, public health activities began to turn more directly toward the prevention of disease in individual people. Organized public health activities moved away from structural protections of food, water, sewage, and housing toward more personal and individual protection through immunization of children. Organized public health activities remained largely local government activities, but there now began to be increasing state government activity in public health as well.

As the twentieth century began to progress, federal government activities grew with regard to specific health problems related to children. The United States Children's Bureau was formed in 1912, and the first White House conference on child health was held in 1919. The Sheppard-Towner Act of 1922 established the federal Board of Maternity and Infant Hygiene; this act provided administrative funds to the Children's Bureau and also provided funds to the states to establish programs in maternal and child health. It also established a pattern of federal-state relationship that was to become standard in later years, with the federal government requiring individual states to develop a plan for providing services, to designate a state agency to administer the program, and to report on operations and expenditures of the program to the federal government. States that did not wish to comply with these regulations were deemed ineligible to receive federal funding, thereby setting the model of the federal practice for establishing guidelines for public health programs and providing funds to the state to implement programs meeting these guidelines.

The Social Security Act of 1935 further expanded the federal government's leadership role in setting national directions for public health; it also further solidified the federal-state partnership with regard to the delivery of public health services in the United States. Under the terms of the Social Security Act of 1935, grants were provided to the states for aiding state and local health departments to provide maternal and child health services as well as the expansion of the work of state and local governments. This marked the first major effort of the federal government to see that a nationwide system of state and local government public health organizations were put into place. By the time that Joseph Moutin issued his landmark report on local public health services in 1946, almost eighty percent of the total United States population had some access to organized local public health services. These services may not have always been of great depth, but at least a national framework of organized local public health services had been established (Moutin, Hankela, & Druzin, 1947).

The period of the New Deal in the 1930s also had a profound effect on the development of governmental public health services, but this effect was unfortunately somewhat negative with regard to the leadership of state and federal government activities. During these times, there was considerable pressure to expand the delivery of personal health services, both curative and preventive, more broadly to the public at large, and there was even some consideration by Franklin Roosevelt's administration of a mandatory, universal health insurance program that would cover the entire population. Because the role of the federal government in so many other areas was aggressively expanding, it was believed that perhaps there might be a similar expansion of governmental role with regard to the direct provision of health services.

Unfortunately, the political backlash against the expansion of the role of the federal government in the direct provision of health services—led primarily by the American Medical Association—was successful in forcing public health officials to assume a more cautious attitude toward the role of government assistance. It became quite clear that there was no strong political support for the expansion of governmental health services, at least in the curative area, and many public health officials limited their activities to those programs and functions that were of a more traditional nature (that is, sanitation, immunization, early detection, and confinement of communicable diseases) rather than risk the wrath of organized medicine. This did not mean that the organized public health efforts of local, state, and federal government were reduced in volume, but it did mean that the governments were much more cautious in expanding the scope of their services, being careful to keep them within the confines of prevention and not venturing into treatment.

Indeed, it should be pointed out that the feeling in the United States was so conservative with regard to the federal government's role in health care that a cabinet-level department focusing on the health of the United States' people was not established until 1953, almost one hundred and eighty years after the establishment of the republic! Various public health activities had been initiated by the federal government over the years, but it was not deemed necessary, or possibly, politically possible, to have a federal "department of health," as health was seen as a personal matter involving private physicians and their patients.

It should be pointed out that this same type of thinking governed our nation's thoughts with regard to education and social welfare: these also were seen as local matters in which the federal government should not be involved, at least not directly. The creation in 1953 of a federal Department of Health, Education, and Welfare (HEW) provided a national focus for developing and implementing federal government policy with regard to these three important areas.

In the period of 1953 to the present, there has been a great expansion of governmental activity focused on the public's health, much of it in the traditional public health areas, but much more in programs and functions related to the provision of personal health services. The passage of the Medicare and Medicaid programs in the mid-1960s is generally not seen as an expansion of the federal government's traditional public health role, but in retrospect, the passage of these financing mechanisms for the expansion of personal health services probably has had as major an impact as any of the previous, more traditional public health activities.

One further important development in public health thinking and theory was the passage of the federal Health Planning and Resource Development Act of 1974 (PL 93-641). Under this law, the federal government provided the funds to individual states for the establishment of a State Health Planning and Development Agency whose purpose was to plan and control the future development of health services—primarily hospitals—in the United States. The thinking behind the passage of this law was that there needed to be a coordinated planning effort to ensure that the proper type and volume of health services were available in equitable fashion throughout the United States, and that this could be carried out only by some type of publicly mandated planning effort to coordinate and regulate the development of these services. Although this national health planning effort was really a public health effort in the broadest sense, it was never fully connected to the already existing public health structures in the country and was never fully accepted as a legitimate public health activity by many formal public health professionals. The implementation of the Health Planning and Resource Development Act of 1974 was complicated and filled with significant controversy throughout the country; the law has since been allowed to lapse on both federal and state levels, and there is presently no direct attempt, by either federal or state governments, to plan the distribution of personal health services.

Lessons from History

What can be learned from this review of the evolution of organized public health efforts in the United States? What important political, social, and cultural trends can be identified that will tell us more about the current and future status of public health in the United States? There are several major points to emphasize.

First, it should be pointed out that organized public health activities in the United States began in local, seaport communities and only gradually expanded to state and federal government agencies. Indeed, the Constitution of the United States reserves to the states all functions (such as health) not specifically earmarked to the federal government. For most of our country's history, public health was an activity that was primarily carried out by a local or state governmental agency, and it was only after World War II that it was perceived as necessary or appropriate to have a federal cabinet-level Department of Health, Education, and Welfare.

In many ways, this development would suggest that our country views public health activities (and perhaps health activities in general) as a local and state matter; federal government involvement developed mostly after World War I, and mostly because of the abundance of federal tax revenues to be redistributed to states and local governments. The continuing efforts to reduce the size and scope of the federal government and to return basic functions (and funds) to local and state governments in recent years may be seen as a continuation of this general idea.

Organized public health activities in the United States began with the quarantine and isolation of potential disease carriers, moved on to the improvement of sanitation in the environment, then went on to focus on immunization of children and control of individuals with contagious infectious disease. Almost all of these activities focused on acute infectious diseases, regardless of their origins. This has given rise to an unofficial and generally unspoken agreement that the primary mission of organized public health efforts in the United States should be toward the prevention and control of acute illness rather than chronic disease.

Organized public health efforts in the United States have focused on outbreaks of illnesses such as diphtheria and polio because of the suddenness and the severity of any outbreaks of these illnesses. In reality, however, the much more serious and major public health problems of the United States are no longer acute infectious diseases, but rather are chronic long-term degenerative conditions such as heart disease, cancer, and stroke. Organized public health efforts throughout the United States have a well-recognized role in protecting the public from outbreaks of infections, but they spend considerably less time and energy on problems of a much more serious and long-term nature, such as cancer, alcoholism, and mental illness. By default, organized public health agencies in the United States have accepted an acute illness prevention role as being appropriate, but they have not accepted a chronic disease prevention role to the same degree of intensity.

Because of the unfortunate political controversies of the 1930s around a possible national health insurance program, it would have to be admitted that there has been a relatively guarded relationship between the private medical sector and organized public health agencies throughout the country. As long as the organized public health agencies kept to the more traditional public health roles of sanitation, immunization, and infectious disease control, their activities were generally supported by the private sector. However, whenever the public health sector became more active in the provision of general health services or in the governance or planning of facilities and personnel in the private sector, considerable opposition arose. As a result of this opposition, organized public health agencies have been rather cautious about expanding their efforts beyond the boundaries of what were perceived as "traditional" public health activities.

This is probably most marked and most obvious in reviewing organized public health's unwillingness or inability to assert any major role in the planning or regulation of the provision of health services in the United States. Although a broad definition of *public health* would certainly include the necessity of ensuring that the public has adequate access to personal health services, this planning or regulatory role has not been one that public health agencies have been willing to assume, or been allowed to assume by other forces in society. As a result, the health care system of the United States is a relatively unplanned and poorly coordinated system compared to most major industrialized countries throughout the world. In these countries, it is assumed that public health must protect the interest of the public in obtaining access to appropriate health services of high quality, but that has not been an accepted role for organized public health in the United States until now.

THE STRUCTURE OF ORGANIZED PUBLIC HEALTH EFFORTS IN THE UNITED STATES

The United States utilizes a very intricate combination of local, state, and federal government public health agencies to accomplish the public sector's responsibilities to the American public. Compared to other countries of the world, the United States has one of the most complex sets of governmental relationships of any country in the world, a set of relationships that reflects the unique social and political values of the people of the United States. To understand how public sector activities in health promotion and disease prevention accomplish their objectives, it is important to understand each of the three elements in the public sector—the local, state, and federal government efforts—and then, after understanding how each segment works, understand the relationships between and among them.

In its important 1988 review of public health in the United States, *The Future of Public Health*, the Institute of Medicine stated that the mission of public health was to assure conditions in which people can be healthy; it further stated that the governmental role in public health was made up of three functions: assessment, policy development, and assurance (Institute of Medicine, 1988). Looked at in another way, these functions could be described as identification of the major public health problems, mobilization of necessary effort and resources, and assurance that vital conditions are in place so that crucial services are received.

With regard to assessment, this heading includes all of the activities involved in community diagnosis, such as surveillance, identifying needs, analyzing the causes of problems, collecting and interpreting data, case finding, monitoring and forecasting trends, research, and evaluation of outcomes. Assessment was seen by the Institute of Medicine committee as inherently a public function because policy formation, in order to be legitimate, is expected to take in all relevant information and to be based on neutral and objective factors. Moreover, public decisions take place in the context of limited resources so that a function of government is to provide a central mechanism by means of which competing proposals can be evaluated with only the best interest of society in mind. A fully developed assessment function is absolutely essential for an ideal public health system: without it, a society's real problems cannot be accurately measured, nor can alternative solutions be objectively evaluated.

Policy development is the process by which a society makes decisions about public health problems, chooses goals and the proper means to reach them, handles conflicting views about what should be done, and allocates resources. The Institute of Medicine asserted that government provides overall guidance in this process, as it alone has the power to give answers that are binding on the entire society. In order to maintain its credibility in this policy development role, the governmental public health agency must pay attention to the quality of the policy development process itself and must raise crucial questions that no one else can raise. To carry out this function effectively, the governmental public health agency must be equipped for its policy role with technical knowledge and professional expertise; this knowledge base of public health can therefore temper the excesses of partisan politics and make for fair social decisions.

The assurance function of governmental public health agencies makes sure that necessary services are provided to reach agreed-upon goals, either by encouraging private sector action, by requiring it, or by providing services directly. The assurance function in public health involves the implementation of legislative mandates as well as the maintenance of statutory responsibilities. It includes regulation of services and products provided in both the public and private sectors, as well as maintenance of accountability to the people by setting objectives and reporting on progress. Carrying out the assurance function requires the exercise of social authority; therefore, this is not a responsibility that can be delegated to the private sector. Members of society expect the government to make certain that they enjoy at least adequate safety and security.

In reviewing the activities of the various governmental levels with regard to public health functions, it will be clear that some levels carry out more of one function than another. For example, the federal government level of public health in the United States has more of an assessment and policy development function than it does an assurance function, whereas state and local government public health activities have more of an assurance and assessment function than they do of policy development.

Federal Government Public Health Activities

The federal government's role in public health was relatively limited until the passage in 1913 of the Sixteenth Amendment to the United States Constitution, which authorized a national income tax. Prior to that time, the federal government's role in much of public life in the United States was relatively limited, particularly with regard to public health because the government had neither statutory nor regulatory authority, nor did it have financial resources available to carry out its will. After the passage of a national income tax in 1913, the resources of the federal government in the United States became so overwhelming that federal government authority in all aspects of life, including public health, became the dominant aspect of governmental activity in the United States. Although local and state governments actually have more formal and official responsibilities placed upon them to carry out public health functions than does the federal government, the federal government has by far the greater financial resources and power to make possible implementation of laws and regulations throughout the country. The federal government, therefore, has the predominant role in public health activities in the United States, not necessarily because of its explicitly assigned public health functions under the United States Constitution, but rather because it has more financial power and authority available to it because of the national income tax.

The federal government's activities in public health in the United States are carried out through the Department of Health and Human Services, a cabinet-level department in the federal government. Although the exact internal organization of the Department of Health and Human Services varies somewhat from Congress to Congress and president to president, there is one descriptive characteristic that seems to remain: the Department of Health and Human Services is composed of a series of relatively separate superagencies that have comparatively little interaction with each other and that relate to quite different specialized constituencies, both public and professional. The Department of Health and Human Services is not a carefully designed and well-integrated organization that was intentionally put together to accomplish very specific functions of the whole organization; rather, it is an historical collection of powerful, individual, specialized agencies that at various times in their history were added into an already-existing federation of superagencies. As a result, the Department of Health and Human Services cannot be seen as functioning as a single, well-coordinated organization with a clear operating agenda that governs all of its parts; rather, the agendas of the individual separate superagencies, taken together, make up the policy of the department itself.

The federal Department of Health and Human Services can most easily be understood as having two major subdivisions, one related to health activities and the other related to human services activities. On the human services side of the department would be organizations such as the Administration on Aging; the Administration for Children, Youth, and Families; and the Social Security Administration (the agency that administers the Social Security program). On the health services side of the department would be health-related organizations such as the Centers for

Disease Control and Prevention; the Food and Drug Administration; the Health Resources and Services Administration; the National Institutes of Health; the Alcohol/Drug Abuse/Mental Health Administration; and the Health Care Financing Administration (now the Centers for Medicare and Medicaid Services). Approximately two-thirds of the total budget of the entire Department of Health and Human Services is devoted to human services activities (and the vast bulk of that is specifically devoted to the Social Security Administration), while approximately one-third of the total Department of Health and Human Services budget goes to health-related activities (and the vast majority of that goes to the Health Care Financing Administration for the Medicare and Medicaid programs). Looked at in another way, more than eighty percent of the total budget of the federal Department of Health and Human Services is absorbed by two major programs, Social Security and Medicare/Medicaid (Institute of Medicine, 1988).

The major activities of the federal Department of Health and Human Services with regard to public health can be described through its eight primary functions: (1) documenting the health status and health situation in the United States through the gathering and analysis of statistical data (National Center for Health Statistics and Centers for Disease Control and Prevention); (2) sponsoring research in both basic and applied sciences (National Institutes of Health and the Alcohol/Drug Abuse/Mental Health Administration); (3) formulating national objectives and policy (Office of the Assistant Secretary for Health); (4) setting standards for performance of services and protection of the public (various agencies within the department); (5) providing financial assistance to state and local governments to carry out predetermined programs (Health Resources and Services Administration); (6) ensuring that personnel, facilities, and other technical resources are available to carry out national policies and goals through support for training, construction, and program development (National Institutes of Health, Alcohol/Drug Abuse/Mental Health Administration, and Health Resources and Services Administration); (7) ensuring public access to health care services by the provision of special health insurance programs (Health Care Financing Administration); and (8) providing limited direct services to certain subgroups of the population (Indian Health Service and the former United States Public Health Services Hospitals for Merchant Seamen).

The major portion of the federal government's health activities are conducted through contracts and grants to states, localities, and private providers and organizations. The federal government acts through financing intergovernmental and interorganizational contracts to encourage various public health initiatives, convening participants around an issue, coordinating activities, and developing state and local provider coalitions. In return for federal funds, states, localities, and private organizations must follow the federal standards and policies set in the contract. In most of its activities, the federal government takes an oversight, policy-setting, and technical assistance role, rather than a direct-provider role. Most contracts to states and localities were initially offered as categorical grants, focusing on particular health issues or populations (such as research training grants for education, nutrition information programs, substance abuse and mental health programs, and family planning programs). In the early 1980s, the federal government grouped numerous categorical grants to states into four major block grants: one in preventive health, one in maternal and child health, one in primary care, and one in alcohol/drug abuse/mental health. The more traditional public health functions of the Department of Health and Human Services are generally channeled through the Health Resources and Services Administration and the Centers for Disease Control and Prevention, but these are by no means the only channels by which federal public health finances and resources are channeled to state and local governments.

It should be noted that one of the federal government's major health activities, the provision of a large volume of direct patient care through the Veterans Administration, has no formal or organizational connection with the Department of Health and Human Services. The Veterans Administration and its extensive network of hospitals and clinics throughout the United States does not operate under the authority or jurisdiction of the Department of Health and Human Services at all.

State Government Public Health Activities

States are the principal governmental entity responsible for protecting the public's health in the United States. In the Tenth Amendment to the United States Constitution, states are designated as the repository of all government powers not specifically designated to the federal government. States carry out most of their responsibilities through their police power—the power to enact and enforce laws to protect and promote the health and safety of the people.

There are fifty-five state health agencies in the United States (the fifty states plus the District of Columbia, Guam, Puerto Rico, American Samoa, and the Virgin Islands). It is probably safe to say that each state agency is somewhat different from all the rest, as there is wide variation in the exact way in which state health agencies are organized. In general, each state agency is directed by a health commissioner or a secretary of health. Each agency also has a state health officer (required to be a licensed physician) who is the top public health medical authority in the state; in many states, the state health officer is the director of the state agency, but in some states, the state health officer works for a nonphysician director who is the administrator of a larger agency or department. In approximately half of the states, there is also some type of state Board of Health or similar appointive body that is charged with the responsibility for approving policy in the public health area and for reviewing the use of public funds. Approximately half the states do not have Boards of Health and operate their public health agencies as administrative units of state government without any outside appointive oversight.

Earlier we described the federal Department of Health and Human Services as a somewhat loose collection of superagencies, each of which operated in a semiautonomous fashion from all the rest. State public health agencies, on the other hand, are relatively compact in the organization of their public health services and function as a single operational unit that is usually fairly well integrated within itself. The variation among state public health agencies, however, is that the public health function may be gathered together with a wide variety of other health-related agencies under some type of superagency or department. In some states, the traditional public health functions, usually gathered together in a single operational unit, are housed in a superagency that also contains organizations that deal with environmental issues, mental health services, services for retarded or disabled individuals, as well as the state Medicaid program. There is no uniform arrangement for these state-level superagencies; thus, the public health unit may stand alone as an organizational unit or may be associated with up to four or five other health-related units in a superagency. In the state of California, for example, the Department of Health Services contains not only the traditional public health functions but also the state Medicaid program, which vastly overshadows the much smaller public health function; in California, the public health agency has the responsibility for certain aspects of environmental issues as they relate to health, but a state environmental agency also has somewhat overlapping concerns in the same area.

Regardless of the organizational arrangement, there are certain functions and activities that seem to be common throughout the fifty-five state public health agencies in the United States. These include the following general functions: (1) collect and analyze health statistics to determine the health status and general health situation of the public; (2) provide general education to the public on matters of public health importance; (3) maintain state laboratories to conduct certain specialized tests that are required by state public health law; (4) establish and police public health standards for the state as a whole; (5) grant licenses to health care professionals and institutions throughout the state and monitor and inspect the performance of personnel and institutions as appropriate; and (6) establish general policy for local government public health units and provide them with financial support as may be appropriate.

In general, state public health agencies nationwide receive half of their financial resources from state taxes, approximately one-third from federal government grants and contracts, and the remainder from special sources such as licensing fees and reimbursements (Institute of Medicine, 1988). In discussing federal public health agencies, we pointed out that the financial resources of the federal public health activities draw on the very large national income tax for the financing of their operations, and at the same time, the federal government agencies have relatively few mandated responsibilities that must be carried out. By contrast, state governments must depend on a less robust state income tax for approximately half of their funding and, at the same time, have many more mandated services that they must provide. In general, state health departments are moderately well funded for the services that they are required to provide but considerably underfunded in terms of the potential health promotion and disease prevention services that they could provide.

If it can be said that the federal government public health agencies focus their energies on the identification of major health problems in the country and the establishment of national policies to attack these problems, state public health departments concentrate their energies on translating national health goals and objectives into state policy and spend a considerable bit of their time seeing that that policy is carried out. Many of these policies are carried out by the state public health agencies themselves, and many of them are carried out by local public health agencies under the direction and supervision of state health departments.

Local Government Public Health Activities

Local health departments are the front line of public health services in the United States. It is here in the local government agencies that the actual daily work of public health takes place, and it is here that the policies and strategies decided upon by federal and state public health agencies must be carried out. It is here where the stress of meeting public health challenges is greatest and where deficiencies or shortfalls are most visible and obvious.

Local health departments carry out their activities under the authority delegated by either their state or their local jurisdictions. Depending upon the interests and the resources of the local government, the local government public health function may either be very broad and energetic or very narrow and restricted. Some local health departments serve a single city or county, while others cover a group of counties. In about one-third of the states, the local health units are actually district offices of state health agencies, and in another one-third, the local health agencies are responsible to both local governments and the state public health agency.

The organization of the local public health agency is generally relatively simple, with the local public health agency responding directly to the local elected authority—either a mayor, county administrator, or board of supervisors. In its operations, however, the local public health authority must depend on state or federal funds for approximately half of its operating budget, so the leaders of the local public health agencies must continuously maintain a dual reporting function, one to their local government and the other to the state and/or federal government that provides them with the bulk of their operating revenues.

A special committee of the American Public Health Association, chaired by Haven Emerson in 1945, defined the six basic functions of a local health department as follows (Emerson, 1945):

1. Vital statistics—recording, tabulating, interpreting, and publishing of essential facts of births, deaths, and reportable diseases
2. Communicable disease control—tuberculosis, venereal disease, measles, hepatitis, and AIDS
3. Sanitation—supervision of milk, water, and eating places
4. Laboratory services
5. Maternal and child health services, including supervision of the health of children in schools
6. Health education of the public

For the most part, local public health departments continue to carry out the vital statistics, communicable disease control, environmental sanitation, and maternal and child health functions even up to the present time. They also, for the most part, maintain active public health education programs, although these efforts have become increasingly endangered by budgetary deficiencies. For the most part, laboratory services are no longer provided by local public health departments but are now provided by state health departments. And for the most part, the local public health department's functions are very immediate and in direct contact with the public: recording births and deaths, trying to maintain control or contact of individual people with serious communicable diseases, inspecting restaurants and other public gathering places to identify sanitary problems, and making sure that newborn infants receive their immunizations for infectious diseases and that children in school have some degree of health supervision. If the federal government's functions can be described as distant, nationwide, impersonal, and related to policy, the local government's public health function can be described as immediate, individual, pragmatic, and personal. The basic operating unit of local government public health only serves to enhance this sense of immediate contact with the public because it is usually represented by the local health center or local public health office; this is usually situated in areas of the greatest public health problems and at locations that provide the easiest access to the most susceptible segments of the population.

Unfortunately, the disconnection between mandated required services and financial resources becomes most apparent at the local public health level. In the United States, local governments are usually the least well financed of the three levels of government, and it is no different for local public health agencies (Institute of Medicine, 1988). It is almost universally the case that local public health agencies are inadequately financed to perform even the minimum functions required by local or state law, let alone to provide an expanded and aggressive public health activity in keeping with the real needs of the public and potential for health improvement (Gordon, Gerzoff, & Richards, 1997). It must be sadly admitted that local public health departments in the United States are probably the weakest link in the public health chain, not because they are inadequately organized or poorly led, but rather because they seldom have the financial resources they need to meet their real potential.

Integrating Public Health Services

From this description, it can be seen that the public portion of our nation's health promotion and disease prevention activities depends upon an intricate collaboration and cooperation between three levels of governmental agencies: federal, state, and local. It involves elaborate transfer of financial resources from the federal government (where the resources are most abundant) to state governments (where resources are less abundant but still sufficient) and through to local public health agencies (where resources are scarcest and responsibilities most intense). The public portion of our nation's health promotion and disease prevention activities is, for the most part, focused first on the protection of the public from potential threats to health and only secondarily on the active promotion of healthier lifestyles.

Although the public health professionals in governmental health agencies know very well that the greatest long-term impact on the health of our nation's people probably depends upon changes in styles of living, those same public health professionals very often find themselves limited in their ability to engage in activities that are directly focused on lifestyle change. Federal, state, and local government public health agencies can create policies and goals to encourage individual personal lifestyle change, but for the most part, the actual implementation of those changes probably rests with the private sector, with the providers of medical care. Governmental public health agencies can go only so far with the resources available to them in creating an atmosphere for major lifestyle change and improvement and, therefore, must depend upon their private-sector colleagues to carry the effort more directly into the homes of individual people. Nevertheless, governmental public health agencies have played a vital role in the protection of the public, in setting strategies and goals for the improvement of the health status of the public, and in motivating the public to move to an even higher level of healthful living.

For that next level of health promotion and disease prevention, however, the full involvement and participation of the private sector is necessary. The importance of the private-sector clinical role was stressed in the United States Preventive Services Task Force Report in 1989 and was reinforced by the United States Public Health Service's major reports, *Healthy People 2000* and *Healthy People 2010*, which set national health promotion and disease prevention objectives for the country (U.S. Department of Health and Hu-

man Services, 2000; U.S. Preventive Services Task Force, 1989; U.S. Public Health Service, 1990).

THE ROLE OF THE PRIVATE SECTOR IN HEALTH PROMOTION AND DISEASE PREVENTION

It is comparatively easy to discuss the role of governmental public health agencies: usually they have been in existence for some time, have clearly defined roles, and have well-documented track records extending over many years. When one approaches the role of the private sector in health promotion and disease prevention, however, discussion becomes more difficult and more diffuse, if no less important. Indeed, in the minds of many individuals, the role of the private sector, particularly the physician in private practice, is increasingly central in creating the major lifestyle changes that are viewed as being so important to the prevention of disease over the long term.

McGinnis and Foege (1993) reviewed the actual causes of death in the United States for the year 1990 and determined that almost half of all of those deaths were attributable to lifestyle and personal actions on the part of individuals, such as tobacco use, improper diet and activity patterns, overuse of alcohol and firearms, unsafe sexual behavior, and vehicular accidents while under the influence of alcohol. They point out that most of these causes of death are only partially amenable to change by broad social or legislative actions and that only individual behavior change will really affect many of them. They also point out that the physician in medical practice is in a key position to influence behavior change because research has shown that individuals are more likely to follow improved health habits if they are encouraged to do so by their usual medical practitioner. The central role of the practicing physician in encouraging and enhancing improved personal life habits has long been acknowledged and must be central to any future national plan of health promotion and disease prevention.

There are two major barriers to the individual physician's assuming the central role in health promotion and disease prevention: (1) the individual physician's willingness and ability to perform these health promotion and disease prevention activities, and (2) the ability of the population to access the services of a private physician.

With regard to the physician's interest in, and ability to perform, health promotion and disease prevention activities, it has long been noted that physicians are generally more interested and more competent in matters related to curative and treatment activities than they are in matters related to health promotion and disease prevention. This may be a reflection of their early medical training, which may have lacked emphasis on health promotion and disease prevention, or it may be related to the physician's natural human tendency to see curative treatment as "doing something" while seeing health promotion and disease prevention as "not doing something." Physicians are by nature activists and are more naturally drawn to the interventions where they are likely to see results in a relatively short period of time as opposed to events where the consequences of their actions will be known only, if at all, many years later.

It should also be pointed out that in the previous era of fee-for-service medicine, physicians were only reimbursed for treatment activities and were usually not reimbursed, either by insurance companies or by individuals paying their own bills, for prevention services. The former methods of payment for medical services encouraged increased active treatment of illness but did not encourage its active prevention. It is only natural, therefore, that physicians in the past should have responded to obvious incentives by spending more of their time and energies on treatment and less on prevention.

Probably a greater barrier to enhancing the role of the private physician in health promotion and disease prevention is the limited access that a significant portion of our population has to medical care. If a significant portion of the United States population is uninsured (estimates run between twelve and fifteen percent at any single point in time) or if a significant portion of the population has very limited insurance with relatively large financial burdens still resting with the individual patient, it is unlikely that individuals will visit a physician on a regular basis (Brown, Valdez, Wyn, Yu, & Cumberland, 1994). If individual people in the United States discover that their insurance plans do not cover health promotion and disease prevention and that they must pay for such tests themselves, they are less likely to use such tests and

procedures and to visit a physician on a regular basis to obtain the counseling and encouragement that might be possible there.

It would seem natural to suggest, therefore, that if our nation wishes to involve the private sector in extensive health promotion and disease prevention activities that reach our entire population, it must be arranged in some fashion for the entire population to have health insurance coverage that ensures adequate access to medical care. Without universal health insurance coverage of some kind, it is an illusion to talk about a nationwide health promotion and disease prevention effort, as a significant percentage of the population (and, perhaps, those at highest risk) cannot access the one place where the most influential health promotion and disease prevention counseling might take place—the office of a private medical practitioner. Universal health insurance coverage, therefore, is central to any nationwide effort of health promotion and disease prevention.

Merely having universal health insurance coverage, however, is not enough if that health insurance coverage does not include financing for health promotion and disease prevention tests, procedures, and counseling. Many of the health insurance plans issued at the present time do not include reimbursement for health promotion and disease prevention, and as a result, individuals who may actually have health insurance coverage of a general nature are not covered for health promotion and disease prevention services. Therefore, it is essential that the design of future health insurance packages include financing for these services. Without such financing, individuals may be actively discouraged from seeking health promotion and disease prevention tests and procedures, as well as advice and counseling, from their primary physician.

The Role of Managed Care in Health Promotion and Disease Prevention

The advent of managed-care health insurance coverage around the United States may present an opportunity to accomplish some of these health promotion and disease prevention objectives, particularly if the specific managed-care plans are those of the health maintenance organization (HMO) type, which reimburse physician groups on a *per capita* basis. The advent of managed care of the HMO type presents opportunities for the expansion of health promotion and disease prevention in ways that have not been previously available (Breslow, 1996).

It is important to note two essential elements of the HMO type of managed-care plan: (1) the official assignment of the long-term responsibility for supervising all aspects of an individual's care to a specific physician or medical group, and (2) the reimbursement of that physician or medical group on a *per capita* basis. Each of these specific aspects of HMO managed care is very supportive of the general long-term thrust in health promotion and disease prevention.

With regard to the first (that is, the assignment of long-term responsibility for an individual's care to a specific physician), HMO managed-care plans require the identification of a specific primary care physician for each person covered by that type of insurance. This puts a particular physician on notice that this individual patient (or family unit) is his/her long-term responsibility. This identification of the individual physician as having an official long-term and continuing responsibility for an individual or a family changes the perspective of the individual physician away from the provision of specific individual services and toward the long-term health of the individual or the family. The designation of an individual physician as a patient's primary care doctor further solidifies the long-term role of that physician in managing the entire health-related set of activities in the minds of both the physician and the patient.

The use of *per capita* reimbursement to the primary care physician further reinforces the long-term nature of the relationship and particularly emphasizes the long-term role of attempting to reach maximum health outcomes, not just providing individual fee-for-service interactions. The HMO *per capita* reimbursement method serves as a reminder to the physician that his/her financial rewards are dependent upon keeping the individual patient as healthy as possible, rather than simply providing a series of individual services to a sick person. The dynamics in the HMO managed-care plan thereby provide more incentives for keeping people healthy.

Managed-care insurance coverage of the HMO type also has a great advantage over the previous fee-for-service type of coverage in that it not only assigns official responsibility to an individual physician or medical group, but it also holds that physician or medical group accountable for what happens to the patient. In the past, no physician or medical group was responsible for reporting to any insurance plan or purchaser of health care about the long-term pattern of services and their results. The individual physician merely provided one service after another on an individual and relatively unconnected basis, and no accountability was ever really required as to how the pattern of individual services eventually affected the overall health of an individual patient.

Under the new forms of HMO managed care, not only is it possible to assign individual long-term responsibility to a specific physician or medical group, but it is also possible, and, indeed, increasingly the rule, to designate specific actions that the physician or group must take during the course of a particular year. It is increasingly common for HMO managed-care plans to outline certain specific services or practices that a physician must follow and also to require documentation of the completion of those services (Schauffler & Rodriguez, 1996).

For example, many HMO managed-care plans require that physicians provide certain health promotion and disease prevention services (such as immunizations for children, provision of mammograms for women over a certain age, blood cholesterol measurements, and the like). Not only are the HMO managed-care plans able to require physicians to provide these services, but they are also able to require the physicians to report that these services have actually been completed.

What this means for the encouragement of health promotion and disease prevention activities on the part of the physician should be obvious. In the future, if it is judged that a certain pattern of health promotion and disease prevention services or activities should be provided to an individual patient during the course of a particular year, that requirement can be written into the contract with the individual physician before he/she is allowed to assume long-term responsibility for the patient. Unwillingness to perform these health promotion and disease prevention actions would bar the physician from being able to contract with the HMO managed-care plan in the first place. The contract language also can ensure that the physician agrees to provide information that will allow the plan to determine whether the services have actually been delivered to the patient as agreed upon.

Many aspects of managed care are cause for concern among thoughtful observers of health care in the United States, but the enhancement of health promotion and disease prevention activities is not one of them. Indeed, one of the major positive aspects of managed care is its potential ability to install an organized, well-financed, and well-documented system of care that emphasizes health promotion and disease prevention. Despite whatever other concerns may exist about managed care, it is clear that the growth of managed-care health insurance coverage offers an opportunity for an entirely new era with regard to the promotion of better health and the prevention of future disease in the United States (Schauffler, et al., 1993, 1994).

SUMMARY

It should be clear from this discussion of health promotion and disease prevention in the United States that this is a shared responsibility between the public (governmental) and the private sectors of health care. Neither sector can do what the other can do, and neither sector can do it alone. For the people of this country to reach their maximum health status, it will be necessary to forge an even stronger public-private partnership that allows both sectors to use their unique roles and advantages to advance the health of the public in ways that have never before been possible.

References

Breslow, L. (1996). Public health and managed care: A California perspective. *Health Affairs, 15,* 92–99.

Brown, E. R., Valdez, R., Wyn, R., Yu, H., & Cumberland, W. (1994). *Who are California's uninsured?* Los Angeles: University of California, Center for Health Policy Research.

Commission on Chronic Illness. (1957). *Chronic illness in the United States:* Vol. I, *Prevention of chronic illness.* Cambridge, MA: Harvard University Press.

Emerson, H. (1945). *Local health units for the nation.* New York: Commonwealth Fund.

Gordon, R., Gerzoff, R., & Richards, T. (1997). Determinants of U.S. local health department expenditures, 1992 through 1993. *American Journal of Public Health, 87,* 91–95.

Institute of Medicine of the U.S. National Academy of Sciences. (1988). *The future of public health.* Washington, DC: National Academy Press.

Leavell, H. R., & Clark, E. G. (1958). *Preventive medicine for the doctor in his community.* New York: McGraw-Hill.

McGinnis, J., & Foege, W. (1993). Actual cases of death in the United States. *Journal of the American Medical Association, 270,* 2208.

Moutin, J., Hankela, E., & Druzin, G. (1947). *Ten years of federal grants-in-aid for public health, 1936–1946.* (Bull. No. 300). Washington, DC: Public Health Service.

Schauffler, H. H., & Rodriguez, T. (1993). Managed care for preventive services: A review of policy options. *Medical Care Review, 50,* 153–198.

Schauffler, H. H., & Rodriguez, T. (1994). Availability and Utilization of Health Promotion and Disease Prevention Programs and Satisfaction with Health Plan. *Medical Care, 32,* 1182–1196.

Schauffler, H. H., & Rodriguez, T. (1996). Exercising purchasing power for preventive care. *Health Affairs, 15,* 73–85.

Shattuck, L. (1850). *Report of the Sanitary Commission of Massachusetts.* Boston: Dutton & Wentworth. (Reprinted by Harvard University Press, Cambridge, MA, 1948).

U.S. Department of Health and Human Services. (2000). *Healthy People 2010.* (2nd ed.). Washington, DC: U.S. Government Printing Office.

U.S. Preventive Services Task Force. (1989). *Guide to clinical preventive services: An assessment of the effectiveness of 169 interventions.* Baltimore: Williams & Wilkins.

U.S. Public Health Service. (1990). *Healthy people 2000: National health promotion and disease prevention objectives* (DHHS Pub. No. PHS 91-50212). Washington, DC: Department of Health and Human Services.

Winslow, C. E. A. (1923). The evolution and significance of the modern public health campaign. Reprinted in: *J of PH Policy, 1*(1); 15–24.

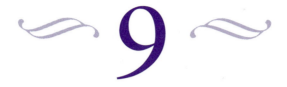

C H A P T E R
9

Ambulatory Health Care Services

Stephen J. Williams

Chapter Topics

- Historical Perspective and Types of Care
- Settings for the Provision of Ambulatory Care
- Ambulatory Practice Settings
- Institutionally Based Ambulatory Services
- Government Programs
- Noninstitutional and Public Health Services
- Organization of Ambulatory Care Systems
- Ambulatory Care and the Challenge of Managed Care
- Summary

Learning Objectives

Upon completing this chapter, the reader should be able to:

- Understand the role of ambulatory care services
- Appreciate the evolution of ambulatory care as a delivery setting
- Review the primary ambulatory care providers
- Outline the organizational role and control mechanisms of ambulatory care services
- Assess the allocation of responsibility for coordination, integration, appropriateness, and rationalization between ambulatory care and other sectors

The evolution of our nation's health care system, particularly trends in the technology of medicine and surgery, and changes in financial arrangements have shifted the focus of the provision and control of health services to the ambulatory care arena. For many years, the hospital was the principal focus of the health care delivery system, but over the past decade, the role of the hospital has eroded while the advantages of shifting control and services to the ambulatory sector have been increasingly recognized by payers and providers alike. The ambulatory arena is more tolerable for the patient as well.

This chapter addresses the historical development and current and future roles of ambulatory care services, placing these services in a broader context that recognizes both the direct provision of care and mechanisms of controlling patients and providers within various payment arrangements. Descriptions of various ambulatory care provider settings, quantitative descriptions of the volume and nature of such services, and the increasingly important role of these services in the coordination and organization of the system are addressed.

The role of ambulatory care services in organizing and rationalizing the health care system has been greatly enhanced by the rapid growth of managed care, by the changing nature and role of hospitals and hospital systems, and by enhancement of the gatekeeper and coordinating function of frontline providers of care. The increasing shift of many services that have been traditionally performed on an inpatient basis such as many surgical services, maintenance-oriented care that is now provided in the home rather than in the hospital, and other practical and technological changes have also heightened interest in ambulatory care. Finally, the increasing consolidation and vertical integration of the health care system is greatly increasing the linkages between ambulatory care and other services.

Tremendous operational and financial pressures have been placed on ambulatory care services over the past couple of years as a result of managed care and other trends in the health care system. Managers of these resources face an increasingly difficult environment. The recent financial difficulties of physician-management companies and of other ambulatory care organizations highlight these pressures. Physician and consumer dissatisfaction with many aspects of managed care, particularly those associated with control of physician practice patterns and behavior, has recently reached a crescendo. Technological advances that increasingly point toward the delivery of services through ambulatory care mechanisms will require organizational responses appropriate to the expanding role of this modality in the provision of care throughout the country.

Many of these changes and trends are discussed in other chapters of this book; their relevance to ambulatory care and ambulatory care's enhanced role in the system is discussed in detail in this chapter. Ambulatory care has long had a central role in health care, a role that is now increasing in scope and importance. An interesting history characterizes the evolution of these services.

Traditionally, ambulatory care services have been viewed as the primary source of contact that most people have with the health care system. Although there are few concise definitions of ambulatory care, these services can be defined as care provided to noninstitutionalized patients. Sometimes ambulatory care is termed care for the "walking patient." Ambulatory care includes a wide range of services, from simple, routine treatment to surprisingly complex tests and therapies.

HISTORICAL PERSPECTIVE AND TYPES OF CARE

Ambulatory care originated with the healing arts themselves. In primitive societies and for many years thereafter, until the advent of institutional care, all care was provided on what might be referred to as an *ambulatory care basis*. Of course, the types of care given then bear little resemblance to today's health care, but the history of civilization demonstrates a consistent commitment to caring for the sick using whatever knowledge has been available at the time. Remarkable forms of medical practice occurred in Greece, Rome, and other relatively sophisticated societies. In fact, many primitive societies had their own indigenous practitioners such as religious healers and medicine men.

In more recent times, ambulatory care was provided in many new settings by a variety of more advanced practitioners. In Europe, and later in the

United States, many of these services were given to wealthy patients in their homes; poor people were cared for in dispensaries and public clinics. With improvements in hospital care, more patients of all social classes received both inpatient and outpatient care in hospital settings. In the United States, the poor have always been more likely than the wealthy to obtain care from the hospital than from private physicians.

In the United States, ambulatory care services were traditionally provided by individual medical practitioners working in their offices and in patients' homes and by public clinics operating primarily for poor and indigent patients. The limited technological armament that physicians required allowed them to travel easily, carrying with them their principal equipment and supplies. Thus, home care was common, especially among wealthier patients. Physicians' offices were frequently located in their homes or in other small buildings, as opposed to today's medical office buildings or large medical centers. The general practitioner who made house calls, provided guidance, and offered available treatments was typical of the primary care provided before World War II.

Since World War II, however, an explosion of medical knowledge has led to increasing specialization, more complex technology, and rapid changes in the setting and nature of services. Fewer physicians are able or willing to travel to the patient's home, and many can no longer carry with them either the equipment and supplies or the specialized personnel available in an office. The growth of technical specialization, in particular, has led to the rapid expansion of new settings for providing care, such as group practices and, more recently, a profusion of specialized facilities. Increased knowledge has also led to the partial phasing out of the traditional general practitioner, although a new form of generalist is now taking hold, encouraged by managed care and concerns over the comprehensiveness of care.

For the poor in both Europe and the United States, care—when available—was often limited to public or philanthropic clinics or dispensaries. Private practitioners may have given their time to serve the poor, but their devotion to the patient was probably limited, as was the availability of care and the facilities in which services were provided.

Early efforts to link ambulatory care services and integrate them formally with inpatient care were promoted in this country and in Europe, in part, through the concept of regionalization. In Great Britain, the concept was presented in the Dawson Report, which eventually led to the National Health Service (United Kingdom Ministry of Health, 1920). In the United States, however, centralization of authority under government of the health care system has not been accepted as a politically viable alternative, a principle most recently affirmed by the rejection of the Clinton health care initiatives discussed later in this book.

The increasing sophistication of insurance mechanisms and the use of ambulatory care services as a control mechanism on the use of all services have led to an increase in the degree of structure of the health care system over the past few years. This increasing structure has primarily occurred in the private, nongovernmental sector. The concept of social and economic regulation of the system through governmental intervention, carried to a high level of sophistication in the Dawson Report, has largely been abandoned, at least for the foreseeable future. Integration of services will focus largely on multiple, independently organized systems of care that are competitive with one another.

The diversity of services, providers, and facilities involved in ambulatory care today is truly amazing and growing all the time. Many of these services and organizations are discussed in this chapter. Particular attention is directed toward rapidly expanding and innovative settings, such as group practice, and integration of settings and services through organized systems of care, especially in managed care. The role of ambulatory care is also discussed in other chapters of this book, especially those dealing with insurance and organizational arrangements.

Levels of Ambulatory Care Services

Ambulatory care services can be differentiated into a number of distinct levels or types of care. Primary prevention seeks to reduce the risks of illness or morbidity by removing or reducing disease-causing agents and opportunities from our society. These activities include efforts to eliminate environmental pollutants that are suspected to cause diseases such as cancer. Other examples of primary prevention include encouraging people to use automobile seat belts, treatment of water and sewage, and sanitation inspections in restaurants. Preventive health services are more direct personal interventions to detect and prevent disease. Examples of these services include hypertension, diabetes, and cancer-screening clinics and immunization programs. The combination of primary prevention and preventive services is our first line of defense against disease.

Medical care that is oriented toward the daily, routine needs of patients, such as initial diagnosis and continuing treatment of common illness, is termed *primary care*. This care is not highly complex and generally does not require sophisticated technology and personnel. The vision of the general practitioner of bygone days, traveling from house to house ministering to the sick, represents the traditional role of primary care, which is replaced in today's society by considerably more skilled practitioners in relatively complex facilities.

In addition to providing services directly, the primary care professional should serve the role of patient advisor, advocate, and system gatekeeper. In this coordinating role, the provider refers patients to sources of specialized care, gives advice regarding various diagnoses and therapies, and provides continuing care for chronic conditions. In many organized systems of care, such as managed-care programs, this role is very important in controlling costs, utilization, and the rational allocation of resources.

The evolution of technology and medicine's increasing ability to intervene in illness have led to greater specialization of health care services. These more specialized services, termed *secondary* and *tertiary care*, are provided in both ambulatory and inpatient settings. The content of secondary and tertiary care practices is usually more narrowly defined than that of the primary care provider. Subspecialists, who provide the bulk of secondary and tertiary care, also often require more complex equipment and more highly trained support personnel than do primary care providers.

In recent years, the evolution of health care services has led to greatly expanded provision of secondary care on an outpatient, or ambulatory care, basis.

Numerous surgical services of increasing complexity have been shifted to the ambulatory arena; recent advances in the use of fiber optic and other technologies suggest that this trend will continue. Diagnostic and therapeutic procedures that used to require hospitalization are also increasingly being performed in ambulatory settings.

There are no clear dividing lines for primary versus secondary and secondary versus tertiary care. Secondary services include routine hospitalization and specialized outpatient care. These services are more complex than those of primary care and include many diagnostic procedures as well as more complex therapies. Tertiary care includes the most complex services, such as open heart surgery, burn treatment, and transplantation, and is provided in inpatient hospital facilities. Most of the care discussed in this chapter involves primary care and those secondary services that can be provided in such settings as office-based practice, hospital out-patient departments, or community clinics.

SETTINGS FOR THE PROVISION OF AMBULATORY CARE

Use of Ambulatory Care Services

Historically, and at the present time, most ambulatory care services are provided in solo and group practice, office-based settings. Institutional settings for care, primarily the hospital, although an important component of the health care system, remain less prominent. Overlap between office-based practice and institutional settings is increasingly common, however, as the dividing lines between various components of the health care system continue to blur. Managed-care programs especially tend to integrate these services.

An indication of the use and sites of ambulatory care visits is contained in Tables 9.1, 9.2, and 9.3, which present survey results on utilization patterns based on national data that are representative of the entire United States population. These data are taken from the National Health Interview Survey (Woodwell, 1999), a national survey of Americans' use of health care services, and they complement the utilization data presented in previous chapters.

Table 9.1. Health Care Visits to Doctor's Offices, Emergency Departments, and Home Visits Over 12 Months by Age: United States, 1998

	Number of Health Care Visits			
Characteristic	None	1–3 Visits	4–9 Visits	10 or More Visits
	Percent distribution			
All persons	15.9	46.8	23.8	13.5
Age Group				
Under 18 years	11.7	54.5	25.6	8.2
Under 6 years	4.9	46.7	36.6	11.8
6–17 years	15.0	58.4	20.3	6.3
18–44 years	21.6	47.7	18.6	12.2
18–24 years	22.6	47.7	18.5	11.2
25–44 years	21.3	47.6	18.6	12.5
45–64 years	15.9	43.6	24.3	16.2
45–54 years	17.2	44.9	22.5	15.4
55–64 years	13.8	41.6	27.1	17.5
65 years and over	7.3	34.1	35.3	23.4
65–74 years	8.4	36.6	34.3	20.8
75 years and over	6.0	30.8	36.5	26.7

Table 9.2. Health Care Visits to Doctor's Offices, Emergency Departments, and Home Visits Over 12 Months, Selected Characteristics: United States, 1998

	Number of Health Care Visits			
Characteristic	None	1–3 Visits	4–9 Visits	10 or More Visits
	Percent distribution			
Sex				
Male	20.7	47.3	21.2	10.8
Female	11.3	46.4	26.3	16.0
Race				
White	15.5	46.8	24.1	13.6
Black	16.4	46.5	23.3	13.8
American Indian or Alaska Native	20.0	39.0	25.1	15.9
Asian or Pacific Islander	21.0	48.2	21.3	9.5
Race and Hispanic origin				
White, non-Hispanic	14.2	47.1	24.6	14.0
Black, non-Hispanic	16.5	46.5	23.2	13.8
Hispanic	24.0	44.8	19.7	11.5
Respondent-assessed health status				
Fair or poor	9.7	23.4	25.3	41.6
Good to excellent	16.6	49.0	23.7	10.8
Poverty status				
Poor	20.9	37.8	22.8	18.5
Nonpoor	13.4	48.6	25.3	12.7

Table 9.3. Interval Since Last Health Care Contact Among Adults, According to Selected Characteristics: United States, 1998

Characteristic	1 Year or Less	More than 1 Year to 3 Years	More than 3 Years
		Percent distribution	
All adults 18 years of age and over	83.1	11.1	5.8
Age Group			
18–44 years	79.0	14.1	6.9
18–24 years	78.9	14.4	6.8
25–44 years	79.1	14.0	6.9
45–64 years	84.6	9.6	5.7
45–54 years	83.8	10.4	5.9
55–64 years	86.0	8.5	5.5
65 years and over	93.3	4.2	2.5
65–74 years	92.2	4.8	3.0
75 years and over	94.7	3.5	1.8
Sex			
Male	76.5	14.7	8.8
Female	89.5	7.6	2.9
Race			
White	83.3	11.0	5.7
Black	84.7	10.3	5.0
American Indian or Alaska Native	77.2	13.0	9.8
Asian or Pacific Islander	78.0	13.6	8.4
Race and Hispanic origin			
White, non-Hispanic	84.3	10.8	5.0
Black, non-Hispanic	84.6	10.4	4.9
Hispanic	76.1	12.9	11.0
Poverty status			
Poor	78.4	12.6	9.0
Nonpoor	85.3	10.3	4.4
Geographic region			
Northeast	86.0	9.3	4.6
Midwest	83.2	11.4	5.4
South	82.7	11.3	6.0
West	71.0	12.0	7.0

Tables 9.1 and 9.2 describe doctor visits experienced by Americans in various demographic categories. The very young and the very old report higher utilization of ambulatory services, and females generally experience higher utilization than males. The lowest-income groups in our population, not coincidentally those of lower health status as well, experience the highest utilization of ambulatory services when the data are examined by income groups. In examining the data by health status, ambulatory services utilization is highest for the less healthy, as would be expected.

Table 9.3, also based on data from the National Health Interview Survey, indicates that most Americans have utilized physician resources in the prior year, with relatively few individuals reporting no utilization for two or more years. Again, females and the poor are more likely to report utilization for one- and two-year periods, and the very young and the very old are also more likely to use services within the prior one or two years.

Use of Office Setting Services

Most utilization data are available from survey research results. To obtain more detailed information on health care use in physician office settings, the federal government has conducted periodic surveys of private, office-based physicians—the National Ambulatory Medical Care Survey (Woodwell, 1999). This survey involves a random sample of the nation's office-based, nonfederal physicians. Physicians are asked to complete a data collection form for each patient treated during a two-week interval.

Tables 9.4 and 9.5 list the most common reasons and the principal diagnoses for all office visits, respectively. The relative prominence of routine care, of follow-up or ongoing care, and of relatively simple primary care is striking and reflects the predominance of routine,

Table 9.4.   Number and Percent Distribution of Office Visits by the Twenty Principal Reasons Most Frequently Mentioned by Patients, According to Patient's Sex: United States, 1997

Principal Reason for Visit	Number of Visits in Thousands	Patient's Sex (Percent Distribution)	
		Female	Male
All visits	787,372	100.0	100.0
General medical examination	59,796	8.0	7.0
Progress visit, not otherwise specified	28,583	3.2	4.2
Cough	25,735	2.8	4.0
Routine prenatal examination	22,979	4.9	—
Postoperative visit	18,861	2.5	2.2
Symptoms referable to throat	17,151	1.9	2.6
Well baby examination	15,526	1.6	2.5
Vision dysfunctions	13,443	1.7	1.6
Earache or ear infection	13,359	1.5	1.9
Back symptoms	12,863	1.5	1.9
Knee symptoms	12,392	1.4	1.8
Fever	12,374	1.1	2.2
Skin rash	12,316	1.4	1.9
Stomach pain, cramps, and spasms	12,078	1.7	1.2
Hypertension	10,875	1.3	1.4
Nasal congestion	10,564	1.3	1.4
Depression	10,488	1.5	1.1
Headache, pain in head	9,589	1.3	1.0
Medication, other and unspecified kinds	9,056	1.1	1.2
Head cold, upper respiratory infection (coryza)	8,965	1.2	1.1
All other reasons	450,380	56.9	57.7

SOURCE: Woodwell, D. A. (1999). *National Ambulatory Medical Care Survey: 1997 Summary.* Hyattsville, Maryland: National Center for Health Statistics.

Table 9.5.   Number and Percent Distribution of Office Visits by Selected Primary Diagnosis Groups, According to Patient's Sex: United States, 1996

Primary Diagnosis Group	Number of Visits in Thousands	Patient's Sex (Percent Distribution)		
		All	Female	Male
All visits	787,372	100.0	100.0	100.0
Acute upper respiratory infections, excluding pharyngitis	31,957	4.1	3.7	4.6
Essential hypertension	29,716	3.8	3.7	3.9
Routine infant or child health check	27,585	3.5	2.8	4.5
Normal pregnancy	22,848	2.9	4.8	0.0
Arthropathies and related disorders	20,860	2.6	3.0	2.2
General medical examination	20,804	2.6	2.6	2.7
Otitis media and Eustachian tube disorders	20,009	2.5	2.0	3.3
Diabetes mellitus	17,878	2.3	2.0	2.7
Malignant neoplasms	16,592	2.1	1.7	2.7
Rheumatism, excluding back	16,415	2.1	2.1	2.0
Dorsopathies	15,831	2.0	1.8	2.3
Chronic sinusitis	13,349	1.7	1.7	1.7
Ischemic heart disease	10,678	1.4	0.9	2.1
Follow-up examination	10,151	1.3	1.4	1.1
Asthma	9,834	1.2	1.1	1.5
Chronic and unspecified bronchitis	9,727	1.2	1.0	1.6
Heart disease, excluding ischemic	9,220	1.2	0.9	1.5
Cataract	9,087	1.2	1.3	0.9
Potential health hazards related to personal and family history	8,355	1.1	1.0	1.2
Allergic rhinitis	7,763	1.0	1.1	0.9
All other	458,713	58.3	59.2	56.8

SOURCE: Woodwell, D. A. (1999). *National Ambulatory Medical Care Survey: 1997 Summary.* Hyattsville, Maryland: National Center for Health Statistics.

day-to-day needs of patients seeking ambulatory care services.

Further understanding of the nature of the visits is obtainable from additional data regarding the services provided to patients and the interactions shared between patients and physicians. Table 9.6 presents the source of payment for patients. The principal sources of payment for patient office visits are private and commercial insurance, Medicare, HMOs, and other managed-care arrangements. The percentage of visits included in this last category likely will increase in future years while managed care grows in popularity. The drugs prescribed during the physician office visits are classified in Table 9.7. The most preva-

lent categories of drugs include cardiovascular and renal, antimicrobial, and pain-relief agents. As technology changes, the classification distribution of various drug categories will likely change in prevalence as well.

Table 9.8 presents the distribution of office visits by the duration of the visit. Relatively few visits require either very short or very long physician contacts. The typical physician office visit requires only about five to thirty minutes of time; nearly three-fourths of all visits require fifteen minutes or less. A high percentage of visits conclude with the recommendation that the patient return at a specified time interval for a follow-up visit.

Table 9.6. Number and Percent Distribution of Office Visits by Primary Expected Source of Payment and Health Maintenance Organization (HMO) Status: United States, 1997

Visit Characteristic	Number of Visits in Thousands	Percent Distribution
All visits	787,372	100.0
Primary expected source of payment		
Private insurance	417,744	53.1
Medicare	163,263	20.7
Medicaid	64,047	8.1
Self-pay	60,869	7.7
Worker's compensation	15,595	2.0
No charge	8,225	1.0
Other	41,000	5.2
Unknown/blank	16,629	2.1
HMO status		
Yes	220,478	28.0
No	488,291	62.0
Unknown/blank	78,602	10.0

NOTE: Numbers may not add to totals because of rounding.

SOURCE: Woodwell, D. A. (1999). *National Ambulatory Medical Care Survey: 1997 Summary.* Hyattsville, Maryland: National Center for Health Statistics.

Table 9.7. Number and Percent Distribution of Drug Mentions by Therapeutic Classification: United States, 1997

Therapeutic Classification	Number of Drug Mentions in Thousands	Percent Distribution
All drug mentions	1,030,897	100.0
Cardiovascular-renal drugs	151,226	14.7
Antimicrobial agents	122,801	11.9
Drugs used for relief of pain	114,583	11.1
Respiratory tract drugs	100,218	9.7
Hormones and agents affecting hormonal mechanisms	98,444	9.5
Central nervous system	90,769	8.8
Metabolic and nutrient agents	58,956	5.7
Skin/mucous membrane	58,756	5.7
Immunologic agents	46,236	4.5
Gastrointestinal agents	43,573	4.2
Ophthalmic drugs	36,369	3.5
Neurologic drugs	25,566	2.5
Hematologic agents	24,556	2.4
Anesthetic drugs	8,361	0.8
Oncolytic agents	7,458	0.7
Otologics	5,614	0.5
Contrast media/radiopharmaceuticals	4,672	0.5
Antiparasitics	4,353	0.4
Other and unclassified	28,386	2.8

SOURCE: Woodwell, D. A. *National Ambulatory Medical Care Survey: 1997 Summary.* Hyattsville, Maryland: National Center for Health Statistics.

Table 9.8. Number and Percent Distribution of Office Visits by Duration of Visit: United States, 1997

Time Spent With Physician	Number of Visits in Thousands	Percent Distribution
All visits	787,372	100.0
0 minutes[a]	25,464	3.2
1–5 minutes	40,523	5.1
6–10 minutes	185,026	23.5
11–15 minutes	247,541	31.4
16–30 minutes	230,656	29.3
31–60 minutes	54,170	6.9
61 minutes and over	3,991	0.5

[a]Visits in which there was no face-to-face contact between patient and physician.

NOTE: Numbers may not add to totals because of rounding.

SOURCE: Woodwell, D. A. (1999). *National Ambulatory Medical Care Survey: 1997 Summary.* Hyattsville, Maryland: National Center for Health Statistics.

The National Ambulatory Medical Care Survey thus provides some insight into the nature of office-based ambulatory care. Much more extensive documentation of the survey and results for various types of services, providers, and patient characteristics is available from the federal government. The survey data are an aid to planning health services in the ambulatory care setting and provide perspectives on national patterns of utilization. The applicability of the data to setting standards of performance in managed-care settings or under contracted agreements for service, however, is limited because of the many variables that could not be adequately measured.

AMBULATORY PRACTICE SETTINGS

Significant differences exist among physician practice settings, and these are discussed in the following sections of this chapter. The two primary noninstitutional settings for the provision of ambulatory care are solo and group practice. Each of these settings may be a component of larger systems of care through such integrating mechanisms as referral arrangements, insurance contracts, and direct ownership of practices. An organized system of care can, in turn, be comprised of various settings or types of ambulatory care providers.

Although the solo practice of medicine has traditionally attracted the greatest number of practitioners, group practice and institutionally based services are now expanding dramatically, continuing a trend that has been building over the past thirty years. Changing lifestyles, the cost of establishing a practice, personal financial pressures on practitioners, contracting and affiliation opportunities under managed care, and the burdens of running a business have enhanced the attractiveness of group practice for many physicians. With sharp increases in the number of physicians beginning practice, the growth of alternative settings, and especially of group practice, has been dramatic. Although solo practice remains an important avenue for providing ambulatory care services, these other settings have rapidly assumed a more prominent and visible role in the health care system, particularly as they provide a further mechanism for the integration, management, and control of health care services.

Solo Practice

Solo practitioners are difficult to uniformly characterize. Early sociological studies focused on specific questions, such as referral patterns or quality of care, and they did not provide a comprehensive picture of what the solo practitioner did. Studies that did contribute to a more complete understanding of the activities of solo practitioners were based on physicians in one geographic area or a particular specialty, and the results of these studies, although interesting and useful, may not be applicable to other practices or areas. In addition, solo practitioners are heterogeneous; they include many types of health care professionals who provide an immense array of services.

Many solo practitioners are subspecialists who provide secondary care primarily on referral from primary care practitioners. Under managed care, these subspecialists are being squeezed by reduced payment for specialty services, by capitation payment for population coverage, and by the increasing trend for gate-keepers to perform services that otherwise might have been referred to subspecialists. Some subspecialists provide both primary and secondary care, since they have insufficient work in their own specialties to achieve desired income levels.

Many solo practitioners, including those trained in general and family practice, internal medicine, pediatrics, and obstetrics and gynecology, provide primary care services. There is some controversy and competition among practitioners concerning which specialists should be providing primary care. The specialty of family practice, in particular, represents a challenge to general internal medicine in providing adult primary care and to pediatrics in providing child care, although the role of family practice is now firmly established, especially in managed care.

Most solo practitioners perform a number of functions in the office, including patient care, consultations, and administration and supervision of office staff. The requirements for administration and for supervision of personnel have been increasing in recent years. Solo practitioners are increasingly affiliating with managed-care networks that help ensure a viable patient population.

Solo practice is often associated with an increased feeling that the provider cares about the welfare of the patient, possibly resulting in a stronger patient-provider relationship than occurs in other settings. There is some evidence that this situation, where it occurs, is a result of the lower level of bureaucracy or organizational complexity in solo practice. Because there is also some evidence that the relationship between patient and physician is related to patient compliance with medical regimens, patients who perceive that they are receiving more personalized care may respond to the care process more positively.

Solo practitioners may not be as restricted in referrals to specialists as providers in some other settings, such as group practice, where organizational loyalties intervene. Managed-care contracts, however, may severely limit referral options.

The solo practitioner may feel a greater identification with the community served, since there is a more direct relationship between patient and provider. Organizational forms, especially managed care, that incorporate solo practitioners into larger systems of care may be decreasing some of this physician-patient bond, especially as providers are forced to discount

fees, increase productivity, and focus on the cost-effectiveness of their practices.

From the provider's perspective, solo practice offers an opportunity to avoid organizational dependence and to be self-employed; there is also no need to share resources or income with other providers. Philosophically, solo practice is most closely aligned with the traditional economic and political organizations that have characterized medicine; younger physicians faced with discounting, contracting, and networks for care, however, may no longer identify with the more traditional perspectives.

All of the increasingly complex problems of administering a practice must be dealt with in solo practice unless a professional manager is hired. Furthermore, competitive pressures in the health care industry are leading many practitioners to question the feasibility and desirability of going it alone. Many solo practitioners are now affiliated with larger entities such as independent practice associations, practice management companies, and other organizations. Thus, solo practice offers distinct opportunities and has philosophical and emotional appeal but is far from devoid of problems and constraints, especially in light of the realities of medical practice today.

Group Practice

Office-based practice includes, in addition to solo practice, group practice. This form of practice has been growing in popularity in recent years, especially as the increasing pressures of practice have led many providers to seek alternative settings in which to work.

Group practice is an affiliation of three or more providers, usually physicians, who share income, expenses, facilities, equipment, medical records, and support personnel in the provision of services through a formal, legally constituted organization. The formal definition of group practice, developed by the American Medical Association and the Medical Group Management Association, is three or more physicians formally organized to provide medical care, consultation, diagnosis, and/or treatment through the joint use of equipment and personnel, and with income from medical practice distributed in accordance with methods previously determined by members of the group. Although definitions of a group practice vary somewhat, the essential element is formal sharing of resources and income.

Traditionally, group practice has meant participation and ownership by physicians. Increasingly, however, as new and more diversified models for the provision of services are developed, other practitioners will participate in group practices. In some communities, for example, group practices of nurse practitioners may be the only sources of health services. Dentists, optometrists, podiatrists, and other specialized personnel are also increasingly developing group practices.

History of Group Practice

Some of the earliest group practices in the United States were started by companies that needed to provide care to employees in rural sites where medical care was unobtainable. For example, the Northern Pacific Railroad organized a practice in 1883 to provide care to employees building the transcontinental railroad. This industrial clinic was one of a number of such clinics founded in the nineteenth century.

Even more significant, however, was the establishment of the Mayo Clinic in Rochester, Minnesota—the first successful nonindustrial group practice. The Mayo Clinic, originally organized as a single-specialty group practice in 1887 and later broadened into a multispecialty group, demonstrated that group practice was feasible in the private sector. The Mayo Clinic also represented a reputable model for group practice in a national atmosphere of fierce independence where group practice was viewed with skepticism and distrust. By the early 1930s, there were about one hundred and fifty medical groups throughout the country, many of which were located in the Midwest. Most included or were started by someone who had practiced or trained at the Mayo Clinic.

In 1932, the Committee on the Costs of Medical Care was established to assess health care needs for the nation (Rorem, 1931). It issued a report that suggested a major role for group practice in the provision of medical care. The committee recommended that these groups be associated with hospitals to provide comprehensive care and that there be prepayment for

all services. The report strongly supported the concept of regionalization that eventually gained wide recognition in the establishment of the British National Health Service, our own military health care systems, and other national models of organized health service systems.

Other constituencies, including some unions, also developed group practices. After World War II, a number of pioneering groups were established. In New York City, the Health Insurance Plan of New York was organized to provide prepaid medical care to the employees of the city—an idea promoted by Mayor Fiorello LaGuardia. On the west coast, the Kaiser Foundation Health Plan was established to provide health care to employees of Kaiser Industries; Kaiser is an affiliation of plans and providers that is now serving millions of Americans across the nation. In Seattle, a revolutionary development included the establishment of the Group Health Cooperative of Puget Sound, a consumer-owned cooperative prepaid group practice. It was founded by progressive individuals who were dissatisfied with the private medical care available to them in the late 1940s.

Developments in medical practice also spurred the group practice movement. Perhaps most notable was the increasing specialization of medicine and the rapid expansion of technology. This increasing sophistication meant that no individual practitioner could provide all the expertise that patients would require. It also meant that more complex and expensive facilities, equipment, and personnel were needed to care for patients. Group practice provided a formal structure for sharing these costs among providers. Many people believed that resources would be used more efficiently in groups. In addition, multispecialty groups, encompassing more than one specialty, could provide patients with more of their health care under one roof and, hence, reduce problems of physical access to care and coordination of services.

Group practice was also thought to promote higher-quality care. Most of the different specialists that a person required would be practicing together and would thus have the opportunity to discuss patient problems among themselves, share a common medical record, and be more able to ensure the quality and continuity of care. Therefore, group practice was viewed by many as being advantageous for the physician—offering opportunities such as easily developed referral arrangements, sharing of after-hours coverage, greater flexibility in working hours, and less financial risk—while also benefiting the patient.

Opposition to group practice occurred mostly for political and philosophical reasons. The American Medical Association and local medical societies have, at times, opposed group practice. Many early group practices had difficulties when physicians were denied admitting privileges in local hospitals. Community-based specialists sometimes refused to treat patients referred by group practice physicians. In more recent years, however, opposition to group practice has lessened dramatically, and restrictive laws have been challenged. The need to form affiliations for contracting under reimbursement programs and for achieving efficiencies in organizing health services more generally has resulted in little remaining formal opposition to group practice.

Survey of Group Practice

The American Medical Association has conducted surveys of physician-oriented medical group practices in the United States on a periodic basis since 1965. These surveys represent the most comprehensive data available concerning the growth and characteristics of group practice in this country. Group practices that qualified within the American Medical Association's definition were identified from a variety of data sources and were then surveyed through a mail data collection instrument. Numerous items of information were collected regarding the nature of the practice and its facilities and relationships to other entities.

The dramatic increase in popularity of practices is reflected in Table 9.9. The number of reporting group practices has more than doubled since 1975. There are now nearly 20,000 group practices in the United States, the majority of which are single-specialty groups.

Even more dramatic is the growth in the number of physicians in a group-practice setting. Over 200,000 physicians in the United States are now working in group practices, which represents a marked increase

Table 9.9. Number of Medical Groups and Number of Physicians in Group Practice, United States, Selected Years

Year	Total Number of Groups	Number of Physician Positions in Group Practice
1969	6,371	40,093
1975	8,488	66,842
1980	10,762	88,290
1984	15,186	139,127
1988	16,495	155,628
1991	16,576	184,358
1996	19,820	206,557

SOURCE: Adapted from *Medical Groups in the U.S., 1999 Edition. A Survey of Practice Characteristics*, by P. L. Havlicek, 1999, Chicago: American Medical Association.

from 67,000 in 1975 and 88,000 in 1980. A higher percentage of all physicians in group practice work in multispecialty-oriented groups as compared to the percentage of total groups that are multispecialty, largely because the average multispecialty group is substantially larger than the average single-specialty group. The average size of all group practices in the United States in 1988 was about nine physicians, an increase from 1980. These data reflect only physician "positions" and exclude other medically related professionals such as nurse practitioners.

Most group practices are professional corporations. The dramatic shift toward professional corporations since 1969 is primarily a result of changes in federal and state laws pertaining to taxation, the increasing size and complexity of the practices themselves, and interrelationships among the physicians participating. Changes in federal tax law may result in further shifts in patterns of legal organizational forms.

Specialty distribution of physicians in group practice has not changed dramatically in recent years. The specialties that account for the largest percentage of physicians participating in group practice include family and general practice, internal medicine, anesthesiology, obstetrics and gynecology, pediatrics, and radiology; many groups are now involved in managed-care contracting.

Table 9.10. Total Groups and Group Physician Positions by Size of Group, 1996

	Groups			Group Physician Positions	
Size of Group	Percent	Number		Percent	Number
3	24.5	4,775		6.9	14,327
4	21.4	4,163		8.1	16,651
5–6	22.9	4,450		11.7	24,096
7–9	12.6	2,449		9.2	19,052
10–15	8.8	1,713		9.9	20,350
16–25	4.8	937		8.9	18,484
26–49	2.7	535		9.1	18,815
50–75	0.8	158		4.6	9,532
76–99	0.4	70		2.9	6,071
100 or more	1.1	218		28.7	59,179

SOURCE: Adapted from *Medical Groups in the U.S., 1999 Edition. A Survey of Practice Characteristics,* by P. L. Havlicek, 1999, Chicago: American Medical Association.

Relatively few groups account for a significant percentage of all physicians in group practice, as presented in Table 9.10. There are relatively few groups that employ more than fifteen physicians. As would be expected, most of the larger groups are multispecialty, while the smaller groups are predominantly single specialty.

The geographic distribution of group practice in the United States is dominated by six states, which account for nearly forty percent of all groups. These states are California, Pennsylvania, New York, Illinois, Florida, and Ohio. The origin, growth, and current distribution of group practice and group practice physicians are not homogeneous throughout the various regions, which reflects a greater acceptance of group practice in some regions as well as a varied distribution of larger urban population centers in the country. As might be expected, physician groups and group-practice physicians are substantially more prominent in metropolitan areas than in nonmetropolitan areas of the country. The development of prepaid group practice also varies by region.

Interestingly, most group practices employed a business manager or administrator, although far fewer had an identifiable medical director. Multispecialty groups were more likely to employ a group administrator, and, as might be expected, larger groups were much more likely to employ administrators and have medical directors than were smaller groups. Nearly all the larger groups did employ an administrator. The market for trained group-practice administrators has grown substantially over the past few years, and its growth is likely to continue as the number of group practices increases.

New Forms of Group Practice

Managed care has led to the development of new forms of group practice to allow physicians alternative settings in which to participate in contracting arrangements such as the independent practice associations (IPAs). Most of this innovation is the result of the need to form contractual arrangements with health systems, managed-care organizations, and insurers. These new organizational forms are continuing to evolve. Smaller practices, in particular, have needed to seek out alliances that facilitate contractual arrangements under managed care. Smaller practices face disadvantages with regard to the availability of capital investment, professional management, and often overhead and other costs. Larger practices and new approaches to creating affiliations of groups facilitate potential economies of scale, efficiencies in management and operations, improved contracting potential and market involvement, and enhanced deployment of capital.

Group practices may be formed by, or affiliated with, larger organizations such as hospitals or health systems. The larger entity may provide capital, management services, patient flows, and contracting assistance to the smaller group. Groups may be affiliated with one another through various mechanisms that may provide management services and contracting potential for solo and smaller group practitioners while preserving a degree of independence for these practitioners. A group practice without walls is another avenue utilized to affiliate practitioners. In essence, practices are merged, but are able to maintain their existing locations with administrative services carried out in a central office or through a contract with a management services organization. There are increasing numbers of for-profit management companies and some not-for-profit entities providing these services to physician groups and, in some instances, actually purchasing groups outright, as well.

From a pragmatic point of view, many of these new forms of group practice are designed to facilitate the participation of solo- and group-practice physicians in the rapidly changing world of managed care where practices must be managed efficiently and have easy access to contracting mechanisms. The specific legal and operational approaches to organizing these integrated forms of group practice vary considerably and are continuing to evolve. Key issues include physician autonomy and involvement in governance and management; sources and uses of capital investment; control over physician clinical practice patterns; extent of control by a larger entity over physician staff, facilities, and daily operation; and relationships with other entities such as hospitals, insurers, managed-care organizations, and, of course, patients. Many physicians and physician practices, as well as other provider organizations, may elect to continue within the more traditional parameters of such managed-care organizations as independent practice associations and preferred provider organizations. Other practices may determine that the assistance available through management-related contractual arrangements warrants the loss of autonomy. Finally, some practitioners may simply sell out to hospitals, health systems, physician management companies, and other organizations and elect to focus on their clinical practice itself.

An Assessment of Group Practice

A critical assessment of group practice yields distinct advantages and disadvantages for both patients and providers as compared to other modalities for providing ambulatory services. Some of these are summarized in Table 9.11. Specific advantages and disadvantages vary from group to group, and Table 9.11 also lists major considerations generally associated with group practice. Some of the topics listed under patient or provider perspectives could readily pertain to both.

The advantages of group practice from the perspective of the provider include shared operation of the practice, joint ownership of facilities and equipment, centralized administrative functions, and, in larger groups, a professional manager. The professional manager can provide expertise in areas often lacking among the providers such as billing, personnel management, patient scheduling, ordering of supplies, negotiating, contracting, and related matters.

Financially, the group relieves the provider of the heavy initial investment often required to establish a practice. In most groups, however, coownership requires that new members buy into the group through purchase of a share of the group's capital over a period of time.

The burden of operating costs is also lessened for any individual member of a group. Rather than having to independently absorb the ups and downs of a practice, as do solo practitioners, those involved in a group practice share the income and expenses within the group, allowing for moderation of those fluctuations experienced in individual practices. For example, a solo practitioner who becomes ill may have no practice income aside from disability insurance, whereas a group member's income may continue during a short period of illness, since other providers are simultaneously generating revenue. However, the

Table 9.11.   Some Advantages and Disadvantages of Group Practice*

Advantages	Disadvantages
From perspective of the provider	
Availability of professional manager	Less individual freedom
Organizational responsibility for patient	Possible excessive use of specialists
Less physician administrative time	Fewer outside consultants
Shared capital expense	Possible reduced identity with patient and community
Shared financial risk	Group rather than individual decision making
Improved contracting and negotiating ability	Sharing of all problems
Better coverage and shared on-call shifts	Necessity of working with others
More flexible working hours	Less individual incentive and more orientation toward security
More peer interaction	Income limitations
Increased access to specialists	Income distribution arguments
Broader array of ancillary services	
Stable income for providers	
No direct financial concerns with patient	
Lower initial investment	
More time for continuing education	
More flexible vacation time	
Generally excellent benefits	
Possible efficiencies of scale	
Use of nonphysician practitioners	
From perspective of the patient	
Care under one roof	Possible lessening of provider-patient relationship
Availability of specialists, laboratories, and so on	Possible overuse of ancillary services
Improved coverage and emergency care	Possible high provider turnover
Central location of medical and administrative records	Heavy patient loads and possible increase in waiting time
Simplified referrals	Less provider incentive for care
Peer interaction among providers	More bureaucracy
Better administration of group	
Possible promotion of efficiency in patient care	

*Some advantages and disadvantages could be included under both provider and patient categories.

provisions of income distribution plans vary substantially among groups.

The participation of physicians in group practice also has a significant advantage in facilitating the development of definitive arrangements for contracting and negotiating. The group can support increased levels of participation, has a knowledgeable group practice administrator to manage the contracts, and can respond to the market with a wider range of services. Even single-specialty groups, with shared on-call services and subspecialization of group members, are able to offer more to the market on a contractual basis than the individual practitioner. Having a professional manager to negotiate on behalf of the group further enhances the relative attractiveness of group practice, particularly for physicians who lack experience in interpreting and negotiating contracts.

Patient care responsibilities are also shared in group practice. This sharing results in greater flexibility of working hours for the provider, as well as more time for vacation and continuing education, without sacrificing the quality of care for the patient. For example, providers cover for each other during vacations and after normal working hours. Although most practitioners in solo practice arrange for patient care coverage, the continuity of care and the extent of coverage are probably greater in group practice, as patients' medical records and the full resources of the group are always available, even if specific providers are not working.

Sharing of patient care may have some other potential benefits. These include more peer interaction as a result of informal discussions and referral of patients among providers. The inclusion of more providers also results in the availability, by necessity, of a wider range of specialists and ancillary services, which represents a convenience for both providers and patients as well as a source of added revenue for the group.

Does the sharing of administrative and patient care activities within group practice produce better care at lower cost? Although many people believe that effective group management uses resources more efficiently than solo practice, the evidence is mixed. Some evidence tends to refute this belief, but more analytical research indicates some economies of scale, or efficiencies, attributable to the grouping of resources for smaller groups, but possibly less so for larger and more bureaucratic groups. The use of personnel may be more advantageous in group than solo practice. Receptionists, medical records specialists, laboratory and radiology technicians, nurses, and other types of personnel may be used more efficiently and in the specialized areas of their training in many medium- and larger-sized groups. In addition, there is some question about whether any savings that are achieved will be returned to consumers or simply represent higher income for providers. Further, the increasing supply of physicians may reduce the desirability of employing mid-level practitioners, except in certain prepaid settings.

The effect of groups on patient care, especially on the quality of care, is an important issue. Sharing of medical records, peer interaction, easy referrals and consultations with specialists, more sophisticated and accessible ancillary services, and more skilled and diversified support personnel are all arguments suggested in support of higher-quality care in group practice. Pressures from managed-care contracts, however, may affect quality-related issues such as use, access, and appropriateness of care.

Group practice also offers advantages to patients and their communities. For the patient, the group offers a wide range of services under one roof so that travel between providers is reduced and access increased. A unified medical record can contribute to continuity of care and less duplication in diagnosis and treatment. Some groups also own or operate hospitals and thus further extend the integration and scope of the services that they provide, an especially important consideration in negotiating with employers and insurers.

Group practices usually offer more accessible care after normal working hours. Some groups also offer emergency services through their own emergency rooms or clinics. Groups with a broader community perspective may even be involved in programs such as school health services and community immunization efforts, and the use of a professional manager should benefit the patient through more efficient scheduling and patient flow and improved overall management of the practice.

On a communitywide basis, group practice may offer a means of attracting providers to areas with inadequate numbers of medical care personnel. By offering peer interaction, support services, and other advantages, groups may increase the appeal of practicing in rural or inadequately served urban centers.

There are also distinct disadvantages to group practice for providers, patients, and communities. From the perspective of the provider, practicing in a group implies less individual freedom, with a variety of restrictions imposed through the sharing of a practice. Ideologically, the limitations of a group in this regard may be difficult for some people to accept because medicine has traditionally been an individualistic enterprise. In addition to reduced freedom, group practice entails sharing responsibilities and problems with others. The interpersonal requirements for working out these responsibilities may not appeal to all practitioners. Older individuals who have been working in solo practice may be especially unlikely to adapt readily to group practice.

The financial advantages for group practice are a trade-off against some restrictions on income generation and the necessity of complying with the group's income distribution and practice pattern requirements.

Thus, there is often more security and less risk but also less incentive and reward for individual initiative and production.

The shift of some patient care responsibilities from the individual practitioner to the group may adversely affect the patient-provider relationship by introducing a degree of impersonalization. If a group has high physician turnover, which is rare, patients may have to change providers frequently. Groups that have too few providers for the number of patients they serve, a common occurrence when excess capacity is being avoided, especially under managed-care financial pressures, also have waiting times for appointments in the office that patients may believe to be excessive. The group may impose greater restrictions on referral practices, consequently limiting the practitioner's willingness to use the expertise of other specialists in the community.

From a community perspective, groups may reduce the geographic dispersion of providers and thus increase difficulties of physical access to care. In addition, groups may reduce competition in the health care marketplace by consolidating what would otherwise be competing providers. Consolidation may eventually reduce the ability of insurers, employers, and other plan sponsors to negotiate favorable terms for contracted care.

The changing organizational structure of the health care system is also changing some aspects of the role of ambulatory care services from the perspectives of providers, consumers, and the community. Ambulatory care is assuming a much greater role in the rationing of care, especially for primary care, and in the control of referrals and use of specialty, laboratory, and other services. These changes are especially notable in managed care and for hospital-sponsored systems of care. Ambulatory care is substantially affecting other provider organizations, especially the hospital, as more and more care is provided on an ambulatory basis. There are important fiscal, organizational, and utilization implications for all components of the system as a result of these changes.

The implications of these structural changes in the provision of health care are profound. Consumers are affected in terms of where and how they receive serv-ices. Providers are affected by changes in their affiliations, referral patterns, incentives, and practice characteristics. And, finally, the community is obviously affected by the changing organization of services, by the formation of alliances, and by shifts in the economic and political clout of various providers.

INSTITUTIONALLY BASED AMBULATORY SERVICES

In addition to solo and group practice in the traditional private sector, many institutions have expanded their involvement in ambulatory care. These institutionally based settings, especially those associated with hospitals, are discussed next.

The hospital has evolved from an institution for poor people who could not be cared for at home to a provider of a full range of health services from primary to tertiary care. As technological advances have brought more services into the hospital and expanded the scope of care provided, the hospital has assumed an especially important role in the provision of highly complex health services. At the same time, an increasing number of people have sought primary care from hospitals, sometimes as a result of the lack of access to other sources of care.

Outpatient and Ambulatory Care Clinics

The increased demands placed on hospitals for care taxed the ability of many facilities to respond with appropriate and adequate resources. The result was overcrowded facilities, the wrong mix of services, equipment, and personnel to respond to patient needs, and extremely dissatisfied consumers and providers. Most hospitals have now successfully responded to these demands by expanding outpatient services and hiring full-time providers to staff redesigned hospital ambulatory facilities.

Traditional hospital outpatient services have been provided in clinics and emergency rooms. In many hospitals, clinics have had second-class status as compared to complex and expensive inpatient services. However, as hospitals have recognized the important role of primary care, especially in managed care contracting, and are seeking to expand the base of patients who are potential users of inpatient and ancillary services, more attention is being directed toward improving clinic operations and services.

Hospital clinics include both primary care and specialty clinics. Many hospitals differentiate between clinics for walk-in patients without appointments and those for scheduled visits. Specialty clinics are usually organized by department and provide services such as ophthalmology, neurology, and allergy care. In teaching hospitals, clinics serve as important settings in which house staff members provide ongoing care to patients and follow-up after hospitalization. Increasingly, clinics also provide an opportunity to expose medical students and house staff to ambulatory care services in order to complement the traditionally more extensive experience with inpatient care. With ambulatory care's increasing role in health services, this trend is significant.

Many hospital primary-care clinics evolved from an orientation of service to the poor and were staffed by physicians who served without reimbursement in exchange for staff privileges. The level of commitment to the patient under such circumstances was—not surprisingly—less than desirable. Many hospitals now employ physicians and other practitioners as full-time clinic staff. Some hospitals have established primary-care group practices to complement other outpatient services and to assume the burden of providing primary care to patients who seek most of their care from the hospital.

The development of a group practice has advantages for both consumers and the hospital by providing comprehensive and accessible care and by removing primary-care patients from facilities that are not designed to serve their needs, such as emergency rooms. Development of these group practices also has the potential of increasing use of the hospital's inpatient and ancillary services, an advantage if occupancy is low. Hospitals with ambulatory care resources can negotiate contracts for providing a wide range of both inpatient and outpatient services. They are subsequently also able to more effectively control the use of services and thus costs. Questions have been raised, however, concerning the ability of hospitals to compete effectively in an arena in which they have not been overly successful in the past. But the increasingly competitive nature of the hospital and the health care marketplace is forcing many hospitals to enter this area of practice even if they are uncertain about doing so.

Ambulatory Surgery Centers

A further innovation in hospital-based care has been the development of ambulatory surgery centers. Originating in hospitals in Washington, D.C., Los Angeles, and elsewhere, these organized hospital units provide one-day surgical care. Patients are usually screened for acceptability by their personal surgeons and then report at an assigned date and time for surgery. The surgeon is supported by the unit's facilities, equipment, and personnel, and the patient is discharged one to three hours after surgery when recovery from anesthesia is sufficiently complete.

In the early 1970s, freestanding ambulatory surgery centers were opened; one of the first was in Phoenix, Arizona. These facilities are independent of hospitals and usually provide a full range of services for the types of surgery that can be performed on an outpatient basis. Community surgeons are granted operating privileges and can perform surgery in these facilities when the patient agrees and when there are no medical contraindications.

Other facilities are also used for ambulatory or outpatient surgery. Many physicians traditionally performed surgery in their offices, although this practice has declined in some specialties as a result of malpractice concerns and the increasing availability of better-equipped and -staffed alternative facilities. Some specialties, such as oral surgery, plastic surgery, and ophthalmology, extensively use office-based facilities.

Freestanding emergency centers have also opened in many cities, paralleling the success of ambulatory surgery centers. These emergency centers sometimes provide a wide range of primary care in addition to responding to urgent problems. The future of specialized ambulatory centers, both in hospitals and as freestanding facilities, will probably include further expansion into other areas of health care, ranging from sports medicine to women's health care.

Even greater innovation has occurred in recent years. Freestanding postsurgical recovery centers for short nonhospital stays of one to three nights are under development to provide a less intensive recovery setting for less complex surgical cases. Mobile diagnostic facilities with sophisticated imaging equipment have been operational for a number of years. Even mobile physician vans are now in use to return the house call to more frequent clinical use by transporting the physician along with his/her office to the patient's home without sacrificing technological capabilities. The challenge for the future remains to identify economically feasible and innovative approaches to providing patient care that expedite the care process and are accepted by consumers, providers, and payers.

Emergency Medical Services

The emergency room, like other hospital departments, has undergone transformation in recent years. The emergency room has expanded in the range of services offered and in complexity. An especially important long-term trend has been the increasing use of the emergency room for primary care. Because the emergency room requires sophisticated facilities and highly trained personnel and must be accessible twenty-four hours a day, costs are high and services are not designed for nonurgent care. To reduce the burden on the emergency room and to meet patient need more effectively, many hospitals treat patients on a triage basis. In this process, often performed by a nurse, the patient's health care needs are determined and the patient is referred to a more appropriate source of care within the hospital. Misuse of the emergency room has received considerable attention over the past twenty years.

Emergency medical services have also been increasingly integrated with other community resources. Included are drug and alcohol treatment programs, mental health centers, and voluntary agencies. Most major urban centers have developed formal emergency medical systems that incorporate all hospital emergency rooms as well as transportation and communication systems. In these communities, people needing emergency care either transport themselves or call an emergency number (such as 911). An ambulance is dispatched by a central communications center that also identifies and alerts the most appropriately equipped and located hospital. In many communities, regional hospital-based trauma centers have been built with extremely sophisticated capabilities. Specialized ambulance services, including mobile coronary care units and shock-trauma vans, are also increasingly prevalent.

GOVERNMENT PROGRAMS

In addition to private sector and institutionally initiated efforts, government programs have been designed to increase the availability of health care resources in many communities. These programs have adapted some of the concepts of private institutional settings, especially those of group practice.

Neighborhood health centers were funded starting in 1965. Originally intended to serve approximately twenty-five million people, this federal program never reached its initial objectives. The program was designed to provide primary medical care with a family orientation. It was targeted for population groups in need of services, as reflected by such indicators as disease prevalence and income level. At the same time, the centers were intended to employ people from the communities they served in positions that would offer opportunities for training and advancement. Responsiveness to community needs was to be ensured by a community board or advisory panel. The centers were to recognize that the broad attributes of a community, such as housing and employment, contributed to health and illness.

Although these health centers were originally intended to serve the poor, changes in federal policy that encouraged them to collect fees from patients and from third-party insurers have broadened the socioeconomic mixture of patients obtaining care. However, the centers still predominantly serve the medically indigent. Sources of funding have been broadened to include local government as well. Pressures for achieving self-sufficiency have been very powerful in recent years.

A related category of provider, the free clinic, evolved from a strong social commitment but has had to face similar financial realities. The combination of former free clinics, neighborhood health centers, public agency clinics, and some hospital clinics and groups now forms an informal safety net of providers for individuals who lack private insurance or access to other sources of care, or who simply need care from an available, sympathetic provider. Many of these providers now contract on their own or in coalitions with other providers to provide care to various individuals under government entitlement programs, sometimes in managed care arrangements, as well.

Other community health centers that have been funded by the federal government include migrant health centers serving transient farm workers in agricultural areas and rural health centers. The National Health Service Corps supported practitioners who were placed in urban and rural areas with shortages of medical resources. Other innovations, such as mobile health vans in rural areas, have also been used to expand the scope of services. The Community Mental Health Center program was established to provide ambulatory mental health services in underserved areas. Community mental health centers were intended to provide outpatient services and emergency care and to work with other community agencies to foster action and concern for mental health.

In recent years, community health centers have evolved into larger practices with multiple sources of support, including increasing reliance on patient fees and private donations. Many of these centers have become more businesslike in their operations. Yet most still face serious problems in attracting adequate financing, in attracting and retaining physicians, and in diversifying their patient mix, especially with regard to patients with insurance or the ability to pay for services on their own. The shift of funding for entitlement programs to prepaid contracts may provide more financial stability for some of these providers in the future. Conflicts exist in some centers over the historical mission of serving the medically indigent versus the need for enhanced fiscal diversity and adopting a more business-oriented approach to operations.

Other Federal Government Programs

The federal government, in addition to supporting a variety of community-based health services organizations, directly operates many health facilities. The Veterans Administration includes the largest health services system under a unified management structure in the United States with more than one hundred and seventy hospitals and clinics. This system provides needed care to millions of veterans throughout the nation. The military services also provide health care to millions of individuals in the armed forces and have developed extensive regionalized facilities throughout the world.

Government has a special responsibility for providing health care to a number of groups within the country. The Indian Health Service is charged with ensuring access to medical care on Indian reservations and in certain other locations. Although the difficulties of operating a largely rural system are immense, the Indian Health Service has succeeded in bringing modern medicine to many people.

NONINSTITUTIONAL AND PUBLIC HEALTH SERVICES

As noted in the introduction to this chapter, there are many ways in which ambulatory and community health services are provided. Although only the most prevalent types of provider and service are discussed here, each helps to meet the many health care needs of a community. The list is nearly endless, and a number of services warrant further discussion.

Home health services are provided by visiting nurse associations, proprietary companies, some hospitals, public health departments, and other agencies. These services allow people to remain in their homes and yet receive essential health services, thereby reducing costs and increasing the quality of life for many.

Rural health care has required unique and innovative solutions in many communities, especially in the absence of adequate supplies of physicians and facilities. In rural Alaska, many towns are served by physicians and other professionals who regularly fly in to treat patients. Satellites are used to facilitate communications with specialists in urban medical centers; even ordinary communications in remote areas may be difficult. Rural health care in many areas remains a challenging test of the ingenuity and resourcefulness of the health services system and community residents.

Other community health services not discussed in detail here include, but are not limited to, school health services, prison health services, vision care, dental care provided by solo, group, and institutionally based practitioners, foot care from podiatrists, and drug dispensing from pharmacists, who often also extensively advise and educate consumers. Voluntary agencies also provide health care services such as cancer screening clinics and health education. Finally, many indigenous health practitioners offer their services in this country and abroad. These practitioners include chiropractors, "medicine men," naturopaths, and others. The supportive and sometimes curative role of these individuals is often underestimated.

Among the most important contributions to reductions in mortality and morbidity in the twentieth century have been such public health measures as the improvement of sanitation, ensurance of potable water supplies, and upgraded housing. In recent years, there has also been an increased awareness of the need to control air and water pollution, to reduce exposure to carcinogens, and to improve and ensure the quality of the environment. The contribution of these efforts to health far exceeds, dollar for dollar, efforts to treat illness once it occurs. Their importance to ambulatory care is mentioned here, however, because public health agencies have responsibility for a remarkable range of relevant services.

And in this context, it is important to emphasize that health care and ambulatory care services also must successfully interact with other aspects of our society. These other areas include social and welfare services, accident prevention in industry and in transportation, protection of the environment, improvement of food and water supplies, and even the general economic well-being of society, as health is directly correlated with employment and income security.

ORGANIZATION OF AMBULATORY CARE SYSTEMS

The changing structure of the health services system has had tremendous implications for ambulatory care services (Ross, Williams, & Schafer, 1997). The increased movement toward integrated systems of care and managed care has led ambulatory care services to assume a central role in the design and operation of many insurance and delivery programs. In addition, those paying for health services, including employers and insurers, have increasingly focused attention on the role that ambulatory care services can provide in improving the coordination and control of care as well as in reducing costs through the reduction of duplication and the shifting of services to lower-cost settings.

Those organizations constructing large-scale, integrated systems of care are continuing to seek existing ambulatory care structures or are building new ones as a means of completing their systems. In particular, insurers, hospitals, and other organizational entities are developing or purchasing ambulatory care resources such as medical practices, clinics, and other existing networks. Government units, such as the military, have long recognized the key attributes of ambulatory care in coordinating and controlling the overall utilization of services and, then, the cost and quality of care. These trends are likely to continue.

There are many key design attributes of ambulatory care that are essential for both the effective operation of ambulatory services and for the full integration of these services into larger systems of care. Ambulatory care is important in providing access to care, particularly within larger integrated systems. Access considerations include scope of services provided and hours of operation as well as distribution of resources throughout a geographic region populated by the target group of consumers. Physical access to the facilities must also be assured, including such considerations as parking, access to public transportation where appropriate, and access to physician facilities for the handicapped.

The scope of services provided must respond to population needs. These needs differ depending on whether the population is enrolled through insurance or entitlement programs or fee-for-service. How the population is served differs substantially in each situation. For both situations, however, decisions must be made concerning the type of care to be provided on an ambulatory versus an inpatient basis.

Marketing advantages can be achieved in the ambulatory care setting by recognizing the special needs of consumers, such as having multilingual staff available where appropriate. The friendliness of the staff and the attractiveness of the physical facilities can have dramatic effects on patient attitudes and satisfaction, not only with the ambulatory care provider but in the larger system of care as well. Thus, ambulatory care provides an influential marketing function in any system of care. Ambulatory care services also generally provide an opportunity for educating the consumer in terms of both health behaviors and appropriate use of the system. This educational role can contribute to cost containment by having patients help in managing their use.

Ambulatory care can provide a key role in the overall provision of coordinated and continuous care. By accepting the gate-keeper role of the primary care physician, using medical records and other administrative tracking of patients, and avoiding duplication of services and unnecessary care, the ambulatory care setting can contribute handsomely to the overall effectiveness of all care provided to the patient. Physician payment incentives can facilitate an enhanced coordinating role for ambulatory care. Centralization of responsibility for patient care thus must be clearly assigned. Mechanisms for monitoring patient and provider behavior to ensure compliance with health system operating guidelines are essential. There is also evidence that more effective continuity of care is associated with higher levels of patient compliance regarding medical regimens, which, in turn, may lead to better health outcomes and eventually lower subsequent utilization rates. Patient satisfaction is generally greater when continuity and coordination of care are achieved—both effective marketing and cost-containment tools.

The quality of care should reflect not only adequate medical skills but also a caring attitude on the part of the provider. Consumers in ambulatory care are capable of detecting some aspects of the technical quality of care, but they are even more aware of provider and system attitudes and behavior. Responding to the consumer is increasingly important in the competitive environment.

AMBULATORY CARE AND THE CHALLENGE OF MANAGED CARE

Ambulatory care services have been, and will continue to be, dramatically affected by the evolution of managed care. Managed care serves to shift considerable risk to practitioners and forces greater efficiencies in the ambulatory care arena. Clinical responsibility in many ambulatory care practices not only for patient care but also for allocation of resources and broader aspects of clinical decision making have also been enhanced by the pressures of managed care. Because managed care is focused on controlling provider and patient behavior, most of that control is being exercised through the ambulatory care arena. These pressures have allowed ambulatory care providers to gain greater power within the health care system, but with enhanced power comes increased responsibility, risk, financial pressures, and frictions with providers, insurers, and patients. Increasingly, the shift of managed care toward organizational forms that are associated with greater controls over resources, providers, and patients is increasing the pressure on those involved in the provision of ambulatory care services. The move toward more integrated health care systems has decreased practitioner autonomy and imposed additional managerial controls and pressures on all participants.

The role of ambulatory care in controlling the patient, particularly through such mechanisms as gate-keepers and various forms of utilization control, places the provider in a more difficult position with regard to patient satisfaction and clinical decision making. Rationing, both directly and indirectly, may result from fiscal pressures and risk shifting under managed care and is exacerbating these pressures. Practitioners in ambulatory care increasingly must face new realities regarding incentives for income and the quality and quantity of the patient's care services.

All of these changes are appreciably affecting the ambulatory care arena and its participants.

At the same time as the financial and clinical practice pressures build, competition in the health care marketplace is requiring ambulatory care practitioners to provide friendly but efficient care that is customer-oriented in a manner that attracts the patient but also controls the resources.

Clinical and managerial information systems have gained increasing importance in ambulatory care. Fiscal reports that reflect costs, expenditures, and other financial indicators are important in light of risk shifting under managed-care contracts. Clinical measures of performance are increasingly utilized to assess physician practice patterns and relative performance among physicians in multispecialty groups. Managed-care organizations and insurers are also utilizing such data for economic credentialing and other assessments of not only clinical but also financial performance on the part of practitioners. These trends concern many observers because access, utilization, quality, and rationing are all affected by use of resources and allocation of services.

The future of health services, particularly with the pressures inherent in managed care and technological advances, will be characterized by further shifts in services from inpatient to ambulatory care settings. Ambulatory care practices will need to respond with appropriate and innovative service delivery options including new equipment, technology, specialized personnel, and facilities. Competition will be driven in managed-care contracting in part by the ability to provide cost-effective care in more innovative and appropriate settings.

Affiliations of provider organizations ranging from direct ownership in integrated systems to loose confederations and affiliations developed through contractual arrangements will enhance integration, coordination, managerial efficiency, and provision of clinical services. All group practices and even solo practitioners must be prepared to participate in various forms of networks, integrated systems, coordinated service-provider organizations, and other innovative approaches to organizing the health care delivery system.

In recent years, the intensity of the financial and delivery pressures placed on ambulatory care providers has increased still further. Managed-care contracting has resulted in tremendous stress due to increasingly cost-conscious negotiations on the part of payers and demands through contractual mechanisms for increased accountability and reporting from ambulatory care providers. Provider, and to an extent consumer, dissatisfaction with these arrangements and their inherent stresses is now leading to a backlash. In some instances, managed-care companies are beginning to back off on their demands for accountability and practice oversight. The trend toward increased provider practice flexibility and independence is starting to accelerate. However, increasing costs in the health care sector continue to erode the foundation for the financial and operational aspects of the relationships between ambulatory care providers and payers. The future of various ambulatory care settings and arrangements will continue to be dependent on payer arrangements that, in turn, are impacted by trends in health care costs, delivery mechanisms and technology, consumer preferences and demands, and government and employer policy development.

SUMMARY

The challenge in ambulatory care is to effectively shift from a traditionally reactive set of providers, attitudes, and operational approaches to the proactive leadership role needed in today's competitive environment. Ambulatory care once meant a largely unaffiliated and unstructured set of small providers responding as business walked in the door. Now ambulatory care is a key element in the structuring of large-scale systems. These systems require financial and contractual arrangements with providers, and these ties are critical to all parties concerned.

The system's structure itself vitally affects the role of ambulatory care services; ambulatory care can, in turn, be vital to the success of the system. In managed-care systems, the ability to control providers and consumers—and hence costs—depends on structuring the system based on the controlling role of ambulatory care and performing needed services through ambulatory delivery vehicles where feasible, while also maintaining quality. Ideally, quality and access will attain acceptable minimum levels under any delivery system, and controls will be built in to monitor both.

From a health care delivery perspective, as opposed to the financial focus of other chapters, the demands on ambulatory care to provide a marketing, integrating, controlling, and organizing function are great. At the same time, services must retain the attributes of high quality, meeting specific patient needs, and offering a stimulating and rewarding environment for the providers as well. This is no small challenge.

References

Havlicek, P. L. (1999). *Medical groups in the U.S., 1999 edition. A survey of practice characteristics.* Chicago: American Medical Association.

Rorem, R. (1931). *Private group clinics.* Chicago: University of Chicago Press.

Ross, A., Williams, S. J., & Schafer, E. L. (1997). *Ambulatory care management* (3rd ed.). Albany, NY: Delmar.

United Kingdom Ministry of Health. (1920). *Dawson report, interim report on the future provision of medical and allied services.* London: His Majesty's Stationery Office.

Woodwell, D. A. (1999). *National Ambulatory Medical Care Survey: 1997 Summary.* Hyattsville, Maryland: National Center for Health Statistics.

CHAPTER
10

Hospitals and Health Systems

William L. Dowling

Chapter Topics

👀 Historical Development of Hospitals

👀 Forces Affecting the Development of Hospitals

👀 Characteristics of the Hospital Industry

👀 Hospitals and Health Systems

👀 Internal Organization of Community Hospitals

Learning Objectives

Upon completing this chapter, the reader should be able to:

- Understand the role of the hospital in today's health care system
- Appreciate the historical trends that have shaped the hospital industry
- Understand the types of hospitals, ownership patterns, and differentiating characteristics of various hospitals
- Comprehend the development of health systems and the role of hospitals in such systems
- Follow the impact of competitive pressures and other developments on the structure and operation of hospitals and health systems
- Understand the internal organizational structure of hospitals

The dramatic advances in medicine around the turn of the last century transformed the hospital into the key resource and organizational hub of the American health care system. Hospitals became central to the delivery of patient care, the training of health personnel, and the conduct and dissemination of health care research. They were built by communities as a collective investment in the sophisticated technology and specialized personnel required to provide modern medical care—a community resource available for the benefit of all. As the repository for the equipment and personnel needed by physicians to support them in providing care, hospitals became the physician's "workshop," ever more the economic and professional heart of medical practice as the pace of advances in medical knowledge and technology accelerated. In recent years, hospitals have expanded beyond their inpatient role to become comprehensive community health centers, often formally linked with physicians, offering a broad range of outpatient, community-based, home-based, and institution-based services. As highly advanced scientific institutions, hospitals manifest the complexity and detached efficiency of a clinical laboratory. As human service organizations, they deal with the emotions of life and death, triumphs and tragedies. Hospitals are frequently the caregivers of last resort for many of the nation's poor who have nowhere else to turn for health care.

Current forces in health care are once again transforming the role of hospitals. Efforts to contain spending for hospital services, declining inpatient volumes, competition from other providers, and outpatient technology have eroded the central role of hospitals. Over the years, however, hospitals have proved to be remarkably resilient to even the most powerful changes in health care.

As we address the role of hospitals in the early part of the twenty-first century, the challenges continue to build. Resources are increasingly being shifted to the ambulatory care arena as technological progress facilitates the performance of many procedures outside of the traditional inpatient arena. Hospitals are increasingly challenged as their acuity of care increases and as cost pressures continue to mount. Yet, at least for the present, the hospital is still an integral component of the nation's health care system and a center of the provision of the most complex services.

Hospitals are big business. Collectively, they are among the largest industries in the United States measured by the dollars they consume or the size of the workforce they employ. One of the largest components of the nation's health care system, hospitals employ nearly half of all health care personnel and consume almost forty percent of the nation's health expenditures.

The magnitude of the hospital industry and the central role hospitals play in the delivery of health services place hospitals at the root of many of the health care system's most pressing problems: rising costs, duplication of services, bed surpluses, overemphasis of specialized services versus primary care, depersonalization of care, and so forth. Furthermore, because the public sees hospitals as community or quasi-public institutions, and because hospitals are heavily dependent on public dollars, hospitals are often targeted by community groups, business coalitions, insurance companies, government agencies, and others as instruments of social change and health system reform.

The hospital industry is a mix of public and private for-profit and not-for-profit institutions. Hospitals range from small institutions in rural areas providing limited basic medical care, to large regional referral centers providing a comprehensive range of sophisticated, highly specialized services. Most hospitals have expanded their roles to include primary care, home care, health promotion, and long-term care services. Hospitals have often reorganized to develop for-profit entities or to sponsor managed-care plans.

While hospitals are traditionally thought of as inpatient institutions, they now play an important role in the provision of outpatient care. Hospitals are often providers of a comprehensive and integrated continuum of health services (Shortell, Gillies, & Devers, 1995). To illustrate, outpatient services—virtually nonexistent until the 1960s—today generate about one-third of the total hospital revenue and exceed inpatient revenue in some situations. Today, nearly all of the nation's community hospitals have organized outpatient departments, emergency departments, ambulatory surgery units, health promotion programs, and many also offer home health services. Many hospitals are also now actively engaged in long-term care and geriatric services.

In recent years, the structure of the hospital industry has changed dramatically in response to the changing health care marketplace and the growth of managed care. Up to the mid-1980s, most hospitals were independent and locally owned. Their focus was mainly on inpatient care. Rarely did they employ or have formal "business" relationships with physicians to share responsibility for patient care. Consolidation of hospitals into local, regional, and even national systems began in earnest with Medicare's switch from cost reimbursement to diagnosis-related group (DRG) payment of hospitals in 1983, because this put great pressure on hospitals to control costs and make up for declining inpatient volumes. Consolidation picked up momentum through the 1990s as a result of the increasing competition among hospitals for the patient volumes controlled by health plans and other purchasers. Consolidation first took the form of horizontal integration—the coming together of independent hospitals into hospital systems—to gain administrative cost savings and economies of scale. More recently, consolidation has increasingly taken the form of vertical integration—the coming together of physicians, hospitals, and other providers into organized delivery systems—in order to contract with health plans and assume financial risk for the care of defined populations.

Changes in the health care environment continue to motivate providers to come together into organized delivery systems, both to increase their negotiating power with health plans and to be able to assume risk for managing care under capitation or other risk-sharing arrangements. The majority of community hospitals are members of systems. Individual providers cannot very well assume risk; this takes an organization of some size. Size also brings economies of scale and the ability to implement information systems and other care management technologies. Delivery systems can also bring all health care resources—physicians, hospitals, long-term care, home care, and so on—into a single organization so as to facilitate coordination of care across the entire range of health services.

Hospitals increasingly seek to form alliances with other delivery organizations and with payors. The recognition in the 1980s and 1990s that the hospital must be part of a larger integrated delivery system and that hospitals and delivery systems themselves must be part of still larger affiliations and financing arrangements continues to define and motivate the evolution of the hospital industry. In some instances, these changes are being implemented through larger and often proprietary chains of hospitals providing services over geographically diverse regions. In other instances, the integration of traditional hospital inpatient and related services to larger delivery systems that are politically integrated or even regionalized is increasingly common. As has been characterized by its history through time, the hospital continues to be challenged and continues to evolve as an institution and in relation to other components of the nation's health care system.

The purpose of this chapter is to characterize the hospital system in the United States, emphasizing major issues and trends. Because the character of the modern hospital reflects its past, the chapter begins with a discussion of the historical development of hospitals. The second section describes the hospital system as it exists today. The third section describes the internal organization of hospitals.

HISTORICAL DEVELOPMENT OF HOSPITALS

The history of hospitals in this country (Figure 10.1) can be traced back to the almshouses and pest houses that existed in some form in most cities of any size by the mid-1700s (MacEachern, 1957). Almshouses, also called *poorhouses* or *workhouses,* were established by city governments to provide food and shelter for the homeless poor, including many aged, chronically ill, disabled, mentally ill, and orphans. Medical care was a secondary function of the poorhouse. In some facilities, however, those who became sick were isolated in infirmaries where care, such as it was before the advent of modern medicine, was provided, typically by other residents. Not until the late 1800s did the infirmaries or hospital departments of city poorhouses

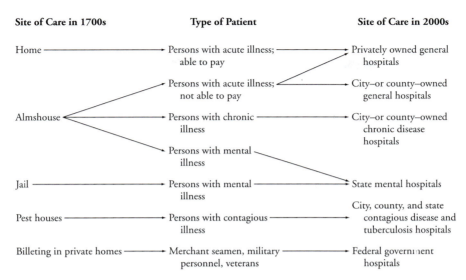

| Site of Care in 1700s | Type of Patient | Site of Care in 2000s |

Home — Persons with acute illness; able to pay — Privately owned general hospitals

Persons with acute illness; not able to pay — City–or county–owned general hospitals

Almshouse — Persons with chronic illness — City–or county–owned chronic disease hospitals

Persons with mental illness

Jail — Persons with mental illness — State mental hospitals

Pest houses — Persons with contagious illness — City, county, and state contagious disease and tuberculosis hospitals

Billeting in private homes — Merchant seamen, military personnel, veterans — Federal government hospitals

Figure 10.1. Evolution of Institutional Care Sites

break away to become medical care institutions on their own—the first public hospitals.

Pest houses were operated by local governments in seaport towns where it was necessary to quarantine people exposed to contagious diseases aboard ship. During epidemics, these institutions were also used to isolate victims of cholera, smallpox, typhus, and yellow fever. Their primary purpose was to control the spread of contagious diseases by removing infected persons from the community. As with almshouses, medical care was a secondary function—in this case, secondary to protecting the community from disease. Pest houses were often established during epidemics and discontinued or closed down when the threat of disease subsided. These institutions were the predecessors of the contagious disease and tuberculosis hospitals that later emerged.

Almshouses and pest houses were maintained for the poor and the homeless and were avoided by everyone else. These institutions were dismal places: crowded, unsanitary, and poorly heated and ventilated. Nutrition was often inadequate, nursing care incompetent, and separation of different types of patients minimal. The contagious, the disabled, the dying, and the mentally ill were often crowded together.

Cross-infection was rampant and mortality high. All those who could afford to were cared for at home or in the homes of neighbors.

The first community-owned or voluntary hospitals in this country were established in the late 1700s and early 1800s, often at the urging of influential physicians who had been trained in Europe and needed facilities to practice obstetrics and surgery in the manner in which they had been taught. These physicians also sought a setting where they could provide preceptor-type instruction for medical students. These early hospitals depended on philanthropy, and contributions were solicited from both private citizens and the local government. Voluntary hospitals generally preceded both religious and public hospitals in the United States, representing a departure from patterns in England and Europe. Voluntary hospitals generally preceded both religious and public hospitals in the United States, representing a departure from patterns in England and Europe. Voluntary hospitals admitted both indigent and paying patients. For example, in its first year of operation in 1751, Pennsylvania Hospital in Philadelphia admitted twenty-four paying patients and forty poor patients. Except in the largest cities where the concentration of poor was too great, the early voluntary hospitals cared for the sick who were unable to pay on a charitable basis. These hospitals relied upon philanthropy and donations of time by the physicians who comprised their medical staffs (MacEachern, 1957; Rosen, 1963).

The first hospitals of this type were the Pennsylvania Hospital, Philadelphia (1751); New York Hospital, New York City (1773); Massachusetts General Hospital, Boston (1816); and New Haven Hospital, New Haven, Connecticut (1826). Voluntary hospitals were established in Savannah, Georgia (1830); Lowell, Massachusetts (1836); and Raleigh, North Carolina (1839). Voluntary hospitals cared for patients with acute illnesses and injuries but did not admit persons with contagious diseases or mental illnesses. Isolation of these unfortunates from the rest of the community was seen as a government responsibility. Therefore, during the same period, a number of city, county, and state mental hospitals were established. These included hospitals in Williamsburg, Virginia (1773); Lexington, Kentucky (1817); Columbia, South Carolina (1829); Worcester, Massachusetts (1832); Augusta, Maine (1834); Brooklyn, New York (1838); and Boston, Massachusetts (1839).

Although voluntary hospitals provided better accommodations and care than had the poorhouses that preceded them, the efficacy of care improved little, and it was not until the late 1800s that hospitals became accepted by persons of all economic strata as the best setting for the care of serious illness and injury. Then, their growth was dramatic. In 1873, there were only 178 hospitals with 35,604 beds in the United States. By 1909, the number of hospitals had increased to 4,359 with 421,065 beds, and by 1929, to 6,665 hospitals with 907,133 beds. This rapid growth was brought about by advances in medical science that rapidly transformed the hospital's role from a custodial institution in which to isolate or shelter the poor to a curative institution in which communities concentrated their health care resources in support of the local physicians for the benefit of all (Corwin, 1946; Rosen, 1963). Starr (1982) has characterized this redefinition of the hospital as a transformation from a social welfare facility to an institution of medical science, from a charitable organization to a business, and from an orientation toward patrons and the poor to a focus on professionals and patients.

FORCES AFFECTING THE DEVELOPMENT OF HOSPITALS

Beginning in the late 1800s and early 1900s, six major developments were particularly significant in transforming hospitals into the institutions of today: (1) advances in medical science increased the efficacy and safety of hospitals; (2) the proliferation of technology and specialization within medicine necessitated the institutionalization of medical care; (3) the development of professional nursing brought about more humane patient care; (4) advances in medical education added teaching and research to the hospital's role; (5) the growth of health insurance provided adequate and certain funding; and (6) government began to exert greater influence over the activities of hospitals (Commission of Hospital Care, 1947; Rosen, 1963; Starr, 1982).

Advances in Medical Science

Most notable in terms of their impact on hospitals were the discovery of anesthesia, followed by rapid advances in surgery, and the development of the germ theory of disease with the subsequent discovery of antiseptic and sterilization techniques. By the early 1800s, enough was known about anatomy and physiology that surgeons were able to perform a variety of fairly complex surgical procedures; however, the inability to deaden pain meant that surgery was extremely traumatic and had to be carried out at great speed. In addition, infection from surgery was common. Ether was first used as an anesthetic in surgery by Long in 1842 and Morton in 1846, and its use then spread rapidly. Great advances in the efficacy of surgery followed.

Before formulation of the germ theory of disease, a few scientists, most notably Holmes in the United States and Semmelweis in Vienna, had observed and reported that fever, infection, and mortality could be reduced through cleanliness. Both concluded that childbed fever, which was the cause of high maternal mortality, was an infection transmitted by physicians, midwives, and medical students to women in labor. In 1861, Pasteur proved that bacteria were living, reproducing microorganisms that could be carried by air or on clothing and hands. It became clear that germs were the cause rather than the result of infection and that germs could be destroyed by chemicals and heat. Lister built on Pasteur's work and, in 1867, introduced carbolic acid spray in operating rooms as an antiseptic to keep air and incisions clean. In 1886, steam sterilization was introduced, providing a means of freeing medical equipment from microorganisms. Surgical infection rates fell. Advances in surgery led to the need for skilled preoperative and postoperative care and well-equipped operating rooms, which could be provided only in an institutional setting. By 1900, forty percent of all hospitalizations were for surgery.

The discovery of sulfa drugs in the mid-1930s and antibiotics in the mid-1940s changed the prevalent causes of death in the United States from infectious diseases to the diseases of old age, particularly heart disease, cancer, and stroke. Hospitals responded slowly to the health care needs of an aging population. Even today, most of the nation's medical resources are still concentrated on curable illnesses that respond quickly to medical treatment rather than on chronic conditions that must be managed over long periods of time. By the mid-1990s, however, hospitals began to broaden their role, adding skilled nursing units, inpatient and outpatient rehabilitation programs, day care, home care, and other services aimed at the elderly and chronically ill.

Advances in medical science today are generating a growing debate about the right balance between cost and improvements in medical diagnosis and treatment. Cost-effectiveness and outcomes research are producing a body of knowledge about the relative value of alternative approaches to care and of new technology. Because hospital care is so costly, much of this research focuses on the effects of shorter stays and of substituting alternative care settings for the hospital. Outcomes research now complements traditional medical research and underpins the development of clinical treatment protocols and utilization parameters that increasingly guide medical practice today.

Development of Specialized Technology

In the late 1800s, medical technology began to proliferate. The first hospital laboratory opened in 1889, and X-ray films were first used in 1896. These developments greatly increased the diagnostic effectiveness of hospitals. The discovery of blood types in 1901 made blood transfusions safe; the electrocardiogram (EKG) was first used in 1903, and the electroencephalogram (EEG) in 1929. In addition to increasing the efficacy of medical care, these advances in technology affected the site and organization of care. As the tools of medicine could no longer be carried in the physician's bag, hospitals became the place where the equipment, facilities, and personnel required by modern medicine were housed. In addition, because physicians could no longer be competent in all areas of medical practice, specialization began to occur within medicine, and new professional and technical occupations began to emerge. Again, the hospital became the place where physicians and support personnel came together to provide patient care.

Developments in specialized technology proceeded at such a rapid pace as to prompt one observer to describe the United States' system as a "medical-industrial complex" (Relman, 1980). Advances in diagnostic imaging and minimally invasive surgery are two hallmarks of late-twentieth century technology breakthroughs. Advances have occurred in administrative as well as clinical technology. Hospital managers now use sophisticated management information systems to analyze costs, utilization patterns, quality, and other dimensions of performance, and to measure and monitor workflow processes. These developments pose economic and political challenges as expenditures for the expensive equipment and highly trained personnel they require drive up hospital costs.

As physicians and the public came to expect that a wide range of advanced technologies would be available in their local hospitals, new discoveries were quickly diffused from large medical centers to smaller institutions. Duplication became commonplace, giving rise to calls to regulate capital expenditures by hospitals. Most states established certificate of need (CON) programs to control capital spending.

Many types of clinical technology—surgical lasers and laparoscopes for ophthalmologic and thoracic procedures, lithotripsy machines for kidney stones, computerized tomography (CT) and MRI units for imaging, and pharmacology agents for behavioral illness—either were developed for use in outpatient settings or reduced the need for all but a few days in the hospital. The emergence of such technology has prompted the shift of many procedures to outpatient settings. Many states have eliminated or weakened their CON programs, relying on market forces rather than regulation to contain spending on new technology (Katz & Thompson, 1996). Today, hospitals increasingly face competition from physician clinics and other freestanding entities that offer high-tech health care services once provided only by hospitals. Thus, recent trends affecting specialized technology have created significant economic and strategic challenges for hospitals.

Development of Professional Nursing

Humane treatment of hospital patients awaited the development of professional nursing. Before the late 1800s, nursing care was provided primarily by Catholic sisters and Protestant deaconesses, who were dedicated but minimally trained. Some religious orders established hospitals, and occasionally were called on by city officials to provide nursing care in public institutions. Almshouses used untrained female residents, and hospitals relied on poorly paid, unskilled labor.

The transformation of nursing into a profession is credited to Florence Nightingale, who completed four months of nurses' training in a deaconess school in Germany. In 1854, Nightingale and thirty-eight nurses were sent by the British government to the Crimea to take charge of nursing care for wounded soldiers. The nurses found conditions deplorable and instituted cleanliness and sanitation, dietary reforms, simple but humane care, discipline, and organization. As a result, mortality dropped dramatically. On her return to England, Nightingale wrote of her experiences in the Crimea and about the contributions of sanitation to the recovery of wounded and ill patients. In 1860, she founded the Nightingale School for Nursing in England.

In the United States, President Abraham Lincoln called on religious orders to provide nursing care for the wounded during the Civil War, but more nurses were needed. Dorothea Dix was appointed Superintendent of Nursing for the Union Army. She began a recruitment program and encouraged a one-month hospital training program for new nurses. By the end of the war, there were two thousand lay nurses in the United States. The first permanent schools of nursing were established at Bellevue Hospital, New Haven Hospital, and Massachusetts General Hospital in 1873. There was some initial reluctance on the part of hospital administrators and trustees to establish nursing schools, but the benefits of good nursing soon became apparent. In addition, student nurses provided better care and were less expensive than the untrained women previously employed to do this work. By 1883, there were twenty-two nursing schools and 600 graduates; by 1898, these totals had grown to 400 schools with 10,000 graduates.

Advances in nursing contributed to the growth of hospitals in two ways: (1) increased efficacy of treatment, cleanliness, nutritious diets, and formal treatment routines all contributed to patient recovery; and (2) considerate, skilled patient care made hospitals acceptable to all people, not just the poor. The public's fear of hospitals began to give way to an attitude of confidence and respect.

There are over two million registered nurses in the United States. About two-thirds of working nurses are employed by hospitals. Developments in nursing today are being shaped in no small measure by the economic pressures on hospitals and by declining inpatient volumes. Nurses may find their professional autonomy in jeopardy. Pressures to contain costs have led to the replacement of professional nurses with less-skilled personnel. In addition, in some hospitals the use of techniques to "reengineer" patient care and achieve process improvements has reduced the demand for professional nurses. Shortages of nurses in some areas have forced hospitals to rely on other personnel or to reduce services.

Contemporary trends in the employment of nurses by hospitals reflect two counteracting forces. On one hand, the increasingly complex case mix of hospital patients as a result of earlier discharge of patients and substitution of outpatient for inpatient care for less complex conditions, combined with the ever more sophisticated technology found in hospitals, has created a demand for more highly trained nurses. Acting to reduce the demand for nurses are declines in patient volumes and pressures to cut costs. The net effect of these forces has been a steady rise in the total number of registered nurses employed by community hospitals.

Advances in Medical Education

Changes in medical education brought about by the Flexner report in 1910 had a major impact on the development of hospitals. Before 1900, great variation characterized the nature and quality of medical education. There were no uniform standards for the academic training of physicians. Most medical schools were proprietary and were not connected with universities. They were dominated by influential practitioners, and most instruction was through didactic (often unscientific) lectures. Apprenticeship practices varied greatly. Clinical and laboratory instruction was minimal, and there was little research.

The Flexner report led to changes in the content and methods of instruction to emphasize the scientific basis of medicine. The standards of education established by the report were widely accepted by both the profession and the public; as a result, medical schools that did not meet the standards were forced to close. State laws were established requiring graduation from a medical school accredited by the American Medical Association as the basis for a license to practice medicine. A four-year course of study at a medical school based in a university became standard, as did clinical training on the wards of a hospital.

These changes expanded the role of the hospital to include education and research as well as patient care. The hospital's role in education became even more prominent as medical specialization led to a proliferation of internships and residencies in the 1920s and 1930s. The requirements of medical education necessitated the expansion of hospital facilities and services and the addition of equipment and personnel. Hospitals were called on to assume a greater role in acquiring and organizing these resources. Quality of care improved through advances in medical education, especially for patients with complex and serious illnesses. On the other hand, specialization led to a fragmentation of care among different physician specialists and ancillary personnel, and decreased interest in chronic, routine, and other "uninteresting" medical conditions.

The growing influence of managed care and the recognition of the oversupply of specialists, however, have gradually led educators, industry representatives, and legislators to shift more training to ambulatory care settings and to increase the number of training slots in the primary care disciplines of family practice, pediatrics, internal medicine, and obstetrics/gynecology. As medical students and residents experience additional community-based education, the traditional focus on the diagnosis and treatment of the individual patient will be balanced by an orientation toward population-based care, health promotion, managed care, physician participation on patient care teams, and patterns of practice consistent with high-volume outpatient settings.

Growth of Health Insurance

The growth of health insurance contributed significantly to the development of hospitals. Private insurance for hospital care expanded rapidly from the end of World War II through the 1960s, increasing both the portion of the population with insurance and the adequacy and scope of coverage. Today, the out-of-pocket cost of hospital care at the time of use is relatively modest for most of the population because most hospital bills are covered by either government or private health insurance.

A variety of factors led to the growth of hospital insurance. From the public's perspective, of course, a hospital stay is sufficiently expensive to warrant the purchase of insurance protection. The hospital industry's interest in insurance began with the Great Depression of the 1930s, when the number of patients who could not pay increased markedly and hospital use declined. The financial solvency of many hospitals was threatened, and the number of hospitals dropped from 6,852 in 1928 to 6,189 in 1937. A study of not-for-profit hospitals in 1935 revealed that on average, total income was three percent less than total expenses. In response, acting through the American Hospital Association, hospitals took the initiative to encourage the development of hospital insurance plans, primarily Blue Cross (Commission of Hospital Care, 1947; Starr, 1982).

The growth of health insurance provided the dollars to finance the great expansion of facilities and services and the prompt implementation of new technology that have characterized the hospital industry since the end of World War II. Insurance also contributed to the increased demand by the public for health services. Because hospital care has been better covered by insurance than care provided in other settings, patients have been reluctant to substitute less-well-insured out-of-hospital services even though they are less costly. This resulted in a bias toward hospital care relative to ambulatory, home, or nursing care settings and a general overuse of hospitals. In recent years, however, concern over the rising costs of hospital care and hospital overuse has given rise to actions to reverse this trend. Insurance plans now actively promote nonhospital alternatives and exercise stringent control over inpatient admissions and lengths of stay. The belief that hospital admissions were often unwarranted was underscored by an influential Rand Corporation study that examined a sample of hospital records from 1974 to 1982. The study concluded that twenty-three percent of the admissions studied were inappropriate and another seventeen percent could have been avoided through the use of ambulatory surgery (Siu, Sonnenberg, Manning, Goldberg, Bloomfield, Newhouse, & Brook, 1986).

The rapid rise in hospital costs through the late 1960s and 1970s was caused in part by cost-based reimbursement, the method of payment adopted by Medicare and Medicaid when these programs were enacted in 1965 following the practice of most Blue Cross plans at the time. Cost reimbursement did not provide hospitals with an incentive to contain costs. The result was inefficiency, duplication of services, and overbuilding. To stem rising hospital costs, public and private payers tried both regulatory and competitive approaches (Luft, 1985). Regulatory approaches—most notably certificate-of-need (CON) review of new hospital beds and equipment, and hospital rate regulation—were initiated by a large number of states in the 1970s. As hospital costs continued to rise, however, economists, businesses, and policy makers began suggesting that market competition would provide greater incentives for controlling health care costs (Havighurst, 1986). The 1980s witnessed a weakening of regulatory approaches to controlling costs and a growing emphasis on market forces. One hallmark of the marketplace model is the buying power of major purchasers of health care such as employer coalitions, managed-care plans, Blue Cross, Medicare, and Medicaid. These purchasers have replaced payment systems based on retrospective costs with payment based on negotiated prices or prospectively set rates.

A major step toward the introduction of economic forces to contain costs occurred with the Tax Equity and Fiscal Responsibility Act (TEFRA) of 1982 (PL 97-248), which converted Medicare reimbursement to a prospective, per-case system based on diagnosis-related groups (DRGs). In turn, many states revised their Medicaid payment methods to pay prospective rates. Additionally, cost-containment pressure has come from health maintenance organizations (HMOs) and other types of managed-care plans that employ financial incentives and utilization controls, as they have rapidly grown to dominate the private insurance market.

While cost-based reimbursement is widely blamed as the root cause of runaway hospital costs, it allowed hospitals to remain current with advances in medical technology and with demands from communities and physicians for ready access to the latest services. In sharp contrast, hospitals now find themselves competing for the growing enrollment of managed-care plans on the basis of price and quality. Quality measures are increasingly used as a tool to assist purchasers and consumers in choosing among health plans and providers, although there is currently little consensus on uniform measures of quality. A fundamental public policy issue yet unresolved is how to assure the poor and disadvantaged access to needed care in a system driven by competitive forces.

Role of Government

Patterns of hospital financing and ownership differ from country to country. Most advanced nations recognize health care as an essential service to which all should have access, and government plays a major role. In Great Britain and many other industrialized nations, government owns and operates most hospitals and employs the physicians who work in them. In other countries, the government limits its role to financing care that is provided by privately owned hospitals and private practitioners. In countries like Canada, where universal health insurance is in effect, hospitals primarily operate on public funds and hence are essentially controlled by the government even though they are not government-owned. In the United States, by contrast, government's role has been generally limited to financing care for needy groups such as the aged, the poor, and the disabled. This role has grown, however, to the point where community hospitals now receive almost half of their income from government sources (primarily Medicare and Medicaid). The rest comes mainly from private health insurance, supplemented by direct payments by patients. In short, the United States has a pluralistic public-private financing system with largely privately owned hospitals. However, as the portion of hospital income financed by the government has increased, so has government's influence.

Government's role in the hospital industry has changed over time. During colonial times, government involvement was mainly at the local level through cities and towns establishing almshouses and pest houses and making grants to help construct and support voluntary hospitals. The initial thrust of federal involvement began in 1935, with federal categorical grants-in-aid to state and local governments to assist in the establishment of public health programs: public health department, communicable disease programs, maternal and child health programs, and public assistance for specific groups such as crippled children, the aged, the blind, the disabled, and poor families with dependent children. These programs were part of the general social reform movement initiated during the Depression with the recognition that state and local government and voluntary efforts alone were not sufficient to meet the needs of out-of-work and vulnerable populations.

Direct federal involvement in the hospital industry began in 1946 with the Hill-Burton (Hospital Survey and Construction) Act. Few hospitals had been constructed during the Depression and World War II, and by the end of the war, a severe shortage of hospitals existed. The Hill-Burton program was enacted to help states and communities plan for and construct hospitals and other health facilities by providing federal grants on a matching basis to supplement funds raised at the community level.

The Hill-Burton program assisted in the construction of nearly forty percent of the beds existing in the nation's short-term general hospitals by 1960 and was the greatest single factor in the increase in the nation's bed supply during the 1950s and 1960s. Another positive impact of the program was that hospital facilities became more evenly distributed across rural and urban areas and high- and low-income states. In retrospect, however, Hill-Burton also contributed to the overbuilding of hospitals and to the preponderance of small rural hospitals that continues to exist today.

From assisting with the financing of hospital construction and promulgating basic life-safety codes for hospitals, government's role expanded to the financing of care with the introduction of Medicare and Medicaid in 1965. In the mid-1980s, the federal government implemented a major policy shift that set the stage for the managed care era by shifting Medicare payment from cost reimbursement to the payment of prospective DRG rates. Resource-based, relative-value rates (RBRVs) were introduced in the early 1990s as the basis for physician payment. By lowering Medicare and Medicaid hospital payments (relative to payments by private insurers), government programs accelerated the introduction of managed care in the 1990s by large private-sector purchasers to counter the practice of cost-shifting by hospitals. The concept of payment based on prospectively set rates, first introduced by the Medicare program, has now been adopted by most state Medicaid programs, private insurance companies, and managed-care plans.

Patterns of Ownership

In the United States, government ownership of hospitals is limited. This is due to several historic factors. First, government was relatively weak in the nineteenth century when hospitals were first established in response to advances in medical science; initiative generally came from private citizens. At that time, the perception prevailed that the needs of the poor could be addressed through charity care financed by philanthropy in private hospitals. In major cities with large concentrations of the poor, however, public hospitals were established to care for the needy.

Second, government responsibility for the health of the public was viewed narrowly before the Depression of the 1930s. Government's job was seen as protecting healthy citizens from persons with contagious diseases and mental illnesses and providing care for special groups such as merchant seamen, military personnel, and the poor. State governments operated hospitals for the mentally ill, and city and county governments in urban areas operated hospitals for the poor and persons with tuberculosis and other contagious diseases. Third, in the United States, government traditionally becomes involved in a sector of activity only when the private sector clearly fails to provide important services. Chronic, psychiatric, and tuberculosis hospital care would have been difficult to finance privately, given the lengthy stays that prevailed and the fact that the incidence of these conditions was greatest among the poor. As a result, care for people with these conditions became a public sector function. The private sector proved better able to finance short-stay hospital care through philanthropy, direct payments, and private health insurance, and government's role here was supplementary.

Current trends in hospital ownership reflect a significant interest on the part of investor-owned companies in the profit potential of efficiently run hospitals (Tables 10.1 and 10.2). As competition increases among hospitals to reduce costs, the emphasis of for-profit hospitals on efficient management, access to capital, and reduced labor costs is being widely imitated in the not-for-profit sector (Reinhardt, 2000). In an industry that remains over capacity in the early 2000s, facilities that do not do well become vulnerable to closure or acquisition by stronger for-profit and not-for-profit systems.

Table 10.1. Hospitals by Type of Ownership and Size of Hospital: United States, Selected Years

Type of Ownership and Size of Hospital	1975	1990	1998
	Number of Hospitals		
All hospitals	7,156	6,649	6,021
Federal	382	337	275
Non-federal	6,774	6,312	5,746
Community	5,875	5,384	5,015
Nonprofit	3,339	3,191	3,026
For profit	775	749	771
State/local government	1,761	1,444	1,218
6–24 beds	299	226	293
25–49 beds	1,155	935	900
50–99 beds	1,481	1,263	1,085
100–199 beds	1,363	1,306	1,304
200–299 beds	678	739	644
300–399 beds	378	408	352
400–499 beds	230	222	183
500 beds or more	291	285	254

Table 10.2.   Hospital Beds and Occupancy Rates by Type of Ownership and Size of Hospital: United States, Selected Years

Type of Ownership and Size of Hospital	1975	1990	1998
	Beds (Number in Thousands)		
All hospitals	1,465,828	1,213,327	1,012,582
Federal	131,946	98,255	56,698
Non-federal	1,333,882	1,115,072	955,884
Community	941,844	927,360	839,988
Nonprofit	658,195	656,755	587,658
For profit	73,495	101,377	112,975
State/local government	210,154	169,228	139,355
6–24 beds	5,615	4,427	5,351
25–49 beds	41,783	35,426	33,510
50–99 beds	106,776	90,394	78,035
100–199 beds	192,438	183,867	186,118
200–299 beds	164,405	179,670	156,978
300–399 beds	127,728	138,938	120,512
400–499 beds	101,278	98,833	81,247
500 beds or more	201,821	195,811	178,237
	Occupancy Rate (Percent of Beds Occupied)		
All hospitals	76.7	69.5	65.4
Federal	80.7	72.9	78.9
Non-federal	76.3	69.2	64.6
Community	75.0	66.8	62.5
Nonprofit	77.5	69.3	64.2
For profit	65.9	52.8	53.2
State/local government	70.4	65.3	62.7
6–24 beds	48.0	32.3	33.2
25–49 beds	56.7	41.3	41.2
50–99 beds	64.7	53.8	54.7
100–199 beds	71.2	61.5	58.4
200–299 beds	77.1	67.1	62.9
300–399 beds	79.7	70.0	64.7
400–499 beds	81.1	73.5	67.3
500 beds or more	80.9	77.3	70.9

CHARACTERISTICS OF THE HOSPITAL INDUSTRY

Hospitals today comprise a complex and diverse industry that is experiencing significant change. As hospitals evolve from the central role in the delivery of health care they occupied in the past to a role as one component of organized networks of providers, they are diversifying services, forming systems, competing for contracts with managed-care plans as an im-

portant source of patients, seeking new sources of capital to finance their transformation to new roles, and expanding linkages with other providers and community-based partners.

Traditionally, hospitals have been classified in three ways: according to length of stay, type of service provided, and ownership. The most common type of hospital is the short-stay, non-federal community hospital, in which the average length of stay is now

Table 10.3. Hospital Admissions and Average Length of Stay by Type of Ownership and Size of Hospital: United States, Selected Years

Type of Ownership and Size of Hospital	1975	1990	1998
	Admissions (Number in Thousands)		
All hospitals	36,157	33,774	33,766
Federal	1,913	1,759	1,133
Non-federal	34,243	32,015	32,633
Community	33,435	31,181	31,812
Nonprofit	23,722	22,878	23,282
For profit	2,646	3,066	3,971
State/local government	7,067	5,236	4,559
6–24 beds	174	95	139
25–49 beds	1,431	870	965
50–99 beds	3,675	2,474	2,265
100–199 beds	7,017	5,833	6,656
200–299 beds	6,174	6,333	6,230
300–399 beds	4,739	5,091	5,021
400–499 beds	3,689	3,644	3,390
500 beds or more	6,537	6,840	7,146
	Average Length of Stay (Number of Days)		
All hospitals	11.4	9.1	7.2
Federal	20.3	14.9	14.4
Non-federal	10.9	8.8	6.9
Community	7.7	7.2	6.0
Nonprofit	7.8	7.3	5.9
For profit	6.6	6.4	5.5
State/local government	7.6	7.7	7.0
6–24 beds	5.6	5.4	4.6
25–49 beds	6.0	6.1	5.2
50–99 beds	6.8	7.2	6.9
100–199 beds	7.1	7.1	5.9
200–299 beds	7.5	6.9	5.8
300–399 beds	7.8	7.0	5.7
400–499 beds	8.1	7.3	5.9
500 beds or more	9.1	8.1	6.5

under seven days (Tables 10.3 and 10.4). In long-term institutions, including chronic disease, psychiatric, and tuberculosis hospitals, the average length of stay can range from two to four months.

A second method of classification is by type of service. General hospitals offer a wide range of medical, surgical, obstetric, and pediatric services, whereas specialty hospitals provide care for a specific disease or population group. Examples of specialty hospitals are children's hospitals and psychiatric hospitals. During the first part of the twentieth century, many specialty hospitals were established by philanthropic support of prestigious physicians who wanted to develop a hospital in their own area of practice. Financial difficulties and advances in medical science eventually made general hospitals more appropriate and efficient, and most specialty hospitals either closed or converted to general hospitals.

Table 10.4. Discharges, Days of Care, and Average Length of Stay in Short-stay Hospitals, According to Selected Characteristics: United States, 1998

Characteristic	Discharges	Days of Care	Average Length of Stay
	Number per 1,000 Population		Number of Days
Total	123.8	611.0	4.6
Age			
Under 18 years	81.9	315.6	3.9
Under 6 years	192.1	645.1	3.4
6–17 years	27.3	152.6	5.6
18–44 years	93.1	380.5	4.1
45–64 years	134.0	678.6	5.2
45–54 years	105.5	530.8	5.2
55–64 years	177.9	906.1	5.2
65 years and over	283.4	1,789.7	6.6
65–74 years	244.6	1,496.6	6.2
75 years and over	333.0	2,160.8	7.0
Geographic Region			
Northeast	252.7	1,814.6	7.4
Midwest	276.6	1,619.0	5.8
South	312.3	2,107.7	6.9
West	285.7	1,493.6	6.2

A third method of classification is according to form of ownership, including private, not-for-profit ownership, government or public ownership, and for-profit ownership. Regardless of ownership, hospitals today face many common challenges, including accessing capital for new ventures, cutting costs to lower prices, and measuring quality and outcomes of care using advanced information systems. And as a result of hospital industry consolidation in the 1980s, 1990s, and early 2000s, many not-for-profit and for-profit hospitals, and even academic medical centers, are now part of large, multihospital systems (Etheredge et al., 1996).

Community Hospitals

Short-stay, general hospitals—whether for-profit, not-for-profit, or public in ownership—are often referred to as community hospitals because they are available to the entire community and meet most community needs for hospital care.

The average length of stay in community hospitals has steadily declined due to several factors, including an increased emphasis on outpatient care; the utilization of management practices carried out by health insurance plans, Medicare, and Medicaid, to reduce unnecessary hospital stays; and the shift to prospective payment by Medicare and other payers. Taken together, community hospitals admitted about 30 million inpatients in 2000, a decrease from 1985. This downward trend in admissions, combined with the shrinking average length of stay, led to a corresponding decrease in total acute care "volume" as measured by inpatient days of care. Traditionally, the major role of community hospitals has been to provide short-term, inpatient care for patients with acute illnesses and injuries; however, the outpatient role of hospitals has been growing in importance.

Community hospitals fall into three ownership categories: private/not-for-profit (owned and operated by community or religious organizations), for-profit (investor-owned), and public (owned by state or local government).

Private/Not-for-Profit Hospitals

Private/not-for-profit hospitals comprise about three-fifths of all community hospitals (Table 10.1). In past years, these hospitals have been pressed to expand their roles to become true community health systems (Goldsmith, 1981). The rationale is that they represent their community's collective investment in health resources financed by a population's insurance premiums. In this view, access to these resources should not be limited to patients who happen to need inpatient hospitalization. Initially, because of limited physician interest, poor reimbursement for nonhospital services, and resistance by nursing homes and other providers, hospitals were slow to expand their roles beyond inpatient care.

More recently, diversification of services has been undertaken by community hospitals to offset declining inpatient revenues, to contain costs by substituting less expensive care settings for expensive inpatient stays, and to respond to community needs. Hospitals are now adding a wide variety of ambulatory care and health promotion services, and a significant proportion have expanded mental health and rehabilitation services as well (Table 10.5). Community hospitals are seeking to play a central role in planning and coordinating the entire range of community health services.

A major trend during the 1980s and 1990s was that of industrywide consolidation, whereby many community hospitals affiliated or merged with other hospitals or joined larger hospital systems. In the 1990s, half of all community hospitals were in systems, with beds in private/not-for-profit systems comprising nearly half of all beds in systems nationally.

Public Hospitals

Public hospitals are owned by agencies of federal, state, or local government. Federally owned hospitals are primarily maintained for special groups of federal beneficiaries: Native Americans, military personnel, and veterans. State governments have generally lim-

Table 10.5. Hospital Outpatient Visits by Type of Ownership and Size of Hospital: United States, Selected Years

Type of Ownership and Size of Hospital	1975	1990	1998
	Outpatient Visits (Number in Thousands)		
All hospitals	254,844	368,184	545,481
Federal	51,957	58,527	63,642
Non-federal	202,887	309,657	481,838
Community	190,672	301,329	474,193
Nonprofit	131,435	221,073	352,114
For profit	7,713	20,110	42,072
State/local government	51,525	60,146	80,008
6–24 beds	915	1,471	4,278
25–49 beds	5,855	10,812	22,694
50–99 beds	16,303	27,582	42,161
100–199 beds	35,156	58,940	107,966
200–299 beds	32,772	60,561	85,494
300–399 beds	29,169	43,699	67,070
400–499 beds	22,127	33,394	49,022
500 beds or more	48,375	64,870	95,508
	Outpatient Surgery (Percent of Total Surgeries)		
Community hospitals	—	50.5	61.6

ited themselves to the operation of mental and tuber-culosis hospitals, reflecting government's early approach to protecting the public by isolating the mentally ill and persons with contagious diseases.

Most local government hospitals are short-stay general hospitals, and most fall into two general types. The first category includes city, county, or hospital district institutions of small or moderate size, with medical staffs consisting of private physicians. Many of these hospitals are located in small cities and towns. They serve both indigent and paying patients. Their costs are met primarily through patient care revenues, and they generally function the same as private, not-for-profit hospitals.

The second category of public hospitals consists of large city or county hospitals in major urban areas. The National Association of Public Hospitals identified sixteen different categories of vulnerable populations among their patients (Andrulis, Acuff, Weiss, & Anderson, 1996). These hospitals serve a wide range of primarily local residents, but concentrate on the poor. The typical large, urban public hospital is staffed mainly by salaried physicians and residents in training. Most are affiliated with medical schools; their operating costs often exceed patient revenues, and deficits are often made up through tax subsidies and Medicare and Medicaid disproportionate-share payments. Large, urban public hospitals play an important safety net role in the health care system. They provide care for all patients regardless of the ability to pay, and offer services that many private hospitals cannot or will not provide, including burn and trauma care, alcohol and drug abuse treatment, psychiatric services, care for persons with communicable diseases, and treatment of persons with AIDS. They are located in inner-city areas where private physicians are often in short supply, and their outpatient departments are often the chief source of ambulatory care for the poor. In addition, public hospitals play a major role in medical education; most are affiliated with a medical school and offer residency training programs. More than half of all practicing physicians receive at least some of their training in public hospitals.

The introduction of the Medicare and Medicaid programs had the potential to reduce the demands on public hospitals by giving the elderly and the poor access to "mainstream" providers. The anticipated shift did not occur, however, in part because private practitioners were in short supply in many inner-city areas; those who were there often limited the number of Medicaid patients they would accept because of low Medicaid payment rates. In addition, cultural and social barriers often discourage the poor from approaching private physicians and hospitals, and as a result, a large proportion of charity care continues to be provided by public hospitals. Given the increasing demands on, and limited financial support for, large, urban public hospitals, their futures are uncertain. Characteristically, these hospitals are old and outmoded, and tend to be underequipped, underfinanced, and understaffed. Administration is often constrained by the bureaucratic red tape of city or county government. Ironically, amid this change, the public hospital has become the darling of several American television dramas over the last ten years.

Many public hospitals offer highly specialized tertiary services such as regional trauma services, burn care, neonatal intensive care, and kidney dialysis for all segments of the population, including privately insured patients. Future strategies recommended for public hospitals include continuing as the regional provider of the most costly, high-technology services for the entire population, shifting nonurgent services to lower-cost community sites, partnering with other public and private agencies to provide health care and social services for the chronically ill, and working with medical schools to adapt clinical training programs to the ambulatory environment (Andrulis et al., 1996).

For-Profit Hospitals

For-profit, investor-owned hospitals are operated to provide a financial return to their owners or shareholders, although spokespersons for the investor-owned hospital companies are quick to point out that profits come from providing good patient care, and satisfying the demands of physicians, patients, and purchasers. At the turn of the century, more than half of the nation's hospitals were proprietary. As late as 1950, there were still over 1,200 proprietary hospitals, but their number declined to under 800 before beginning to rise in recent years. An important underlying shift took place during this period: large, national, investor-owned corporations acquired proprietary hospitals formerly owned by single individuals or partnerships. In recent years, the growth of these companies has been mainly through the purchase of not-for-profit and public hospitals—often those in financial difficulties because of declining inpatient volumes, high debt, and an inability to compete successfully for contracts with managed care plans.

The investor-owned hospital companies assert that their institutions are able to earn profits while maintaining quality by operating more efficiently than not-for-profit hospitals. In addition, investor-owned systems often respond first to strategic opportunities such as population shifts because of their ability to raise capital quickly. They point to the availability of management specialists, the application of modern management techniques, cost savings in construction, economies of scale, and group purchasing as key factors enabling them to control costs without compromising quality.

For-profits have expanded outpatient volumes. For-profit hospitals report lower average lengths of stay, fewer personnel, and lower expenses per inpatient stay than their not-for-profit counterparts. Critics claim, however, that these apparent efficiencies and the profits they generate are actually attributable to admitting patients with less serious medical conditions, not offering expensive services that do not pay for themselves, and concentrating on those patients able to pay the full costs of hospitalization. Critics also note that the profits derived from these cost savings are passed on to shareholders rather than to the community in the form of lower prices. By not admitting uninsured patients, for-profit hospitals can avoid charity care and bad debts, which may run as high as ten percent of total expenses in not-for-profit and public hospitals in certain locations. By not admitting seriously ill patients, for-profit hospitals can avoid providing expensive or unprofitable services. The for-profits reply that they provide community benefits through the taxes they pay, and that these taxes often exceed the amount of charity care provided by tax-exempt not-for-profits.

Do for-profit hospitals really act any differently than not-for-profits? The literature comparing the two supports a number of inferences. Not-for-profits do provide more charity care than for-profits, although the differences are often small. Not-for-profits generally treat a higher portion of Medicaid patients. Not-for-profits are more involved in education and research, and more frequently offer high-cost, unprofitable services such as neonatal intensive care units (NICUs), transplant surgery, burn care, and trauma centers. They are more likely to be located in lower-income areas and to provide community services such as free clinics, HIV/AIDs care, and outreach workers. Few hospital studies have looked carefully at quality of care in relation to ownership, although for-profit hospitals have equal or higher rates of accreditation than not-for-profit hospitals. Studies of nursing homes, however, consistently find more quality problems in for-profit homes. And for-profit nursing homes and home care agencies are more likely to select patients based on their ability to pay.

Perhaps most surprising, given the constant claim of the for-profits that they are more efficient than not-for-profits, is a growing body of evidence suggesting that the opposite is true. Several studies have compared costs, productivity, revenues, and profits in not-for-profit and for-profit hospitals, adjusting these measures for case-mix complexity and outpatient activity. For-profits were found to have higher profit margins and higher gross and net revenues per case-mix adjusted patient stay. Not-for-profits, however, had lower costs per adjusted stay, even after crediting for-profits for the taxes they pay. Efficiency and productivity were not found to differ significantly between the two types of hospitals. In short, the higher profits earned by the for-profits were due to higher prices and "revenue management" rather than better management of costs or productivity (Shukla & Clement, 1997).

A very important current issue, given the health care industry's shift toward market-oriented reform, is whether health care purchasers place enough value on the availability of charity care, needed but unprofitable services, and other community benefits to contract preferentially with hospitals or systems that provide these services. It does not appear that this is the case. This could be due to the current preoccupation with price. It could also be due to the lack of unequivocal measures of community service. Some purchasers are even wary of providers that give substantial community service, fearing that the costs of these services will be shifted to them in higher prices. Purchasers do weigh the overall reputation of hospitals, and they are beginning to look at Health Plan Employer Data Information Set (HEDIS) and patient satisfaction measures, but these measures focus mainly on a plan's members, not on benefits provided to the community as a whole. There is little to suggest that purchasers place much value on a comprehensive range of services, on health promotion, on serving all segments of the population, or on actions aimed at optimizing the community's overall health. Perhaps, as economists suggest, not until competition has forced down the prices of all providers and narrowed the price differences among them will other factors be given more weight (Dowling, 1996).

Small and Rural Hospitals

Small and rural hospitals constitute a large part of the United States hospital industry. Most small hospitals are located in rural communities. The preponderance of small hospitals is a legacy of the Hill-Burton program, which channeled funds to the thinly populated rural areas least able to finance hospital construction without outside help.

In general, small hospitals care for less seriously ill patients than do larger hospitals; their average length of stay is shorter and their care less specialized. The national average daily census for community hospitals with fewer than one hundred beds has declined rapidly over time.

Small and rural hospitals face a number of problems that threaten their future viability. Several hundred hospitals have closed since the early 1970s, and many have become part of for-profit or not-for-profit multihospital systems. In general, small hospitals cannot afford as broad a range of services as their larger urban counterparts and find it difficult to keep abreast with developments in medical technology. In addi-

tion, labor requirements are high in small hospitals for the services offered, and small hospitals tend to operate at far less efficient occupancy levels than larger hospitals. On the other hand, the few studies that have examined quality in relation to size suggest that small hospitals that treat only conditions they are equipped to handle can achieve equally good outcomes as larger hospitals.

Small and rural hospitals have historically been strongly affected by Medicare and Medicaid funding, due in part to less adequate private health insurance coverage in rural areas and a higher elderly population. In the 1980s, the Medicare Prospective Payment System effectively penalized rural hospitals because the low-wage scales in rural areas resulted in low DRG payment rates. Coupled with the depressed economies of some of these communities, these pressures caused a number of small hospitals to incur operating losses and threatened the survival of many.

Strategies employed by rural hospitals focus on linking with other local and regional hospitals, joining managed-care contracting networks, and seeking additional resources by broadening their role in the communities they serve. The key to the future of small and rural hospitals would appear to lie in regional networking, especially because managed care organizations favor wide geographic availability of health care services for their enrolled populations (Brown, 1996). These arrangements should encourage referral of patients to the institutional setting most appropriate to their needs. Rural communities are also seeking to strengthen their hospitals by entering into contractual relationships with their physicians that unify the interests of the two.

Strategic relationships between urban and rural providers today range from informal agreements to formal affiliations, joint programs, and the merger of institutions into multihospital systems. The objectives of such relationships include: (1) a two-way flow of patients, with patients referred to larger hospitals for specialized services and returned to smaller communities for long-term, follow-up, and home care; (2) participation in the continuing educational programs of the larger hospital; (3) management assistance from the larger hospital; (4) consolidation of services; and

(5) group purchasing. Many rural hospitals have begun to collaborate with urban health care systems in "telemedicine" programs that provide clinical support and educational programming across great distances. The success of regional networks depends on community support, collaboration between management and physicians, and synchronized financial incentives. The number of examples of effective regional relationships involving hospitals, public health departments, physician groups, and even school districts is growing. In the long run, community and regional networking may preserve rather than threaten the independence and viability of smaller hospitals.

Academic Medical Centers

Academic medical centers (AMCs) are university-owned hospitals. They are typically large, urban institutions. AMCs' patient care activities are included in the overall statistics for community hospitals. Despite significant strategic challenges facing AMCs today in the form of increased competition and reduced financial support, these institutions are largely responsible for the major advances in twentieth-century American medical treatment, technology, and training.

Historically, AMCs have performed several distinct functions simultaneously: they operate as tertiary-care referral centers offering state-of-the-art technology for the diagnosis and treatment of the most complex medical problems; they function as the primary clinical teaching site for their medical schools; they house much of the nation's medical research; and they care for a large portion of the poor in the areas where they are located. Care in AMCs is primarily provided by faculty and residents whose patient care activities are administered by faculty practice plans. Many patients are enrolled in clinical trials run by faculty researchers.

The expansion of AMCs in number and degree of sophistication roughly parallels a fifty-year period of substantial investment in medical research by the federal National Institutes of Health. AMCs were given an additional boost by Medicare and Medicaid reimbursement. In the early 1980s, however, with Medicare's introduction of the DRG prospective payment system to contain Medicare spending, the fortunes of many

AMCs began to change. AMCs in general have been slow to respond to the cost-cutting incentives implicit in prospective payment and managed care.

Historically, teaching hospitals relied heavily on public subsidies in the form of Medicare and Medicaid payments for direct and indirect medical education costs, and "disproportionate share" payments in recognition of the high portion of poor patients they serve. These subsidies are seriously threatened by cutbacks in public health care spending and by market pressures to contain private spending. Teaching hospitals have also been able to cost-shift some of their higher costs to private insurers in the form of higher rates. In addition, like all hospitals, many teaching hospitals are experiencing declines in admissions and lengths of stay (Carey & Engelhard, 1996).

Because AMCs have depended on Medicare payment supplements to help cover the costs associated with teaching, they are especially vulnerable to payment cuts. In addition, AMCs must compete with community hospitals to be included in the provider networks of managed-care health plans. Hence, they are under great pressure to reduce costs, but given their salaried physician staffs and relatively high operating costs, this transition will be difficult.

The societal pressures that led AMCs to expand expensive teaching and research programs and acquire advanced technology have reversed course, and now challenge AMCs to compete for contracts with managed-care plans and other purchasers based on competitive prices. As a result, many AMCs that in the last two generations built national and international reputations through the growth of state-of-the-art technology are now trying to adapt by developing primary care delivery networks, revising teaching programs, downsizing, and aligning with not-for-profit or for-profit systems in order to be better positioned in the new medical marketplace.

HOSPITALS AND HEALTH SYSTEMS

Consolidation of hospitals and other providers into networks and systems—first in the form of hospitals coming together into multihospital systems, and more recently, in the form of hospitals, physicians, and other providers consolidating into integrated health care systems—has been a dominant trend in the health care industry since the early 1970s. Consolidation is fundamentally changing the landscape of the nation's health system and, even more significantly, is reshaping the relationships among purchasers, health plans, providers, and the people they serve. Consolidation can take many organizational forms: acquisition of one entity by another, the merger of two or more entities to create a new organization, or the formation of more loosely structured alliances and networks.

Consolidation in the health care industry is of two basic types: horizontal integration and vertical integration. Horizontal integration refers to the coordination or consolidation of facilities or services that are at the same stage of the patient care "production process." Examples include the coming together of hospitals into multihospital systems (which is the focus of this chapter), the joining of individual physician practices into medical groups, and the merger of a number of home care agencies into a single, larger home-care organization. The primary goals of horizontal integration are economies of scale, elimination of redundant or underutilized facilities, group purchasing, streamlining operations, and, in recent years, strengthening the resulting system's hand in competing for and negotiating contracts with health plans.

Vertical integration refers to organizing the production of patient care so that the sequential stages in the process are carried out or coordinated by a single organization (Gillies, Shortell, Anderson, Mitchell, & Morgan, 1993; Mick & Conrad, 1988). Comprehensive integration would entail coordinating the entire range of services for protecting, maintaining, and restoring peoples' health, from disease prevention and health promotion at one end of the spectrum to treatment and rehabilitation at the other. Coordinated provision of a full continuum of services, in turn, would require coordination of the work of physicians, one or more hospitals, long-term care facilities, home-care agencies, and a variety of other providers. The goals of vertical integration are cost-effectiveness, continuity and quality of care, and better positioning of the providers comprising the integrated health care system to compete, assume risk, and manage the care of the population served.

Two fundamental motives propelled the multihospital system movement of the 1970s and 1980s that so dramatically changed the character of the hospital industry: organizational survival and organizational growth. For many freestanding hospitals, the increasingly complex, fast-changing, demanding, even hostile health care environment made survival problematic. Competition, financial pressures, regulation, and other external forces were so threatening that hundreds of hospitals turned to systems for the strength to survive, albeit under different ownership. For the systems, acquisition of additional hospitals provided a means to grow—to add new services, enter new markets, establish new referral patterns, or build more financial and political power.

Nonfederal multihospital systems, defined as corporations that own, lease, or manage two or more acute care hospitals, account for about half of the nation's community hospitals. Multihospital systems have religious affiliations, are secular not-for-profit, or are investor-owned. The investor-owned systems tend to be large.

The growth of horizontally integrated hospital systems began in earnest in the late 1960s, spurred by the entry and expansion of investor-owned systems in response to the improved financial climate for hospitals following the enactment of Medicare and Medicaid. Not-for-profit system growth picked up in the mid-1970s. Today, hospital acquisitions, mergers, and affiliations are aimed at better positioning the participants to compete for market share. Because health care markets are local in nature, local or metropolitan groupings of hospitals have gained in importance, and large multistate systems have tended to plan their strategies and investments on a market-by-market basis, even divesting hospitals in markets where they have a limited presence.

How well have multihospital systems actually performed? Shortell's (1988) seminal review of the evidence on system performance, based on the handful of then-available studies and on comparative data from nearly one thousand system and freestanding hospitals, concluded that "there is little support for any of the alleged advantages of system hospitals relative to their nonsystem counterparts. . . . Little if any economic or service 'value added' appears to be present." Areas of performance examined by Shortell included the following:

- costs, economies of scale, efficiency, productivity
- prices
- financial performance, profitability
- access to capital
- charity care provided
- services offered
- managed-care involvement
- quality patient-care outcomes

Shortell hypothesized that the unimpressive performance of systems was largely due to the fact that many systems had formed mainly as a defensive reaction to the increasingly hostile health care environment. Systems were seeking security rather than lower costs or greater community health benefits. Nor did most systems really behave like systems in the sense of "operating as an organic whole with a strategic intent." Shortell's findings undoubtedly also reflected the fact that in the mid-1980s, many systems were in the formative stages, and most saw themselves as horizontally integrated hospital systems, not as vertically integrated delivery systems.

Vertical Integration

The pressures to transform today's fragmented financing and delivery structures into rationally designed, integrated health care systems come from the growth of managed care and the movement toward health care reform. These forces are giving rise to two new realities: (1) Medicare, Medicaid, and private purchasers are curtailing their spending to the point that the flow of dollars into health care will not sustain the delivery system as it exists today, and (2) capitation-based payment is ending the separate flow of payments to each category of provider and putting providers at financial risk. But today's fragmented nonsystem of still largely independent physicians, hospitals, and health plans is not structured to manage care within fixed-dollar limits or to deploy resources more rationally.

There is growing recognition that changing financial and market pressures call for a restructuring of the way health care is delivered. Providers are responding by coming together into organized delivery systems able to accept responsibility for the health of enrolled populations, manage care across the full spectrum of services, reduce fragmentation and redundancy, and do so within fixed financial resources increasingly determined by purchasers. This model is generally referred to as a *vertically integrated delivery system.* An extreme form of vertical integration intended to capture patients at the source (that is, when they choose a health insurance plan) entails integration of the delivery and financing functions. A number of delivery organizations are starting health plans or contracting with a health plan to be the plan's exclusive or preferred provider resource. At the same time, a number of health plans are approaching this from the other direction and assembling their own provider networks through selective contracting. The integrated delivery system is clearly an idea whose time has come, although most providers are just beginning to assemble all the elements (Dowling, 1995).

The generic elements or properties that characterize a vertically integrated delivery system include the following (Dowling, 1995; Shortell et al., 1995):

1. *A broad range of facilities and services*—prevention, promotion, primary care, specialty care, acute care, long-term care, home care—under a single organizational umbrella. This facilitates coordination and continuity of care and the use of the sites of care most appropriate to each patient's needs.
2. *A group or network of primary care physicians* formally linked with the delivery system through arrangements that align the interests of both parties. The primary care physicians should be organized to manage care and promote health within available resources. They should be geographically located to provide access to the system throughout the area served. Economic incentives and organizational loyalties should be structured so that the primary care physicians share responsibility with the system for costs, outcomes, and system performance.
3. *Specialists* and other providers formally linked with the delivery system through arrangements and incentives that align the interests of both par-

ties and encourage the delivery of cost-effective, quality care.

4. *Mechanisms for coordinating/integrating care* across the entire spectrum of services that facilitate cost-effective, quality care and reduce fragmentation, duplication, and redundancy. Examples include primary care physicians as care managers, clinical nurse specialists in care coordination roles, coordination by interdisciplinary teams, case management, treatment guidelines, an integrated information system, a single medical record, and discharge coordinators/social workers in both inpatient and outpatient settings.

5. *Health promotion services* that prevent or reduce the risks of illness and injury. Examples include immunizations and other prevention services, health education, lifestyle change programs, fitness programs, self-care education, and occupational health and safety programs. Mechanisms for identifying high-risk people and bringing them into specially tailored health maintenance programs are especially important.

6. *Information systems* that enable planning, monitoring, evaluating, and publicly reporting on cost-effectiveness, quality, and outcomes. Information systems should be able to track populations/patients over time and across providers/sites, integrate data from all settings, and relate outcomes to treatment. Information systems should be able to support the management of patient care as well as the management of financial risk. Information should enable the profiling of both providers and treatment patterns.

7. *Integrated strategic planning, resource allocation, and assessment of system performance* facilitated by cross-functional management and organizational structures. Systematic assessment and deployment of new technologies.

8. *Unified marketing and contracting* such that the delivery system approaches the market as a single entity.

9. *Integration of financing and delivery* through common ownership and/or exclusive or preferred relationships with health plans.

The growth of managed care has made integration of financing and delivery especially important. Previously, insurers paid for the services rendered by whatever providers individuals chose. Few providers were excluded. With the advent of HMOs, PPOs, and selective contracting, insurers and health plans began to contract only with selected providers and to employ financial disincentives to discourage their enrollees from using other providers. Hence, health plans became the providers' source of patients. Integration of finance and delivery gives providers a direct link to the source of patients. It also enables the delivery system to (1) align incentives, (2) rationally deploy resources internally (which is almost impossible if insurers pay each provider independently and often in a contradictory manner), and (3) benefit financially from being efficient. A few major integrated health care systems like Kaiser and Group Health Cooperative of Puget Sound own their own health plan; most systems contract to assume the financial risk for the care of the enrollees of health plans they do not own. The delivery system's goal, however, is to be in the position to control the methods and levels of payment to its providers; that is, to manage the capitation dollar.

System leaders believe vertical integration can cut costs substantially through improved cost-effectiveness of care, lower admissions, lower service utilization, shorter lengths of stay, economies of scale, greater volumes, and increased productivity. Reductions in length of stay and service utilization are widely reported to result from the use of clinical treatment guidelines, case management, discharge planning, coordination of posthospital services, and filling gaps in the availability of services. Where systems are at financial risk as a result of capitated contracts for the health of a defined population, greater emphasis is placed on health education, health promotion, and prevention. Vertical integration, driven by capitation and guided by population-based planning, also tends to lead to efforts to achieve a better fit between a system's resources and the needs of the populations it serves. Attention focuses, for example, on the balance between primary care physicians and specialists. Hospital beds are eliminated in favor of outpatient facilities and long-term care beds. The matching of system resources to the needs of the population served has come to be called *rightsizing* (Coddington, Moore, & Fischer, 1996).

Consolidating a substantial portion of an area's providers into a single system can greatly strengthen the system's bargaining power with purchasers. In some cases, this has gone so far as to raise antitrust questions. It may be that many systems first pursue integration mainly to cut costs and/or to gain market power. But once the elements of integrated service delivery are assembled, systems faced with increasing pressures from purchasers to cut costs may then turn their attention to the efficiencies achievable through better coordination of care. Coddington et al. concluded from a study of ten integrated health care systems that the strategies pursued by these organizations were primarily aimed at gaining competitive advantage. "However, when properly implemented . . . these strategies also enable organizations to increase the value added they bring to their customers and communities" (p. 181).

Many observers see the hospital- or hospital system-sponsored integrated delivery system as the ideal organizational form and inevitable end point toward which health care delivery is transitioning. Hospitals have capital, community ties, and management leadership, and most have already diversified vertically into a broad range of services. Some enjoy dominant market positions.

Competition for the central role in reorganizing delivery is coming from increasingly aggressive purchasers. As meaningful information on costs, efficacy, and customer satisfaction becomes more readily available, and as the oversupply of hospital beds and physicians in many markets gives purchasers alternative providers from which to choose, purchasers will be in a position to selectively contract with whatever providers they believe give them the most value. In short, purchasers will be able to put together their own provider networks.

Between the provider-sponsored and purchaser-sponsored models lies a third model: a long-term, bilateral contract between a provider network or system and an intermediary who plays the role of exclusive distributor of the providers' health benefits product to one or more purchasers. A group model HMO marketed by a single insurer or health plan approaches this model. Typically, the intermediary is in the driver's seat in this model. A fourth candidate for the central role in integrating the delivery of care and controlling the flow of dollars is the conglomerate of medical groups. Such "supergroups" can pursue contracts with health plans on behalf of their participating physicians and accept financial risk, often for hospital as well as physician services.

Hospital Responses to Competition and Cost-Containment Pressures

In addition to the trend toward consolidation, hospitals are actively adapting to the new competitive environment in other ways. Prospective payment and price competition create a strong incentive for hospitals to achieve more efficient staffing levels, as labor represents approximately fifty-four percent of the average hospital's costs. Hospitals are looking at ways to utilize nurses more efficiently by re-engineering how patient care is provided, and many hospitals are substituting less highly trained support personnel for professional nurses. Total Quality Management and Continuous Quality Improvement (TQM/CQI) techniques have been applied to streamline work processes and restructure the way ancillary departments support nursing and other direct patient care departments. Hospitals are also attempting to increase the productivity of their workforce by cross-training employees to fill multiple positions. Unfortunately, this emphasis on cost containment and productivity is likely to create new conflicts between hospitals, nurses, and labor unions.

Hospitals are investigating other methods of increasing their efficiency and competitiveness, including product- or service-line management. The practice of analyzing hospital programs and services as strategic business units (SBUs) in order to identify and enhance profitable services and turn around or eliminate unprofitable services is being advocated by many as a more businesslike approach to hospital management. The concern is that some hospitals may discontinue services that are unprofitable but needed by the community. Still, a positive aspect of product-line management is the development and organization of services to meet the special needs of specific subgroups in the population. Examples include diabetes programs, women's programs, and sports medicine clinics. It can be argued that competition is forcing hospitals to be much more sensitive to the needs and desires of people for convenient, specially tailored services (Cunningham, 2001).

Under Medicare's DRG payment system, there is a strong incentive for hospitals to discharge patients as soon as medically warranted, and this has done a great deal to foster the effectiveness of discharge planning. The role of the discharge planner is critical in ensuring that patients receive proper care after leaving the hospital. For elderly patients in particular, rehospitalizations may result unless proper discharge instructions and support services are provided. In many instances, the elderly patient cannot be discharged from the hospital until placement in a nursing home is secured or arrangements are made for home care. This has heightened the interest of many hospitals in operating their own skilled nursing units and home care programs. A major concern of the Medicare program is that hospitals not discharge patients too soon. Hospitals are under great pressure to deliver exactly the right amount of care to Medicare patients; too much care may result in reimbursement denials and too little care can result in penalty assessments or lawsuits. As a result, hospitals are placing more emphasis on complete documentation of patient care in medical records.

INTERNAL ORGANIZATION OF COMMUNITY HOSPITALS

From the outside, hospitals appear as cohesive organizations with a united sense of purpose and a clear goal of providing high-quality patient care. From the inside, however, hospitals are comprised of several different components, each of which has distinct goals and roles. The management team is responsible for the efficient operation of the institution as a whole; the medical staff is responsible for the quality of patient care provided by physicians; and the governing board sets institutional policy and goals and has the responsibility for the fiscal health of the organization (see Figure 10.2).

Each party has distinct responsibilities. The governing board is ultimately responsible for everything that goes on in the hospital, both administratively and clinically. The board's role is often described as one of stewardship for the institution. It carries out this responsibility by adopting policies and plans to guide the hospital's operation; selecting and delegating management responsibilities to a chief executive and supervising the chief executive's performance; and appointing physicians to the medical staff, approving the medical staff's organization for governing itself and for supervising the professional activities of its members, and delegating responsibility to the medical staff for the provision of patient care.

In reality, boundaries between areas of authority among triad members are not always clear. For example, while it might seem there is a clear distinction between governance and the medical staff's responsibility for patient care, courts have concluded that hospitals have a corporate responsibility or legal liability for ensuring that patients receive high-quality patient care. Thus, the governing board must make sure that only qualified physicians practice in the hospital and that quality assurance mechanisms are established and working, yet only the medical staff has the expertise to assess qualifications and judge the care provided by individual physicians.

Although the medical staff is legally subordinate to the governing board's authority over the affairs of the institution, physicians are partially autonomous from the board through the structures set forth in the medical staff bylaws. And from an economic perspective, physician independence from the hospital exists because most are in private practice and are not employed by the institution. On the other hand, physicians in most specialty fields need access to the hospital to practice modern medicine, and only the governing board has the power to grant the privilege of practicing in a hospital. The unique relationship between physicians and hospitals is not without stresses and strains, and it makes the governance and management of hospitals a challenging responsibility.

In delineating the roles of the board and management, distinctions are not always clear between the board's responsibility for adopting policies to guide the hospital and management's responsibility for implementing these policies and managing the hospital's activities on a day-to-day basis. Problems can arise when the governing board becomes involved in

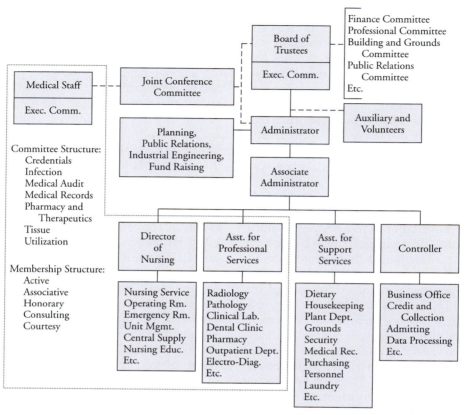

Figure 10.2. Prototypical Hospital Organization Chart

SOURCE: Reprinted with permission from *A Primer for Hospital Trustees,* Chamber of Commerce of the United States, 1974, Washington, DC: Author.

administrative matters. On the other hand, management may make decisions that overreach specific (or implied) board policies. Teamwork and communication are necessary to avoid conflict or misunderstandings.

Hospital executives have developed significant expertise in recent years in dealing with the increasingly complex operational, market, and regulatory issues confronting hospitals. But because the internal triad does not always agree on directions and priorities, hospitals often experience internal tensions and find it difficult to respond in a systematic way to environmental conditions and changing community needs. Given the challenges within today's health care in-

dustry, it is more imperative than ever that hospital leadership work as a team.

The Governing Board

The governing board of the community hospital has evolved in function and structure as the hospital itself has developed new roles. During the late 1800s and early 1900s, when advances in medical science were transforming hospitals from custodial institutions for the sick poor to sources of effective and safe care for the entire community, board members were often wealthy benefactors who gave money to establish and equip the hospital and meet its deficits. The primary function of the board at that time was trustee-ship; that is, preserving the assets that they and others like them donated. The trustees' job was seen as providing the facilities and equipment the medical staff needed to care for patients with little direct involvement in medical matters. Administrative duties were divided among board members; the hospital manager often functioned as a clerk.

After World War I, the complexity and size of hospitals exceeded the ability of board members to personally handle day-to-day administration. Business managers were employed to handle administrative and financial matters; the business manager and superintendent of nurses reported to the board, and the board coordinated their work. As operational complexity and the competence of hospital managers increased, they gradually assumed administrative responsibility for nursing and all of the hospital's departments, so that only one person reported directly to the board. The business manager's title evolved to "superintendent."

The governing board's role changed further as hospitals became ever more complex and as philanthropy yielded to patient revenue as the primary source of financial support. The board's role became one of overall policy making and planning, and board membership was used to augment and supplement the skills of the administrative staff. Hospital boards included fewer philanthropists and more individuals with specific management skills, including business executives, attorneys, bankers, architects, and contractors. Reflecting these areas of expertise, board decision-making tended to focus on finance, personnel, and physical plant matters. Boards typically deferred to the medical staff regarding physician qualifications and patient care.

Since the 1960s, several major trends have brought further change in the governing board's role. Continuing advances in medical science, the proliferation of medical technology, and the rapid growth in hospital sophistication have given hospitals a central role in the United States health care system while also creating public concern about the cost of hospital care. Public expectations regarding hospitals' responsibility to the community have also changed, so that hospitals are now viewed as community resources with obligations to address community needs. In addition, the regulation of hospital construction, costs, quality, and use, as well as labor relations, have become more stringent, particularly following the establishment of Medicare and Medicaid. Finally, court decisions have clearly established the concept of corporate or institutional responsibility for ensuring the quality of patient care. As a result of these forces, the governing board's role has broadened and become more demanding.

Boards have become quite active in monitoring the changing environment, becoming knowledgeable about community concerns and external trends, and interpreting the significance of these trends for the hospital. External competitive pressures have forced hospitals to reexamine their priorities and programs, and boards have found it necessary to provide clearer direction and stronger leadership in strategic planning. Boards have expanded community representation within their membership and assumed the role of mediating between the demands on the hospital from the community, the medical staff, employees, and interest groups. Board members often take the lead in discussions with other hospitals about an alliance and merger, and boards assume the central role in exploring system opportunities. Finally, boards have been forced to take a more active role in quality control, rather than abdicating this responsibility to the medical staff. Although the function of quality monitoring is still delegated to the medical staff, boards are more actively involved in scrutinizing how well this function is carried out.

Research on the topic of effective hospital governance has suggested several success factors for effective performance. These include a clearly defined mission for the organization, a decision-making process based upon continuing education, an efficient board structure with clear priorities, and a communication and reporting system for clear information.

The board is responsible for ensuring that the mechanisms for evaluating the credentials of physicians and monitoring the care they provide are established and working. Courts have held the board and the hospital responsible in malpractice cases in which reasonable precautions were not taken to ensure the careful selection of the medical staff, establishment of high standards of care, and enforcement of policies, rules, and regulations. In practice, direct board control over medical staff performance is limited and depends more on the medical staff's commitment to quality than on formal sanctions such as suspending or terminating a physician's hospital privileges. As governing boards have become more actively involved in medical and patient care matters, an increasing number have added physicians to their membership. More than half of all community hospital boards now include physicians.

Governance functions and structures in multihospital systems are important issues for the hospital field. Several models for structuring governance in multihospital systems have been developed. In the parent holding company model, governing bodies exist at both the system and institutional levels. Some systems have adopted a variation of the parent holding company model in which there is a system-level governing board and boards at the institutional level that serve in an advisory rather than governing capacity. The corporate model exists when a single system-level governing board carries out all governance activities for both the system and the individual institutions that make it up. In all three models, the corporate-level board is likely to retain responsibility for decisions regarding the transfer or sale of assets, formation of new companies, purchase of major assets, changes in hospital bylaws, and appointment of local board members. The corporate model has the advantage of structural simplicity and clear lines of authority, while the holding company model provides for greater input and involvement at the community level. In general, the more decentralized the governance model, the more likely it is that activities such as service development, strategic planning, capital and operating budget, medical staff privileges, and appointment and evaluation of the hospital chief executive officer will be under local board control.

Today, governing boards are being challenged as never before. They are called on to oversee system and institutional costs and effectiveness in meeting community, patient, and purchaser demands in an environment of constant change. They seek to balance the institution's overall mission, quality, and community benefit, while also seeking to compete effectively.

Hospital boards are increasingly required to understand the long-term implications of significant business decisions, such as physician practice acquisitions or the signing of managed-care contracts. The boards of investor-owned systems are also concerned about profits and the financial return to the company's shareholders. This shift in trustees' roles is a significant adjustment from traditionally passive asset management and short-term financial oversight. Some boards are clearly rising to the new challenges. They are being more selective in choosing members, they are educating themselves more fully, and they are streamlining board structures to expedite decision making.

Management

Hospital, and more recently, health system management has grown in importance as hospitals have grown in size and sophistication and combined into multihospital systems. The job of implementing board policy and the responsibility for day-to-day operations are delegated by the board to the chief executive officer. The chief executive officer has direct responsibility for the management team, the institution's finances, acquiring and maintaining equipment and facilities, planning and implementing new services, and hiring and supervising personnel. A key aspect of the job is to coordinate and serve as the channel of communication among the governing board, medical staff, and hospital departments. Even more critical today is strategic planning to position the hospital to compete effectively in the managed-care marketplace.

In addition to financial, personnel, and physical plant matters, the management team plays an important role in patient care. It is responsible for coordinating the work of the patient care and support departments, ensuring that departments are adequately equipped and staffed and functioning smoothly. Under the chief executive, the management team is actively involved in planning for new patient care services and in ensuring that the hospital meets accreditation, licensure, and regulatory standards. Because the medical staff is normally not employed by the hospital, the chief executive must establish a cooperative working relationship with physicians to accomplish tasks that involve both administrative and clinical considerations. The management team acts as the liaison with the community and with external agencies, both bringing information from these sources into hospital decision-making and planning processes, and representing the hospital to outside parties. Because of the increasing impact of external and regulatory pressures on hospitals, this latter role has become one of the most important aspects of hospital managers' jobs.

Medical staff relations have, in the last decade, become a critical area of concern for management. Although the nature of physicians' hospital practice has historically been voluntary, today numerous alliances and joint ventures between hospitals and physicians are being formed, including physician-hospital organizations (PHOs) for joint contracting with health plans. Many hospitals and integrated delivery systems are actively pursuing the acquisition of physician practices and entering into contractual relationships with medical groups to be better positioned to compete for contracts with health plans, assume risk, and manage care for contracted populations. In these scenarios, the arrangements between the hospital and physicians resemble a business partnership more than the traditional hospital–medical staff relationship.

Historically, hospital administration has advanced rapidly as a profession, moving from business manager in the 1920s, to management coordinator in the 1950s, to the modern-day corporate chief executive with authority for directing all aspects of the hospital's strategy and operations. As professional management has broadened from hospitals to ambulatory care, long-term care, home care, health plans, medical groups, and other organizations, the title "hospital administration" has given way to "health care administration," and the chief executive's title is commonly "president" or "chief executive officer" rather than "administrator." To survive the challenges encountered in today's competitive environment, the successful chief executive and management team must continuously develop new skills, including the ability to articulate a clear and compelling vision for the organization, formulate and execute strategies, empower the organization's people, innovate, prac-

tice value-based management, satisfy consumers and purchasers, and accept increasing levels of entrepreneurial risk.

Hospital Medical Staff

The governing board delegates responsibility for assuring high-quality patient care to the medical staff, which is formally organized to carry out this responsibility and is accountable to the board for it. Unlike in many advanced countries, where hospital medical staffs are composed of salaried physicians, the medical staffs of most hospitals in the United States are composed of private practitioners who are not employees of the hospital. The relationship between the hospital and its medical staff is a mutually dependent and sometimes stressful one. The hospital is dependent on the medical staff to admit and care for patients and monitor the quality of patient care. In a sense, physicians are the clients of the hospital because they admit patients, decide how long they will stay, order tests and procedures, and direct the care provided by the hospital's staff. On the other hand, physicians are dependent on the hospital because, in order to practice modern medicine, they must have access to its diagnostic and therapeutic services. Thus, a *quid pro quo* relationship exists: physicians agree to abide by hospital policies and medical staff rules and to devote time to the medical staff's quality assurance functions (in the past, they also contributed time to care for indigent patients), in return for the privilege of using the hospital to care for their patients. This traditional relationship is under intense pressure today, however, as the competitive, managed-care marketplace has created an alphabet soup of physician-hospital arrangements for contracting with health plans and has intensified competition between physicians.

In carrying out its responsibility for ensuring the quality of patient care, the medical staff organizes and governs itself, establishes qualifications for appointment to the staff and for clinical privileges, establishes standards of care and rules and regulations to guide the provision of care, and supervises the professional performance of its members. These duties are accomplished in accordance with the medical staff bylaws, which set forth the form, functions, and responsibilities of the medical staff. Bylaws must be approved by both the medical staff and the governing board.

Different categories of appointment to the medical staff carry different privileges and responsibilities. *Active medical staff* members have full hospital privileges and provide most of the medical care in the hospital. They are responsible for the governance and administrative activities of the organized medical staff. The *associate medical staff* consists of physicians and dentists who are being considered for advancement to the active medical staff; *courtesy medical staff* members meet the qualifications for active membership but admit patients to the hospital only occasionally (usually because they are on the active staff of another hospital); and the *consulting medical staff* includes physicians and dentists who are recognized for their professional expertise and who act as consultants to the hospital medical staff physicians, although they primarily practice in other hospitals. Finally, the *honorary staff* consists of physicians recognized for their past service to the hospital; and *residents* are employed as the house staff of hospitals with formal teaching programs, functioning under the supervision of attending physicians.

The administrative head of the typical community hospital's medical staff organization is the president or chief of staff. The chief of staff (1) acts as liaison among the governing board, the chief executive, and the medical staff; (2) chairs the executive committee of the medical staff and serves as an ex officio member of all medical staff committees; (3) enforces governing board policies and medical staff bylaws; (4) maintains standards of medical care in the hospital; and (5) provides for continuing education for the medical staff. Although the chief of staff is usually elected by the medical staff, this position is also in a sense part of the hospital's administrative structure, directly accountable to the hospital's governing board. Larger hospitals often employ a full-time salaried medical director to augment the chief of staff in linking administrative and medical staff activities, to direct the administrative infrastructure that supports quality assurance and utilization review, and to participate with the governing board and management team in strategic planning and program development. This trend is growing rapidly in light of the challenges inherent in

integrating physicians and hospitals to assume quality care and be better positioned for managed care.

Most of the organizational responsibilities of the medical staff are carried out by committees. The *executive committee* is the key administrative and policy-making body of the medical staff. It governs the activities of the medical staff, and all other committees are advisory to it. It is typically composed of the chief of staff, the chiefs of the clinical departments, and a number of at-large members elected by the active medical staff. The *joint conference committee* is the formal liaison between the governing board and medical staff and includes members from both groups plus the chief executive. This committee is a forum for discussing medical administrative matters of mutual concern. The *credentials committee* reviews the qualifications of applicants to the medical staff and makes recommendations regarding appointments, annual reappointments, and clinical privileges. Recommendations are transmitted through the medical staff executive committee to the hospital's governing board, which has final authority over medical staff membership and privileges. Other medical staff committees oversee specific functional areas or departments (for example, emergency room, nursing, pharmacy, special care, and surgery) and manage important quality assurance and monitoring activities, including medical audit, utilization review, and tissue review.

Under pressure from managed-care organizations and other purchasers of health care services, hospitals have moved rapidly in the 1990s and early 2000s to gain greater control over the appropriateness and cost-effectiveness, as well as quality, of the care provided within their walls. Shifts in reimbursement toward prospective payment have significantly changed the financial incentives for hospitals. To a greater extent than ever before, hospitals now must ensure that hospital admissions are justifiable, that lengths of stay do not exceed accepted norms, and that treatment regimens are medically appropriate. As an extension of their traditional responsibility for quality, it is critical that medical staff now share in the process of evaluating utilization, particularly under health plan contracts in which there is fixed reimbursement. Evidence-based practice guidelines, continuous quality improvement (CQI) techniques, and other quality/cost-management tools have become commonplace with hospital medical staffs. Hospitals have also been faced with health plans' and purchasers' interest in quality report cards and outcomes measurement.

The growing pressure on hospitals to exercise greater influence over physician behavior to control costs and utilization and improve outcomes represents a significant threat to physician autonomy and can result in increased conflict between hospital management and the medical staff. Methods used by hospitals to influence physician behavior include direct appeals, adding physicians to the governing board, establishing medical director positions, joint ventures between medical services and technology, "economic credentialing," and the employment of physicians. Additional approaches include education, peer review and feedback, administrative rules, participation in developing treatment guidelines, and incentives (Grieco & Eisenberg, 1993).

In heavily managed-care–driven markets, hospitals and physicians are pursuing a variety of strategies depending on the leverage that managed-care organizations have in the selection of providers and pricing of managed-care contracts. In some markets, integrated physician/hospital arrangements have been formed as a vehicle for sharing the benefits and risks of health plan contracting, while in other markets intense competition for ambulatory care services and health plan contracts has left hospitals struggling to utilize excess capacity while their physicians migrate to other facilities, or consider selling their assets to practice management companies.

The responsibilities of the hospital medical staff (credentialing, appointing, privileging, reviewing, and reappointing) and its formal structure (officers, committees, departments, and links to the governing board and management), as commonly defined and practiced are often referred to as the "Joint Commission Model" (White, 1997). This is because of the great influence the standards and accreditation process of the Joint Commission on Accreditation of Healthcare Organizations (JCAHO) has had over the years on the quality assurance activities of medical staffs. Even hospitals that do not seek accreditation tend to adhere to the JCAHO's prescriptions as the best "conventional wisdom" about how medical staffs should work. The influence of the JCAHO goes beyond what

might be expected of a voluntary accreditation process because accreditation is accepted by the federal Medicare program as meeting its standards for participation (and payment), and by most states as meeting their hospital licensure requirements. Over the years, the standards spelled out in successive versions of the JCAHO's *Accreditation Manual for Hospitals* have essentially defined (some would say dictated) what is considered good practice with regard to the design, roles, and functions of the organized hospital medical staff.

The Joint Commission Model, however, evolved during the years before competition, managed care, and the resulting consolidation of providers into networks and systems. Today, physicians and hospitals are joining together to form physician-hospital organizations (PHOs) or even larger vertically integrated delivery systems to better position themselves to compete for contracts with health plans and public purchasers, and to be able to assume risk and manage the care of the populations for which they contract. Many believe the realities of the new medical care marketplace make the Joint Commission Model an anachronism.

Without question, many of the characteristics of the competitive marketplace differ from the assumptions that underlie the Joint Commission Model. In contrast to the tradition of an open hospital medical staff, with privileges dependent only on clinical qualifications, health plans, networks, and systems typically select only a subset of the community's physicians, with selections based on economic as well as quality criteria. Managed-care organizations also have a strong preference for primary care physicians versus specialists. Some hospitals are actively downsizing their medical staffs to more closely fit the size of the population for which they contract to care. Health plans and provider organizations often do their own credentialing, no longer relying on the hospital. Further, as hospital utilization is closely scrutinized and admissions discouraged, care is shifted to the clinic or physician's office, away from the reach of hospital credentialing and peer review. In addition, purchasers are demanding "report cards" that call for outcome measures of quality quite different from the structural measures traditionally emphasized by the JCAHO. And perhaps most important, as physicians increasingly compete with each other as participants in rival provider organizations, is it reasonable to expect them to dispassionately judge each others' credentials and patient care as members of the same hospital medical staff? In short, as medical groups and provider organizations position themselves for a more competitive marketplace, these organizations are taking over functions historically performed by hospital medical staffs. In addition, adherence to treatment guidelines and utilization parameters may subsume chart-by-chart peer review. Despite all of these trends, as of today, many hospital medical staffs continue to take their traditional quality assurance responsibilities seriously. It would seem, however, that new structures, more suited to the changing marketplace, will emerge as hospitals face the future.

SUMMARY

The early years of the new century have witnessed a degree of resurgence in hospital financial viability and success, especially as pertains to the for-profit sector and publicly held hospital management companies. But throughout the hospital industry challenges continue to mount. These include both short term issues such as constantly changing Medicare rules and reimbursement levels and longer term concerns, particularly the aging of the population (Lubitz, Greenberg, Gorina, Wartzman, and Gibson, 2001). Changing technology, which heavily affects the nature and quantity of services provided in hospitals, and especially in the inpatient arena, further complicates long term planning. Access to capital, complex issues pertaining to the organization and role of the medical staff, nursing needs, an increasingly complicated legal environment and the constant threat of litigation of all types, and pressures from managed care insurers, government, and other contracting organizations further muddies the water. Yet in this excruciating environment, our population continues to enjoy access to the best hospital care in the world, an incredible achievement for the industry and a continuing challenge for the future.

References

Andrulis, D. P., Acuff, K. L., Weiss, K. B., & Anderson, R. J. (1996). Public hospitals and health care reform: Choices and challenges. *American Journal of Public Health, 2,* 162–165.

Brown, M. (1996). Mergers, networking, and vertical integration: Managed care and investor-owned hospitals. *Health Care Management Review, 1,* 29–37.

Carey, R. M., & Englehard, C. L. (1996). Academic medicine meets managed care: A high impact collision. *Academic Medicine, 8,* 839–845.

Coddington, D., Moore, K., & Fischer, E. (1996). *Making integrated health care work.* Colorado: Center for Research in Ambulatory Health Care Administration.

Commission of Hospital Care. (1947). Expansion of hospitals, 1840–1900. In *Hospital care in the United States* (pp. 454–526). Cambridge, MA: Harvard University Press.

Corwin, E. H. (1946). *The American hospital.* New York: Commonwealth Fund.

Cunningham, R. (2001). Hospital finance: Signs of "pushback" amid resurgent cost pressures. *Health Affairs, 20,* 233–240.

Dowling, W. L. (1995). Strategic alliances as a structure for integrated delivery systems. In A. Kaluzny, H. Zuckerman, & T. Ricketts, III (Eds.), *Partners for the dance: Forming strategic alliances in health care* (pp. 139–175). Ann Arbor, MI: Health Administration Press.

Dowling, W. L. (1996, Summer). The community-oriented integrated health care organization: How viable? *Frontiers of Health Services Management, 12*(4), 58.

Etheredge, L., Jones, B. J., & Lewin, L. (1996). What is driving health system change? *Health Affairs, 4,* 93–104.

Gillies, R. R., Shortell, S., Anderson, D., Mitchell, J. B., & Morgan, K. L. (1993, Winter). Conceptualizing and measuring integration: Findings from the Health Systems Integration Study. *Hospital and Health Services Administration, 38*(4), 467–489.

Goldsmith, J. C. (1981). *Can hospitals survive?* Homewood, IL: Dow Jones-Irwin.

Grieco, P. J., & Eisenberg, J. M. (1993, October 1). Changing physician practices. *New England Journal of Medicine, 329*(17), 1271–1273.

Havighurst, C. C. (1986). Changing the locus of decision making in the healthcare sector. *Journal of Health Politics, Policy and Law, 11,* 697–735.

Katz, A., & Thompson, J. (1996). The role of public policy in health care market change. *Health Affairs, 2,* 77–91.

Lubitz, J., Greenberg, L. G., Gorina, Y., Wartzman, L., & Gibson, D. (2001). Three decades of health care use by the elderly, 1965–1998. *Health Affairs, 20,* 19–32.

Luft, H. S. (1985). Competition and regulation. *Medical Care, 23,* 383–400.

MacEachern, M. T. (1957). *Hospital organization and management* (3rd ed.). Chicago: Physicians Record Company.

Mick, S., & Conrad, D. (1988). The decision to integrate vertically in health care organizations. *Hospital and Health Services Administration, 33*(3): 345–360.

Reinhardt, U. E. (2000). The economics of for-profit and not-for-profit hospitals. *Health Affairs, 19,* 178–186.

Relman, A. S. (1980). The new medical-industrial complex. *New England Journal of Medicine, 17,* 963–970.

Rosen, G. (1963). The hospital: Historical sociology of a community institution. In E. Freidson (Ed.), *The hospital in modern society* (pp. 1–36). New York: The Free Press.

Shortell, S. (1988, Fall). The evolution of hospital systems: Unfulfilled promises and self-fulfilling prophesies. *Medical Care Review, 45,* 177–214.

Shortell, S. M., Gillies, R. R., & Devers, K. J. (1995, Summer). Reinventing the American hospital. *The Milbank Quarterly, 73*(2), 131–160.

Shukla, R. K., & Clement, J. (1997, Spring). A comparative analysis of revenue and cost-management strategies of not-for-profit and for-profit hospitals. *Hospital and Health Services Administration, 42*(1), 117–134.

Siu, A. L., Sonnenberg, F. A., Manning, W. G., Goldberg, G. A., Bloomfield, E. S., Newhouse, J. P., & Brook, R. H. (1986). Inappropriate use of hospitals in a randomized trial of health insurance plans. *New England Journal of Medicine, 315,* 1259–1266.

Starr, P. (1982). *The social transformation of American medicine.* New York: Basic Books.

White, C. H. (1997). *The hospital medical staff.* Albany, NY: Delmar Publishers.

CHAPTER

11

The Continuum of Long-Term Care

Connie J. Evashwick

Chapter Topics

- What Is Long-Term Care?
- Who Needs Long-Term Care?
- How Is Long-Term Care Organized?
- Service Categories
- Financing
- Integrating Mechanisms
- Public Policy Issues
- The Long-Term Care Continuum of the Future
- Summary

Learning Objectives

Upon completing this chapter, the reader should be able to:

- Describe who uses long-term care and under what circumstances
- Explain the role and scope of services included in long-term care
- Articulate how long-term care services are organized, operated, financed and integrated
- Evaluate model delivery systems approaches to long-term care for the future
- Articulate national policy issues pertinent to long-term care

Long-term care is one of the greatest challenges facing the health care delivery system. In terms of population need, consumer demand, resource consumption, financing, and system organization, long-term care will be a dominant issue during the twenty-first century. The components of long-term care have grown during the past decades. Integration is beginning to occur. In order for the limited available resources to meet increasing demand, the system that currently exists—an unevenly financed array of fragmented services—must evolve into a well-organized, efficient, client-oriented, cost-effective continuum of care.

A case study illustrates an extreme of the issues and current challenges of long-term care.

Mrs. Jackson is a sixty-six-year old widow, a successful librarian, still working, who lives alone in a third-story suburban apartment in a small Midwestern town. She is generally healthy but has mild hypertension and is diabetic. One night during the winter, she slips on the ice while carrying groceries up the front steps of her building and breaks her hip. A neighbor calls the 911 emergency number, and eventually an ambulance arrives. The ambulance takes Mrs. Jackson to the emergency room of the nearest hospital. Mrs. Jackson cannot be admitted because she does not have proof of insurance, her Medicare card, credit cards, or even her checkbook on hand, and her condition is determined not to be life-threatening. She is thus transferred to another hospital. Mrs. Jackson's only physician is an internist who cannot handle a fracture, so Mrs. Jackson is operated on by the surgeon on call.

After the surgery, Mrs. Jackson spends two weeks in the hospital, one on the surgical floor and one on a step-down unit. Her physician stops by to visit, but her care is the responsibility of the surgical residents who change on an undetermined schedule. Her employer has recently reduced the health benefits that the group policy covers. Her insurance covers only the first thirty days of hospital care, and Medicare, as a secondary payer, picks up some of the uncovered expenses. Because she has a daily copay, she is anxious to be discharged as quickly as possible.

The physician recommends that Mrs. Jackson go to a rehabilitation hospital. The nearest one, however, is in the next town. Instead, Mrs. Jackson agrees to spend a week or two at a nursing home until she is able to move about more easily.

Mrs. Jackson finds that the majority of patients in the nursing home are quite elderly, most in their late eighties

and most suffering from Alzheimer's or some other form of dementia. There is little independence. Mrs. Jackson is glad when she feels strong enough to go home. The nursing home orders a walker for her before she leaves so that she can get around her apartment on her own.

At home, Mrs. Jackson must recuperate before she is able to ambulate easily. She has no way to get down the stairs, let alone to the grocery store, post office, or pharmacy. A neighbor who is a nurse arranges for a homemaker from a local agency to come in three days a week for two hours to help her. She is not quite ill enough to qualify for home health care as defined by the regulations of her health insurance or Medicare (that is, "homebound") thus she pays the homemaker directly. A colleague from work offers to stop by the pharmacy to pick up prescriptions for her. As a widow, Mrs. Jackson never cooked much for herself. A friend arranges for Meals on Wheels to deliver a hot meal at lunch and a cold snack for dinner. However, no food comes on the weekends. Meanwhile, bills begin to flood in from the emergency room, the hospital, the nursing home, several different physicians, and the home health agency. She is not sure what her private insurance will pay, what Medicare will pay, and what she must pay herself.

Mrs. Jackson returns to the hospital outpatient department for rehabilitation therapy, but she must depend on one of her neighbors being at home to help her get up and down the stairs. She cannot drive, so she calls a cab, which does not always come to the suburbs on time and is expensive. The therapists at the outpatient department are different than those in the hospital or at the nursing home, and Mrs. Jackson feels as though no one quite knows her clinical history or recent condition. Her insurance does not cover outpatient rehabilitation, but the office clerks tell her that Medicare Part B may cover the services.

Mrs. Jackson struggles along for several weeks and eventually is able to return to work. She believes that the medical care and therapy she received have been good quality. She comes out of the experience, however, with huge bills and negative feelings about the impersonality of the health care system, the high costs and low insurance coverage for long-term care, the fragmentation of services and payment, and the frustrating helplessness of professionals in mobilizing resources to facilitate the simple functions of daily living. She realizes that if she were twenty years older, were no longer covered by her employer's insurance or Medicare, had spent much of her savings, and lived in an isolated two-story house in a rural area rather than in an apartment complex filled with friends and neighbors, her experience would have been far worse. 🌸

The implications? The existing formal system of providing care to persons with long-term, complex problems is both complicated and fragmented. With some notable exceptions, the long-term care system functions because of individual expertise and informal relationships. On a broad scheme, it is highly regulated, costly, and occasionally arbitrary, with access to services limited by place, patient characteristics, and knowledge. Most of all, the extant system of long-term care does not consistently meet the needs of consumers, providers, or payers.

As described in the following text, the demand for long-term care will grow exponentially during the first half of the twenty-first century. The Baby Boom generation will begin to swell the population of older adults with chronic illnesses and those caring for family members with chronic illnesses, and thus consumer interest in arranging long-term care services will likely soar. The size of the younger disabled population will also grow. The combined consumer-based demand for well-organized long-term care will exacerbate the forces of managed care and integrated health care delivery systems that are already prompting change in the organization and financing of the health care delivery system.

This chapter describes the various facets of long-term care as they exist at the outset of the twenty-first century and presents a conceptual framework for understanding how the many pieces of long-term care can be molded into a rational system for the future.

WHAT IS LONG-TERM CARE?

Long-term care refers to health, mental health, social, and residential services provided to a temporarily or chronically disabled person over an extended period of time with a goal of enabling the person to function as independently as possible.

Long-term care has the following characteristics:

- The conditions causing the need for long-term care may be physical or mental, temporary or permanent.
- The need for care is due to functional disabilities.
- The goal is to promote or maintain health and independence in functional abilities and quality of life.

For those who are terminally ill, the goal is to enable them to die peacefully and with dignity.

- The multiple services required, the professions involved, and the settings of care span broad spectrums.
- Care is multifaceted, recognizing all spheres of a person's life: physical, mental, social, and financial.
- Care is orchestrated around the unique needs of each individual and family, and thus the patterns of care vary.
- Service delivery can be expected to change over time as the client's and family's needs change.

WHO NEEDS LONG-TERM CARE?

The primary consumers of long-term care are people who have chronic and/or complex health problems accompanied by functional disabilities. Clients may require care for a relatively short period of time, such as several months, or for an extended or indefinite period of time.

The first group includes those who have relatively short-term problems that require orchestration of a complex set of community-based services. This group includes those with acute injury or illness who ultimately will achieve complete recovery or independence but who require an extended period of convalescence or treatment, such as persons suffering from cancer, head trauma, hip fracture, or stroke.

The second group comprises those who have ongoing (chronic) and multiple health and/or mental health problems and who are unable to care for themselves (functionally disabled) and thus require nursing or supportive health care for a prolonged or indefinite period of time. The paths leading to the use of formal or informal long-term care services are complex, as shown in Figure 11.1.

Definitions

Chronic connotes permanent, or at least indefinite. For technical data collection purposes, chronic is defined by the National Health Interview Survey as any condition that lasts three months (or ninety days) or more (Adams & Marano, 1995). Chronic conditions

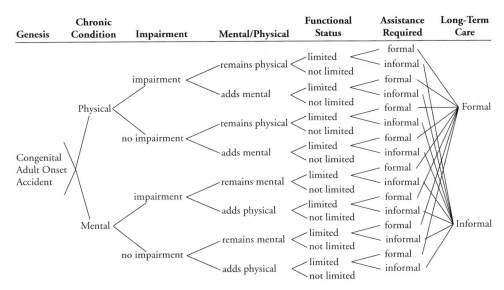

Figure 11.1.   Progression of Chronic Illness

may be derived from physical or mental conditions. Over the progression of a disease, both may occur. Chronic conditions may be as life-threatening as coronary artery disease or as harmless as mild arthritis. In 1995, an estimated 99 million people had some type of chronic condition (Hoffman & Rice, 1996). By 2020, a projected 134 million people will have a chronic condition, and this number will grow to 167 million by 2050 (Hoffman & Rice, 1996). Figure 11.2 shows the projected growth in the prevalence of chronic illness.

Chronic illnesses vary by age and other patient characteristics. For example, asthma is most common among children; arthritis is most common among seniors. Table 11.1 shows the prevalence of the top twelve physiological chronic conditions and shows the difference in prevalence between the total adult population and those age sixty-five and older.

Chronic conditions vary in the extent to which they are stable and the extent to which they require formal care. Some conditions, such as stroke, may have a progressive improvement over time; some conditions have episodic flare-ups; yet others are stable but require daily attention indefinitely.

An *impairment* is defined as "a chronic or permanent defect, usually static in nature, that results from disease, injury, or congenital malformation. It represents a decrease in or loss of ability to perform various functions" (Adams & Marano, 1995). Permanent impairments, such as limb amputation or blindness, may require an initial adjustment and are then more or less stable.

Disability is a general term that refers to any long- or short-term reduction of a person's activity as a result of an acute or chronic condition (Adams & Marano, 1995). The National Health Interview Survey compiles data on the "ability to perform major activity." Major activity is defined according to age: playing for young children up to age five, attending school for school-age children five to seventeen, working or keeping house for adults age eighteen to sixty-nine, and self-care and independence for people age seventy or older (Adams & Marano, 1995). In 1994, approximately fifteen percent of the United States population had some

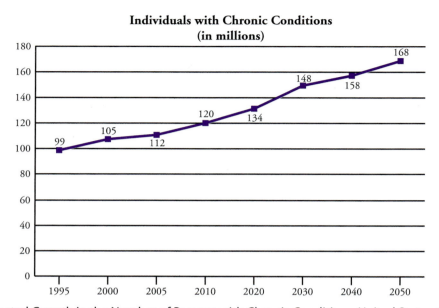

Figure 11.2. Projected Growth in the Number of Persons with Chronic Conditions: United States, 1995–2050

SOURCE: From "Projected Growth in the Number of Persons with Chronic Conditions, United States, 1995–2050," by C. Hoffman and D. Rice, 1996, *Chronic Care in America: A 21st Century Challenge*, p. 9. Copyright 1996 by Robert Wood Johnson Foundation. Reprinted with permission.

Table 11.1. The Twelve Most Prevalent Physical Chronic Conditions, for Total Adult Population and Adults Age 65+

	Total Adult Population	**Adults Aged 65+**
	Per 1,000	**Per 1,000**
Sinusitis	134	151
Arthritis	129	502
Orthopedic impairment	120	166
Hypertension	109	364
Allergies without asthma	101	80
Hearing impairment	86	286
Heart conditions	86	325
Asthma	56	51
Bronchitis	54	61
Migraine headache	43.4	48.1
Visual impairment	33.1	82.2
Diabetes	29.9	48.1
Total U.S. population, 1994: 259,634,000; total ages 65+: 31,026		

SOURCE: "Current Estimates from the National Health Interview Survey, United States, 1994," National Center for Health Statistics, 1995, *Vital and Health Statistics* (Series 10, No. 193), Tables 57, 62, 78.

Table 11.2. Percent Distribution of Persons by Degree of Activity Limitation Due to Chronic Condition, by Age

| Age in Years | Percent Distribution | | | |
	No Activity Limitation	Some Limitation	Limited in Major Activity	Unable to Do Major Activity
All people	85.0	15.0	10.3	4.6
Under 18	93.3	6.7	4.9	0.7
18–44	89.7	10.3	7.1	3.2
45–64	77.4	22.6	17.1	9.2
65+	61.8	38.2	22.6	10.7

SOURCE: "Current estimates from the National Health Interview Survey, United States, 1994," National Center for Health Statistics, 1995, *Vital and Health Statistics* (Series 10, No. 193), Table 67.

degree of activity limitation due to a chronic condition (Adams & Marano, 1995). Table 11.2 shows the percentage of the population, by age, who experience activity limitations due to chronic conditions.

In addition to the measure used by the federal government of ability to perform major activity, a much more common indicator of disability is *functional ability*. Functional ability has been described as a person's ability to perform the basic activities of daily living. Initially defined by Katz and colleagues, years of research have produced commonly accepted measures and scales of functioning. These are referred to as activities of daily living (ADL) (Katz, Ford, & Moskowitz, 1985) and instrumental activities of daily living (IADL) (Lawton & Brody, 1969). Activities of daily living include the ability to eat, dress, perform personal care and grooming, transfer from bed to chair, bathe, walk, and maintain bowel and bladder continence. The instrumental activities of daily living include handling monetary affairs, telephoning, grocery shopping, housekeeping, doing chores, and arranging for transportation. Functional ability declines with age. Table 11.3 shows the level of functional ability among the older population. However, estimates are that as many as 50 million people need help with the basic activities of daily living, and forty-two percent of these are under age sixty-five (McNeil, 1992).

Functional disabilities may be due to physical or mental problems, and over time, both may occur. Alzheimer's disease is one example. Estimates are that twenty-five percent of those age eighty-five

Table 11.3. Functional Disability Among Older Adults

Age	Needs Help With One or More Activities of Daily Living (Percent)	Needs Help With One or More Instrumental Activities of Daily Living (Percent)
65–69 years	14.7	19.9
70–74 years	21.1	24.7
75–79 years	24.1	29.2
80–85 years	34.4	40.0
85+	49.8	55.2

SOURCE: Adapted from "Aging in the Eighties: Functional Limitations of Individuals 65 and Over," by D. Dawson, G. Hendershot, & J. Fulton, June 10, 1987, *Advance Data* (No. 133), National Center for Health Statistics.

and older have Alzheimer's or a related dementia (Alzheimer's Association, n.d.). Alzheimer's begins by affecting mental functioning and behavior. Ultimately, it affects a person's physiological systems as well. Approximately 4 million people suffer from Alzheimer's disease (Alzheimer's Association, n.d.). The number of persons with Alzheimer's disease will increase as the population ages, to as many as 14 million by 2050 (Evans, 1989).

Chronic illness, impairments, and functional disabilities are interrelated. Of those with chronic conditions and/or impairments, some portion will be limited in activity. Of those who are limited, some will nonetheless be independent, and some will be limited in functional activities of daily living. All of those who are unable to perform the basic activities of daily living need help from devices, from informal sources, or from formal sources. Regardless of their physical or mental limitations, those most likely to need assistance from formal sources are people who are very old, have multiple chronic conditions, live alone, and have minimal or no support system of family and/or friends. Figure 11.2 shows the multiple paths to needing assistance. Those requiring the assistance of formal long-term care services are the primary users of the services described in this chapter.

Understanding Demand

In brief, the users of long-term care represent a mosaic of sub-segments of the population. Projecting the demand for long-term care requires an understanding of the definitions and subsets of the population with chronic illnesses, impairments, functional disabilities, and the portending growth of each, tempered by projections of advances in biomedical technology, pharmaceuticals, and assistive devices, as well as changes in the workforce, demographic trends, and social policies.

Using conservative parameters, Spector, Fleishman, Pezzin, & Spillman (2000) conservatively estimate the number of adults age eighteen and older who used long-term care services during the mid-1990s to be about 9.4 million. The total number of people of all ages who will be unable to go to school, to work, or to live independently due to chronic conditions is projected to reach 17 million by the year 2020 (Hoffman & Rice, 1996). Many of these people will need long-term care from informal and/or formal sources at some point during their lives, if not indefinitely.

Because there is no single identifier or uniform pattern of long-term care users, long-term care services can be organized on various dimensions: demographic characteristics (for example, age, gender, economics), affinity (for example, veterans), disease category/diagnosis (for example, mental status, AIDS/ARC), or impairment (for example, the blind).

Public policies that regulate providers and fund services tend to have evolved over the years around the specific target groups rather than with a more comprehensive approach. Examples of the subsets of potential users of long-term care illustrate the array of conditions leading to long-term care and the basis of fragmented service organization, financing, and regulation. Separate systems of long-term care services have developed for each major subset of users. The groups highlighted below also warrant attention because of their magnitude and because of the policy and financing issues likely to arise in the future to address their demands.

The Aged

As shown in Tables 11.1 and 11.2, chronic illness and functional disabilities increase with age. Of persons age sixty-five and older, eighty percent have at least one chronic health problem, and the majority have multiple problems. As shown in Table 11.3, of those age sixty-five to sixty-nine, less than one in six, or fifteen percent, experience functional ADL disabilities, while half of those age eighty-five and older suffer functional disabilities.

The changing demographic composition of the United States will make long-term care an increasingly significant aspect of the health care system. The number of people over the age of sixty-five will increase from 33.5 million in 1995 to 70 million in 2030 (American Association of Retired Persons, 1996). As shown in Figure 11.3, older adults will increase from under thirteen percent of the United States population in 1990 to twenty percent of the total population by the year 2030 (American Association of Retired Persons, 1996). The very old, or those over age eighty-five, are increasing the most rapidly in terms of percentage. As stated previously, the very old suffer the most functional disabilities and thus are those who most need long-term care. As the number of old and very old people increases, the need for long-term care will rise.

The Young Disabled

The total demand for long-term care also includes younger people who have disabilities. Hoffman and Rice (1996) estimate that of the 99 million with chronic conditions in 1996, seventy-five percent were younger than age sixty-five. The 1994 Disability Sup-

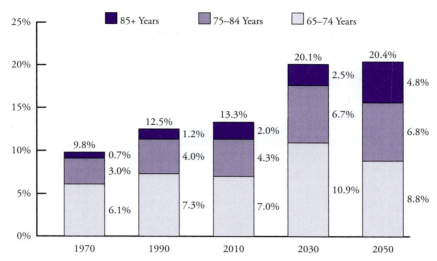

Figure 11.3.   Projected Growth in the Older Population as a Percentage of U.S. Total Population, 1970 to 2050

Note: Details may not sum to totals because of rounding.

SOURCE: Georgetown University IHCRP based on Hobbs and Damon, 1996; data from the U.S. Bureau of the Census.

plement to the National Health Interview Survey identified more than 3.5 million people between the ages of eighteen and sixty-four who were disabled to the point that they required long-term care services, and an additional one-half million adults under age sixty-five receive care through the mental health system (Spector et al., 2000). Moreover, as noted earlier, forty-two percent of those with functional disabilities are under age sixty-five.

Younger people who require long-term care include those with neurological diseases or degenerative neurological conditions, accidents resulting in paralysis, debilitating strokes, end-stage cancer, blindness, early Alzheimer's disease, a variety of mental conditions, AIDS/ARC, and children with birth defects and congenital abnormalities.

Because of advances in biomedical technology, people who would previously have died due to trauma or degenerative diseases now live, but with disabilities. The number of children and adults under age sixty-five needing long-term care will thus continue to grow until advances in biomedical technology that result in prevention or cure of chronic illness exceed advances that prolong the lives of those with chronic disabling conditions.

Veterans

Because women outnumber men among the very old, long-term care is often associated with women. However, men, too, need long-term care. The Department of Veterans Affairs is facing the challenge of caring for aged veterans, the vast majority of whom are men (General Accounting Office, 1987; Levenstein, 2001; U.S. Department of Veterans Affairs, 1989). By 2000, 8.9 million, or thirty-seven percent of veterans were seniors, and by 2020, 7.7 million, or forty-five percent of living veterans, will be age sixty-five or above (Keenan, 1989). The Department of Veterans Affairs, which has its own health care services, faces the same challenge as the public and private sectors in trying to construct an efficient, integrated system to care for those with multifaceted, chronic illnesses and functional dependencies (Levenstein, 2001).

AIDS/ARC

The Autoimmune Deficiency Syndrome (AIDS) epidemic was first recognized in the United States in the early 1980s. In 1999, the number of people in the United States reported to be HIV positive—the precursor to

AIDS—was estimated to range from 650,000 to 900,000 (CDC, 2000). As many as one in 300 people may be HIV positive, but many are not aware of their condition.

By the late 1990s, considerable progress had been made in preventing and treating the disease. However, the sudden and rampant expansion and the initial deadliness of the disease brought national attention to the care needed by those suffering from AIDS and AIDS-Related Conditions (ARC). Special programs with special funding, exemplified by the federal Ryan White CARE Act, have been established throughout the nation to meet the extended care needs of the AIDS/ARC population.

Mentally Ill

Approximately 66 million adults over the age of eighteen are estimated to suffer from some form of mental illness in a given year (National Institute of Mental Health, 1999). Depression is the most common condition, affecting more than 19 million adults annually. Between three and five million people have a severe mental disorder, and about three-fourths of these are limited in daily functioning by their mental condition (Kraus, Stoddard, & Gilmartin, 1996). Among school-age children, attention deficit hyperactivity disorder (ADHD) affects three to five percent. Definitive counts of people with mental retardation are not available, but the number may be more than 3 million (Kraus et al., 1996). Many of those with mental conditions, whether permanent or temporary, are limited in their ability to perform basic ADLs or IADLs, and thus need help from informal or formal sources.

The Blind and Visually Impaired

Millions of Americans of all ages suffer from vision problems. Approximately 120,000 people are blind. An additional 3 million report severe vision impairment, defined as vision deficiencies that cannot be corrected by glasses or other medical or surgical interventions (The Lighthouse, 2000). Among people age forty-five to sixty-four, fifteen percent are visually impaired. This proportion increases with age: of those age sixty-five to seventy-four, seventeen percent, and of those age seventy-five and older, twenty-six percent, are visually impaired (The Lighthouse, 2000). Even among children under age eighteen, nearly one percent are blind in one or both eyes or have difficulty seeing, even with glasses.

Many adaptive technologies have been developed to help those who have difficulty seeing, ranging from the widespread use of Braille on elevator buttons, to books in large print or on tape, to computers with large fonts and special color-contrast screens. Nonetheless, the blind and visually impaired may require assistance with the functions of daily living on a regular basis or at some point in time, and, when ill, require even more help.

Caregivers

The demand for long-term care extends beyond those suffering directly from some type of disability. Caregivers, family members, and employers are also affected—and have the potential to impact the system for providing long-term care.

People with functional disabilities need help to perform the ADL and the IADL. The majority of care, perhaps as much as ninety percent, is provided by family and friends on an informal basis. Thus, the consumer demand for long-term care must include caregivers and employers, as well as the disabled themselves. Caregiving became recognized as a health care issue during the 1980s. For the first time in history, the average American family had more parents than children. Women in the United States are estimated to spend an average of seventeen years of their lives caring for children and eighteen years caring for their parents (The Daughter Track, 1990). More than one-fourth of the adult population provides care to a family member or friend during any given year (National Alliance for Caregiving, 1997). In 1996, this represented more than 54 million caregivers.

The most recent survey on caregivers was conducted by the National Alliance for Caregiving (1997) and the American Association of Retired Persons. It revealed the following: Nearly three-fourths of caregivers (seventy-two percent) are women. About half are spouses, and one-third are children of the disabled person. More than one-third are caring for two or more older relatives or friends at the same time. Forty percent are caring for children under eighteen at the same time as older relatives or friends. The average caregiver provides eighteen hours of care per week, but in 4.1 million households the caregiver provides forty or more hours of care per week.

Caregivers are susceptible to health problems. The physical and emotional demands of caregiving can be extensive. Caregivers who can no longer meet the needs of functionally disabled persons often turn to nursing homes. The health care system has begun to accommodate by organizing services for caregivers, such as respite, educational programs, counseling, and support groups. Trends for an increasing number of women working and smaller families mean that, in the future, the United States will face a significant decline in available family caregivers at the same time that the population in need of help increases dramatically. The formal health care system must do whatever it can to support those who are willing and able to be informal caregivers in order to maximize their involvement with the functionally disabled.

Employers

Employers have long recognized that caregiving adds to their costs both in the health consequences for caregivers and the days of work lost due to caregiving responsibilities. Travelers Company was one of the first to study the prevalence of caregiving. In a 1985 survey, they found that twenty-eight percent of their employees age thirty or older cared for an aged parent an average of ten hours per week (The Daughter Track, 1990). The productive time lost by employees in caring for elderly relatives is estimated to cost American businesses billions of dollars each year.

As a result of the attention given during the 1980s to the effect of caregiving on work productivity, employers have set up programs to facilitate caregiving. These range from education to access to national networks of case managers. These reduce stress and time lost while enabling employees to fulfill their responsibilities to their family members. A well-organized system of long-term care is thus sought not only by those suffering from complex chronic illnesses but

also by families, friends, employers, providers, and payers.

Terminology

Users of long-term care are referred to variously as *patients, clients, participants,* and *residents,* depending upon the perspective of the service provider. This chapter uses the terms *patients* and *clients* as general terms and uses specific terms as appropriate for individual services.

HOW IS LONG-TERM CARE ORGANIZED?

Most long-term care is provided by friends and family. The formal system of providing long-term care has no single structure or financing. As previously noted, to the extent that "systems" exist, they have been established around a specific target population, and thus each long-term care system is different. Moreover, just as each person requires care for a unique set of conditions, each community has its own combination of available resources, funding sources, and organization. A distinct arrangement is made for each individual and is usually more informal than formal. A major dilemma in long-term care is the incongruity between the ideal long-term care system and the current system.

As described previously, long-term care is designed for people who require multiple and ongoing health, mental health, and social support services over an extended period of time and whose needs are likely to change. The ideal system is one that provides comprehensive, integrated care on an ongoing basis and offers various levels of intensity that change as a client's needs change. The goal is to provide the health and related support services that enable a person to maximize functional independence. This contrasts with the goal of acute care, which is to "cure" the patient of an illness. Many clients may use only select components of the system and may remain involved with the organized system of care for a relatively short period of time; others may use only a limited and stable set of services over a prolonged period of time.

This ideal system of long-term care is referred to throughout the remainder of this chapter as the *continuum of care*. A continuum of care is defined as:

> a client-oriented system composed of both services and integrating mechanisms that guides and tracks patients over time through a comprehensive array of health, mental health and social services spanning all levels of intensity of care. (Evashwick, 1987)

The continuum of care concept extends beyond the definitions of long-term care. A continuum of care is a comprehensive, coordinated system of care designed to meet the needs of patients with complex and/or ongoing problems efficiently and effectively. A continuum is more than a collection of fragmented services. It includes mechanisms for organizing those services and operating them as an integrated system.

The goal is to facilitate the client's access to the appropriate services at the appropriate time, quickly and efficiently. Ideally, a continuum of care does the following:

- It matches resources to the patient's condition.
- It monitors the client's condition and changes services as the needs change.
- It coordinates the care of many professionals and disciplines.
- It integrates care provided in a range of settings.
- It enhances efficiency, reduces duplication, and streamlines patient flow.
- It maintains a comprehensive record incorporating clinical, financial, and utilization data.

A true continuum of care should have two major priorities: (1) achieving cost-effectiveness by maximizing the use of resources, and (2) enhancing quality through appropriateness and continuity of care.

Service Categories

Over sixty distinct services could be identified in the complete continuum of care. For simplicity, the services are grouped into seven categories: (1) extended care, (2) acute inpatient care, (3) ambulatory care, (4) home care, (5) outreach, (6) wellness, and (7) housing. In brief, the seven categories represent the basic types of health care assistance that a person would need over time, through periods of both wellness and illness. Table 11.4 lists the major services within these categories.

This chapter approaches the continuum of care from the perspective of health care. In theory and in practice, even more services that affect health status or health care use could be included, such as retirement planning, social activities, and guardianship.

Extended Inpatient Care

This is for people who are so sick or functionally disabled that they require ongoing nursing and support services provided in a formal health care institution, but who are not so acutely ill that they require the technological and professional intensity of a hospital. The majority of extended care facilities are referred to as nursing facilities, although this is a broad term that includes many levels and types of programs. Subacute units, rehabilitation units, and intermediate care facilities also offer extended inpatient care.

Acute Inpatient Care

This is hospital care for those who have a major and acute health care problem. For the majority of people, a typical hospital stay of four to eight days is the intensive aspect of a longer spell of illness, preceded by diagnostic testing and succeeded by follow-up care.

Ambulatory Care Services

These are provided in a formal health care facility, whether a physician's office or the outpatient clinic of a hospital or an adult day care program. They include a wide spectrum of preventive, maintenance, diagnostic, and recuperative services for people who manifest a variety of conditions, from those who are entirely healthy and simply want an annual checkup to those with major health problems who are recuperating from hospitalization to those with chronic conditions who need ongoing monitoring.

Table 11.4.   Services and Service Settings of the Continuum of Care

Extended Care	Home visitors
Skilled nursing facilities	Home-delivered meals
Step-down units	Homemaker and personal care
Swing beds	
Nursing home follow-up	*Outreach and Linkage*
Intermediate Care Facilities for the Mentally Disabled	Health Fairs
	Screening
Acute Care	Information and referral
Medical/surgical inpatient unit	Telephone contact
Psychiatric inpatient unit	Emergency response system
Rehabilitation inpatient unit	Transportation
Interdisciplinary assessment team	Senior membership program
Consultation service	
	Wellness and Health Promotion
Ambulatory Care	Disease Management Programs
Physicians' offices	Educational programs
Outpatient clinics	Exercise programs
Interdisciplinary assessment clinics	Recreational and social groups
Day hospital	Senior volunteers
Adult day care	Congregate meals
Mental health clinic	Support groups
Satellite clinics	
Psychosocial counseling	*Housing*
Alcohol and substance abuse programs	Continuing care retirement communities
	Independent senior housing
Home Care	Congregate care facilities
Home health—Medicare	Adult family homes
Home health—private	Group homes
Hospice	Assisted living
High technology	Short-term housing for families and/or patients
Durable medical equipment	

SOURCE: Adapted from "Definition of the Continuum of Care," by C. Evashwick, in *Managing the Continuum of Care*, edited by C. Evashwick & L. Weiss, 1987, Gaithersburg, MD: Aspen.

Home Care

This category represents a variety of nursing, therapy, and support services provided to people who are homebound and have some degree of illness or functional disability, but who are able to satisfy their needs by bringing services into the home setting. Home health programs range from formal programs of high-technology drug therapy or high-touch skilled nursing care to relatively informal networks that arrange housekeeping for friends.

Outreach Programs

These make health and social services readily available in the community rather than within the formidable walls of a large institution. Health fairs in shopping centers, senior membership programs, and emergency response systems are all forms of outreach. They are targeted at the healthy who are living in the community for the purpose of keeping them connected with the health care system.

Wellness Programs

These services are provided for those who are basically healthy and want to stay that way by actively engaging in disease prevention and health promotion. Wellness programs include health education classes, exercise programs, health screenings, and disease management programs.

Housing

Housing for frail populations increasingly includes access to health and support services and, conversely, recognizes that the home setting affects health. Housing incorporating health care ranges from independent apartments affiliated with a health care system that sends a nurse to do weekly blood pressure checks to assisted living with nursing and social services provided around-the-clock on site.

The categories are for heuristic purposes only. The order of the categories and the services comprising them can vary. The categories can be appropriately reordered on the basis of the dimension being considered: duration of stay, intensity of care, stage of illness, disciplines of professionals, type of facility, availability of informal support, and primary payer. Within each category are health, mental health, and social services, potentially provided by professional clinicians, provider organizations, families, and/or clients themselves. A more accurate diagram would be a multidimensional matrix showing the interrelationship of all of these factors in caring for a single individual and family. Such a matrix would be dynamic, not static, for the relationships would be different for each individual client and would change over time as the client's needs changed.

Within the categories as well as between them, the services of the continuum are distinct. Each has different regulatory, financing, target population, staffing, and physical requirements. Each has its own admission policies, patient treatment protocols, and billing system. Each organization has its own referral and discharge networks. In addition, each has its own measures of quality and choice of accreditation body. A primary reason for organizing services into a continuum is to achieve integration, yet the differences among services make unified planning and operations quite difficult. One challenge faced by administrators in the initial creation of a continuum of care is that each service must be dealt with separately and brought into a cohesive whole.

The continuum of care is so extensive that it is unlikely that any single organization can offer a complete continuum for all of its clients. The goal of the provider should be to facilitate access for clients to the services they need. In brief, an organization need not have all services under its direct ownership or control; rather, it may have a variety of formal and informal relationships with other providers in the community. The purposes of organizing into a continuum of care model are to increase the efficiency of client flow, maximize use of resources, enhance quality through greater continuity of care, and improve market share by offering a desirable product.

The trend in the 1980s was for organizations to broaden the scope of the services provided and lay the groundwork for the continuum of care to be created during the 1990s. Some organizations bought others, some started new entities, and some simply added new staff and new divisions. The 1990s saw the further expansion of long-term care services and the recognition that fragmented services do not meet the needs of those with multifaceted, chronic conditions nor the needs of providers or payers to achieve cost-effective, efficient care, particularly under managed-care and at-risk arrangements. Private entities, including hospitals, medical groups, and managed-care companies, began disease-management programs. Public entities, led by state governments, launched models of pooled financial and eligibility programs. This context of service availability, consumer demand, and provider and payer financial attention is a prerequisite for a continuum of care.

Integrating Mechanisms

By definition, a continuum of care is more than a collection of fragmented services; it is an integrated system of care. To gain the system benefits of efficiencies of operation, smooth patient flow, and quality of service, integrating mechanisms are essential. Four integrating management systems are required: interentity structure, care coordination, information systems, and financing.

Interentity Structures

This means that management arrangements and operating policies are in place to enable services to coordinate care, facilitate smooth client flow, and maximize the use of professional staff and other resources. Examples include product line management organization, joint planning and operating committees, transfer arrangements, and joint budgeting.

Care Coordination

This refers to the coordination of the clinical components of care, usually by a combination of a dedicated person and established processes that facilitate communication among professionals of various disciplines at multiple sites. Case management, extended-care pathways, interdisciplinary teams, and single-access referral are all techniques for achieving care coordination.

Integrated Information Systems

Ideally, one client record should combine financial, clinical, and utilization information being used by multiple providers and payers across multiple sites, with automatic updating of information.

Integrated Financing

This approach removes barriers to continuity and appropriateness of care by having adequate financing for long-term care as well as acute care, preferably paid by a capitated or pooled system to allow maximum flexibility of service arrangement.

SERVICE CATEGORIES

This section presents basic information about the major services comprising the continuum of long-term care. As shown in Figure 11.4, most services have grown substantially in numbers during the past two decades, indicating both greater availability and expanded demand for long-term care. Note that the total number of community hospitals has decreased while the number of nursing homes has remained stable, indicating the greater affordability and consumer preference for non-institutional services.

One of the challenges long-term care presents for administrators, policy-makers, clinicians, and families is that information about long-term care services is not available in a single location. Data about service availability or operation are not necessarily comparable, if indeed available at all. Each service is unique, reflecting the differing forces that guided service development and explaining the difficulties faced in creating a cohesive system.

Each service is described briefly, followed by a profile of national capacity, operating characteristics, and clients. Extensive data, presented in previous editions of this book, are not included because of the relative ease of obtaining complete and current data from the Internet. Rather, key Internet sites having additional information are given for each service.

Hospitals

Long-term hospitals are defined by Medicare as hospitals that have an average length of patient stay greater than twenty-five days. The nation has fewer than 150 official long-term hospitals, but some states have special categories for chronic or long-term stay hospitals. Long-term hospitals recognized by Medicare are paid by a different system than DRG-based payment.

Psychiatric hospitals comprise about two-thirds of the long-stay hospitals in the nation, or about 650 institutions. Many psychiatric hospitals and psychiatric units within hospitals are integral parts of a community's continuum of care for the mentally ill.

Rehabilitation hospitals serve those who need additional therapy to recover from acute trauma, ranging from automobile accidents involving the young to strokes among the old. In addition, rehabilitation services are provided to thousands of people each year in rehabilitation units of general hospitals, subacute units, skilled nursing facilities, outpatient clinics, or through home care agencies—any or all of which may be part of an acute care or specialty hospital.

Service Growth

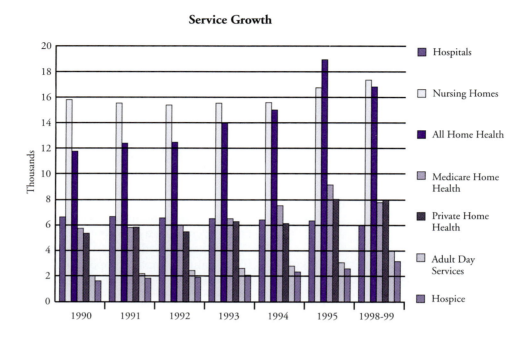

Figure 11.4. Service Growth

SOURCE: The Center for Health Care Innovation, CSULB, Long Beach, CA.

Federal hospitals, short-stay as well as long-stay, include *Department of Veterans Affairs (DVA) facilities.* The DVA operates its own continuum of care for veterans, which is "the largest coordinated system of health and long-term care services in the world" (U.S. Department of Veterans Affairs, 1986). DVA complexes often include short-stay hospitals, long-stay hospitals or units within the acute hospital, geriatric evaluation units (GEUs), skilled nursing facilities or units, adult day care, hospice, home health, residential care homes, and respite. The DVA has also been on the forefront of developing geriatric research, education, and clinical centers (GRECCs). Since 1975, the DVA has established twenty-two GRECCs, which are based in DVA hospitals throughout the nation. In previous times, the largest proportion of the DVA health care budget was for hospital care. By 2020, however, forty-five percent of veterans will be age sixty-five or older. Thus, in the future, the proportion of the DVA

health care budget spent on long-term care will increase dramatically.

General community hospitals provide many of the services in the continuum of long-term care. Nationwide surveys conducted in 1981 (Evashwick, Rundall, & Goldiamond, 1985) and 1985 (Hospital Research and Educational Trust, 1986) demonstrated that, even before the portending increase in demand due to the baby boom maturation, hospitals provided a wide array of long-term care and geriatric services to reach clients and families before and after a stay in the inpatient unit. Table 11.5 shows select geriatric and chronic care services offered by hospitals.

The rationale for hospitals of all types to be involved in long-term care is clear. Nationally, thirty-five percent of hospital admissions and forty-five percent of all inpatient days are for people age sixty-five and older (American Hospital Association, 2000). One in four older adults is admitted to the hospital each

Table 11.5. Geriatric and Long-Term Services Offered by Hospitals

Adult day care
Arthritis treatment center
Assisted living
Burn treatment
Cancer screening, diagnosis, and treatment
Case management
Congregate care
End-of-life services
Geriatric assessment
High-tech home therapy
Home health
Hospice
Intermediate nursing care
Meals on Wheels
Retirement housing
Rehabilitation therapies
Respite
Skilled nursing care

year, and of those admitted, more than fifty percent are re-admitted at least once (Health Data on Older Americans, 1993). As noted earlier, the health problems of seniors are characterized as chronic and multifaceted. For hospitals to provide high-quality care to seniors, they must address the needs of these patients beyond the few days spent in the hospital. As the older population grows in number and proportion, the hospital will be faced with an increasing demand for comprehensive, coordinated, continuing care by senior consumers and their families.

The trend toward outpatient care also contributes to the hospital's role in providing long-term care. As hospitals move more and more of their services to an outpatient basis, those who are admitted are increasingly those with multiple and/or complex, long-term conditions who need multifaceted, continuing care.

A third reason prompting hospital involvement in the continuum of long-term care is financial. In 1995, nearly fifty-one percent of community hospitals' revenues came from Medicare (American Hospital Association, 2000). Hospitals thus have a high financial stake in caring for older people, the majority of whom have chronic conditions. Conversely, hospitals are the largest recipients of Medicare funds, receiving approximately forty percent of the Medicare budget each year. This subjects the hospital to policy changes brought about as Congress responds to the demands of seniors and competing forces, such as balancing the federal budget.

As managed-care systems evolve, the acute hospital finds it advantageous from a financial standpoint and essential from a marketing standpoint to provide a spectrum of services. To ensure viable financial performance, particularly under capitated arrangements, the hospital must manage access to services beyond those of acute inpatient care. Diversification of owning and operating multiple levels of service may also contribute to the hospital's revenues.

Operating Characteristics

Table 11.6 summarizes basic information about hospitals. Hospitals may have those with chronic conditions as inpatients for the shortest duration of the condition. However, from a systems perspective, hospitals are the high-cost service and are the greatest single locus of expensive health care resources. They thus have a dominant role in building a cost-effective continuum of care.

Table 11.6. Service Snapshot: Hospitals

Number of facilities	About 6,000
Number of beds	About 1 million
Number of admissions	About 32 million per year
Charges	$1,200/day room cost, minus ancillaries
Major payers	Medicare, commercial insurance
Licensure	State department of health
Certification	Medicare, Medicaid
Accreditation	Joint Commission on Accreditation of Healthcare Organizations

SOURCE: Table adapted from Paone, D. (2001). Hospitals. In C. Evashwick (Ed.), *The continuum of long-term care.* (2nd ed.). Albany, NY: Delmar Thomson Learning.

Clients

About 32 million admissions to hospitals occur each year. This figure excludes newborns but includes those who may be admitted more than once. Even subtracting those with multiple admissions, hospitals are clearly the most frequently used of all of the services of the continuum of care.

The most common reasons for admission vary with age. The top diagnoses listed as a reason for admission to acute hospitals are chronic or long-term conditions: heart condition, cancer, stroke, fracture (primarily hip), pneumonia, and psychosis (U.S. Department of Health and Human Services, 2000).

Sources of Information

The single most extensive and complete source of information about hospitals is the American Hospital Association (AHA), which conducts an annual survey of all United States hospitals. Their data are proprietary and must be purchased. Data on hospitals can also be found through the Health Care Financing Administration Web site and the Joint Commission on Accreditation of Healthcare Organizations (JCAHO).

National Profile

The common vision of the acute hospital is one of complicated machines, bustling staff, and patients arriving and departing quickly, cured of their ailments. In reality, the hospital plays a significant role in providing the continuum of long-term care.

Of the more than 6,000 hospitals in the United States in 1999, almost all served patients with long-term needs. Of the top leading causes for admission to community hospitals, most are associated with chronic conditions. Most community general hospitals also offer select services for people with chronic conditions. Some hospitals specialize in serving patients with long-term conditions. Long-term, tuberculosis, rehabilitation, orthopedic, chronic disease, and psychiatric hospitals all serve patients with long inpatient lengths of stay.

Nursing Homes

Nursing home is a broad term that encompasses a wide spectrum of facilities ranging from small privately-owned, community-based facilities to twenty-bed units of acute community general hospitals to twelve-hundred-bed government-operated institutions. *Convalescent home, retirement center, long-term care facility, health center, nursing facility,* and other similar terms have no specific meaning nationally. *Skilled nursing facility* and *intermediate care facility for the mentally disabled* are terms that have specific definitions under Medicare and Medicaid regulations.

Nursing homes may be freestanding units of hospitals or integral parts of campus care retirement centers of multilevel housing complexes. Many facilities have a combination of skilled nursing care and personal care beds. The common feature is that a person who is not able to remain at home alone due to physical health problems, mental health problems, or functional disabilities resides at the facility. These people are called *residents* rather than *patients.* Residents may stay for a short period of days or an indefinite period of time.

Each state licenses long-term care facilities and each has its own licensing requirements, reimbursement policies, governing regulations, classification systems, and terminology. As part of the regulatory process, each state establishes its own definitions of nursing homes and related long-term care institutions.

National Profile

The federal government periodically conducts a survey of nursing facilities across the nation. For data collection purposes in 1997, the National Center for Health Statistics defined a nursing home as "a facility with three beds or more that is either licensed as a nursing home by its state, certified as a nursing facility under Medicare, identified as a nursing care unit of a retirement center, or determined to provide nursing or medical care" (NCHS, 2000). The 1997 nationwide survey reported 17,000 nursing facilities with over 1.8 million beds (Gabrel, 2000). Occupancy averaged 88 percent, with over 1.6 million residents at any given time. During the year, nearly 2.37 million people were admitted (see Table 11.7).

Nursing homes contrast with hospitals markedly in some ways. About two-thirds are proprietary. The majority are ninety-nine beds or less, and ninety-two percent are less than 200 beds. More than half are owned by a multifacility organization (chain). Nursing homes are unevenly distributed throughout the nation, by state as well as by census region.

Operating Characteristics

The Service Snapshot in Table 11.8 summarizes additional information about nursing home operations. The average cost of nursing home care ranged from $2,000 to $5,000 per month in 1997, varying by state and type of facility. Payment for nursing home care is made primarily by Medicaid (more than half) and by private individuals and families. Medicare pays only about eight percent of the annual national costs of nursing home care, which comprise only about four percent of the Medicare annual budget. The Department of Veterans Affairs, private insurance, and other payers account for the remainder. The heavy dependence on state Medicaid payments poses a financial challenge for nursing homes. In some states, the expenditure for the nursing home component of Medicaid is the largest single expense in the state budget. As states look for ways to control their budgets, funding for nursing home care is heavily scrutinized. States have used certificate-of-need authorities to limit the number of nursing home beds allowed in the state and thereby limit state spending.

Payment methods for nursing homes vary by state. Several payment systems have been tried. Most states have some form of cost-based per diem rates. Rates

Table 11.7. Characteristics of Nursing Homes, 1997

	Number	Percent
Total	17,000	100.00
Ownership		
Proprietary	11,400	67.1
Nonprofit	4,400	26.1
Government	1,200	6.8
Bed Size		
Less than 50 beds	2,200	12.9
50–99 beds	6,300	37.2
100–199 beds	7,200	42.2
200 beds or more	1,300	7.7
Certification		
Medicare & Medicaid	13,200	77.7
Medicare only	800	4.7
Medicaid only	2,300	13.6
Not certified	700	4.1
Census Region		
Northeast	2,900	17.3
Midwest	5,800	34.2
South	5,400	31.8
West	2,900	16.8
Affiliation		
Chain	9,600	56.3
Independent	7,400	43.2

SOURCE: Gabrel, C. (2000). An overview of nursing home facilities; Data from the 1997 National Nursing Home Survey. Advance data from *Vital and Health Statistics*, No. 311. Hyattsville, MD: National Center for Health Statistics.

Table 11.8. Service Snapshot: Nursing Homes

Number of facilities	17,000
Number of beds	1.8 million
Number of residents (census)	1.6 million
Charges	$2–5,000 per month (free-standing rate)
Major payers	Medicaid, Private out-of-pocket
Licensure	State Department of Health
Certification	Medicare, Medicaid
Accreditation	Joint Commission on Accreditation of Healthcare Organizations

SOURCE: Gabrel, C. (2000). An overview of nursing home facilities: Data from the 1997 National Nursing Home Survey. Advance data from *Vital and Health Statistics*, No. 311. Hyattsville, MD: National Center for Health Statistics. Table adapted from Evashwick, C. (Ed.). (2001). *The continuum of long-term care*. Albany, NY: Delmar Thomson Learning.

may be adjusted for case mix, and ancillary costs, such as physical therapy, may be included in the per diem rate or paid separately. With the Balanced Budget Act of 1997, the federal government instituted a case-mix payment system for those nursing facilities that received payment from Medicare. For the top ten diagnoses, Medicare established a case-mix prospective rate. This new method of Medicare payment for nursing facilities is being revamped and implemented during the early years of the new century.

Nursing homes are highly regulated. Concern about quality is juxtaposed with the limited budgets of state Medicaid agencies and private families. In the mid-1980s, the Institute of Medicine produced a report criticizing the quality of care in nursing facilities. Many of its recommendations were subsequently implemented by the federal government. The 1987 Nursing Home Reform Act, incorporated into the Omnibus Budget Reconciliation Act of 1987 (OBRA), made significant changes in how nursing homes operate and how they are evaluated (Coleman, 1991). The survey process was changed from one focusing on physical and task criteria to one focusing on the caring process, resident feelings, and patient care outcomes. The minimum data set (MDS) was required to be completed for all residents, initiating standardization of record-keeping and providing a basis for comparison of patient status and case-mix-based reimbursement methodologies. In 2000, the Institute of Medicine published another report on the status of quality care in nursing facilities (Institute of Medicine, 2000), potentially fostering further changes in nursing home quality control.

Nursing facilities can choose to be accredited by the Joint Commission on Accreditation of Healthcare Organizations (JCAHO). However, only about five percent elect to do so, in contrast to the nearly ninety-five percent of hospitals that seek accreditation from JCAHO.

The majority of employees of nursing homes are unskilled or low-skilled: nurses' aides, housekeeping and maintenance employees, and food service workers. Even in skilled nursing facilities that meet Medicare requirements, a facility of ninety-nine beds or less is required to have a registered nurse on duty only eight hours per day. On evening and night shifts, the highest professional staff may be a licensed vocational nurse. Other health care professionals who work with nursing homes include physicians, pharmacists, dietitians, occupational, physical, speech, and respiratory therapists, and medical social workers. Except in very large homes, these professionals will work on a part-time contract basis rather than as employees. The number of full-time equivalents (FTEs) per 100 beds serving all three shifts has increased over time, from 41.2 in 1973 to 54.7 in 1995, but nonetheless remains quite low (Strahan, 1997).

Clients

Table 11.9 characterizes nursing home residents. Nursing homes primarily serve the very old and frail. Of the 1.6 million residents in 1997, more than ninety-one percent were age sixty-five and older; forty-six percent were eighty-five and older. Three out of four residents were women, and nearly nine out of ten were white.

The primary diagnoses of nursing home residents are circulatory system disorders, mental disorders, and diseases of the nervous system. Functional dependence is high. Eighty-six percent of those age sixty-five and older require assistance with at least one ADL. Many have suffered debilitating strokes and have not fully recovered mentally or physically. As many as two out of three residents have some type of mental disorder, most often organic brain syndrome or Alzheimer's disease.

The reasons people are admitted to nursing homes tend to be functional dependency rather than diagnosis alone. Past research has shown that for every person in a nursing home, two equally ill people reside at home, cared for by family and friends (Spector et al., 2000). Admission to a home usually occurs because friends and family can no longer provide the level of support required. Night wandering and incontinence are two problems that frequently stress a family beyond its caregiving capacity and result in admission of the frail person to a nursing home. People who are single and do not have strong social support systems are also more likely to be in nursing homes.

The lifetime chance of ever being in a nursing home is about one in two (Kemper & Murtaugh,

Table 11.9. Characteristics of Nursing Home Residents by Age, Sex, and Race, 1997

	Number*	Percent
All Ages	**1,608,700**	100.00
Age		
Under age 65	136,740	8.5
65–74 years	197,870	12.3
75–84 years	527,654	32.8
85 years and older	738,303	45.9
Unknown	6,435	0.4
Sex		
Female	1,161,481	72.2
Male	447,219	27.8
Race		
Caucasian	1,401,178	87.1
African American	167,305	10.4
Other	22,522	1.4
Unknown	17,696	1.1

*Numbers not in bold derived from percent distribution.

SOURCE: Gabrel, C. (2000). An overview of nursing home facilities: Data from the 1997 National Nursing Home Survey. Advance data from *Vital and Health Statistics*, No. 311. Hyattsville, MD: National Center for Health Statistics.

1991). The likelihood of nursing home admission, however, increases with age. Of people age sixty-five to seventy-four, only one in ten is in a nursing home at any given time. Of those age eighty-five and above, twenty percent reside in a nursing home.

Duration of stay in a nursing home spans a wide range. Half of all those admitted are discharged within one year; thirty percent within ninety days. Nineteen percent of women and twelve percent of men stay in a nursing home more than five years (Kemper & Murtaugh, 1991).

The widespread use of nursing homes will continue at least during the first half of the twenty-first century. The *rate* of use of nursing homes may decline as more community-based housing and service options are available, as the technological ability to provide care at home expands, and as biomedical technology is able to cure or prevent the physical and mental decline that causes functional disability. However, as the population grows older, including the ex-

ceptionally numerous baby boom generation, there will be greater numbers of those who need the care offered by nursing homes.

Sources of Information

Two associations are excellent sources of extensive information about long-term care facilities: the American Association of Homes and Services for the Aged (AAHSA), which represents not-for-profit organizations, and the American Health Care Association (AHCA), which represents for-profit facilities. The American College of Health Care Administrators (ACHCA) is the professional association for administrators of nursing homes and senior housing complexes. The Health Care Financing Administration has data on nursing facilities, but only those that are certified to participate in the Medicare and Medicaid programs. States typically have data on the facilities they license.

Home Health

Home health care is one of the oldest components of the continuum of care. A number of home health agencies across the nation have celebrated their centennials. Home care consists of several types of services: skilled nursing care and therapies, homemaker/personal care/chore services, high-technology home therapy, durable medical equipment, and hospice. The services may all be provided by one agency, or an agency may specialize in only one. However, high-technology home therapy and durable medical equipment (DME) companies are likely to be distinct organizations, and hospice may be provided by organizations from a variety of venues, so these are discussed separately.

Skilled home health services include the following:

- nursing care, provided by registered nurses or a licensed vocation nurse, ranging from basic nursing procedures to highly complex care
- physical therapy
- occupational therapy
- speech therapy
- respiratory therapy

- medical social services
- case management
- nutrition assessment and counseling
- patient education
- medications management

Homemaker/personal care includes these services:

- dressing and personal care
- bathing and grooming
- meal preparation
- shopping
- transportation
- light housekeeping
- select household chores
- other tasks that do not require trained health care professionals

Often several services are provided to a single patient by a multidisciplinary team. A combination of skilled and unskilled service providers may be engaged. Each provider, however, may visit the patient at a different time, and several distinct agencies may be involved.

National Profile

The agencies providing home health and homemaker care are differentiated by those that are Medicare-certified and those that are not. Medicare-certified agencies must comply with the conditions of participation specified by the Medicare program and clients must meet Medicare criteria for reimbursement (delineated later in this section). Comprehensive data are available on the certified agencies through the Medicare program. Data on agencies that are not certified are less complete because there is no single regulatory or financing source that requires reporting. However, noncertified agencies are quite similar to certified agencies in services provided, clients, and fees; the differences are primarily in organizational characteristics, payment systems, and proportion of clients with skilled versus unskilled needs.

Home care agencies take an array of organizational forms. The Health Care Financing Administration (HCFA) has developed a classification system that involves ownership, control, and tax status. The categories follow.

Freestanding

Visiting nurses associations—voluntary, nonprofit organizations governed by a board of directors and usually financed by tax deductible contributions as well as earnings. (The term earlier had a more specific meaning and referred to home care agencies that were named Visiting Nurse Associations and shared a common history.)

Public agencies—government agencies operated by a state, county, city, or other unit of local government, such as public health departments, having a major responsibility for prevention of disease and for community health education.

Proprietary agencies—freestanding, for-profit home care agencies. These range from single agencies owned by individuals to large nation-wide chains.

Private non-profit—not-for-profit freestanding agencies that are privately developed, governed, and owned.

Other—freestanding agencies that do not fit one of the other categories for freestanding agencies.

Facility-based

Hospital-based—operated as an integral part of a hospital, such as a department or unit. Agencies that have working arrangements with a hospital or are owned by a hospital but operated as separate entities are classified under one of the freestanding categories.

SNF—agencies based in skilled nursing facilities.

Rehabilitation—agencies that are based in rehabilitation hospitals or outpatient clinics.

Formal home care organizations were first opened in the 1880s. By 1963, 1,100 agencies existed. By 2000, the number had mushroomed to over 20,000 (National Association for Home Care, 2000). Medicare agencies by type are shown in Table 11.10. A major trend has been for proprietary and hospital-based agencies to increase and VNA agencies to decrease. Medicare agencies peaked in number in 1997 at 10,444, and declined in number in the next few years due to the changes in reporting and reimbursement required by the Balanced Budget Act of 1997.

Table 11.10. Medicare-Certified Home Health Agencies, by Auspice, 1967–1999

	1967	1999
VNA	642	487
Government	939	918
Proprietary	0	3,192
Private nonprofit	0	621
Hospital-based	133	2,300
SNF-based	0	163
Rehabilitation-based	0	1
Other	39	65
Total	1,753	7,747

SOURCE: Adapted from National Association for Home Care, *www.nahc.org*, March 2000.

Non-certified agencies numbered approximately 10,000 in 2000. This number has been stable since the mid-1990s. These agencies, which do not depend upon Medicare funds, were not affected by the reimbursement changes in Medicare and thus did not experience the trend in closures affecting the Medicare-certified agencies. The majority of non-certified agencies are proprietary and for-profit, including large national and regional chains.

Operating Characteristics

Operating characteristics of home care agencies are highlighted in the service snapshot in Table 11.11. In 1998, approximately $41 billion dollars of total national health expenditures were spent by the United States on home care services (NAHC, 2000). This represents about three percent of personal health care expenditures.

Of the $41 billion, $14 billion was spent on Medicare home care. In 1997, about nine percent of the annual Medicare budget was spent on home care. Medicare is the single largest payer for Medicare-certified home health agencies. In an effort to control the rising costs of the Medicare program, Congress implemented radical changes as part of the Balanced Budget Act of 1997. Payment for Medicare-certified providers of all types is in flux at the time of this writing, and is likely to remain so for several years, particularly for home health agencies. Reimbursement for home care was changed from a per-visit basis to a per-beneficiary limit, and restricted to the agency's lowest allowable costs. These costs were pegged to a new case-mix system, implemented through an interim payment system (IPS), and calculated on a new required information system (OASIS). As a result of these changes, the Medicare payment for home care services dropped from $14 billion to $9.5 billion in 1999, and from nine percent to four percent of the total Medicare budget (NAHC, 2000).

Medicaid, the Older Americans Act, Title XX Social Services Block grants, the Department of Veterans Affairs, CHAMPUS, Workers' Compensation, county mental health departments, commercial insurance companies, and managed-care health plans all also fund limited amounts of home care.

Meanwhile, non-certified home health agencies continue to charge on a per-hour basis. In 1998, the rate was about $90 per hour for a visit by a Registered Nurse, and about $45 per hour for a home health aide. For lower-priced hourly services, such as personal care, agencies often have a two- or four-hour minimum. Although not eligible for Medicare payment, non-certified agencies may be paid by other government programs, as well as by private insurance, managed care, and direct client fees.

Staffing of Medicare-certified agencies complies with federal regulations, and professionals are typically full- or part-time employees. In contrast, most non-certified agencies hire staff on an hourly or per diem basis, enabling them to staff according to client demand.

Licensing by the state department of health is typically required of Medicare-certified agencies due to their capacity as providers of skilled health care services. Non-certified agencies may be required to be licensed by the health department if they provide skilled services, but may only be required to have no more than a business license if they provide only personal care support services.

Medicare-certified agencies can receive accreditation by either the Joint Commission on Accreditation of Healthcare Organizations (JCAHO) or the Community Health Association Program (CHAP). Home care agencies not certified by Medicare can

Table 11.11.   Service Snapshot: Home Health Care

	Medicare-Certified	Private
Number of agencies	9,655	~10,000
Number of clients	3.4 million	4.6 million (est.)
Total visits	270,000	NA
Charges	$96/visit (RN)	$90/hr (RN)
Major payers	Medicare	Out-of-pocket
	Medicaid	Government programs
	Out-of-pocket	Private insurance
Licensure	State department of health	Business license
Certification	Medicare, Medicaid	May have Medicaid or other government certification
Accreditation	JCAHO, CHAP	CHAP, NHC, NLN*

Note: Data for 1998. Comparative data on private agencies not available for 2000.

*CHAP is Community Health Accreditation Program, NHC is National Homecaring Council, NLN is National League of Nursing.

SOURCE: National Association for Home Care, *Home Care Statistics,* 1999.

seek accreditation from the National League of Nursing, National Homecaring Council, or CHAP (see Table 11.11).

Clients

Skilled home care clients are those who are recovering from an acute episode of illness, require rehabilitation, suffer from chronic illnesses that need ongoing monitoring or intense attention, are undergoing special short-term therapies, and/or are in the last stages of life. To be eligible for the skilled services paid for by Medicare, a client must be a Medicare enrollee and be certified by a physician to meet several criteria: to be homebound (i.e., unable to go out of the home independently), be capable of improvement, require only intermittent care rather than continuous care, and require either nursing or physical therapy care. Home health aide care, occupational therapy, medical social work, and select other services can be paid for by Medicare only to those who first require nursing or physical therapy. All services must be prescribed by a physician and are limited in duration, based on the assumption of the client's prognosis to improve. The most frequent source of referrals is people being discharged from an acute hospital stay.

Those who use home care services not requiring skilled care are typically people who are functionally impaired on a short-term or permanent basis and who require assistance with the activities of daily living (ADLS) or instrumental activities of daily living (IADLs). Services may be provided indefinitely. Depending upon the payment source, private home care does not necessarily require a physician's prescription, and clients thus come from many sources.

In 1996, 7.2 million people, or nearly three percent of the U.S. population, used home care services (NCHS, 2000a, 2000b). As shown in Table 11.12, almost two-thirds of the users were women, and almost two-thirds were age sixty-five or older. In general, home care is widely used, regardless of race, age, marital status, income level, geographic area, or any other characteristics.

Users of home care have a variety of conditions. Diseases of the circulatory system and heart conditions account for more than one-third (thirty-five percent) of the primary diagnoses and neoplasms account for another sixteen percent (Haupt, 1998). Homebound status and the inability to perform self-care are the underlying similarities among all home care users.

High-Technology Home Therapy

High-technology home therapy appeared in the early 1980s as new technologies emerged. Cost-containment initiatives squeezing hospitals and advances in drug

Table 11.12. Characteristics of Home Health Users by Age, Sex, and Race, 1996

	Percent: 100.00
Age	
Under age 45	19.5
45–54	5.9
55–64	8.4
65–69	10.8
70–74	13.2
75–79	12.5
80–84	14.2
85+	15.4
Sex	
Female	63.5
Male	36.5
Race	
Caucasian	62.8
African American	7.4
Other	2.6
Unknown	27.2
Marital Status	
Married	37.0
Widowed	24.6
Divorced or separated	5.0
Single	18.4
Unknown	15.0

SOURCE: Haupt, B. (1998). An overview of home health and hospice care patients: 1996 National Home and Hospice Care Survey. Advance data from *Vital and Health Statistics*, No. 297. Hyattsville, MD: National Center for Health Statistics.

and equipment made it possible to deliver services in the home that had formerly been available to patients only in hospitals. A major advantage of providing high-technology therapy in the home is that it is much less expensive than providing the same care in a hospital or nursing home.

The expansion of ambulatory care, especially ambulatory surgery, beginning in the late 1980s and continuing into the 1990s has further abetted the trend to move services out of the hospital and into home settings. High-technology services now provided in the home include those that are listed here:

- intravenous antibiotics
- oncology therapy
- pain management
- parenteral and enteral nutrition
- ventilator care
- high-risk pregnancy monitoring
- infant monitoring

High-technology home therapy typically involves pharmaceuticals and equipment that are expensive, require special staff expertise to use and monitor, and are available only from select sources. The total volume of patients requiring high-technology care is small, and the protocols can vary on an individual basis much more than for basic home care.

High-technology home therapy is provided by many Medicare-certified and private home health agencies. In addition, some agencies specialize only in providing high-technology home care. The cost for each patient can be quite high, and reimbursement is often negotiated with the insurance company or health plan on an individual basis. Companies with the requisite expertise have found that they can thrive just by specializing in this one component of home care. Hence, continued growth in the high-technology arena is likely in the future.

Durable Medical Equipment

Durable medical equipment (DME), ranging from walkers to electric beds, is frequently provided in conjunction with home health care. The home health agency often assumes responsibility for arranging for equipment, and may have a formal or informal affiliation with a local durable medical equipment company to provide the needed equipment. If the equipment is to be paid for by Medicare, it must be prescribed by the client's physician.

During the 1980s, the durable medical equipment business boomed as a fast-growing area of home health care less regulated and more lucrative than other areas of health care delivery. Many joint ventures were initiated: multihealth care systems acquired or started DME businesses, and home health conglomerates were tried, bringing all aspects of home health care together into one parent company. In the mid- and late-1980s, Medicare tightened its regulatory and payment policies. The DME field has since stabilized, and DME remains an essential, but distinct, component of home health care.

Sources of Information

The National Association of Home Care (NAHC) is a major source of data and information about all aspects of home care, with a Web site updated annually: *www.nahc.org*. In addition, the National Center for Health Statistics conducts a series of surveys that produce data on home care on intermittent bases.

Hospice

Hospice is an agent that provides care for the terminally ill. It began as a formal program in Great Britain, under the leadership of Dr. Cecily Saunders, and spread to the United States during the 1970s. The philosophy of hospice is that terminally ill people should be allowed to maintain life during their final days as free of pain and in as natural and comfortable a setting as possible. Every attempt is made to enable the client to remain at home; other services are brought in as needed. All aspects of hospice emphasize quality, rather than length, of life.

Elements common to all hospices include those that follow (Lack, 1978; U.S. Department of Health and Human Services, 1991):

- service availability, including medical and nursing care, to home care patients and institutional inpatients, on a twenty-four-hour-per-day, seven-day-per-week, on-call basis
- a full complement of skilled and homemaker home care services
- inpatient care as needed in an acute hospital or nursing home
- respite care for the family provided in the home, hospital, or nursing home
- control of physical symptoms, including use of palliative drugs

- psychological, social, and spiritual counseling for patient and family
- physician direction of services
- central administration and coordination of services, and collaboration among provider organizations (home health agencies, hospitals, nursing homes)
- multidisciplinary team of care providers
- use of volunteers as an integral part of the health care team
- treatment of the patient and family together as a unit
- bereavement follow-up for family and friends

National Profile

The concept of hospice and its implementation received considerable national attention during the late 1970s and 1980s. Federally funded demonstration projects tested the impact of hospice on patient and family quality of life and cost-effective use of resources. Ultimately, Medicare established the Hospice Benefit in 1983, specifying certification criteria and a payment system for organizations and eligibility criteria for beneficiaries.

In 1999, the United States had an estimated 3,140 formal hospices (National Hospice and Palliative Care Organization, 2001). Hospice is an approach to care, and as such, can be offered through a variety of organizational settings. The National Hospice and Palliative Care Organization (NHPCO) reports that forty-four percent of hospices are independent organizations, thirty-three percent are operated by hospitals, seventeen percent are operated by home health agencies, and four percent are offered by nursing homes or under other auspices. A few hospices have distinct inpatient facilities separate from any other health care provider facility. Three-fourths (seventy-six percent) of hospice programs are nonprofit, eighteen percent are for-profit, and four percent are operated by units of government.

Operating Characteristics

Operating characteristics of hospices are given in the service snapshot in Table 11.13. Data are representative of the field, but not complete because many hos-

Table 11.13. Service Snapshot: Hospice

Number of organizations (est.)	3,140
Number of clients (est.)	700,000
Average length of stay	48 days
Major payers	Medicare
	Private insurance
	Medicaid
Medicare payment rate	$101.84 day for routine home care
	$453.04 per day for inpatient care
Certification	Medicare, Medicaid
Licensing	State department of health (44 states)
Accreditation	JCAHO
	CHAP

SOURCE: Facts and Figures on Hospice Care in America, National Hospice and Palliative Care Organization, *www.nhpco.org*, 2001.

pices are organized informally. Medicare is the major payer for hospice care, covering about two-thirds of the participants. Private insurance, Medicaid, and a mix of other sources also contribute payment for hospice care. Medicare requires rather stringent conditions of participation and has a unique payment system that pays differentially for routine daily care, hospital episodes, and other aspects of care.

Clients

The number of people using hospice has increased from less than 200,000 per year in 1985 to an estimated 700,000 clients in 1999 (NHPCO, 2001). Of the 2.5 million people who died in 1999, nearly one in three (twenty-nine percent) were receiving hospice care at the time of death. In a 1999 survey, twenty-two percent of those people who experienced the terminal illness of a friend or family member within the past year reported using hospice services. Eighty percent of the respondents did not know the meaning of the term (NHCOP, 2001).

Hospice clients have a variety of conditions. Cancer is the most common primary diagnosis. Those age sixty-five and older comprise about three-fourths of hospice users; about ten percent are between the ages

of eighteen and forty-nine (NHPCO, 2001). Men represented fifty-two percent of hospice clients in 1995. Eighty-three percent of 1995 clients were Caucasian non-Hispanic, eight percent were African American, three percent were Hispanic, and six percent were identified as "other," indicating a greater proportion of use by Caucasians than people of other racial groups (NHPCO, 2001).

Sources of Information

The National Hospice and Palliative Care Organization and the National Association of Home Care are the organizations that represent hospice programs; both maintain data. In addition, the federal government Health Care Financing Administration has data on hospice programs certified for participation in Medicare. The National Center for Health Statistics, also a unit of the federal government, conducts periodic surveys on special topics and has in the past gathered information specifically about hospice programs and users.

Adult Day Services

Adult day services are a daytime program of personal care, skilled care, supervision, socialization, and assistance with the ADLs that enables frail, often older people to remain in the community. By attending adult day care, people who are functionally disabled due to physical or mental disorder and/or moderately ill but not in need of twenty-four-hour nursing care can remain in their homes at night with their families and friends while receiving the care that they need during the day. Adult day services participants may attend on an indefinite basis or just while recovering from an acute episode of illness. The goal is to foster the maximum possible health and independence in functioning for each client, as well as to provide respite and support for each caregiver and family. For many, adult day services programs provide an alternative to nursing home care.

No comprehensive reporting system captures national data on adult day services. The characteristics described next in this text are believed to represent the field, but exact numbers and precise documentation are not available. Those attending are called *participants*, rather than "patients" or "clients."

National Profile

Adult day services have proliferated during the past two decades. Before 1975, fewer than 100 centers were identified; by 1985, the number had grown to 1,200 (Von Behren, 1986). By 1989, over 2,100 adult day care centers existed, providing care to nearly 42,000 people each weekday (Zawadski & Von Behren, 1990). Recent estimates are of more than 4,000 adult day service centers (National Adult Day Services Association, *www.ncoa.org/nadsa,* 1996).

The services offered by adult day programs are categorized in a levels-of-care framework developed by the National Adult Day Services Association (NADSA, 1996). The services offered in each of the three levels are shown in Table 11.14. The levels-of-care framework is relatively new and still evolving.

Operating Characteristics

Key operating characteristics of adult day services programs are shown in the service snapshot in Table 11.15. Adult day services may be freestanding (about one-third) or sponsored by a parent organization (about two-thirds), such as a hospital, nursing home, multi-purpose senior center, community social services agency, government agency, or church. The majority are not-for-profit. Many adult day care centers cannot cover their costs; they depend heavily on philanthropy, volunteers, and in-kind contributions.

The services offered by a given program are designed to meet the needs of the target population served by that center. Similarly, the physical space, staff, and financing of the center vary with the services offered. Most adult day services programs operate Monday through Friday during typical working hours. The physical facility is typically one or two large rooms, a kitchen, and one or two smaller rooms that can serve alternate purposes.

The average daily cost of attending an adult day care center is $43, but charges vary depending upon the range of services offered, number of days attended per week, and various other factors. Many centers use a sliding fee scale for private pay patients to accommodate family incomes.

Despite the fact that most of the participants are over age sixty-five, Medicare does not pay for adult day services because they are deemed to be maintenance, rather than acute recovery. (Rehabilitation services provided as part of adult day services programs may be billed for separately under Medicare Part B, but only with proper documentation that the participant is recovering from an acute episode and has the potential to improve.) Medicaid is the largest single payer. Fees paid directly by participants and families are the second largest source. Most adult day care centers patch together funds from several sources, including Title III of the Older Americans Act, Title XX social service block grants, Veterans Affairs contracts, state and local mental health and developmentally disabled programs, United Way, long-term care insurance, private foundations grants, and fundraising activities (National Adult Day Services Association, 1996).

Adult day services are defined and regulated by states. Unlike services paid for by Medicare, there is no federal definition, delineated conditions of participation, or data base. Thirty-four states license adult day services, but the remaining sixteen do not. Each state thus defines adult day services and establishes its own licensing requirements.

In 1999, the Commission for the Accreditation of Rehabilitation Facilities (CARF) initiated an accreditation program for adult day services. The accreditation standards use the levels-of-care framework established by the National Adult Day Services Association.

Clients

Those who attend adult day services programs are typically in fragile mental or physical condition, or both. Clients range from those who have only physical problems, such as stroke victims with compromised mobility, to those who are physically able but have cognitive impairments, such as Alzheimer's disease or developmental disabilities, to individuals with both physical and mental impairments. The common characteristic is the inability to manage ADLs or IADLs independently.

About half of adult day services participants suffer from cognitive impairment; an additional one-third have Alzheimer's disease or related disorders (National Adult Day Services Association, 1996). Nearly sixty percent require assistance in two or more activi-

Table 11.14. Services Provided by Adult Day Services Programs

Services	Models		
	Core	**Enhanced**	**Intensive**
Assessment and individualized plan of care	X	X	X
Therapeutic recreational activities	X	X	X
Assistance with ADLs	X	X	X
Health-related services: health care coordination, illness prevention, and health education not requiring licensed health care professional	X	X	X
Social services • Referral to community services • Individual or group counseling	X	X X	X X
Nutrition/food services • Meals and/or snacks • Screening, assessment, development, and monitoring of nutrition plan of care by professional	X	X	X X
Transportation: arranging or providing	X	X	X
Emergency care: procedures for responding to participant's need for emergency care	X	X	X
Nursing services • Assessment, monitoring, and intervention on moderate basis • Medications management • Nursing services of a more intensive nature, including skilled nursing services		X X X	X X X
Physical, occupational, and speech therapy • At a functional maintenance level • At a restorative or rehabilitative level		X	X X
Other specialized supportive services as needed (e.g., psychiatric evaluation and consultation)			X

SOURCE: *Standards and Guidelines for Adult Day Services*, NADSA, NCoA, 1997.

ties of daily living. One-fourth rely on a cane or walker; many are wheelchair-bound.

The majority of participants come for an indefinite period of time; however, some come only during the recuperative period of an acute episode of illness until they have regained independence in physical or mental functioning. Clients may attend every day of the week or just select days, depending upon the caregiver's needs.

The average age of participants is seventy-six years (National Adult Day Services Association, 1999). Two-thirds of all participants are women. Two-thirds of participants live with a spouse, adult children, or other family or friends; one-fourth live alone.

Table 11.15. Service Snapshot: Adult Day Services

Number of centers	4,000 (est.), located in all 50 states
Capacity	160,000 total enrollees (est.)
Average enrollment/center	40
Average daily attendance	22
Average daily charges	$43; range $30–$90
Major revenue sources	Medicaid, private fees, grants, philanthropy
Licensure	State health or social services department
Certification	Medicaid (in select states)
Accreditation	Commission on Accreditation of Rehabilitation Facilities (CARF), initiated in 1999

SOURCE: Tedesco, J. (2001). Adult day services. In C. Evashwick (Ed.), *The continuum of long-term care.* (2nd ed.). Albany, NY: Delmar Thomson Learning.

Those served by adult day services include families as well as the participants themselves. Adult day services make it possible for many people to maintain their loved ones in their home the majority of the time, while having the assistance they need to be able to work, manage family responsibilities, and have a moment of respite.

Sources of Information

The National Adult Day Services Association (NADSA) is the national association compiling data and information on day care services. It is a unit of the National Council on Aging (NCOA).

Housing

Housing is an integral component of the continuum of long-term care (Pynoos, 2001). The physical features of housing affect the ability of the occupants to care for themselves and maintain their independence. Conversely, the housing environment can create an enabling or an at-risk circumstance for those whose ability to manage the activities of daily living is compromised.

Housing that incorporates services and that is purposely designed to be supportive to those with functional disabilities has become increasingly available and important. As federal and state regulations for Medicare and Medicaid reimbursement have limited the accessibility of nursing facilities, supportive housing facilities have evolved as lower-cost, lower-intensity alternatives.

National Profile

Supportive housing is manifested by a variety of physical facilities and service arrangements, ranging from free-standing single family homes located in communities catering to older adults to small rooms in family-run board and care homes. The goal of supportive housing is to enable residents to maintain independence; services and physical environment are designed to accomplish this goal.

Supportive housing typically does not offer medical services, except for multi-level complexes that include skilled nursing units. Rather, it tends to offer physical or personal assistance to those who need help performing the ADLs or IADLs, as well as opportunities for socialization and recreational activities. Table 11.16 lists the range of housing types and the independence level of residents.

There is no single source of data on supportive housing, and even aggregating data that do exist overlooks many facilities. Rough estimates indicate that at least six million people reside in supportive housing—four times the number who reside in nursing homes.

Operating Characteristics

Housing types vary so greatly that a single service snapshot is not helpful. Table 11.17 highlights characteristics of different types of housing.

For any type of independent housing, physical adaptations and on-site services may be few or many—but they are the responsibility of the individual and family,

Table 11.16.   The Continuum of Housing

Housing Options for Seniors	Level of Functional Ability								
	Independent			Semi-independent			Dependent		
Community-based single family housing	X	X	X	X	X				
Community-based apartment dwelling	X	X	X	X	X	X			
Granny Flat/Echo Housing/Accessory Unit		X	X	X	X				
Shared housing		X	X	X	X				
Retirement community (age 55+)	X	X	X	X	X				
Age-segregated apartment dwelling		X	X	X	X				
Continuing Care Retirement Community (CCRC)			X	X	X	X	X	X	X
Congregate housing (20+ units)			X	X	X	X			
Board and care home					X	X			
Assisted living (personal care) complex					X	X	X		
Foster care					X	X			
Intermediate nursing care							X		
Skilled nursing care								X	X

SOURCE: Pynoos, J. (2001). Housing. In C. Evashwick (Ed.), *The continuum of long-term care* (2nd ed.). Albany, NY: Delmar Thomson Learning.

Table 11.17.   Typical Characteristics of Multiunit Supportive Housing

Type of Housing	Residents	Payment Sources	Typical Cost per Month	Services Available On-Site

Independent
  Private
  Public
	Wide mix
	Low-income
		Tenant
		Tenant,
		  HUD subsidies
			Full range
			30% of income
				Very limited or none
				Service coordination, limited services

Congregate Housing Services Program	Moderate ADL and IADL dependency	Tenant, HUD subsidies	30% of income	Service coordination, meals, transportation, homemaker
Assisted Living	High levels of ADL dependency and cognitive impairment	Tenant, Medicaid waivers	$1,400–2,500	Medication management, personal care, meals, housekeeping, unscheduled assistance, preventative care, transportation
Continuing Care Retirement Communities	Middle to upper income	Tenant	$800–2,000 plus buy-in	Medical services, meals, building maintenance, housekeeping, social activities, transportation

SOURCE: Pynoos, J. (2001). Housing. In C. Evashwick (Ed.), *The continuum of long-term care* (2nd ed.). Albany, NY: Delmar Thomson Learning.

both to organize and to pay for. In the past few years, "smart homes" have become very creative in incorporating a wide array of in-home modifications and creative designs to facilitate independent functioning.

Housing options designed specifically for those with functional disabilities include categories such as assisted living, congregate care, group family homes, and board and care homes. These environments typically offer meals, housekeeping, laundry, transportation, twenty-four-hour security, social and recreational activities, and emergency call assistance. Medication management and personal assistance for ADLs or IADLs are also offered by many. Services may be included in the basic monthly charge, or may be added as specific fees based on the resident's needs. Although some homes have licensed health care personnel such as registered nurses, the majority do not offer services required to be delivered by licensed staff. Staffing is therefore modest.

Unlike health services, many forms of housing are not licensed or regulated by government, except with regard to construction. States may license supportive housing under categories other than health care, such as residential care, under the department of social services. However, each state or locality establishes its own definitions and regulations.

Most housing is also paid for by the individual. The Department of Housing and Urban Development (HUD) supports 20,000 housing complexes throughout the United States, some of which are targeted for seniors or those with disabilities. However, HUD's primary function is to support the availability of housing for low-income residents, not those requiring long-term care. HUD is precluded from offering services in its facilities. It does, however, offer rent subsidies. Select other federal programs and various state programs also provide rent subsidies or low-income housing that may be used by those who need long-term care.

Clients

The residents of housing are as varied in their needs as the types of housing in which they reside. The commonality is that those who need other services of the continuum of long-term care must consider their physical environment as an integral part of their long-range plan of care. The environment can be adapted to help a person with functional disabilities to maintain his or her independence. Alternatively, a poor environment can result in injury or incapacitation, causing an individual to require hospital or nursing home services.

Sources of Information

The American Association of Homes and Services for the Aging (AAHSA) and the American Health Care Association (AHCA) are the trade associations that represent, respectively, not-for-profit and for-profit nursing homes and supportive housing facilities. Assisted Living Facilities of America (ALFA) is a trade association for assisted living complexes. Each of these associations has extensive information available. The American College of Health Care Administrators (ACHCA) is the professional association for executives who head supportive housing and nursing facilities.

FINANCING

Financing is one of the primary problems inhibiting the provision and organization of long-term care on a coordinated, continuing basis. To understand the challenges of changing long-term care financing to facilitate the ideal continuum of care, an understanding of current financing is essential. Long-term care is not a single category of service, so singular and complete data are not readily available.

National Health Expenditures

Table 11.18 shows National Health Expenditures for 1998. The United States spent $1.15 trillion on personal health care expenditures (NCHS, 2000a). Of personal health care expenditures, more than one-third ($383 billion) was spent on hospitals, and about twenty-two percent ($230 billion) was spent on physicians. Medication was the third largest category, at $122 billion. The amounts spent on nursing home care and home health care were, respectively, $88 and $29 billion.

Table 11.18. National Health Care Expenditures, by Category, 1998 (numbers in millions, rounded)

Category	$ in Million	Percent
All expenditures	$1,149	100.0
Health services and supplies	1,114	96.9
Personal health care	1,019	88.7
Hospital care	383	33.3
Physician services	230	20.0
Dentist services	54	4.7
Nursing home care	88	7.6
Other professional services	67	5.8
Home health care	29	2.5
Drugs	122	10.6
Vision products	16	1.3
Other personal health	32	2.8
Program administration	58	5.0
Public health	37	3.2
Research and construction	35	3.1
Research	20	1.7
Construction	16	1.3

SOURCE: National Center for Health Statistics (2000). *Health, United States, 2000.* Hyattsville, MD: Public Health Service.

Payers

As with understanding the clients of long-term care or the array of formal long-term care services, describing the financing of long-term care is another mosaic of varied pieces. Much long-term care is provided *by friends and families*, and no consensus prevails about how to calculate the costs of these services. (Studies about the cost to employers of labor lost by caregivers are the most precise.) Many services are also paid for privately, and data on these costs are difficult to obtain, typically relying upon the client or family member's memory. *Nursing homes and home health care agencies* are assumed to provide a high proportion of long-term care clients, so data about these services are often used as proxies for long-term care expenditures. Although Medicare only covers acute care, those age sixty-five and older have many chronic conditions, so Medicare data present insights into the financing of

care for a segment of the population that extensively uses long-term care. Medicaid, although limited to those low in income, covers long-term nursing home care and home care, so these data, too, contribute to the overall picture. Table 11.19 shows the disparate amounts paid by the primary payers for four major categories of personal health care expenditures.

The following highlights dollars spent in recent years. Later in the chapter, the section on policy discusses the policy implications of long-term care financing.

Public Programs

As noted above, Medicare is the primary payer for those age sixty-five and older who are major users of both acute and long-term care. Medicare expenditures for 1998 totaled $213 billion (NCHS, 2000a, 2000b). Of the Medicare expenditures, only six percent were spent on nursing home care, and less than three percent on home health care.

Expenditures for Medicaid, the federal program for low-income people that is matched by state funds, were a market contrast. Of the $142 billion spent in 1998 by Medicaid, nearly twenty-nine percent of expenditures were for skilled nursing and intermediate care facilities, and an additional two percent were for home health care (NCHS, 2000a, 2000b). In some states, Medicaid nursing home care is the largest single item in the state budget.

Other federal programs that pay for long-term care services include the Older Americans Act, the Veterans Affairs health and housing programs, and Social Security Title XX. Numerous states and local programs also support long-term care.

Payment for long-term care is complicated by the fact that each state has its own payment system. Even within federal programs such as Medicaid and Title XX, each state decides which services it will pay for and what type of payment system to use. The most progressive systems base payment on client acuity levels. As states move toward Medicaid managed care, flat capitated rates are being implemented. Within a given state, payment may also vary from one locality to another.

Table 11.19. Expenditures on Hospital Care, Nursing Home Care, Physican Services, and All Other Personal Health Care Expenditures, 1998

	Percent Distribution of Expenditures				
	Hospital	Nursing Home Care	Physician Services	Other Personal Health Care	Total
Out-of-pocket payments	3.4	32.5	15.6	38.4	19.6
Private health insurance	30.8	5.3	50.5	30.8	33.1
Other private funds	5.0	1.8	2.0	4.0	3.7
Government					
Total	60.8	60.4	31.9	26.8	43.6
Medicaid	15.9	46.3	6.5	13.5	33.7
Medicare	32.4	11.9	21.5	8.4	9.9
Total dollars in billions	$383	$88	$230	$319	$1,019

SOURCE: *Health, United States 2000.* (DHHS Pub. No. 00-1232, Table 119), National Center for Health Statistics, July 2000, Hyattsville, MD: Public Health Service.

Private Insurance

Standard commercial health insurance and managed-care health plans are oriented primarily to cover acute care services and/or have a cap on the amount of extended care that is covered. Long-term care insurance is designed specifically to cover the services needed by those with long-term disabilities.

By the end of the twentieth century, approximately six million of the 256 million U.S. residents owned long-term care insurance policies (Health Insurance Association of America, 2000). Although the overall proportion is quite small, the increase in policyholders during the last few years of the 1990s was exponential. Long-term care insurance has been available since the early 1980s. However, policies were very expensive and very constricted in coverage. During the latter part of the 1990s, policies became broader and more flexible in coverage, and sales to groups, rather than individuals, contributed to lower administrative costs and greater outreach, including to younger markets.

The long-term actuarial projections on which the premiums for long-term care insurance are based do not necessarily reflect a health care system in flux, and the relatively few people using benefits mean that experience is light. The structure and costs of long-term care insurance will likely change as the long-term care system itself changes in the availability and affordability of services and as insurance companies acquire more experience on which to base premium calculation.

Service Payment Sources

Accessing the funds required for the long-term care support for any given individual requires expertise in merging complex payment streams. Similarly, managing long-term care services, whether individually or as part of a continuum, involves dealing with multiple payer organizations. As shown in Table 11.19 and the service snapshots, each of the major services of the continuum of care is paid by different configurations of multiple sources. Each payer has its own payment system, client eligibility requirements, and payment rate.

Several issues are noteworthy. First, although Medicare is limited by law primarily to acute care, it is a major source of funding for major long-term care services. Second, combining services into a single efficient operation presents a significant administrative challenge when the financing is so varied. Third, when so much care is paid for by public programs that are governed by strict and often inconsistent regulations, achieving the flexibility and options needed by an individual client and family may be extremely difficult.

INTEGRATING MECHANISMS

For a continuum of care to function as a system of care rather than as a collection of fragmented services, integrating mechanisms are essential. As described earlier, these include (1) an internal organization that coordinates the operations of various services; (2) a management information system that integrates clinical, utilization, and financial data and follows clients across settings; (3) a case management/care coordination program that coordinates care across services; and (4) a financing mechanism that enables the flexibility of funds across services. These integrating mechanisms are in various stages of development; few comprehensive systems that include all of these components exist. Considerable advancement was made, however, during the decade of the 1990s. The Balanced Budget Act of 1997 caused a temporary setback. However, the need for integration from the client's perspective remains.

Interentity Structure

Interentity planning and administration must be structured both within an organization and across organizations. Client services are not likely to be coordinated unless the units that are providing the services are coordinated administratively, particularly when budgeting and financial issues arise. A person with a hip fracture may be cared for by the emergency room, acute care inpatient unit, skilled nursing facility, rehabilitation hospital or unit, home health agency, and durable medical equipment company. Even when all of these services are within the same parent organization, the client fills out admissions papers six different times, deals with six different sets of clinicians and administrators, and receives bills from six distinct provider entities.

Administrative structures are necessary for a continuum of care to (1) ensure channels of commu-

nication and cooperation; (2) establish clear lines of authority, accountability, and responsibility for client services; (3) negotiate budgets and financial trade-offs; (4) address issues of risk management and liability; and (5) present a cohesive, consistent message in interactions with external agencies and the community.

Administrative mechanisms within an organization that promote seamless functioning of a continuum of care include those listed below:

- a designated senior administrator responsible for decisions that affect several different departments or units
- an integrated budget that recognizes the contribution of each unit to the performance of the whole, including losses in one unit that produce larger gains in another unit
- interdepartmental/interentity planning teams and committees that cut across service areas
- interdisciplinary and interdepartmental task forces focusing on specific short-term issues
- product line management or a matrix structure that spans internal and external service units organized as a continuum of care

The organizational issues inherent in operating an efficient continuum of care began to be articulated during the late 1980s and 1990s (Evashwick, 1997; Rundall & Evashwick, 2001). Experts studied health care systems and physician groups (Coddington, Moore, & Fischer, 1994; Gillies, Shortell, Anderson, Mitchell, & Morgan, 1993). National associations delineated criteria for integration (The Catholic Health Association, 1993, 1995). The Joint Commission on Accreditation of Healthcare Organizations added a segment on integration to its organizational analysis. The National Chronic Care Consortium (NCCC) arose as a cooperative of members that spearheads initiatives regarding integrating financing and organization between acute and long-term care. The NCCC has developed the SASI (Self-Assessment for Systems Integration) tool for measuring an organization's structural and process readiness for integration (National Chronic Care Consortium, 1996).

Today's organizations that exemplify continuum structure are ones that have evolved over time with gradual modifications. Only as research and evaluation entities have articulated requisite administration structures and as the other three integrating mechanisms have evolved to the stage of being practical realities have organizations realized that they must consciously implement internal management structures in order to maximize the benefits of comprehensiveness, continuity, and integration offered by a continuum of care.

Integrated Information Systems

Integrated information systems are necessary for efficient management of the continuum. In order to implement quality assurance and utilization review programs, assess efficiency of operations, track and aggregate client experiences, and calculate the long-term costs of care, comprehensive and integrated data systems and accompanying management reporting systems are imperative. Many health and social service organizations still maintain separate clinical, financial, and utilization data systems. During the late 1990s, hospitals began to develop data systems to integrate the multiple components of inpatient and outpatient records. Nursing homes were forced to computerize patient records due to reporting requirements specified in the Omnibus Budget Reconciliation Act of 1987 (OBRA 1987). Home health agencies were required by Medicare to computerize their records as part of the Balanced Budget Act of 1997. However, many small organizations—particularly social service agencies, small community-based agencies, and housing facilities—still do not have computerized clinical records. Despite the advances in technology, very few health care organizations maintain data on clients as they move from one service to another, such as from acute hospital care to home care.

The ideal information system for a continuum of care was conceptualized in the mid-1980s (Zawadski, 2001). However, the computer technology to make such a system feasible and affordable depended on (1) the development of new computer chips with expanded capacity and networking capability, which occurred during the latter part of the 1980s, and (2) on the establishment of the Internet, which became widely available in the latter half of the 1990s. The proliferation of search engines and the move to open architecture made interface of existing systems possible. Figure 11.5 schematically shows an ideal integrated patient record (Zawadski, 2001).

Today, information systems that combine the financial, clinical, or utilization aspects of a client's care across settings have been designed and are slowly being implemented. Payers and utilization review companies have enhanced their databases and tracking programs to evaluate the cost of caring for a client through an episode of illness. And evaluators have specified criteria for quality that depend upon tracking client data over time and on a community-wide basis. Nonetheless, a host of barriers to integrated information systems remain, ranging from the high cost of search engines to issues of patient confidentiality to human resource training.

Care Coordination

The clinical care for a person in the continuum must be coordinated over time, across settings, and among various professionals. Several techniques have evolved for doing so: case management, interdisciplinary teams, clinical liaisons, single-entry access points, extended care pathways and disease-management programs are among the most common.

The most common form of care coordination is case management. This is also referred to as a service coordination or care management, and occasionally by other terms. The purpose of case management is to work directly with clients and families over time to assist them in arranging and managing the complex set of resources that the client requires to maintain health and independent functioning. Case management seeks to achieve the maximum cost-effective use of scarce resources by helping clients get the health, social, and support services most appropriate for their needs at a given time. It guides the client and family through the maze of services, matches service need with funding authorization, and coordinates with clinicians and provider organizations.

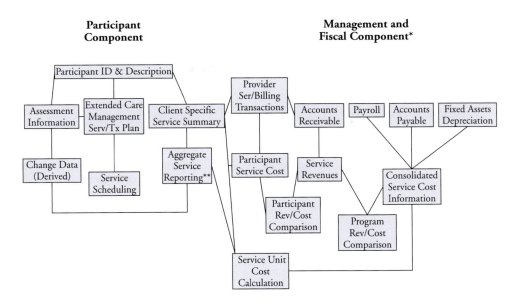

Figure 11.5.   Model Integrated Information System for a Chronic Care Organization

SOURCE: Zawadski, R. (2001). Information Systems. In C. Evashwick, (Ed.), *The continuum of long-term care* (2nd ed.). Albany, NY: Delmar Thomson Learning. Reprinted courtesy of Delmar Thomson Learning.

Case management is defined as a process (White & Gundrum, 2001). The components are:

- assessment
- care planning
- arranging services
- monitoring
- reassessment

Assessment is usually done by a multidisciplinary team that includes a nurse, a social worker, a physician, and other professionals as indicated by the conditions of the particular client. When possible, assessment includes evaluation of the home environment and family situation. Based on the results of the assessment, the team concurs on a specific plan of action and recommends an array of appropriate services.

The ongoing case manager may be a nurse, social workers, or health care professional trained specifi-

cally as a case manager. The case manager is responsible for arranging the services ordered by the team and maintaining contact with the client and the service providers to confirm that services are being delivered and are meeting the client's needs. Reassessment of the client's status occurs either according to a regularly scheduled checkup with the clinicians or when the case manager detects a change that warrants reevaluation. Long-term case management is distinguished from short-term service arrangement by intensity, breadth of services encompassed, and duration (Applebaum & Austin, 1990).

Table 11.20 shows the characteristics of different types of case managers and illuminates the dimensions that categorize case management programs: funding/reimbursement, targeting, gatekeeping, and organizational auspices (White & Gundrum, 2001).

The authority of the case manager to arrange service use varies. Three basic models exist: broker, service

Table 11.20. Summary of Case Management Types and Key Characteristics

Type	Population	Setting	Focus	Financing
Medical				
Primary Care	Patients	Dr. office; clinics	Prevent; diagnose; treat; monitor	Private pay; insurance; Medicare; Medicaid
Acute Care	Patients	Hospital; acute, subacute facilities	Facilitate flow of care; discharge; prevent readmission	Private pay; insurance; Medicare; Medicaid
Other Medical (including home health)	Medically dependent, complex or problems facility	Skilled nursing facility; home, special	Treat; monitor; supervise; prevent; rehabilitate	Private pay; insurance; Medicare; Medicaid
Managed Care	Enrollees; high risk, high cost	Primary/acute settings	Authorize, verify services and utilization; manage benefits/costs	Private pay; employer; Medicare; Medicaid
Long-Term Care Insurance	Enrollees	Home; assisted living; skilled nursing facility	Authorize, verify services and utilization; manage benefits/costs	Private pay
Non-Medical				
Community/ In-Home	Community functional/ cognitive disability	Non-institutional	Coordinate wide range of non-medical care; keep independent	Private pay; waiver funds; grants/ contracts
Nursing Facility	On-going need for care, supervision; chronic problems	In-home, community or facility	Monitor, prevent decline; link to needed resources	Private pay; some insurance; waiver funds; grants/contracts
Mental Health	Complex, chronic psychiatric problems	In-home community-based group home	Education; life skills, adaptation; compliance monitoring	Private pay; some insurance; some Medicare; Medicaid; grants/contracts
Other	Usually well; need advice, counseling	Community	Resource/service information, referrals	Private pay; grants/ contracts

SOURCE: White, M. & Gundrum, G. (2001). Case management. In C. Evashwick (Ed.), *The continuum of long-term care* (2nd ed.). Albany, NY: Delmar Thomson Learning.

management, and managed care (Applebaum & Austin, 1990). Under the broker model, case managers identify needed services and make referrals but have no authority over service delivery. With service management, the case manager has authority over payment but usually has a capitated or predetermined cap

limiting how much can be spent. Managed care places the provider at risk, and thus the case manager has no set cap but clear financial incentives to use resources carefully and wisely.

A case manager can handle twenty to eighty active clients, depending on the breadth and intensity of the program, the dependence level of the clients, and the organizational resources supporting the care coordination operations.

The fee for case management is $50 to $150 for an initial assessment, and then a lesser fee for ongoing monthly service or follow-up consultation. Medicare does not pay for care coordination except under home health or as a physician activity. A case management program may be paid for entirely or partially by certain state government programs, such as Medicaid, Title XX, mental health, or Older Americans Act funds; demonstration grants; private moneys, such as grants, foundations, or donations; select insurance companies who now cover this as a benefit; or directly by clients or families.

During the past decade, the providers and payers of health care have recognized the need to develop a cost-effective means of dealing with the complexity of a clients' ongoing needs for comprehensive, continuing care. Case management has the potential to coordinate an array of resources, both within a given organization and externally in other community agencies, and to make astute use of a variety of financial resources to maximize the care affordable by the client. The trend to recognize the distinct role of a case manager/care coordinator is further enhanced by the expansion of health care organizations into continuums of care, with more than a single type of service available within the same organization and with a pool of funds for health and social support services to be spent at the discretion of the provider.

Case management is likely to become even more prevalent in the future as part of the expansion of integrated health care delivery systems and capitated managed-care arrangements. Its cost-effectiveness will likely continue to be examined, and refinement and streamlining of the models will likely continue to occur.

Integrated Financing

Comprehensive, flexible, and adequate financing is a goal of the ideal continuum. This is the single component of the continuum of care most critical and most challenging in the twenty-first century. As with many other areas of health care, delivery system changes will be driven by financial incentives. The problems of fragmented financing were previously highlighted in the chapter. For a continuum to achieve the desired access to the full spectrum of long-term care services, financial barriers must not dominate placement and resource allocation decisions. Several trends and demonstrations offer hope that the financing of long-term care is moving in the direction required for the continuum.

The number of seniors enrolled in HMOs continues to increase. In 1990, 2,138,000 people, or approximately 6.7 percent of seniors, were enrolled in HMOs (Office of Prepaid Health Care Operations and Oversight, 1991). By 1999, 6.5 million seniors were enrolled in 273 Medicare-certified health plans, for a total of thirteen percent of those age sixty-five and older (Health Care Financing Administration, 1999; National Center for Health Statistics, 2000b). Many people under age sixty-five with chronic illnesses are also enrolled in HMOs, and the enrollment of younger adults also continues to increase.

As currently structured, HMOs are not required specifically to offer a comprehensive continuum of care nor to provide ongoing services for chronic problems. Nor do they coordinate care and monitor use as ideally as they might. However, many offer a fairly broad array of services. And, as evidenced by the experience of the S/HMOs described below, they do have a structure that can be expanded into an integrated continuum when the market and financial incentives are right.

Social HMOs, or S/HMOs, were begun in 1985 by the HCFA as a demonstration project. The purpose of the S/HMO was to examine the utilization and relative cost-effectiveness of a capitated payment system that includes chronic and extended benefits as well as medical services. The HCFA described the model as follows (Health Care Financing Administration, 1991a):

> The S/HMO model includes four basic organizational and financing features. First, a single organizational structure provides a full range of acute and long term care services to voluntarily enrolled Medicare beneficiaries. Beneficiaries pay a monthly premium for services. In addition to the basic Medicare

benefits, services include nursing home, home health, homemaker, transportation, drugs, and others. Second, a coordinated case management system is used to authorize long term care services for those members who meet specific disability criteria, within a fixed limit of about $6,000–$12,000 per year. Third, the S/HMOs are designed to serve a cross-section of the elderly population, including both the functionally impaired and unimpaired elderly. Fourth, financing is accomplished through prepaid capitation by pooling funds from Medicare, Medicaid and member premiums. The initial financial risk was shared by the S/HMOs and HCFA. After 30 months of the demonstration, the S/HMO sites assume full financial risk for service costs.

Three of the four original S/HMOs have endured into the twenty-first century: Kaiser Permanente in Portland, Oregon; Metropolitan Jewish Geriatric Center in Brooklyn, New York; and Senior Health Action Network (SCAN) in Long Beach, California. In the mid-1990s, the demonstration was extended and authorized to add new sites, with revised formulae for calculating payments. As of this writing, the six newly authorized sites have not yet opened, and the payment structure continues to be highly complex.

Rigorous evaluation of the S/HMOs has been minimal. In brief, the experiment by the federal government of funding both acute and long-term care through a single health plan remains more demonstration than norm.

The Program of All-Inclusive Care for the Elderly (PACE) is another program initially funded by HCFA. It began as a demonstration during the early 1990s to test a variation of a capitated payment program linked with a service system for the chronically ill. PACE attempts to replicate On-Lok, a program serving the Chinese community of San Francisco that centers around adult day care. On-Lok and its replicated sites organize a continuum of care for an extremely frail elderly population at considerably less than the cost of care for a comparably ill population which is not part of an organized system of care. The HCFA described the original model as follows (Health Care Financing Administration, 1991b):

[It] includes as core services the provision of adult day health care and multi-disciplinary team case management through which access to and allocation of all health and long term care services are arranged. Physician, therapeutic, ancillary, and social support services are provided on site at the adult day health center whenever possible. Hospital, nursing home, home health, and other specialized services are provided extramurally. Transportation is also provided to all enrolled members who require it. Financing is accomplished through prospective capitation of both Medicare and Medicaid payments to the provider.

PACE differs from the S/HMO in that it focuses only on frail, elderly people who are eligible for nursing home placement, while the S/HMO attempts to get a representative population over which to spread the risk of service use. Each PACE site serves 120–325 people, compared to the 5,000–10,000 served by each S/HMO. The provider network of PACE is smaller, more tightly controlled, and focuses around adult day care. Finally, the financial arrangements are different. PACE receives a capitated amount from Medicare and Medicaid for a frail, high-use population and may also charge private pay clients on a sliding scale basis. The S/HMO functions more like an HMO, charging enrollees premiums and negotiating with Medicare and Medicaid for capitated payments based on a healthy population. The Balanced Budget Act of 1997 authorized PACE as a reimburseable service under Medicare, thereby moving the program from demonstration to permanent status.

Both S/HMOs and PACE are efforts to combine acute care and long-term care funding into an integrated system that enables a care manager to allocate resources according to need, rather than by the constraints of fragmented financing.

Long-term care insurance emerged during the late 1980s as another way to fund long-term care. By 1994, 121 companies offered some type of long-term care product (Health Insurance Association of America, 2000). The number of people who had purchased policies grew from 815,000 in 1987 to over 1.65 million in June 1990 and to 6 million by 2000. A major trend has been to market long-term care insurance to younger adults as part of employer-sponsored benefit packages. Long-term care insurance aids the development of comprehensive financing for a continuum of services. For those who have Medicare Part A and Part B or indemnity insurance to cover acute services, long-term care insurance offers complementary coverage for the long-term, ongoing services.

When long-term care insurance policies began to be sold in the early 1980s, they reflected acute care health insurance by paying based on diagnosis and use of limited services, specifically either nursing homes or home health. By the early 1990s, the policies had changed to be based on functional disability and to pay on a per diem basis. Payout of such policies is typically based on being functionally disabled, not having a specific disease. The recipient can spend the daily allotment to pay for whatever services they choose to use, including skilled nursing facilities, home health, homemakers, assisted living, or other formal or informal home support services.

Although reaching only a very small number of people, the public programs and trends in private insurance and HMOs portend positively for future financial flexibility that will enable a continuum of care to integrate services according to client need rather than categorical funding.

Continuing Care Retirement Communities (CCRCs) offer a housing-based model of a continuum of care. Financing is integrated from private sources: buy-in fees, ongoing monthly payments, fee-for-service charges, and possibly long-term care insurance or annuity payouts, with an underlying base of an insurance model.

Typically, residents who have little or no need for assistance with ADLs or IADLs buy in to a housing unit of the CCRC, which may range from a house to a full apartment to a modified apartment. A monthly fee is charged in addition to the buy-in. Services are arranged by the housing provider and are increased as a resident's needs increase. For example, the CCRC may have its own home health agency and could provide in-home skilled care or support services as needed. Different levels of housing are available on the same campus, so a resident may move into smaller quarters as his or her need for services increases. Additional fees may or may not be charged as service and housing levels change.

The CCRC coordinates both care and financing. Because CCRCs are private pay, no external authorities regulate eligibility for services or restrict the flow of funds. Except for acute hospital care, most types of care are provided on the same campus, so continuity of staff and records is relatively easy to achieve.

The CCRC model is complex in that it involves housing, hospitality, health, and social services, a combination of insurance and fee-for-service payments, and business as well as care regulatory scrutiny from state and local authorities. CCRCs provide evidence that continuum of care models do exist that have achieved integration of services in a cost-effective manner while enabling those needing long-term care to maximize their independence and remain in a home setting.

PUBLIC POLICY ISSUES

The public policy issues related to long-term care are complex, reflecting the diversity and breadth of the field. The United States has no single national policy on long-term care. Many policies have resulted from the advocacy of a specific client group and relate only to the needs of that group. The legislative thrust of policies tends to be one of four types: financing, direct service provision, regulation, or resource generation. Public policies are implemented by units of government, and they tend to apply only to the unit governed (although some federal policies involve state application). In brief, a comprehensive description of public policy would cover the issues pertaining to each target group, service and integrating mechanism at federal, state, and local levels for financing, regulatory, resource, and service arenas. Table 11.21 lists major federal legislation pertaining to long-term care. Note the varied foci of the laws.

This section highlights critical policy issues that should be considered by those involved in creating or managing a continuum of long-term care.

This section highlights fundamental policy issues that should be considered by those involved in creating or managing a continuum of long-term care.

The resolution of the issues identified in the following text is likely to take place gradually. Great impetus for major change may await the explosion of

Table 11.21. Major Federal Legislation Pertaining to Long-Term Care

Social Security Act, 1935
Veterans Administration, 1963, 1972, 1975, 1980
Mental Health Acts, 1963, 1967, 1971, 1986
Title XVIII (Medicare), Social Security Act, 1965
Title XIX (Medicaid), Social Security Act, 1965
Older Americans Act, 1965
Housing and Urban Development Act, 1965, 1974
Developmental Disabilities Services and Facilities Act, 1970
Title XVI (Supplemental Security Income), Social Security Act, 1972
Rehabilitation Act, 1973
Title XX, Social Security Act, 1974
Omnibus Budget Reconciliation Act, 1987
Medicare Catastrophic Coverage Act, 1988 (repealed, 1990)
Americans with Disabilities Act, 1990
Patient Self-Determination Act, 1991
Family Medical Leave Act, 1993
Health Insurance Portability and Accountability Act, 1996
Balanced Budget Act, 1997
National Caregiver Support Act, 2000

demand that will accompany the graying of the Baby Boom generation. In either case, managers must be aware that legislation and regulations may appear in any or all of the following areas, pertaining to any subset of the target population, and directed at any individual type of service provider or payer.

Financing

Financing is one of the primary challenges to providing long-term care on a coordinated, continuing basis. The definition of a continuum of care assumes: (1) adequate financing available to provide clients with an array of needed health, mental health, and social services; (2) access to such financing; and (3) the flexibility to apply funds in a variety of ways as needed by a given individual. At national and local levels, the current mechanisms of financing inhibit the operation of a continuum of care.

- The federal government does not have a national policy or program that funds long-term care.

- The cost of a universal long-term care program paid for by government funds is likely to prohibit a national policy from being developed in the foreseeable future.

- States fund a great deal of long-term care through Medicaid, Title XX, the Older Americans Act, and state programs, but funds are categorical, and each state creates its own program of services, eligibility, and payment systems.

- Most providers do not have control over all the pertinent financing streams, thus limiting their ability to pool funds and allocate resources from an internal process to match a client's needs with appropriate care.

- Much of the long-term care is paid for by individuals. In effect, the national policy on long-term care is to leave care to the responsibility of individuals and families with states, primarily through Medicaid, as a backup.

In outlining the considerations for a national health policy that would cover long-term care, the Pepper Commission of 1989 estimated the cost at $43 billion (U.S. Bipartisan Commission on Comprehensive Health Care, 1991). This represented about half of the total amount spent by Medicare in 1990 and ten times the amount Medicare spent on nursing home and home care. The amount was viewed as prohibitively expensive for a nationwide program. The Medicare Catastrophic Care Act of 1988 approached the long-term care arena by incrementally expanding select Medicare benefits. Funding relied on taxing the older population. The opposition by seniors was so great that the law was quickly repealed. In the early 1990s, the costs of long-term care were dealt a further blow by being excluded from President Clinton's proposal for national health reform. Although the total reform initiative failed, the fact that long-term care had been dropped before the program got to its final stages further indicates the high cost, the uncertainty, and the general preference of the nation that long-term care remain the responsibility of states and individuals. This is reinforced by the health priorities of the Bush administration, which focus on Medicare pharmaceutical costs and Social Security reform, with no mention of long-term care.

Fragmentation

As is evident from the discussion of services, the continuum of care consists of a myriad of different services provided by many organizations, each governed by several different public and/or private sources. To provide any type of comprehensive, continuous care requires achieving cohesion. At the same time, flexibility must be maintained in order to tailor the program to the unique needs of each individual. Individual service providers and agencies must cooperate and share common goals. Although this is readily acknowledged, establishing the mechanisms to achieve such cooperation and sharing requires overcoming history and learned preference, state, local, and federal regulations, and a myriad of other operational barriers.

Funding for long-term care services comes from health, mental health, social service, public welfare, social security, and housing programs, to mention only the main public funding sources. Individuals, families, employers, and a variety of insurers and managed-care companies represent the private side. Each payer, whether private or public, has distinct requirements. Administration of long-term care services, particularly those that are paid for by public sources, reflects the financing fragmentation. For example, four or five different state agencies may be involved in paying for home health services. Regulation, including state licensure, is similarly divided among multiple government authorities. Fragmentation of delivery is likely to continue as long as the regulatory authorities and funding streams remain fragmented.

The intent of the continuum of care is to be able to pool funding streams and service availability in order to provide the care required by an individual. Putting in place the mechanisms to do this is the leading challenge of the twenty-first century. Several states have initiated programs to combine funds at the state agency level. Wisconsin and Minnesota are among those that have pooled dollars and authorities at the state level. As states move their Medicaid recipients into managed care, additional opportunities may arise to pool funding streams for long-term and acute care. Trends toward capitated financing for both Medicaid and Medicare are encouraging as eventual platforms for achieving integrated financing, which will facilitate the integration of long-term care services.

Availability and Accessibility

For years, the cry in the community-based, long-term care arena was that services were simply not available. During the 1980s, the nation made great progress in this area. As can be noted from the earlier section on individual services, the number of providers grew during the 1980s and 1990s: home health agencies doubled, adult day care centers grew in profusion, hospice became a common and integral component of the system, and hospitals added services specifically for older adults and those with chronic conditions. In general, most urban areas now have a wide array of community-based services for those requiring long-term care.

Nonetheless, not all services are available to everyone when needed. Affordable homemaker and unskilled home support remains one of the services for which demand exceeds supply. Nursing home beds are in short supply in some areas because the state, in an attempt to limit Medicaid spending, has not allowed the construction of new beds. Transportation presents a major barrier to access even when services are available. State Medicaid waivers may eliminate financial barriers to community-based services for those who qualify as low-income, but do nothing to minimize costs for those who are just above poverty-level income. Rural areas continue to suffer a lack of many services, not just health care. The operation of a continuum of care assumes the availability and accessibility of key services. To the extent that public policy and funding limit service access or availability, the continuum of care will be abbreviated and patient flow inhibited accordingly.

Staffing and Expertise

The majority of staff in formal organizations providing long-term care are low-skilled workers. They receive low pay and have tasks that are physically and emotionally demanding. A high proportion are recent immigrants whose native language and customs differ from those of the majority of frail people for whom they care. Turnover is high, reaching as much as 100 percent annually in some nursing homes and home health agencies. Aides are particularly difficult to find and keep. Long-term care providers face a major challenge in trying to provide quality care when they do not have the resources to attract and retain quality staff.

A shortage also exists of experts in chronic care, geriatrics, and rehabilitation. Physicians, nurses, social workers, and rehabilitation therapists who specialize in the care of the elderly or chronically ill are in great demand and short supply. For example, in 1999, physicians certified as having a subspecialty in geriatrics numbered fewer than 9,200 and only 6,515 held their primary certification in rehabilitation medicine (American Board of Medical Specialties, 2000). These numbers are not adequate to meet the needs of the nation's 37 million seniors or 99 million people with chronic conditions.

Payment discourages many health care professionals from going into long-term care. Pay scales are lower than in acute settings. Physicians do not get reimbursed adequately for the time it takes to go to a nursing home or make a home visit, compared to what they get paid for seeing patients in their office. The average pay wage for nurses in nursing homes is lower than the average wage for nurses in a hospital.

Attitudes are also an obstacle to attracting and keeping both skilled and unskilled providers in long-term care. United States society is one that values youth. Despite attempts to change the image of older adults, many young people still have a negative stereotype of older people. In addition, health professionals, who are trained to cure, find it difficult to accept chronic illness and an orientation toward maintaining functional independence rather than recovery.

Federal, state, and private organizations have addressed the issues of long-term care manpower shortages. Educators as well as providers have also sought to change attitudes through improved knowledge of the aged and the aging process. Many health care provider organizations now conduct aging sensitivity training as part of their orientation and ongoing in-service education. Nonetheless, developing an adequate pool of health manpower for long-term care remains one of the challenges of changing the health care delivery system for the future.

THE LONG-TERM CARE CONTINUUM OF THE FUTURE

Do continuums of long-term care exist? Is it possible to overcome the problems of fragmentation, financing, and access to create an effective, efficient, consumer-oriented, high-quality system of care? Few, if any, complete continuums of long-term care are now in operation. The success of components of a complete continuum of care, however, has been ably demonstrated. Select programs throughout the nation provide encouragement for the future. In contrast to Mrs. Jackson's experience described at the beginning of this chapter, how do extant and future continuums provide long-term care? The following scenario already occurs in exemplary organizations.

Mrs. Smith is an eighty-year-old widow who lives alone. She slips in the bathtub and breaks her hip. She uses her voice-activated emergency response system necklace to call for help. When received, the call automatically asks what the problem is, then calls both a neighbor and emergency assistance. The neighbor comes over to be with Mrs. Smith, having agreed in advance to help in times of emergency.

The paramedics also arrive within minutes, stabilize Mrs. Smith, and take her to the hospital. Mrs. Smith belongs to the hospital-sponsored senior membership program, Silver Services, which was notified automatically via computer when the call came in. A laminated barcoded ID card from Silver Services gives the paramedics and the doctors in the emergency room all the basic administrative and clinical information they need to initiate treatment. The card also contains identification numbers that enable the clinicians to access Mrs. Smith's fully integrated, current medical record through the Internet to obtain more detailed information about her clinical condition, recent treatment history, and advanced directives.

While in the hospital, a care coordinator, with whom Mrs. Smith talked when she enrolled in Silver Services, visits her and reassures her that whatever services she needs will be arranged. When Mrs. Smith has recovered enough to be discharged from acute service, she is transferred to a rehabilitation-oriented skilled nursing facility. Mrs. Smith never liked the idea of being in a "nursing home," but she does not feel negative about this one because the ambiance is positive, the staff are pleasant and encouraging, and she is confident that her physician and care coordinator will arrange her transfer home.

Indeed, two weeks later Mrs. Smith goes home with home health nursing and rehabilitation. The social worker at the hospital has arranged for Meals on Wheels to bring a hot meal daily, and a homemaker comes in twice a week to help with personal care, shopping, mail, and housekeeping. The emergency response system gives Mrs. Smith the security to remain alone at night, and she knows that she can call the Silver Services number at any time if she has questions or needs non-emergency assistance. Mrs. Smith also knows that her physician is regularly informed of what is happening to her through automated daily updates to her clinical record from all providers.

After several more weeks, Mrs. Smith is steady enough to leave her second-story apartment and go for additional outpatient therapy. The therapists have automated and immediate access to all of her records through the health system's computerized comprehensive patient record, and thus they know exactly what exercises the home health staff has recommended that she continue.

Mrs. Smith's total spell of illness cost her very little out-of-pocket. The health care providers she used were all participants in the Medicare HMO in which she was enrolled. She made regular monthly payments somewhat above those required for Medicare Part B, and she acknowledged the HMO as her Medicare Part A and B provider. The care coordinator explained to Mrs. Smith that as long as she did not exceed the lifetime allowance and used the providers within the HMO network, she could use whatever levels of institutional or community-based services her physician and care coordinator felt necessary.

Mrs. Smith also had the peace of mind of knowing that she had organized her legal and financial affairs well in advance, just in case anything serious happened. A lawyer from Silver Services had helped her prepare a will, designate a sibling to assume durable power of attorney for health care, and execute an advanced directive to express her preferences to her physician and family about the use of life-sustaining measures. ❧

SUMMARY

Long-term care in the United States has undergone major changes in the last thirty years. It has evolved from an insular, isolated potpourri of services bifurcated around nursing homes and social service agencies to a broader, more extensive network of many services available at many locations throughout the community. Its financing sources, coordinating mechanisms, and general outlook have changed greatly as public awareness of its importance has increased.

Long-term care will continue to change as demand grows. Ideally, the twenty-first century will see the basic structure of the long-term care delivery system shift from one of fragmented services to a comprehensive continuum of care. The future for the continuum of care, while challenged by the forces facing health care in general, is impressive and exciting.

References

Adams, P. F., & Marano, M. A. (1995). Current estimates from the National Health Interview Survey, 1994. National Center for Health Statistics. *Vital Health Statistics, 10*(193), 81.

American Association of Retired Persons. (1996). *A profile of older Americans.* Washington, DC: Author.

American Board of Medical Specialties. (2000). *Annual report handbook.* Evanston, IL: American Board of Medical Specialties.

American Board of Medical Specialties. (2001). Available: *www.abms.org.*

American Hospital Association. (2000). Available: *www.aha.org.*

Applebaum, R., & Austin, C. (1990). *Long-term case management.* New York: Springer.

The Catholic Health Association. (1993). *A handbook for planning and developing integrated delivery.* St. Louis,

MO: The Catholic Health Association of the United States.

The Catholic Health Association. (1995). *A workbook on long-term care in integrated delivery.* St. Louis, MO: The Catholic Health Association of the United States.

Centers for Disease Control. (2000). Available: *www.cdc.gov/hiv/stats.*

Coddington, D., Moore, K., & Fischer, E. (1994). *Integrated health care: Reorganizing the physician, hospital and health plan relationship.* Englewood, CO: Center for Research in Ambulatory Health Care Administration.

Coleman, B. (1991). *The Nursing Home Reform Act of 1987: Provisions, policy, prospects.* Boston: University of Massachusetts.

The daughter track. (1990, July 16). *Newsweek,* p. 53.

Evans, D. (1989). Prevalence of Alzheimer's disease in a community population of older persons: Higher than previously reported. *Journal of the American Medical Association, 262*(18), 2551–2556.

Evashwick, C. (1987). Definition of the continuum of care. In C. Evashwick & L. Weiss (Eds.), *Managing the continuum of care: A practical guide to organization and operations* (p. 23). Gaithersburg, MD: Aspen.

Evashwick, C. (1997). *Seamless connections.* Chicago: American Hospital Publishing.

Evashwick, C. (Ed.). (2001). *The continuum of long-term care.* New York: Delmar Publishers, Inc.

Evashwick, C., Rundall, T., & Goldiamond, B. (1985). Hospital services for older adults: Results of a national survey. *The Gerontologist, 25*(6), 631–637.

Gabrel, C. (2000). *An overview of nursing home facilities: Data from the 1997 National Nursing Home Survey.* Advance data from *Vital and Health Statistics 311.* Hyattsville, MD: National Center for Health Statistics.

General Accounting Office. (1987). *VA health care: Assuring quality care for veterans in community and state nursing homes* (Pub. No. GAO/HRD-88-18). Washington, DC: Author.

Gillies, R. R., Shortell, S. M., Anderson, D., Mitchell, J. B., & Morgan, K. L. (1993). Conceptualizing and measuring integration: Findings from the health systems integration study. *Hospital and Health Services Administration, 38*(4), 467–490.

Haupt, B. (1998). *An overview of home health and hospice care patients: 1996 National Home and Hospice Care Survey.* Advance data from *Vital and Health Statistics* (No. 297). Hyattsville, MD: National Center for Health Statistics.

Health Care Financing Administration. (1991a). *Social health maintenance organization demonstration.* Baltimore: HCFA Office of Demonstrations and Evaluation.

Health Care Financing Administration. (1991b). *Program of all-inclusive care for the elderly (PACE).* Baltimore: HCFA Office of Demonstrations and Evaluation.

Health Care Financing Administration. (1999). *Managed care in medicare and medicaid fact sheet.* Baltimore, MD: HCFA Office of Research and Administration.

Health data on older Americans: United States, 1992. (1993, January). In *Vital and Health Statistics* (DHHS Pub. No. HS 93-1411, Series 3, No. 27).

Health Insurance Association of America. (2000). Available: *www.hiaa.org/.*

Hobbs, F. & Damon, B. (1996). U.S. Census Bureau *www.census.gov/.*

Hoffman, C., & Rice, D. (1996). *Chronic care in America: A 21st century challenge.* Princeton, NJ: The Robert Wood Johnson Foundation.

Hospital Research and Educational Trust. (1986). *Emerging trends in aging and long-term care services.* Chicago: Author.

Institute of Medicine. (2000). *Building a safer health system* [On-line]. Available: *www.iom.edu.*

Katz, S., Ford, A. B., & Moskowitz, R. W. (1985). Studies of illness in the aged. The index of ADL: A standardized measure of biological and psychosocial function. *Journal of the American Medical Association, 94.*

Keenan, M. (1989). *Veterans and the demand for long-term care.* Washington, DC: American Association of Retired Persons.

Kemper, P., & Murtaugh, C. (1991). Lifetime use of nursing home care. *New England Journal of Medicine, 324,* 595–600.

Kraus, L., Stoddard, S., & Gilmartin, D. (1996). *Chartbook on disability in the United States, 1996.* National Institute on Disability and Rehabilitation Research (No. H133D50017). Washington, DC: U.S. Department of Education.

Lack, S. A. (1978). *The first American hospice: Three years of home care.* New Haven, CT: The Connecticut Hospice.

Lawton, P., & Brody, E. (1969). Assessment of older people, self-maintaining and instrumental activities of daily life. *The Gerontologist, 9,* 179–186.

Levenstein, M. (2001). The Department of Veterans Affairs. In C. Evashwick (Ed.), *The continuum of long-term care.* Albany, NY: Delmar.

The Lighthouse. (2000). Available: *www.lighthouse.org.*

McNeil, J. M. (1992). *Americans with disabilities: 1991–92. Survey of income and program participation.* Washington, DC: U.S. Bureau of the Census.

National Adult Day Services Association. (1996). *Adult day services funding fact sheet.* Washington, DC: National Council on Aging.

National Alliance for Caregiving. (1997). *Family caregiving in the U.S.* Bethesda, MD: Author.

National Association for Home Care. (2000). Available: *www.nahc.org.*

National Center for Health Statistics. (1996, June). *Health, United States, 1995* (DHHS Pub. No. PHS 96-1232, 6-0250). Hyattsville, MD: Public Health Service.

National Center for Health Statistics. (2000a). *Health, United States, 2000.* Hyattsville, MD: National Public Health Service.

National Center for Health Statistics. (2000b). Health maintenance organizations (HMOs). *Health, United States, 2000.* Hyattsville, MD: National Public Health Service.

National Chronic Care Consortium. (1996). *Self-assessment for systems integration tool.* Bloomington, MN: Author.

National Hospice and Palliative Care Organization. (2001). *Facts and figures on hospice care in America.* [On-line]. Available: *www.nhpca.org.*

National Institute for Mental Health. (1999). Available: *www.nimh.nih.gov.*

Office of Prepaid Health Care Operations and Oversight. (1991). *Monthly report Medicare prepaid health plans.* Rockville, MD: Health Care Financing Administration.

Pynoos, J. (2001). Housing. In C. Evashwick (Ed.). *The continuum of long-term care.* Albany, NY: Delmar Publishers, Inc.

Rundall, T., & Evashwick, C. (2001). Organizing the continuum of long-term care. In C. Evashwick (Ed.). *The continuum of long-term care.* Albany, NY: Delmar Publishers, Inc.

Spector, W., Fleishman, J., Pezzin, L., & Spillman, B. (2000). *The characteristics of long-term care users* (AHRQ Publication No. 00-0049). Rockville, MD: U.S. Department of Health and Human Services, Public Health Service.

Strahan, G. W. (1997). *An overview of nursing homes and their current residents: Data from the 1995 National Nursing Home Survey* (DHHS Pub. No. PHS 97-1250 7-0122). *Vital and Health Statistics* Advance Data (No. 280). Hyattsville, MD: National Center for Health Statistics.

U.S. Bipartisan Commission on Comprehensive Health Care. (1991). *A call for action, executive summary.* Washington, DC: U.S. Government Printing Office.

U.S. Department of Health and Human Services. (1991). *Medicare hospice benefits* (Pub. No. HCFA 02154). Washington, DC: U.S. Government Printing Office.

U.S. Department of Health and Human Services. (2000). *Health, United States, 2000.* Hyattsville, MD: National Center for Health Statistics.

U.S. Department of Veterans Affairs. (1986). *VA in brief* (VA Pamphlet No. 06-83-1). Washington, DC: Author.

U.S. Department of Veterans Affairs. (1989). *Annual report, 1988.* Washington, DC: Author.

Von Behren, R. (1986). *Adult day care in America: Summary of a national survey.* Washington, DC: National Institute on Adult Day Care, National Institute on the Aging.

White, M., & Gundrum, G. (2001). Case management. In C. Evashwick (Ed.). *The continuum of long-term care.* Albany, NY: Delmar Publishers, Inc.

Zawadski, R. (2001). Information systems. In C. Evashwick & L. Weiss (Eds.), *Managing the continuum of care.* Gaithersburg, MD: Aspen.

Zawadski, R., & Von Behren, R. (1990). *The national adult day center census—'89.* San Francisco: University of California Institute for Health and Aging.

C H A P T E R

12

Mental Health Services

Mary Richardson
Sharyne Shiu-Thornton

Chapter Topics

- Incidence and Prevalence of Mental Disorders
- Early Views on Mental Illness
- Understanding Mental Illness in the United States
- Shaping Mental Health Policy
- Delivering Mental Health Services
- The Changing Mental Health Service System
- Patterns of Mental Health Service Utilization
- Mental Health Personnel
- Financing Mental Health Care
- Managed Mental Health Care
- Summary

Learning Objectives

Upon completing this chapter, the reader should be able to:

- Understand the basis for defining mental health services
- Appreciate the history of mental health
- Understand the various settings and arrangements for delivering mental health services
- Appreciate the financing issues in mental health
- Assess the complex personnel issues in mental health
- Assess policy alternatives in mental health

An estimated thirty to forty percent of American adults experience one or more psychiatric disorders in their lifetimes (Robins, Locke, & Regier, 1991). Twenty percent have an active disorder during any given year (USDHHS, 1999). Twenty-one percent of children ages nine to seventeen receive mental health services in a year (USDHHS, 1999). Data developed by the Global Burden of Disease study, conducted by the World Health Organization, the World Bank, and Harvard University, report that mental illness, including suicide, ranks second in the burden of disease in established market economies such as the United States (Murray & Lopez, 1996).

Over the last several decades, societal perspectives of mental illness have changed. Mental health research, expanded treatment options, and the civil rights movement have all contributed to a more enlightened social response and greater acceptance of mental health services as a treatment rather than a custodial function.

This chapter describes the development of mental health services in this country, the users and reasons for use, the organization and financing of services, recent trends, and the challenges of providing care. Although related issues of utilization and financing are discussed in other chapters, the unique nature of mental health services is presented in detail in this chapter.

INCIDENCE AND PREVALENCE OF MENTAL DISORDERS

The 1978 President's Commission on Mental Health set the stage for the development and implementation of two epidemiological studies of the prevalence of mental illness: the Epidemiologic Catchment Area (ECA) Program and the National Comorbidity Survey (NCS). The ECA involved interviewing household and institutional residents older than eighteen and was conducted at five sites around the country between 1980 and 1985. More than 20,000 adults were asked about their need for seeking and obtaining mental health services. The NCS, conducted between 1990 and 1992, interviewed a stratified national sample of more than 8,000 adults, using the Composite International Diagnostic Interview. Both studies concluded that during a one-year period, twenty-two to twenty-three percent of the U.S. adult population have diagnosable mental disorders according to established, reliable criteria. In general, nineteen percent of the adult U.S. population have a mental disorder alone, while three percent have both mental and addictive disorders, and six percent have addictive disorders alone. Consequently, about twenty to thirty percent of the population have either a mental or addictive disorder (Regier et al., 1993b; Kessler et al., 1994). Approximately three percent of the population experience co-occurring disorders in one year and are more likely to experience a chronic course and to utilize services than are those with either type of disorder alone (Kessler et al., 1996; Regier et al., 1993c).

In 1999, the first White House Conference on Mental Health was held and the first Surgeon General's Report on Mental Health was published. This report was a product of a collaboration between the Substance Abuse and Mental Health Services Administration (SAMHSA) and the National Institutes of Health (NIH) through its National Institute of Mental Health (NIMH). The report summarizes more than 3,000 research articles and other materials, providing an up-to-date review of scientific advances in the study of mental health and mental illnesses. Among its more important conclusions, the report emphasizes that there are a variety of treatments of well-documented efficacy that exist for the array of clearly defined mental and behavioral disorders that occur across the life span. However, the report also points out that many obstacles remain that limit the availability and accessibility of mental health services, noting that the stigma associated with mental illness remains as one of the most powerful barriers.

Mental illness affects people differently, depending on age, sex, and marital status. Ninety percent of all people with psychiatric disorders report the onset of first symptoms by the age of thirty-eight, while the median age of onset of the first symptom was sixteen. Men experience higher rates of psychiatric disorder over a lifetime than women (thirty-six percent versus thirty percent), but they experience about the same rate of active disorder over the course of any single year (thirty percent). The most common disorders, in general, are phobia and alcohol abuse, but their prevalence differs markedly between men and women. The most frequent diagnosis for men aged eighteen to sixty-four is alcohol abuse/dependence followed by antisocial personality, with severe cognitive impairment becoming the most prominent diagnosis for men ages sixty-five and over. Somatization disorders are the most common diagnosis reported for women of all ages, followed by obsessive compulsive disorders. Women between the ages of twenty-five and forty-four often cite major depressive episodes. The rates of mental disorders, except for cognitive impairment, drop after age forty-five for both men and women (Howard et al., 1996).

Ethnicity and socioeconomic status appear to be correlated to prevalence, but are confounding factors. Persons of color are overrepresented among those in the lowest socioeconomic groups. Blacks generally have a higher lifetime rate of reported psychiatric disorder (thirty-eight percent) than whites or Hispanics. Other differences in lifetime rates, related to socioeconomic status, include people who fail to complete high school (thirty-six percent), are unemployed (forty-eight percent), or are working as unskilled laborers (forty-one percent). Unemployed individuals report higher rates of mania, schizophrenia, and panic disorder. The lowest rates of psychiatric disorder are among people who are married and have never divorced or separated (twenty-four percent lifetime and thirteen percent active). Unmarried persons report a higher prevalence of drug abuse, mania, and antisocial personality disorders.

Diagnosing Mental Illness

The American Psychiatric Association classifies mental illness within several general categories, including impairment of brain tissue, developmental disorders, and disorders where the clinical cause is unknown. A major trend in psychiatric diagnosis is to use more objective, rather than subjective, standards for classification, replicable from one observer to the next. The Diagnostic and Statistical Manual (DSM-IV) published by the American Psychiatric Association contains the classification system used extensively in diagnosing mental illness (Robins et al., 1991). These

classifications are generally used in studies of incidence and prevalence of mental disorder.

In addition, the Epidemiologic Catchment Area (ECA) Program developed a system for assessing mental and addictive disorder prevalence, incidence, and service use rates (Regier et al., 1984). An interview schedule, the Diagnostic Interview Schedule (DIS), was developed for use by lay interviewers to assess the presence, duration, and severity of symptoms in study participants according to DSM-IV diagnostic criteria. Interviews were subsequently scored by computer according to diagnostic algorithms specified by DSM-IV and other diagnostic systems.

Classification of mental retardation is based on another system, entitled *Mental Retardation: Definition, Classification, and Systems of Support, Special Ninth Edition, 1992.* Unique to this classification system is the use of functional rather than clinical definitions and a focus on the interaction between the person, the environment, and the intensities and patterns of needed supports.

Finally, diagnosing mental illness can be further complicated by societal views of mental illness. Defining the overlap between social problems and mental illness is difficult. Are deviations such as delinquency or criminal behavior a mental health problem? What about poverty, discrimination, and unemployment? Mental health caregivers and advocates for persons with mental illness often seek to be inclusive with definitions in order to advocate for societally sanctioned interventions, while others with a more conservative bent are more likely to attribute such social issues to immorality rather than to illness. Under this more conservative approach, individuals are held accountable for the consequences of their illnesses, and society is expected to punish or confine them. Where to draw the line is the fodder for much political debate.

EARLY VIEWS ON MENTAL ILLNESS

Societies have always defined and classified human behavior in ways that differentiated between what was acceptable and what was not. Value systems, which shape social and cultural perspectives, also determine what constitutes deviant behavior. Societal tolerance of deviant behavior partially determines what a particular society believes to be mental illness. Although society now views mental illness in the context of biologic, sociologic, political, and cultural frameworks, there is a history of thought about mental illness and deviant behavior that predates current scientific thought.

During the Middle Ages, aberrant behavior was attributed to demonic influences, evil spirits, and the like. In an agrarian feudal society, people who could not work and sustain themselves were regarded as "mad." Society tolerated such people, who were allowed to wander if they were not too troublesome (Levine, 1981). Communities were able to offer them some basic support; if they became troublesome, they were driven away. With the rise of a mercantile society in Europe and a breakdown of feudal estates, major social and political upheavals occurred, leaving many people homeless and with no means of support. Groups of unemployed, including disbanded soldiers, wandered the countryside joining the ranks of those viewed as mad or insane. Thus, a larger social grouping was formed and included people who were considered to be socially destitute. Community resources were quickly overwhelmed.

In England, the Elizabethan Poor Laws of 1601 heralded a recognition of the responsibility of government to society as a whole in addressing the problems of the destitute and the ill. In each community parish, overseers were assigned to provide care for the sick and disaffected members of society. Later, lunatic hospitals were opened throughout England, although their purpose had more to do with protecting society from the misfits than with providing care. Conditions were abominable, and inmates were often chained and provided only the barest essentials of survival.

In 1656, the French Parliament authorized the construction of the Hôpital Génerale, where people who were poor, sick, or insane were confined in rather dismal circumstances. The eighteenth century, however, ushered in the Age of Enlightenment. Scientific thought began to replace magic and religion, creating a secular basis for societal debate. In France, Philippe Pinel introduced the idea of mental illness as a medical condition (Weiner, 1979). Pinel, often credited with unchaining the inmates and introducing humanistic treatment, actually worked with Jean Baptiste Pussin, the governor of mental patients who had himself been a patient at the Hospice de Bicetre in Paris. It was Pussin who advocated much of the improved treatment introduced by Pinel. The ideas of both Pinel and Pussin spread throughout Europe and, later, to the United States.

The development of American psychiatry in the nineteenth century was strongly influenced by Dr. Benjamin Rush, long considered the father of American psychiatry. Dr. Rush was also a pioneer in hospital reform. Before the nineteenth century, formal treatment centers in America were nonexistent. Private physician services were available to those with money. The rest faced imprisonment or hospitalization, with one not much different from the other. The hospital reform spearheaded by Pinel in the late 1700s in France was paralleled in this country by Rush's activities. The American Psychiatric Association was started through the efforts of affiliated hospital superintendents who, like Rush, were concerned with hospital conditions. Even into the twentieth century, treatment of mental illness based on medical/clinical approaches occurred in state-supported hospitals that were often located in remote areas and functioned as large human warehouses.

As the scientific revolution gained momentum, Kraepelin, a German physician working in the late 1800s, outlined a concise system of classification establishing mental illness as a separate and distinct disease entity subject to the rules that applied to physical or somatic illness. His work legitimized psychiatry as a branch of medicine. Kraepelin described in detail the symptoms, course of the disease, and prognosis of dementia praecox and manic depressive psychoses. The disease concept, however, implies that the patient can become "well."

Sigmund Freud introduced the psychological view of mental illness, describing the deterministic nature of mental illness, and relating it to disturbances and distortions created by unconscious developmental difficulties, psychic growth and maturation, and conflicts over sexual and self-destructive instincts. His work became the basis for the development of psychoanalysis. The Freudian model leads to long-term and intensive psychotherapy, requiring substantial and expensive therapeutic resources. Thus were born both the biomedical and psychological fields of mental health study and treatment, which continue to exist in a parallel fashion but are not well integrated.

UNDERSTANDING MENTAL ILLNESS IN THE UNITED STATES

Biomedical Advances

The advance of biomedical research in the twentieth century incorporated mental health research, producing substantial evidence for organic causes of mental illness. The discovery of the spirochete that causes syphilis, general paresis, and discoveries of chromosomal aberrations in mental retardation were cited as evidence. Studies of schizophrenia, defined as a diagnosis by Bleuler in the early 1900s (replacing dementia praecox), and manic depressive syndromes have suggested possible familial tendencies. For example, ten percent of children of schizophrenic patients are also diagnosed as schizophrenic, possibly indicating a genetic basis for this illness. Transcultural studies of mental illness have demonstrated remarkably uniform prevalence rates for schizophrenia in different countries and cultures.

With the rapid technological sophistication of genetic and other biomedical research, there promises to be substantially more sophisticated mental health research that may assist in determining the relationship between biomedical and social/cultural factors affecting mental illness.

In 1990, the U.S. Congress declared the Decade of the Brain. During this period, our understanding of the manner in which biological, psychological, and sociocultural factors affect both health and illness has been advanced by research on the causes, or etiology, of mental illness. Researchers now believe that several susceptibility genes interact with each other and with environmental factors to influence the risk of developing a particular mental or physical disorder.

Research in basic neuroscience, behavioral science, and genetics has contributed greatly to our understanding of the complex workings of the brain. Newer approaches to neuroscience are correcting the commonly held misperception that the mind and body are somehow "split" and that mental health and mental illnesses are unrelated to physical health. Modern integrative neuroscience links research on the broad aspects of brain function with the remarkably detailed tools and findings of molecular genetics. The sequencing of the human genome during the past decade will improve our ability to identify the genetic risk factors for a variety of conditions, including mental illness. Moreover, advancements in genetic understanding will improve our ability to effectively manage many forms of mental illness through improved therapeutics and prevention strategies.

Social Psychiatric and Behavioral Perspectives

During the twentieth century, there has been increasing acceptance of pluralistic determinants of mental illness, including biologic and sociologic factors. Harry Sullivan was the first American psychiatrist to develop a theory stressing the importance of interpersonal relations in disease etiology. Concurrent with the development of social psychiatric definitions were psychological and behavioral concepts of mental illness. Carl Jung broke away from the Freudian approach and formed the field of analytic psychology. Erich Fromm, a psychoanalyst never trained in medicine, and others applied anthropologic and sociologic concepts to Freud's theories. Later, John B. Watson discarded Freudian theory and developed behaviorism, which recognized only observable behavior as critical to the diagnosis of mental illness. He believed that all behavior was predictable on the basis of environmental stimuli. Psychologists introduced classic conditioning and learning theory to psychiatrists and other psychopathologists.

Reliance on the disease concept of mental health was reduced. A greater understanding of personality development in the context of social and cultural influences set the stage for the development of a biopsychosocial model. This model recognizes the interaction of biology and psychological development within the context of culture. The development of humanistic psychology had origins in the behavioral movements. The Freudian approach was considered too pessimistic and the behavioral approaches too mechanistic. Carl Rogers developed the technique of client-centered therapy, which recognized the client's role in effecting his or her own rehabilitation. According to this approach, client behavior is compared to expected behavior for the culture or environment of the client.

Cultural Concepts of Mental Health

During the 1960s, and continuing throughout the following two decades, a growth in the literature on the significance of culture to the understanding of mental health and illness occurred, reflecting multidisciplinary research contributions from anthropology, psychology, social work, and psychiatry. Various labels have been used to describe these disciplines' focus on the intersection of culture and health/mental health: transpersonal psychology, cross-cultural psychology/psychiatry, and medical and psychological anthropology, to name a few. While the methodological approaches varied, a shared research focus across these disciplines included the description, documentation, and interpretation of mental illness and suffering across cultural groups and languages. Symptom manifestations were described within the larger cultural patterns of kinship, gender roles, health beliefs and practices, child rearing, and religious/spiritual world views.

Transcultural psychiatry (or cultural psychiatry) incorporates a biopsychosocial approach to understanding the culturally constructed meaning of suffering and illness. The recognition of the complex interplay of biologic, sociologic, and environmental circumstances and the cultural context that shapes and frames meaning stimulated changes in how symptoms need to be interpreted, diagnoses made, and treatment plans developed (Kleinman, 1988; Kleinman & Good, 1985; Sue & Sue, 1990). Juxtaposed with this awareness of the role of culture in symptomatic expressions of illness and suffering was the channeling of funding in the late 1980s to an increased emphasis on the brain and the biological underpinnings of mental illness.

Thus, most of the mental health research and practice remains dominated by the mainstream (Eurocentric) perspective of mental illness with the resultant interpretation of what is abnormal or deviant (pathological) behavior a reflection of the values, norms, and belief system of the mainstream. African American patients are more likely to be diagnosed with schizophrenia and substance abuse than similar Caucasian patients (Strakowski et al., 1995) and receive more psychiatric medication and higher antipsychotic dosages than patients of other races (Bender, 1996). The comorbidity of drinking, depression, and suicide among American Indian populations challenges first assessment, secondly diagnosis, and then meaningful intervention when decontextualized by the diagnostic categories of the DSM-IV (Maser & Dinges, 1992). Mental health services to refugee populations dramatically reflect the challenges of assessment, diagnosis, and treatment and the limitations of mainstream, Western conceptualizations of mental illness as reflected in the DSM-IV when applied with no understanding of the cultural context of the patient. The mainstream provider who is either ignorant or blatantly dismissive of cultural explanations of spirits, ghosts, or ancestors as responsible for one's illness places the provider and the patient at odds at the onset of any encounter. Thus, issues of access and utilization, much less assessment and diagnosis, cannot be fully understood outside the context of a patient's culture (Gong-Guy, Cravens, & Patterson, 1991; Westermeyer, 1985).

SHAPING MENTAL HEALTH POLICY

Deinstitutionalization

Before World War II, few outpatient mental health facilities existed. Growing federal interest, coupled with advances in psychopharmacology and changing social perspectives of mental illness, began to spur the creation of outpatient facilities. The development of psychopharmacology in the 1950s had a profound impact on the field of mental health. The prognosis for the thousands of patients in mental hospitals—many of whom suffered from schizophrenia, depression, and mania—remained dismal. However, the use of antipsychotic medications for schizophrenia, antidepressants for depression, and lithium in the treatment of mania rapidly improved the prognosis for these patients. Psychotropic drugs led to dramatic breakthroughs in the treatment of mental illness and enabled thousands of patients previously considered incurable to be effectively treated on an outpatient basis.

The use of psychotropic drugs created a climate that encouraged the development of various innovative therapeutic approaches, leading to a radical decline in hospital lengths of stay for patients with psychiatric diagnoses. Patients now could control their behavior through the use of drugs and, it was hoped, with continuing therapeutic support, function within the community. Thus, a mental health system previously based primarily on inpatient facilities had to develop new approaches to serving patients who no longer needed to be hospitalized. The general public, however, remained distrustful of, and misinformed about, the nature of mental illness, and there was little advocacy for improvement except from mental health advocates and professionals. Nevertheless, there was a dramatic increase in outpatient clinics from 400 before World War II to 1,234 by 1954 (Rumer, 1978).

The National Mental Health Act of 1946 (PL 79–487) signified an increased federal interest in the plight of the mentally ill. The law created the National Institute of Mental Health (NIMH) and increased appropriations for therapy and research. In addition, recognition of the psychological problems of soldiers during World War II motivated Veterans Administration (VA) hospitals to provide expanded mental health services.

Civil Rights and Advocacy

Beginning in the late 1950s, mental health services in the United States have been profoundly shaped by a series of important court cases stimulated by the civil rights movement. Three areas of legal change have had major effects on the chronically mentally ill. They include substantive and procedural alterations in civil commitment laws, the limited implementation of a constitutionally based right to treatment, and the partial recognition of a right to refuse treatment (Lamb & Mills, 1986).

Deinstitutionalization and the way it was implemented were significant factors in the development of civil commitment laws. The influx of previously hospitalized mentally ill people into the community and the lack of consistent residential and treatment services created a large group of people whose lifestyles varied significantly from those of the general population. Philosophical debates raged on the right of an individual to choose this "alternative lifestyle," and the responsibility of society to ensure that individuals who appear unable to care for themselves have protection under the law. Civil commitment laws, initially general in definition, became more definitive and embodied criteria specifying the danger to self or others, or the incapacity to care for self, with the presence of mental illness as a requisite for commitment. Laws also became specific regarding the duration of commitment, and the length of time was generally brief. Finally, individuals committed under these laws had rapid access to courts, public defenders, and other elements of the judicial system which ensured due process. Implementation of laws in most states became quite literal, and danger to self or others often became the deciding criterion. Yet, findings suggest that irrespective of commitment criteria, eighty-five percent of those committed are not dangerous. This emphasis may significantly reduce the number of people who could be helped by commitment and, some would argue, contribute to the increase of urban homeless people (Kleinman & Good, 1985).

The right to treatment was first addressed in 1952 in civil commitment cases relating to sexual psychopaths. *Rouse v. Cameron* in 1966, based on arguments of cruel and unusual treatment and the right to due process, found that people judged criminally insane had the right to treatment. Because early cases did not define criteria for treatment but merely stated that some effort was required, there was little immediate impact. A decision by Judge Frank Johnson of Alabama in 1972, based on a class-action suit (*Wyatt v. Stickney*) related to conditions in state hospitals, required that right to treatment be enforced and implemented. Various courts have subsequently specified minimum standards for treatment. In 1975, the Supreme Court cast significant doubt on a constitutionally derived right to treatment by deciding the case of *Donaldson v. O'Connor* on the narrowest possible grounds. Donaldson, a patient in a Florida hospital for fourteen years, sued for damages and demanded his release. The narrowness of the ruling limited the potential impact of the right-to-treatment litigation on increased support for the chronically mentally ill (Kleinman & Good, 1985).

The right to refuse treatment often raises conflicting interests among society, mental health providers, and patients. The implications of behavior control through the use of behavior therapies, drug therapy, and psychosurgery create problems that have been addressed by the judicial system and by mental health professionals. The first of two right-to-refuse cases considered by the court was *Mills v. Rogers,* a class-action suit brought by patients at Boston State Hospital. In the years since, clinicians have been confronted with a bewildering set of pronouncements from the courts (Applebaum, 1983). Evidence suggests that the right to refuse treatment has significantly increased both use of seclusion and transfers to maximum-security hospitals for chronically mentally ill individuals (Kleinman & Good, 1985). In *Stensuad v. Reivil* (Reivil et al., 1985), the court ruled that the purpose of commitment is custody, care, and treatment, and that such treatment reasonably includes psychotropic medication. Confidentiality has long been central to the role of mental health care providers.

Over the last decade, exceptions to confidentiality rules have been developed when the life of a third party is endangered by a patient (Eth, 1990). The American Psychiatric Association has proposed a model statute limiting psychiatrists' liability for their patients' violent acts and, at the same time, suggesting that confidentiality may be breached in the context of treating an individual who is infected with the human immunodeficiency virus (HIV) (Westermeyer, 1985). Advocacy for individual rights and the well-being of society is a continuing challenge in the mental health field.

In the late 1980s, the federal government passed legislation requiring that states that accept federal funds for mental health services create programs for protecting and advocating the rights of the mentally ill. This legislation is patterned after similar legislation in the field of developmental disabilities. Protection and advocacy agencies for individuals with developmental disabilities are mandated in each state and funded through federal appropriation. Advocates for persons with developmental disabilities have generally been regarded as very successful pioneers in advocacy movements, although their success has met with mixed enthusiasm from professionals and policy makers in the field of developmental disabilities. They remain a significant and powerful force. Legislation establishing similar advocacy systems within mental health built on the developmental disabilities protection and advocacy system by integrating the two.

The decade of the 1990s saw new civil rights legislation as well. In 1990 the Americans with Disabilities Act (PL 101–336) was passed. This civil rights bill is intended to promote the rights of more vulnerable citizens, including those with mental illness. Primarily it addresses employment and public access, ensuring the rights of discrimination and access to all public facilities, whether for transportation, recreation, or other similar activities. It generally does not address access to health and mental health care, although it does prohibit employers from providing differential coverage or denying coverage based on disability.

Impact on Policy

In 1955, the National Mental Health Study Act (PL 84–182) was passed, which authorized $750,000 for a three-year study of the entire mental health system. The result was the Action for Mental Health Report, published in 1961, after President John F. Kennedy had taken office. His continuing interest and support of this new policy direction was responsible for many subsequent changes. Although this report covered many issues in the provision of mental health services, the primary emphasis of the legislation that followed, during the Kennedy administration, was on outpatient services. Concern was increasingly focused on providing comprehensive mental health services to people not requiring hospitalization as well as to those not previously having access to mental health services. The Mental Retardation Facilities and Community Mental Health Centers Construction Act of 1964 (PL 88–164) provided construction monies for community mental health centers that were to serve designated catchment areas of

74,000 to 200,000 people. The five basic services that the centers were required to provide included inpatient, outpatient, emergency, day treatment, and consultation and education services. Significantly, the legislation mandated that services be provided regardless of the patient's ability to pay.

Many centers were built with the newly available funding for construction, but money for staffing and operations continued to be scarce. Finally, in 1967, an amendment to the legislation provided the necessary operations money on a matching basis, with funding for each center declining over an eight-year period. This was the "seed money" concept, and it was hoped that the construction and development of a community mental health center would encourage the community to gradually assume financial responsibility for services. Because catchment areas varied in their ability to provide matching funds, the subsidy for services in different areas also varied considerably. And although there was an allowance for poorer communities, the capability to readily obtain local matching funds was a distinct advantage for some centers.

In retrospect, the whole notion of matching local funds ignored the inability of some communities to assume the associated financial burden, especially in the areas of greatest need. Since many centers faced closure or significant reduction in services, additional legislation (PL 94–63) was passed in 1975. This law included the provision for a one-year distress grant at the end of the eight years of operational support if alternate funding was not obtained. This legislation was designed to overhaul the community mental health center network and to increase the original five required services to twelve, including care for drug abuse problems, children, and the aged, as well as screening, follow-up, and community living services. Planning and evaluation of local community mental health services were mandated, and two percent of each center's budget was to be used for these purposes. Community mental health centers were also required to operate under the authority of a board of directors structured to represent the local community. These boards, however, were often composed of well-educated, upper-middle-income people who frequently were health care providers, despite the location of many mental health centers in lower-income communities.

Concern for the inadequacies of the mental health system led President Jimmy Carter to establish the President's Commission on Mental Health in 1977. The president's wife, Rosalyn, served as honorary chairperson, continuing an active interest in mental health services that began in Georgia during Carter's tenure as governor. The report produced by this commission influenced policy formation and, in many ways, became the heart of the Carter administration's Mental Health Systems Act, passed by Congress in 1980 (PL 96–398) (Levine, 1981). Although the act authorized continuation of provision to establish additional community mental health centers and authorized spending for many new initiatives, it was never implemented. Under the conservative administrations of Ronald Reagan and George Bush, monies authorized were never appropriated.

Although the Mental Health Systems Act was never implemented, the national plan, also called for by the President's Commission on Mental Health, was produced and underwent limited distribution (Koyanagi & Goldman, 1991). Titled "Toward a National Plan for the Chronically Mentally Ill," the plan focused on federal mainstream resources, especially those available under the Social Security Act.

Although mental health policy underwent fiscal conservatism during the 1980s, mental health advocates, linked to a doctrine of increased state responsibility, went into action. The National Institute of Mental Health's Community Support Program (CSP), a demonstration program for the care of people with severe mental illness, survived the decade despite repeated attempts by the Reagan administration to eliminate it. In 1986, the State Comprehensive Mental Health Services Plan Act of 1986 (PL 99–660) built on the CSP system by calling on each state to work with the Medicaid agency and prepare a detailed plan for the care of individuals with serious mental illness (Rumer, 1978).

As categorical mental health funds were organized into state block grants, advocates also set about to improve funding in mainstream resources (Rumer, 1978). The four programs upon which these efforts were focused included Supplemental Security Income, Social Security Disability Insurance, Medicaid, and Medicare. The national plan became the blueprint for incremental change. Structural changes were made in each of the four programs that expanded benefits to individuals with mental illness, although full benefit of these changes has yet to be realized.

Mental health policy in the 1990s has been shaped by continuing battles over the role and survival of entitlement programs as well as categorical programs aimed at special populations, such as the mentally ill. In addition, as federal policy makers implement incremental changes in health care financing, mental health services are directly affected as well.

One of the most significant trends to impact treatment for persons with mental illness during the 1990s has been the rapid shift toward managed care as a means of controlling costs. Mental health services, including drug and alcohol treatment, offer an easy target for managed care because they have traditionally been provided in institutions with longer lengths of inpatient stay than is the case for medical care, and costs have, indeed, been reduced at a faster pace. However, as a result, there has been an increased democratization of care as levels of treatment have been adjusted so that each individual receives approximately the same amount of care regardless of the severity of the illness.

In 1996, the Mental Health Parity Act (PL 104–204, MHPA) was passed. Under this law, a plan providing both medical and surgical benefits and mental health benefits could not impose aggregate lifetime or annual expenditure limits on mental health benefits if it did not impose such limits on substantially all medical and surgical benefits. At the time the law was passed, five states had mental health parity laws. Subsequently, four states introduced some form of parity legislation in 1997, and nineteen states adopted some form of parity legislation by the end of 1999. Access to care declined during this period, however, and more individuals with probable mental health disorders lost insurance between 1996 and 1998 than gained it and more reported decreases in health benefits. This may be due, in part, to the fact that employers may be dropping health care coverage altogether, or dropping mental health benefits, in an effort to avoid any increased costs that might occur as a result of the parity legislation.

DELIVERING MENTAL HEALTH SERVICES

Prior to 1955, most mental health services were provided in state or county mental hospitals, generally located away from areas of any population density. The policy of deinstitutionalization has created a dramatic reduction in episodes of inpatient treatment since 1955 and a shift away from the use of state and county mental hospitals. Between 1955 and 1980, the resident census of state and county mental hospitals declined from 559,000 to 138,000, or to one-quarter of the previous census (Goldman, Adams, & Taube, 1983). Of the state mental hospitals remaining in operation in the mid-1980s, thirty were exclusively for children, twelve were security hospitals for the criminally insane, nine were teaching hospitals, and the remaining facilities were not designated for a special program goal or specific clientele.

Despite vigorous efforts at deinstitutionalization, state and county mental hospitals continue to be a locus of care for a wide variety of patient groups, serving as the "floor" of the mental health system, as they are the "source of last resort." They provide acute inpatient treatment to persons who have been unresponsive to treatment in other settings or who have exhausted their financial or other resources. Patient profiles have changed over the years, however. Previously, such hospitals were populated by long-stay, predominantly middle-aged and elderly persons with schizophrenia, but now they are serving more young males with schizophrenia, females of all ages with schizophrenia, and elderly females with organic brain syndromes (Holcomb & Ahr, 1987).

Role of the Nursing Home

As long-stay patients were relocated from state and county mental health hospitals, nursing homes became a substitute, providing long-term custodial care functions. Of slightly more than 1.5 million people over the age of eighteen living in nursing homes or personal care homes, approximately sixty percent have some type of mental disorder (Lair & Lefkowitz, 1990). Approximately twenty-nine percent have dementia only, including chronic or organic brain syndrome, and 13.7 percent have dementia in combination with one or more mental disorders. The remainder have a mental disorder but no dementia.

Concern over the numbers of people with mental illness and mental retardation living in nursing homes was the basis for the congressional passage of new laws governing nursing homes as part of the Omnibus Budget Reconciliation Act of 1987 (OBRA 1987). Under these provisions, nursing homes must screen all residents to determine their mental status. If placement in the nursing home is related only to mental status and not justified by the level of nursing care required, the individual is to be moved into a more appropriate treatment setting. In the event an individual is mentally ill with nursing care needs requiring nursing home placement, the nursing home is required to provide treatment appropriate to the mental needs of that patient in addition to the nursing care provided. Great controversy arose with the enactment of the law, and regulatory action has been the subject of considerable lobbying, affecting full implementation of the act.

Deinstitutionalization is undergoing a second-generation effort. During this second phase, court decisions focus on institutions where deinstitutionalization efforts may have already taken place (Geller, Fisher, Wirth-Cauchon, & Simon, 1990). It is likely more difficult to sustain remaining patients in the community, even when adequate services are available. Age, specifically age over sixty, appears significantly related to longer community tenure and a lower likelihood of readmission. The other most consistently significant predictor is prior hospitalization history. Geller and associates found that many people who have displayed a tendency toward frequent hospitalization will persist in that pattern even in the presence of community-based resources.

Questions still remain about whether further reductions in institutional populations are feasible (Gottheil, Winkelmayer, Smoyer, & Exine, 1991). Also of interest is the path by which deinstitutionalization is accomplished. If contrasts are drawn between mental health and mental retardation, two areas of service that were initially integrated in federal policy and funding, it is interesting to note their divergence in practice as goals of deinstitutionalization were pursued. Providers of services to individuals with mental retardation and other developmental disabilities argue vehemently that independence, choice, and personal dignity are directly related to living at home in the community. This strongly held belief has been the basis for the development of a network of community-based services over the past three decades, largely financed through state and private sources.

The mental health system, on the other hand, created federally sponsored community mental health centers, intended to form the backbone of community services for persons with severe mental illnesses. As federal funds began to disappear, mental health centers had to seek funding from states and other sources somewhat later in the game. Although financing has become more local in origin, program focus appears to remain heavily oriented toward promoting and preserving federal support. Perhaps coincidentally, the mental health service system continues to place less emphasis on developing natural community supports for integrated living experiences as the disability system is doing. Moreover, mental health services, unlike developmental disabilities services, continue to exist under the influence of medical approaches to treatment, whereas the disability movement has shifted toward education and habilitation models of intervention.

The Homeless Mentally Ill Person

One of the more challenging problems created by deinstitutionalization has been the number of persons released from state and county mental health hospitals who end up on the streets. Critics of the implementation of deinstitutionalization, noting inadequate funding, the failure to develop needed community services, and difficulties in maintaining continuity of care after hospital discharge, cite growing numbers of persons with chronic mental illness among the homeless population. Persons with mental illness make up a substantial percentage of the homeless population of the United States, with estimates ranging from twenty to forty percent of the total (Klebe, 1991). Although difficult to quantify, estimates in recent years place the number of homeless people in a range from a quarter million to five million. Consensus has settled on a survey conducted by the Urban Institute in March 1987 over a one-week period, which resulted in an estimate of 496,000 to 600,000 homeless people in the United States. The Urban Institute further estimated that if 600,000 people were homeless during one week, more than one million were homeless at some time during the entire year.

Other studies estimate that twenty to forty percent of the homeless population suffer from such serious mental illnesses as schizophrenia, manic-depressive illness, or severe depression. The Urban Institute study indicates that mental illness is most prevalent among single homeless adults, male or female, and is less evident among the typical homeless family of a woman with children, although the prevalence of mental illness among such homeless families is above the average for the general United States adult population. The annual report of the Interagency Council on the Homeless notes that the higher prevalence of mental illness in the homeless population, and, conversely, the rate of homelessness among those who are mentally ill, is not surprising. Noninstitutionalized mentally ill people are less likely to find employment, housing, or other benefits, or assistance to help keep them from becoming homeless than those who are not mentally ill. Mentally ill people in the community are not only less likely to be able to function or work, but they are also less aware of the services available to them and less willing to seek help. They face frequent discrimination from employers and landlords, and they often face shortages of treatment facilities and housing opportunities in their communities as well. Abuse of alcohol and other drugs has also been a constant problem among the homeless population, often among the same individuals who suffer from mental illness.

The National Institute on Alcohol Abuse and Alcoholism (NIAAA) estimates that thirty-five to forty percent of the homeless population suffers from chronic alcohol problems (Reivil, 1985). The same agency, in conjunction with the National Institute on Drug Abuse (NIDA) and others, estimates that ap-

proximately ten percent to twenty percent of the homeless population have chronic problems with drugs other than alcohol. Data from the Urban Institute study indicates that almost half of all severely mentally ill homeless people also have problems with alcohol and other drugs.

There has been quite a bit of talk, but little definitive action, on behalf of homeless persons who are mentally ill (Eth, 1990). In 1984, the American Psychiatric Association (APA) published the results of a Task Force on the Homeless Mentally Ill, and described homelessness as but one symptom of the problems faced by chronically mentally ill people in the United States (Lamb, 1990). The APA Task Force Interagency Council called for a comprehensive and integrated system of care for chronically mentally ill people in order to address the underlying problems that cause homelessness. The task force's recommendations called for an adequate number and range of supervised, supportive housing settings; a well-functioning system of case management; adequate, comprehensive, and accessible crisis intervention in the community and in hospitals; less restrictive laws on involuntary treatment; and ongoing treatment and rehabilitative services, combined with assertive outreach programs when necessary. With few exceptions, these recommendations have not been implemented. In addition to funding problems, a fundamental civil rights issue is being debated. Do the homeless mentally ill have a basic right, irrespective of their mental status and lack of competence, to refuse treatment and appropriate housing and to live on the streets instead? Or does this "right to choice" translate into a life characterized by deprivation, victimization by predators, and the development of life-threatening health care problems or other cruel interpretations of the basic principles of civil rights (Koyanagi & Goldman, 1991)?

THE CHANGING MENTAL HEALTH SERVICE SYSTEM

The mental health service system is divided into public and private sectors. Public sector services are directly operated by government agencies such as state and county governments or are financed with government resources such as Medicare and Medicaid.

Private sector services include those directly operated by private agencies as well as services funded through private sources such as employer-provided insurance coverage. Publicly financed services can be provided by private organizations: that is to say, a private facility may also receive a portion of revenue from public sector funding sources.

The total number of mental health organizations in the United States increased steadily from 3,005 in 1970 to 5,284 in 1990. Within that total number, inpatient state and county mental health facilities declined in number, representing only a third of all psychiatric beds in 1990 as compared to four-fifths in 1970. Ironically, despite a major effort to substantially reduce the size and numbers of inpatient state and county mental health facilities, the number of organizations with inpatient settings doubled from 1,734 to 3,430 between 1970 and 1990. Figure 12.1 depicts the increase in organizations with inpatient or residential facilities. This occurred largely as a result of an increase in numbers of private psychiatric hospitals, separate psychiatric services of nonfederal general hospitals, residential treatment centers for emotionally disturbed children (RTCs), and other organizational types with psychiatric beds. Veterans Administration medical centers with psychiatric centers remained relatively unchanged during this same period (Redick, Witkin, Atay, & O. Manderscheid, 1994).

The private psychiatric hospital is generally categorized as either nonprofit or for-profit, although few, if any, nonprofit hospitals have been founded in decades. Nonprofit hospital financing comes from a variety of sources, including fees, endowments, grants, government contracts, and private donations. Of the for-profit hospitals, approximately ninety percent are owned by corporations (Bittker, 1985). The for-profit groups have been characterized by the development of corporate chains. The growth of private psychiatric hospitals and RTCs is believed to be due, in part, to expanded psychiatric hospitalization benefits by a number of insurance carriers. As benefits expanded, the number of inpatient admissions increased between 1970 and 1990 from 1,282,698 to 2,035,245, although the average daily inpatient census in mental health organizations underwent a general decline, dropping from 471,451 in 1969 to 226,953 in

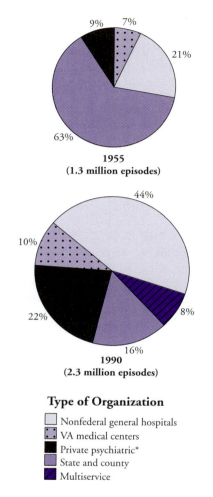

1955
(1.3 million episodes)

1990
(2.3 million episodes)

Type of Organization

☐ Nonfederal general hospitals
▦ VA medical centers
■ Private psychiatric*
▨ State and county
▨ Multiservice

*Includes residential treatment centers for emotionally disturbed children

Figure 12.1. Inpatient and Residential Treatment Care Episodes in Mental Health Organizations, 1955, 1990

SOURCE: *Mental Health, United States, 1994* (DHHS Pub. No. SMA 94–3000), edited by R. W. Manderscheid & M. A. Sonnenschein, Washington, DC: U.S. Government Printing Office.

1990 (U.S. Public Health Service, 1980). This is indicative of shorter lengths of stay but higher rates of readmission.

Trends began to change in the 1990s, however, with the implementation of managed care. The number of staffed beds at psychiatric hospitals and in psychiatric units of acute care hospitals, for example, de-

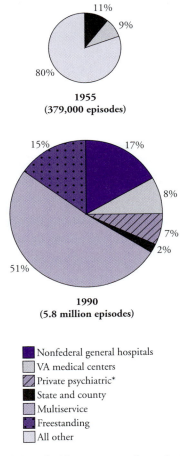

11%

9%

80%

1955
(379,000 episodes)

15%   17%

8%

7%

2%

51%

1990
(5.8 million episodes)

■ Nonfederal general hospitals
□ VA medical centers
▨ Private psychiatric*
■ State and county
▨ Multiservice
▨ Freestanding
□ All other

*Includes residential treatment centers for emotionally
disturbed children

Figure 12.2. Outpatient Episodes in Mental Health
Organizations, 1955, 1990

SOURCE: *Mental Health, United States, 1994* (DHHS Pub. No. SMA
94–3000), edited by R. W. Manderscheid & M. A. Sonnenschein,
Washington, DC: U.S. Government Printing Office.

clined 13.1 percent between 1997 and 1999, with a corresponding increase in the average number of annual outpatient visits of 6.8 percent. Since 1993, there has been a total reduction in staffed beds of 20.7 percent and median length of stay has fallen by 30.3 percent (Galloro, 2000).

Psychiatric outpatient services now constitute a large part of the total mental health services delivery

system in the United States, accounting for 74 percent of the total services provided in 1990 as compared to 1955 when 77 percent of mental health services were provided in inpatient settings, nearly the reverse (see Figure 12.2). There also has been consistent growth in numbers of organizations providing outpatient services between 1970 and 1990 (1,734 to 3,430), and partial care services (778 programs in 1970 and 2,340 programs in 1990).

PATTERNS OF MENTAL HEALTH SERVICE UTILIZATION

Today, mental health services are organized into separate but overlapping sectors that include both inpatient and ambulatory components. The ECA and NCS data are collected and organized by classifications of service types and include the following sectors: the specialty mental health and addictive disorders (SMA), general medical/nursing home (GM), other human service professionals (HS), and, explicitly recognizing the role of a person's social network, the voluntary support network (VSN) of self-help groups, family, and friends (Regier et al., 1993).

Information on patterns of use of mental health services is reported from NIMH's ECA and NCS epidemiological studies. Thus, data are obtained from two instruments: the ECA's Diagnostic Interview Schedule (DIS), and the NCS's Composite International Diagnostic Interview. The DIS is an instrument for assessing and categorizing mental health problem information for study purposes. The Composite International Diagnostic Interview is based on DSM-IV-TM™ diagnoses and includes more categories than the DIS. However, they both provide data unbiased by diagnostic customs of practitioners (Howard et al., 1996).

According to recent national surveys, a total of about fifteen percent of the U.S. adult population use mental health services in any given year. Eleven percent receive their services from either the general medical care sector or the specialty mental health sector, in roughly equal proportions. In addition, about five percent receive care from the human services sector, and about three percent receive care from the voluntary support network. (The overlap across these latter two sectors accounts for these figures totaling more than fifteen percent.) (USDHHS, 1999).

Ambulatory Services

Using ECA Program data, Narrow and colleagues (1993) estimated that during a one-year period, 22.8 million persons made 326 million outpatient visits to professional or volunteer sources of care for mental health or substance abuse reasons. Of the 22.8 million persons using these services, 12.4 million (fifty-four percent) met full DIS/DSM-IV criteria for a current mental or addictive disorder during the one-year time frame. An additional 37.4 percent did not have a one-year diagnosis, but met criteria for lifetime psychiatric disorder or a subthreshold condition. Persons with mental health or substance abuse problems using outpatient services averaged 14.3 visits per person per year. The majority (eighty-five percent) were seen in a professional service, although only sixty percent of the visits were accounted for in this sector. Nearly forty percent of the visits were in the VSN sector, although this sector accounted for only twenty-nine percent of persons seeking help. The VSN sector, thus, averaged more visits per person (19.8 versus 10.1) than did the professional sector. SMA sector services accounted for 38.4 percent of all treated persons, and 37.5 percent of the visits. The GM sector accounted for forty-four percent of people seeking treatment, but only 11.1 percent of all mental health/substance abuse visits.

Of the total 22.8 million persons using outpatient services, 3.4 million persons had a substance use disorder and utilized 56.3 million visits during one year. Eighty-three percent of these people were seen in at least one professional setting, while thirty-six percent made use of voluntary services. Approximately 1.9 million were persons with a comorbid mental and addictive disorder. More than sixty-two percent of the 56.3 million visits made by persons with a substance use disorder (35.1 million visits) were made by persons who also had a comorbid mental disorder. More than fifty-one percent of people with comorbid disorders were seen in the specialty mental health sector, and eighty-seven percent were seen in at least one of the professional settings (Geller et al., 1990).

There were 6.7 million persons with affective disorder, accounting for 120.2 million visits with an overall annual visit rate of eighteen visits per person.

Ninety percent were seen in the professional sectors, and more than twenty-eight percent were seen in the VSN sector. More than forty-eight percent were seen in the GM sector, accounting for 12.3 percent of total mental health and addictions visits to this sector. Bipolar disorders affected 1.1 million persons who utilized 16 million outpatient visits, with more than eighty percent of these visits made to professional sectors, including fifty-five percent to the GM sector.

Persons with anxiety disorders (6.4 million people) utilized 98 million visits, averaging 15.4 visits per person, with 87.3 percent used in the professional sector and twenty-nine percent in VSN. Somatization disorders accounted for only 231,000 people utilizing outpatient mental health services during a one-year period, making 5.2 million visits, or 22.3 visits per person. Nearly all visits (96.4 percent) were in the professional sector. There were 688,000 persons with antisocial disorder who made 18.2 million visits, averaging 26.4 visits per person. Those with antisocial disorders, similar to persons with substance abuse disorders, used the VSN sector more frequently, where 35.9 percent of treated persons used 54.7 percent of the total visits in this category. Persons with antisocial disorders accounted for only thirty-two percent of ambulatory visits in the SMA sector, and 4.1 percent to the GM sector.

In contrast, persons with severe cognitive impairment, 658,000 persons, were among the highest users of the GM sector where forty-five percent received treatment. A total of 11.2 million visits were made by persons with severe cognitive impairment, with the majority of total visits in a year made to the professional sector (83.6 percent), and 27.5 percent to the VSN sector.

More than one million persons with schizophrenia accounted for 16.7 million visits in one year. Approximately ninety-eight percent of people with schizophrenia received treatment in professional sectors, accounting for seventy-nine percent of the visits. Persons with schizophrenia were high users of psychiatric outpatient clinics, with 10.6 percent of all visits made to this setting. Use of services in the GM sector was similar to use by persons with other disorders, but use of the VSN settings was significantly lower.

Inpatient Services

Narrow and colleagues (1993) also report on inpatient service utilization. Approximately 1.4 million people were admitted to an inpatient facility in one year, with 1.1 million having a current DIS/DSM-IV mental disorder at some point in the year. Of the remaining 300,000 persons, nearly all had a lifetime psychiatric disorder or significant psychiatric symptoms. The majority of persons were admitted to general hospitals (43.3 percent), with an additional 35.2 percent admitted to state and county mental hospitals. Private psychiatric hospitals accounted for 10.8 percent of admissions, while VA hospital psychiatric units accounted for 7.1 percent. The remainder were admitted to community mental health center inpatient services (4.2 percent) and alcohol/drug treatment units (7.2 percent).

Persons with substance abuse were particularly high users of general hospital settings, with more than twice as many admitted to general hospitals rather than state and county mental hospitals (50.2 percent versus 21.4 percent), as were persons with nonalcoholic drug use disorders (84.7 percent versus 6.0 percent). The differences between admissions for persons with substance abuse disorders in general were not reported as statistically significant by the authors, while the differences for persons with nonalcoholic drug use disorders were found to be significant.

Persons with severe cognitive impairment were admitted to state and county mental hospitals more of the time (67.9 percent) followed by persons with schizophrenia (45.2 percent), phobia (42.3 percent), and unipolar major depression (38.7 percent). Persons with bipolar mental disorder were admitted only 13.4 percent of the time.

The GM sector in the mental health service system continues to grow in importance. In addition, a large number of people support networks of friends, relatives, and self-help groups which also are of substantial importance. The use of the GM sector underscores the importance of adequate preparation for recognizing, appropriately referring, and treating mental health and addictive disorders within all parts of the health and mental health care systems. Although general hospitals continue to play a major role in providing inpatient mental health services, state and county mental hospitals are still an important sector, serving persons with the most severe mental illness. This is worthy of special concern as the health care system advances toward managed care, leaving state and county mental health hospitals to compete for limited public dollars while serving the most challenging population.

Unmet Needs

In the ECA Program, more than seventy percent of persons with a recent mental health or addiction disorder received no services, and only thirteen percent reported that they obtained treatment from a mental health professional. The NCS study reported seventy-nine percent of individuals with a recent disorder who obtained no services, and only about twelve percent of persons with a recent disorder had obtained some service from a mental health professional during the previous year. Persons with a major depression were the most likely to receive services, and particularly from a mental health professional, while persons with a substance abuse disorder were the least likely to obtain services. Other disorders with wide variation included anxiety disorders for which thirty-three percent sought services overall, but considerable variation in source of care was reported within the category. Persons with phobia only reported service utilization approximately one-third of the time while respondents diagnosed with a panic disorder reported use of services almost sixty percent of the time (Lair & Lefkowitz, 1990).

Other Factors Affecting Use Patterns

People elect to seek mental health services for a variety of reasons including those associated with degree and impact of illness, education, marital status, age, and race (Lair & Lefkowitz, 1990). Other factors contributing to seeking help include consultation with informal help sources, referral by medical providers, supportive family members and friends, and ability to overcome the stigmatization society often places on mental illness. Financial and geographic access to services also affects utilization. The concepts of utilization variables and data assessment are relevant to understanding and interpreting mental health data, while specific aspects of use of mental health services are presented in this section.

Table 12.1 describes the relationship between demographic variables and making a visit to a mental health professional. People with higher education and income are more likely to seek services, although education and income are inversely related to the

Table 12.1. Lifetime Probability of Making a Mental Health Visit Given the Presence of a Diagnosis

Demographic Variable	At Least One Diagnosis in Lifetime	At Least One Visit in Lifetime (Given a Diagnosis)
Gender		
Male	.382	.201
Female	.348	.254
Education		
Grammar school or less	.470	.110
Some high school	.389	.202
High school graduate	.314	.246
Some college	.311	.351
College graduate	.289	.432
Marital status		
Married	.314	.209
Widowed	.362	.101
Separated or divorced	.491	.347
Never married	.375	.273
Race		
White	.329	.274
Nonwhite	.426	.165
Income (in dollars)		
< 10,000	.411	.205
10,000–14,999	.350	.230
15,000–19,999	.331	.250
20,000–24,999	.327	.309
25,000–34,999	.313	.297
> 35,000	.285	.371
Age (in years)		
18–20	.309	.246
21–30	.390	.263
31–40	.398	.367
41–50	.377	.335
51–60	.361	.238
61+	.330	.096

Data from the Epidemiologic Catchment Area survey from 1980 to 1984.

SOURCE: *Mental Health, United States, 1994* (DHHS Pub. No. SMA 94–3000), edited by R. W. Manderscheid & M. A. Sonnenschein, Washington, DC: U.S. Government Printing Office.

likelihood of experiencing mental health and addictive disorders. Women are slightly more likely to seek services, although men are more at risk for mental health and addictive disorders over the course of a lifetime. As suggested by utilization patterns, professional intervention for persons with mental health and addiction disorders is substantially influenced by informal help sources and social networks. Medical care providers are another important source of referral to mental health services as well as for the provision of services directly. The degree to which general medical providers are adequately trained to recognize and appropriately intervene in the case of mental illness or substance abuse is still debated. With the growing influence of managed care, help-seeking will be affected by the use of primary care physicians as gate-keepers. It will fall to them to appropriately assess, refer, or intervene. This may prove challenging if they are not trained to conduct and interpret mental health status and psychosocial assessments.

MENTAL HEALTH PERSONNEL

There are many different types of professionals providing mental health services. They involve a number of interesting and complex issues, mostly unique to the mental health field. The number of full-time equivalent (FTE) staff employed in specialty mental health organizations in the United States rose from 375,984 in 1972 to 563,619 in 1990, with the largest increase attributed to professional patient care staff (from 100,886 to 273,374) (U.S. Public Health Service, 1980). This increase can be attributed in large part to the increase in the number of mental health organizations during this same period. The number of FTE administrative, clerical, and maintenance staff, however, increased by a relatively small amount over the same period, dropping from thirty-six percent to twenty-six percent of all FTE staff.

Staff patterns varied among the different mental health organizations, due to such factors as differences in types of service programs offered, caseload mix, budgetary factors, and differentials in the supply and accessibility of specific types of staff. For example, in 1986, thirty-five percent of the FTE staff in state mental hospitals were classified as "other mental health workers" (holding less than a B.A. degree); by contrast, in other mental health organizations, the proportion of FTE staff in this category ranged downward, from twenty-two percent in RTCs to two percent for freestanding psychiatric outpatient clinics. Conversely, state mental hospitals had the smallest percentage of FTE professional patient care staff (thirty percent) (Redick et al., 1991).

The role and influence of the general medical sector is growing, and approximately 116,642 primary care physicians report that they provide mental health services (Lair & Lefkowitz, 1990). They further report spending twenty-three percent of their work-week doing so. Overall, primary care physicians, psychiatrists, social workers, and psychologists provided fifty-three percent, nineteen percent, fifteen percent, and thirteen percent of all mental health services, respectively (Knesper & Pagnucco, 1987). This invites further exploration as to the nature and degree of services provided and the preparation for doing so.

The traditional providers of mental health services in the specialty mental health sector, however, continue to be psychiatrists, psychologists, psychiatric nurses, and social workers. The scope of practice amongst the various professionals has changed substantially over the years as social workers and nurses, in particular, have taken over clinical areas of practice previously claimed by psychiatry. Psychiatry has shifted more toward practice that encompasses the underlying medical issues within mental health practice.

Psychiatrists

Psychiatry is the medical specialty dealing with mental disorders. Traditional psychiatry offers medical/clinical definitions of mental illness. Social psychiatry, in contrast, is concerned with the environmental and societal phenomena involved in mental and emotional disorders and the use of social forces in the treatment of such disorders. Much of the scientific work of social psychiatry has been in the area of epidemiology, particularly estimation of the incidence and prevalence of mental illness in community and hospital settings. Growing concern for the environment in large mental hospitals during and after World War II also added impetus to the social psychiatric movement, and as early as 1946, the American Psychiatric Association adopted a rigid set of standards for mental hospitals and appointed a Central Inspection Board for enforcement of these standards. Social psychiatry, in an effort to transform these large institutions from custodial care to treatment centers, developed the concept of the therapeutic community, the fundamental tenet of which is that patients can assist in their own rehabilitation as well as in the rehabilitation of other patients. Social psychiatry also includes transcultural and community psychiatry. Transcultural psychiatry studies the incidence and prevalence of mental disease across societies and delineates the social forces that affect the manifestations of these illnesses. Community psychiatry has been described as "social psychiatry in action" (Lipton, Sabatini, & Katz, 1983) and is involved in the development, planning, and organization of community mental health programs and consultation to local agencies.

The number of psychiatrists in the United States increased from approximately 7,000 in 1950 to more than 32,000 by 1985, including those working primarily in administration. By 1994, approximately 44,255 psychiatrists were reported in practice.

Psychologists

Psychology, which struggled to create its own professional identity in the early years of this century, has emphasized scientific research in academic settings. Beginning as a philosophy, psychology has become firmly established as a social science, and psychologists have promoted and conducted research on the functioning of the human mind, especially through development of scientifically validated testing instruments. Beginning in the early twentieth century, psychological testing began to be used in conjunction with psychiatric treatment. Research by psychologists in classic conditioning and behavior theory also aided psychiatrists, who still provided most therapeutic care.

During World War II, psychologists began to be seen in an increased role in clinical practice. With the expansion of mental health services in VA hospitals, the training of clinical psychologists began in earnest. In 1946 the Veterans Administration, in conjunction with the American Psychological Association, began the Veterans Administration Psychology Training Program, which is still a major source of training for clinical and counseling psychologists. The professional application of psychology received further endorsement at the American Psychological Association Vail Conference of 1973, which emphasized the continued training of clinicians and scientists in psychology. Psychologists are licensed or certified in all states and the District of Columbia. In almost all states, the training required for licensure is a doctoral degree, although a few states allow limited licensure for graduates of master's degree programs; however, independent private practice is prohibited. Licensure is not required for practice in some settings, however, and unlicensed psychologists most often practice in school or community mental health facilities.

The American Psychological Association reported a 1986 membership of 63,000. A more recent study reports 56,000 working in the specialty mental health sector specifically (Lair & Lefkowitz, 1990). There are likely more than 70,000 master- and doctorate-level psychologists if nonlicensed psychologists are included (President's Commission, 1978). The pool of clinically trained women psychologists, for the most part, tends to be younger and more diverse in terms of racial and ethnic minority representation. In fact, participation by women in psychology has increased in many ways. Within the practice-oriented subfields, women account for fifty-seven percent of all new 1989 Ph.D.s, compared to twenty-one percent in 1965. By the early 1990s, sixty-two percent of all full-time students in doctoral, clinical, counseling, and school psychology programs were women.

Psychiatric Nurses

The professional training of nurses in this country began in the 1860s and consisted primarily of apprenticeships. The first training program that prepared nurses to care for the mentally ill was started in 1882 at McLean Hospital, a private psychiatric facility in Waverly, Massachusetts. Although there was a growing appreciation of nurses who received this type of training, poorly funded psychiatric hospitals continued to employ lesser-trained aides at very low pay.

Whatever nursing care did exist in these hospitals consisted mainly of custodial care focusing on the physical needs of the patient, and the nurse continued to practice in a dependent relationship with a physician. The development in the 1930s of somatic treatments for mental illness, such as insulin shock therapy, psychosurgery, and electroshock therapy, required the services of highly skilled nurses and established a more significant role for nurses in psychiatric treatment. The advent of the therapeutic community in psychiatric hospitals broadened the role of the nurse even further. As the twenty-four-hour care necessary for developing and maintaining the therapeutic milieu was recognized, the nurse became a valuable member of the therapeutic team. The involvement of nurses in group psychotherapy after World War II resulted in federal appropriations for training nurses. Despite the recognition of psychiatric nursing as a legitimate nursing role, however, the exact function of the nurse in mental health care remained only vaguely delineated.

Nursing education has become much more academically based over the past thirty years as the need for college-level training programs and nursing research was recognized. Graduates of nursing schools obtained an increasingly strong professional and academic education, often training side by side with psychiatrists, psychologists, and social workers. Nurses who earned advanced degrees were often recruited for teaching, however, and the two-year associate degree and diploma nurses were more prevalent in clinical practice. As nurses began to move into the role of psychotherapists, partially in response to the shortage of psychiatrists in most hospitals, interprofessional conflicts developed. But the exploding demand for therapists further legitimized the nurse's role in therapy, and by the late 1960s, the clinical specialty of psychiatric nursing was firmly established. The first organization to certify clinical specialists in psychiatric nursing, in 1972, was the New Jersey State Nurses Association.

Nursing education includes training in psychiatric nursing at all academic levels. The associate degree nurse with two years of training in an academic program and the diploma nurse trained in a hospital program most often provide clinical services.

Baccalaureate- and master-level nurses often work in supervisory positions or in teaching, and doctorate-level nurses usually teach rather than provide clinical services. In 1984, approximately 10,034 master's-prepared psychiatric nurses were working in nursing positions (Bittker, 1985), although one study suggests only 3,000 nurses are working in the specialty mental health sector (Knesper & Pagnucco, 1987). A declining number of nurses are entering psychiatric nursing relative to other specialties such as pediatrics and medical surgical nursing. Ninety-six percent of master's-prepared psychiatric nurses are female. As with all mental health professions, psychiatric nursing reflects serious underrepresentation of minorities in its membership. Approximately ninety-six percent of all female master's-prepared psychiatric nurses are white; only about two percent each are black and Hispanic, and less than one percent are Asian, Pacific Islander, or Native American.

Social Workers

The history of social work dates back to the late nineteenth century and the volunteer mothers who provided disadvantaged persons with charitable aid through the Charity Organization Societies. Social work began to develop as a profession during the early twentieth century. Reform-minded women struggling for equality became social workers and began working in medical and psychiatric settings, schools, and correctional institutions. The development of social psychiatry also prompted the formation of a professional identity for social workers. Adopting the Freudian psychoanalytic model of many psychiatrists, social workers struggled for increased responsibility in the treatment of mental and emotional disorders.

The practice of psychotherapy expanded the social workers' domain from providing charitable assistance to the poor to providing a therapy that was viewed as legitimate by the middle and upper classes. Because psychoanalysis and psychotherapy remained medical specialties, social workers were less successful in developing a separate professional identity, and their practice continued in the shadow of psychiatry.

Training includes two-year associate degree programs graduating human service workers, baccalaureate programs in social work currently recognized as the beginning professional level, master's-level degrees in social work, and doctoral programs. In addition to the basic training of the discipline, social work education offers specialized training in mental health and in human services administration. The National Association of Social Workers lists about 129,092 members (Bittker, 1985). Of this total, 81,737 are master- or doctoral-level social workers. Eighty-one percent are in full-time practice, and 45,000 are reported to be active within the specialty mental health sector (Lair & Lefkowitz, 1990). Social workers are predominantly female (seventy-two percent). Social workers are found in the public sector, including health and mental health services, public welfare, and child welfare, and in the private sector, including employee assistance programs and private practice.

Other Mental Health Personnel Concerns

Professionals with expertise in mental health concerns are practicing an increasingly wide range of disciplines. Schools of education are training counseling and guidance personnel as well as special education teachers who work in schools and other settings. The special needs of people recovering from mental and emotional disabilities have been recognized by such professional groups as occupational and recreational therapists and vocational counselors. Practitioners in marriage and family counseling, in art, music, and dance therapy, and in religion provide counseling and therapy in many mental health settings, as do professionals receiving master of arts (MA) degrees in behavioral sciences with an emphasis on counseling skills.

Training for allied professionals varies tremendously. These personnel serve as mental health workers, alcohol and drug abuse counselors, day care workers, board and home care providers, foster parents, patient advocates, and hospital psychiatric aides. In some mental health centers, half of the positions are filled by these individuals. Community volunteers are another important component of the mental health work force. Thousands of people offer their time and services, performing tasks ranging from assisting with clerical needs to working directly with patients.

Indigenous healers are rarely recognized by traditional mental health service providers. The significance of their role is often poorly understood, underestimated, disparaged, or simply unknown to conventional providers. Depending on the specific culture, healers may be assigned various labels in the literature, for example, indigenous, traditional, or ritual healer; spirit doctor; medicine man/woman; or shaman. These indigenous or traditional healers are distinct from informal caregivers or natural helpers who are found in diverse cultural groups and/or settings. Such individuals may include elders in a community, "natural" leaders, community volunteers, or other individuals who are recognized for particular gifts of helpful caring and compassion.

The extent to which traditional healers and natural helpers may be involved in the care of mentally ill patients varies greatly. Patients and their families may utilize both conventional, mainstream mental health services and traditional healing without the awareness of mainstream providers due to fears that the patients will offend their mainstream provider or will lose the services of their mainstream provider. Providers may be completely unaware of the traditional health beliefs and practices of culturally diverse patients or, if they are aware, lack the understanding and skills to integrate the patient's beliefs into their treatment plans. A survey of Canadian family physicians inquiring about the degree to which they supported First Nation patients' utilization of Native healing practices and medicines revealed that while the notion of utilization was broadly accepted, they had limited understanding of how to integrate these practices with their own. Furthermore, the more serious the illness as perceived by the physician, the less likely the physician was to support it using other treatment approaches (Zubeck, 1994). There is growing recognition that patients utilize multiple healing approaches along with the conventional, mainstream health system formally available to them. The challenge for integration, much less acceptance, is complex and involves overcoming language barriers, gaining cultural knowledge and information, acquiring skills to broker systems of beliefs between provider and patient, balancing patient safety and well-being, and considering medical, legal, and financial responsibilities.

FINANCING MENTAL HEALTH CARE

Mental health services have historically been financed through the public sector, first by states and their support of state and county mental hospitals and, later, by the federal government with the advent of Medicaid, Medicare, and other federally sponsored mental health programs such as the community mental health centers. Psychiatric insurance under other forms of insurance has traditionally been inconsistent and less comprehensive than coverage for general medical conditions. Coverage for mental illness has been characterized by limitations in the form of caps on total coverage available and higher coinsurance and deductibles. Since the 1970s, however, major United States employers have become increasingly aware of the need to give greater priority to emotional problems (Goldbeck, 1983). The image of the American worker as being able to cope with any problem drowned in a sea of reports on growing rates of alcoholism, drug abuse, and legal, marital, and financial problems (Howard et al., 1996). Mental health benefits became more explicitly defined, and benefits were designed and structured in employee assistance programs (EAPs), emphasizing early intervention, particularly when such intervention was viewed as cost-effective. Employee assistance programs, originally focused on alcohol treatment, expanded in scope. Corporate mental health programs began employing staff psychiatrists, psychologists, and social workers. Simultaneously, insurance plans, in general, began to focus more on prevention and early intervention as a means of reducing absenteeism, increasing worker productivity, and managing costs.

Total per capita expenditures for mental health services increased from $3.3 billion in 1969 to $69 billion in 1996. Spending for direct treatment of substance abuse was almost $13 billion and for Alzheimer's disease and other dementias was almost $18 billion. Between 1986 and 1996, mental health expenditures grew at an average annual rate of more than seven percent. Because of the changes in population, reimbursement policies and legislative and regulatory requirements during the 1990s, the share of mental health funding from public sources grew from forty-nine percent to fifty-three percent. Overall, the rate of growth in the public sector was slightly more than eight percent per year while the private sector increased a little more than six percent. Figure 12.3 depicts mental health expenditures by payer in 1996.

In the 1950s, state psychiatric hospitals accounted for eighty to ninety percent of expenditures for mental illness care. By the 1970s and 1980s, the introduction of Medicare and Medicaid, coupled with changing federal policy vis-à-vis the community mental health care system, broadened the funding base. Medicare and Medicaid, however, paralleled the principles and coverage typical of health insurance and covered only acute psychiatric inpatient care in general hospitals in the same manner as medical conditions, limiting care in public or private psychiatric hospitals. Outpatient coverage was severely restricted. The greater availability of inpatient coverage skewed the growth of mental health services such that general hospital psychiatric services increased during the period 1960–1980, leaving the financing of state mental hospital systems to state governments. Congress felt that states should continue their responsibility for care of the chronically mentally ill and not shift this cost to the federal government.

In the 1980s, federal dollars accounted for nineteen percent of expenditures for both office-based care and other organized mental health settings as compared to twenty-nine percent in the general health sector. The reductions in federal support have been absorbed by state and local government, which funded thirty-three percent of the total, about three times the corresponding percentage in the health sector. Private insurance and direct patient payments accounted for fifty-two percent of mental health expenditures. The federal share of the mental health bill was primarily divided between Medicare and Medicaid. Medicaid payments were more than triple those made through Medicare. In 1986, estimated Medicare mental illness payments were $1.7 billion; about sixty-three percent of this total was paid to general hospitals and nineteen percent to psychiatric hospitals, for a total of

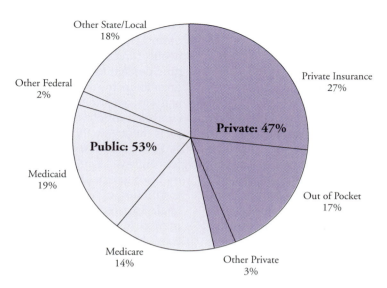

Figure 12.3. Mental Health Expenditures by Payer, 1996 (total = $69 billion)

SOURCE: USDHHS. (1999). Mental Health: A Report of the Surgeon General, Rockville, MD. US Department of Health & Human Services, Substance Abuse and Mental Health Services Administration Center for Mental Health Services, National Institutes of Health, National Institute of Mental Health.

eighty-two percent in hospital inpatient settings. In 1983, Medicaid paid $3.4 billion for mental illness care, with approximately thirty percent going toward hospital inpatient care, fifty-one percent toward intermediate care/skilled nursing facilities, and the remainder to outpatient services (Bittker, 1985).

As America entered the 1990s, health care costs continued to spiral, and the federal government responded by legislating an end to the cost-reimbursement system for Medicare providers predominant in the 1960s and 1970s. Rather, the federal payment for health care became based on payer-determined prices. Psychiatry, however, was excluded from the capitated reimbursement plan under Medicare diagnosis-related groups (DRGs), introduced gradually beginning in 1983. Hospitals defined as rehabilitation, long-term, pediatric, or psychiatric continued to be paid under a cost-based reimbursement system with limits on rate of growth. The exemptions were based on uncertainty about how well a DRG-based payment system would work for specialized facilities and units. Another initiative to contain national health care costs was the resource-based relative value scale (RBRVS) Medicare fee schedule, phased in over a five-year period begin-

ning in 1992, although it had limited impact on psychiatric practice.

As health care costs continued to rise dramatically in the 1990s, outpacing the rate of inflation, employers and insurers found evidence that mental health/substance abuse costs were actually rising faster than were medical surgical costs. Some employers reported twenty-five percent or more of their total health care claim dollars were spent toward payment of their mental health/substance abuse claims, which accounted for only seven percent of total claims made (Theis, 1994; Winegar & Bistline, 1994). The cost per employee rose from $163 in 1987 to $318 in 1992 (Redick et al., 1991). By the early 1990s, reports estimated that as much as forty percent of all psychiatric hospitalization was inappropriate (Strumwasser, Paranjpe, & Udow, 1991).

The implementation of managed care during the 1990s was viewed by some as an opportunity to control the costs of mental health services while improving access, thereby promoting parity between general medical care services and mental health services (Sturm & Wells, 2000). Several approaches to managing mental health services emerged within private insurance, public insurance, and public direct-service programs, including carve-out strategies whereby mental health and substance abuse services are separated from other types of health care services and managed by a specialty vendor who may assume some level of financial risk. These arrangements occur at different levels of the system including with payers, health plans, and group practices, and within the public and private sector. By 1999, almost 177 million people (seventy-two percent) with health insurance were enrolled in some form of managed behavioral health care (Hay Group, 1998). Managed-care strategies have resulted in dramatic savings in the cost of mental health services (Goldman, McCulloch, & Sturm, 1998; Ma & Maguire, 1998).

MANAGED MENTAL HEALTH CARE

Prepaid health plans such as health maintenance organizations (HMOs), utilization review organizations (UROs), and comprehensive case management all began to emerge as organizational types in response to reducing costs and improving the integration of the differing parts of the health care system. Insurers and employers have also collaborated with fee-for-service practitioners and hospitals to create preferred provider organizations (PPOs) and exclusive provider organizations (EPOs) intended to offer care at a discounted rate. These types of comprehensive prospective payment systems have begun to play an important role in the delivery of psychiatric services, often termed behavioral health care within these new arrangements.

By 1994, half of the membership of the National Association of Psychiatric Health Systems (representing private sector psychiatric systems) utilized some form of capitated payment, and twenty percent reported risk-sharing arrangements (Covall, 1995). Within the public sector, at least thirty-five states have implemented some form of capitated payment system for Medicaid clients with severe mental illness, and the Health Care Financing Administration (HCFA), which oversees the Medicaid program, has awarded more than seventeen waivers allowing states to change the types of services provided, the method of delivery, and the population to be served (Shera, 1996).

Implemented on a state-by-state basis, Medicaid managed-care strategies vary. For example, some states have integrated people with severe mental health problems into the total population under management while others have elected to use a managed-care carve-out. Others have devised their own systems or utilized reinsurance mechanisms to minimize the financial risk of provider organizations (Durham, 1994).

Psychiatric practice in HMOs, concurrently the most common model of prospective payment, has been shown to be cost-effective, and differing models of mental health service delivery have emerged. Psychiatric services, or behavioral health care services, are often included in other alternative provider organizations, although often with modest coinsurance payments and strict limits on the duration of services.

Improved integration between medical care and psychiatric services or behavioral health care is growing in importance for several reasons. Possibilities for costs offsets, created by new models incorporating medical and psychiatric care, provide an impetus, as does the growing role of medical providers and the general health sector in mental health service utilization. Mental health problems may present initially as somatic complaints. Reasons for somatization may include: (1) culturally held perceptions that less stigma is attached to a medical encounter as compared to a mental health encounter, (2) culturally shaped expressions of emotional or psychological distress that are reflected in body/physical sensations, and (3) the legitimization of the medical visit over the mental health visit where the medical encounter is financially covered.

Improved integration also increases the likelihood of identifying and effectively treating comorbidities between physical and mental disorders. Effective integration, however, requires a broad spectrum of service choice and flexible financing mechanisms in order to meet the needs of people with both mild and severe mental illness. HMOs have shown the ability to manage mental health care with significant cost savings, but enrolled populations traditionally have not included those with the most severe mental illness (Mechanic, 1994). It remains to be seen how effectively and efficiently people with severe mental illness will fare under such arrangements.

Integrating persons with severe mental illness into managed financing and care schemes is a daunting task. The chronicity of the condition and the likelihood that its severity will affect individual ability to seek and appropriately utilize care are significant challenges within a system that emphasizes outpatient treatment and aims for short-term recovery. These conditions are exacerbated by high rates of poverty and dependence among this population. Durham (1994) cautions that within managed-care systems that view capitation financing mechanisms as a "quick fix" for out-of-control budgets, persons with severe mental illness are at risk for inappropriate, perhaps naive, approaches to care. The emphasis, rather than on financing, should be on informed and well-supported clinical providers, flexible service networks, clinical guidelines and outcome measurements specifically addressing the care needs of persons with severe mental illness, and financial incentives that do not put physicians at odds with pursuing care that is in the best interest of the patient (Durham, 1994).

As the management of care more closely links mental health and the larger health services system, concerns for patient care and treatment are raised. Confidentiality, considered an essential component of the therapeutic process, may be compromised as computer-based patient record systems become more widespread and access to records becomes expanded (Parsi, Wislade, & Corcoran, 1995). The contractual relationship between managed-care organizations and their enrollees has been called into question. Psychiatrists and other providers express concern that clinical goals and concern for the patient will become subsumed by organizational concerns and cost-reduction goals, promoting reduced utilization of care in situations where such reductions are not warranted, and may produce ill-intended consequences. These concerns have become heightened with the rapid expansion of for-profit managed-care systems and the emphasis on shareholder return.

Courts have ruled, however, that cost-containment methods that adversely impact a physician's medical judgment and result in injury to a patient may result in liability (*Wickline v. State*, 1986). Breach of contract (*Williams v. HealthAmerica*, 1987), breach of warranty (*Boyd v. Albert Einstein Medical Center*, 1988), and fraud have all been successfully litigated (Chittenden, 1991; Hall, 1994; Manderscheid & Sonnenschein, 1990).

Recent research has shown that outcomes of care can be improved through effective system and service integration, however. Von Korff and Simon (1996), reporting on a study of 25,916 enrolled members of a large, nonprofit HMO, found significant improvement in patients with major and minor depression when provided a redesigned, more structured intervention and follow-up program, although initial costs of care were reported to be higher (Theis, 1994). They hypothesize that nonprofit HMOs are particularly suited for improving the management and outcome of patients with mental illness because of their public domain research capabilities, in addition to their experience in organizing and managing integrated care. Wagner, Austin, and Von Korff (1996) suggest the following guidelines, based on experiences in developing and implementing clinical guidelines for common psychological disorders: a need for structured treatment programs; provider training programs; automated case registries; restructured primary-specialty care relationships; new assessment and care technologies; and care incentives that reward optimal long-term outcomes and proactive follow-up (Goldbeck, 1983).

SUMMARY

The mental health system is working vigorously to catch up with current knowledge and philosophy, but its efforts are warped by a confusing mixture of economic and political constraints. Previous philosophy that heralded the ability of all people to live in the community has not been realized. Many people who need mental health services and have no financial or social resources find only limited, or possibly no, services. Mental health services for those who do have resources have expanded and changed considerably, leaving even greater evidence of a two-tiered system of care. Despite the many problems that remain in the system, mental health professionals, citizen advocates, and consumers continue to labor toward greater access to financial resources, more and improved services, and less stigma for mental illness. Custodial treatment still exists, but we are learning how to use all of our treatment resources better. Many people do go unserved or inappropriately treated, but the problems of the mentally ill continue to receive attention and concern. In short, the mental health system continues to gain credence and legitimacy as a significant and important part of health care.

References

American Association on Mental Retardation. (1992). *Mental Retardation: Definition, classifications, and systems of support* (special 9th ed.).

Applebaum, P. (1983). Refusing treatment—The uncertainty continues. *Hospital and Community Psychiatry, 34,* 11–12.

Bender, K. J. (1996, September). Study finds higher antipsychotic dosages given to blacks. *Psychiatric Times,* 3–4.

Bittker, T. (1985). The industrialization of American psychiatry. *American Journal of Psychiatry, 142,* 149–154.

Chittenden, W. A. (1991). Malpractice liability and managed health care: History and prognosis. *Tort and Insurance Law Journal, 26,* 451–496.

Covall, M. (1995). Fine-tuning psychiatric health care. *Health Systems Review, 29*(4), 30–34.

Durham, M. (1994). Healthcare's greatest challenge: Providing services for people with severe mental illness in managed care. *Behavioral Sciences and the Law, 12,* 331–349.

Eth, S. (1990, April). Psychiatric ethics: Entering the 1990s. *Hospital and Community Psychiatry, 41*(4), 384–386.

Galloro, V. (2000). Behavioral health outpatient figures up. *Modern Healthcare, 30*(46), 48–49.

Geller, J. L., Fisher, W. H., Wirth-Cauchon, J. L., & Simon, L. J. (1990, August). Second-generation deinstitutionalization, 1: The impact of Brewster vs. Dukakis on state hospital casemix. *American Journal of Psychiatry, 147*(8), 982–987.

Goldbeck, W. (1983). Psychiatry and industry: A business view. *Psychiatry Hospital, 13,* 11–14.

Goldman, H., Adams, N., & Taube, C. (1983). Deinstitutionalization: The data demythologized. *Hospital and Community Psychiatry, 34,* 129–134.

Goldman, W., McCulloch, J., & Sturm, R. (1998). Costs and use of mental health services before and after managed care. *Health Affairs, 17,* 40–52.

Gong-Guy, E., Cravens, R. B., & Patterson, T. E. (1991, June). Clinical issues in mental health service delivery to refugees. *American Psychologist,* 642–648.

Gottheil, D., Winkelmayer, R., Smoyer, P., & Exine, R. (1991, July). Characteristics of patients who are resistant to deinstitutionalization. *Hospital and Community Psychiatry, 42*(7), 745–748.

Hall, R. C. W. (1994). Legal precedents affecting managed care: The physician's responsibilities to patients. *Psychosomatics, 35,* 105–117.

Hay Group. (1998). *Health care plan design and cost trends— 1988 through 1997.* Arlington, VA: Hay Group.

Holcomb, W. R., & Ahr, P. R. (1987). Who really treats the severely impaired young adult patient? A comparison of treatment settings. *Hospital and Community Psychiatry, 38,* 625–631.

Howard, K. I., Cornille, T. A., Lyons, J. S., Vessey, J. T., Lueger, R. J., & Saunders, S. M. (1996, August). Patterns of mental health service utilization. *Archives of General Psychiatry, 53*(8), 696–703.

Kessler, R. C., McGonagle, K. A., Zhao, S., Nelson, C. B., Hughes, M., Eshleman, S., Wittchen, H. U., & Kendler, K. S. (1994). Lifetime and 12-month prevalence of DSM-III-R psychiatric disorders in the United States: Results from the National Comorbidity Survey. *Archives of General Psychiatry, 51,* 8–19.

Kessler, R. C., Berglund, P. A., Zhao, S., Leaf, P. J., Kouzis, A. C., Bruce, M. L., Friedman, R. M., Grossier, R. C., Kennedy, C., Narrow, W. E., Kuehnel, T. G., Laska, E. M., Manderscheid, R. W., Rosenheck, R. A., Santoni, T. W., & Schneier, M. (1996). The 12-month prevalence and correlates of serious mental illness. In R. W. Manderscheid & M. A. Sonnenschein (Eds.), *Mental health, United States, 1996* (DHHS Publication No. (SMA) 96- 3098, pp. 59–70). Washington, DC: U.S. Government Printing Office.

Klebe, E. R. (1991, April 12). *Homeless mentally ill persons: Problems and programs.* CRS Report for Congress (Pub. No. 91-344). Washington, DC: Library of Congress.

Kleinman, A. (1988). *Rethinking psychiatry: From cultural category to personal experience.* New York: Free Press.

Kleinman, A., & Good, B. (1985). *Culture and depression.* Berkeley, CA: University of California Press.

Knesper, D. J., & Pagnucco, D. J. (1987). Estimated distribution of effort by providers of mental health services to U.S. adults in 1982 and 1983. *American Journal of Psychiatry, 144,* 883–888.

Koyanagi, C., & Goldman, H. H. (1991). The quiet success of the national plan for the chronically mentally ill. *Hospital and Community Psychiatry, 42*(9), 899–905.

Lair, T., & Lefkowitz, D. (1990, September). Mental health and functional states of residents of nursing and personal care homes. In *Agency for health care policy and research. National Medical Expenditure Survey research findings 7* (DHHS Pub. No. 1990-3470). Washington, DC: U.S. Government Printing Office.

Lamb, H. R. (1990, May). Will we save the homeless mentally ill? *American Journal of Psychiatry, 147*(5), 649–651.

Lamb, H., & Mills, M. (1986). Needed changes in law and procedure for the chronically mentally ill. *Hospital and Community Psychiatry, 37*, 475–480.

Levine, M. (1981). *The history and politics of community mental health.* Oxford: Oxford University Press.

Lipton, F., Sabatini, A., & Katz, S. (1983). Down and out in the city—The homeless mentally ill. *Hospital and Community Psychiatry, 43*, 817–821.

Ma, C. A., & McGuire, T. G. (1998). Costs and incentives in a behavioral health carve-out. *Health Affairs, 17*, 53–69.

Manderscheid, R. W., & Sonnenschein, M. A. (Eds.). (1990). *Mental health, United States, 1990* (DHHS Pub. No. ADMI 90–1708). Washington, DC: U.S. Government Printing Office.

Maser, J. D., & Dinges, N. (1992). Comorbidity: Meaning and uses in cross-cultural clinical research. *Culture, Medicine, and Psychiatry, 16*, 409–425.

Mechanic, D. (1994). Integrating mental health into a general health care system. *Hospital and Community Psychiatry, 45*(9), 893–897.

Mechanic, D. (1995). Management of mental health and substance abuse services: State of the art and early results. *The Milbank Quarterly, 73*(1), 19–55.

Mechanic, D., & McAlpine, D. D. (1999). Mission unfulfilled: Potholes on the road to mental health parity. *Health Affairs, 18*(5), 7–21.

Murray, C. J. L., & Lopez, A. D. (Eds.). (1996). *The global burden of disease. A comprehensive assessment of mortality and disability from diseases, injuries, and risk factors in 1990 and projected to 2020.* Cambridge, MA: Harvard School of Public Health.

Narrow, W. E., Regier, D. A., Rae, D. S., Manderscheid, R. W., & Locke, B. Z. (1993, February). Use of services by persons with mental and addictive disorders. *Archives of General Psychiatry, 50*(2), 95–107.

National Institutes of Health. (1997). Report of the National Institute of Mental Health's Genetics Workgroup, Bethesda, MD: NIMH.

Parsi, K. P., Wislade, J. D., & Corcoran, J. D. (1995). Does confidentiality have a future? The computer based patient record and managed mental health care. *Trends in Health Care Law, 10*(1/2), 78–82.

President's Commission on Mental Health. (1978). *Final report Vol. II, Task panel reports.* Washington, DC: U.S. Government Printing Office.

Redick, R. W., Witkin, M. J., Atay, J. E., & Manderscheid, R. W. (1991, April). *Staffing of mental health organizations, United States, 1986 (Mental Health Statistical Note No. 196).* Washington, DC: U.S. Department of Health and Human Services, U.S. NIMH.

Redick, R. W., Witkin, M. J., Atay, J. E., & Manderscheid, R. W. (1994). Highlights of organized mental health services in 1990 and major national and state trends. *Mental Health* (U.S. NIMH Rep. No. 77–99).

Regier, D., Myers, J., Kramer, M., Robins, L. N., Blazer, D. G., Hough, R. L., Eaton, W. W., & Locke, B. Z. (1984). The NIMH epidemiological catchment area (ECA) program: Historical context, major objectives and study population characteristics. *Archives of General Psychiatry, 41*, 934–941.

Regier, D. A., Narrow, W. E., Rae, D. S., Manderscheid, R. W., Locke, B . Z., & Goodwin, F. K. (1993a, February). The de facto US mental and addictive disorders service system. *Archives of General Psychiatry, 40*(2), 85–94.

Regier, D. A., Narrow, W. E., Rae, D. S., Manderscheid, R. W., Locke, B. Z., & Goodwin, F. K. (1993b). The de facto US mental and addictive disorders service system: Epidemiologic Catchment Area prospective 1-year prevalence rates of disorders and services. *Archives of General Psychiatry, 50*, 85–94.

Regier, D. A., Farmer, M. E., Rae, D. S., Myers, J. K., Kramer, M., Robins, L. N., George, L. K., Karno, M., & Locke, B. Z. (1993c). One-month prevalence of mental disorders in the United States and sociodemographic characteristics: The Epidemiologic Catchment Area study. *Acta Psychiatrica Scandinavica, 88*, 35–47.

Reivil, S. R. et al. No. 84-C-383-S (W.D. Wis., Jan. 10, 1985).

Robins, L. N., Locke, B. Z., & Regier, D. A. (1991). An overview of psychiatric disorders in America. *Psychiatric disorders in America.* New York: Free Press.

Rumer, R. (1978). Community mental health centers: Politics and therapy. *Journal of Health Politics, Policy and Law, 3*, 531–558.

Shera, W. (1996). Managed care and people with severe mental illness: Challenges and opportunities for social work. *Health and Social Work, 21*(3), 196–201.

Strakowski, S. M., Lonczak, H. S., Sax, K. W., West, S. A., Crist, A., Mehta, R., & Thienhaus, O. J. (1995, March). The effects of race on diagnosis and disposition from a psychiatric emergency service. *Journal of Clinical Psychiatry, 56*(3), 101–107.

Strumwasser, I., Paranjpe, N. V., & Udow, M. (1991). Appropriateness of psychiatric and substance abuse hospitalization. *Medical Care, 29*(Suppl.), AS77-AS90.

Sturm, R., & Wells, K. (2000). Health insurance may be improving—but not for individuals with mental illness. *Health Services Research, 35*(1), 253–262.

Sue, D. W., & Sue, D. (1990). *Counseling the culturally different* (2nd ed.). New York: Wiley.

Theis, G. A. (1994). Considerations under capitated behavioral health care services. *Medical Interface, 7*(10), 123–129.

U.S. Department of Health and Human Services. *Mental health: A report of the surgeon general.* Rockville, MD: U.S. Department of Health and Human Services, Substance Abuse and Mental Health Services Administration, Center for Mental Health Services, National Institutes of Health, National Institute of Mental Health, 1999.

U.S. Public Health Service, U.S. Department of Health and Human Services Steering Committee on the Chronically Mentally Ill. (1980). *Toward a national plan for the chronically mentally ill.* Washington, DC: Author.

Von Korff, M., & Simon, G. (1996). *Mental illness in the general medical sector: Prevalence, burden, utilization, management and outcomes.* Washington, DC: National Institute of Mental Health.

Wagner, E. H., Austin, B. T., & Von Korff, M. (1996). Improving outcomes in chronic illness. *Managed Care Quarterly, 4,* 12–25.

Weiner, D. B. (1979). The apprenticeship of Philippe Pinel: A new document, "Observations of Citizen Pussin on the Insane." *Psychiatry, 736,* 1128–1134.

Westermeyer, J. (1985, July). Psychiatric diagnosis across cultural boundaries. *American Journal of Psychiatry, 142*(7), 790–805.

Winegar, N., & Bistline, J. L. (1994). *Marketing mental health services to managed care.* New York: Haworth.

Zubeck, M. (1994, November). Traditional native healing. *Canadian Family Physician, 40,* 1897–1903.

PART

4

Nonfinancial Resources
for Health Care

CHAPTER

13

Pharmaceuticals*

Chapter Topics

- Progress Against Disease
- Drug Research
- Regulatory and Legal Issues
- Drugs and Health Services
- The Pharmaceutical Marketplace
- The Role of Government
- Summary

Learning Objectives

Upon completing this chapter, the reader should be able to:

- Understand the nature of the pharmaceutical industry
- Appreciate the role of pharmaceuticals in promoting health
- Understand the drug discovery process
- Appreciate the complex legal and regulatory issues facing the industry
- Understand the role of government and public policy with regards to pharmaceuticals

*From Pharmaceutical Research and Manufacturers of America (PhRMA), *Industry Profile 2000,* Washington, DC: PhRMA. Copyright 2000 by PhRMA. Adapted with permission.

Breakthrough medicines and vaccines have played a central role in the unprecedented progress in the treatment of fatal diseases. Leading causes of death have been eliminated, and Americans of all ages enjoy vastly increased life expectancy and improved health. Antibiotics and vaccines figured importantly in the near eradication of syphilis, diphtheria, whooping cough, polio, and measles. Likewise, cardiovascular drugs, ulcer therapies, and anti-inflammatories have had a major impact on heart disease, ulcers, emphysema, and asthma. While much progress has been made, many challenges remain.

Major diseases such as AIDS, Alzheimer's, arthritis, cancer, depression, diabetes, heart disease, osteoporosis, and stroke still afflict millions of Americans and cost society more than $645 billion annually. Advances in biomedical science are helping researchers develop novel approaches to attack infectious, chronic, and genetic diseases. New knowledge and novel research techniques in biochemistry, molecular biology, cell biology, immunology, genetics, and information technology are transforming the process of drug discovery and development. As the human genome is mapped, a myriad of potential new targets for pharmaceutical innovation will be identified. Currently, only about 500 distinct targets exist for drug interventions. That figure is expected to increase six- to twenty-fold, to 3,000 to 10,000 drug targets, in the near future. Already, more than sixty new biological therapeutics and vaccines have been approved by the Food and Drug Administration (FDA) and are on the market. And more than 60 million patients worldwide have been helped by medicines produced through biotechnology. Three hundred and fifty biotechnology medicines—produced by 140 pharmaceutical and biotechnology companies—are in development.

The role of the pharmaceutical industry in addressing the challenges of disease and illness is the subject of this chapter. The history, function, priorities, and regulation of the industry are addressed. At the beginning of the twenty-first century, Americans are riding a wave of unprecedented growth, prosperity, and health into the new millennium. Spurred by technological advances, productivity is up, unemployment is down, and, in health care, progress is ac-

celerating against disease. People are living longer, healthier, and more productive lives as a result, in considerable part, of the efforts of the research-based pharmaceutical and biotechnology industries in discovering new medicines to prevent, treat, and cure disease. And, as the pace of scientific and medical progress quickens, the best is yet to come with more precise, more effective new cures and treatments with fewer side effects.

PROGRESS AGAINST DISEASE

Breakthrough medicines and vaccines have played a central role in this century's unprecedented progress in the treatment of fatal diseases. Leading causes of death have been eliminated, and people of all ages enjoy vastly increased life expectancy and improved health (Figure 13.1). Advances in biomedical science and revolutionary new research techniques are helping to develop novel approaches to attack infectious, chronic, and genetic diseases. By unraveling the underlying causes of disease, today's research holds the promise that tomorrow's medicines will move beyond the treatment of the symptoms of disease to the prevention or cure of the disease itself (Figure 13.2).

Improvements in life expectancy are due in large part to historic discoveries of anti-infective therapies. Introduction of the first sulfa drug in 1935 stimulated interest in pharmaceutical research and set the stage for the successful development of penicillin. The fifteen years between 1938 and 1953 became known as "The Age of Antibiotics" as the result of the introduction of an unprecedented number of new anti-infective agents. Antibiotics and vaccines played a major role in the near-eradication of many major diseases of the 1920s, including syphilis, diphtheria, whooping cough, measles, and polio. Since 1920, the combined death rate from influenza and pneumonia has been reduced by eighty-five percent. Despite a recent resurgence of tuberculosis (TB) among the homeless and immunosuppressed populations, antibiotics have reduced the number of TB deaths to one-tenth the levels experienced in the 1960s. Before antibiotics, the typical TB patient was forced to spend three to four years in a sanitarium and faced a thirty to fifty percent chance of death. Today, most patients can recover in six to twelve months with a full and proper course of antibiotics. Lack of compliance among the homeless and the subsequent emergence of drug-resistant strains of TB remain a challenge to public health officials.

Pharmaceutical discoveries since the 1950s have helped to cut death rates for chronic as well as acute conditions (Figure 13.3). From 1965 to 1996, cardiovascular drugs such as beta blockers and ACE inhibitors contributed to a seventy-four percent reduction in the death rate for atherosclerosis. Similarly, H2 blockers, proton pump inhibitors, and combination therapies cut the death rate for ulcers by seventy-two percent. Anti-inflammatory therapies and bronchodilators helped to reduce the death rate from emphysema by fifty-seven percent and provided relief for those with asthma. Similarly, since 1960, vaccines have greatly reduced the incidence of childhood diseases—many of which once killed or disabled

thousands of American children. Over the past decade, a new vaccine has helped to cut the incidence of hepatitis B, a leading cause of liver cancer in the United States. According to the Centers for Disease Control and Prevention, more than one million Americans are chronically infected with hepatitis B.

Such progress against disease has been made possible by advances in scientific understanding and technology that have enabled pharmaceutical researchers to target successively more complex diseases (Varmus, 1995). Researchers studied the effects of natural products and derivatives on tissue biochemistry to provide insights that led to the development of antibiotics. As antibiotics enabled people to survive to more advanced ages, researchers concentrated on receptors and enzymes to develop anti-inflammatory and cardiovascular treatments. More recently, they began using genetic engineering to develop biotechnology medicines. Scientists are currently employing cell

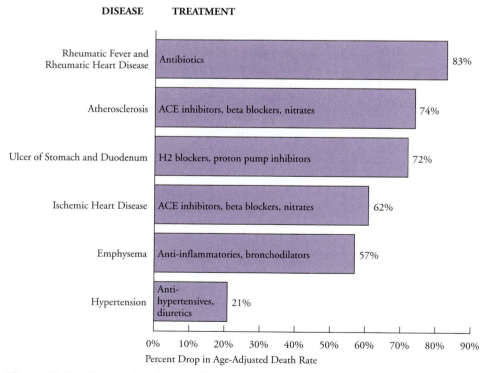

Figure 13.1. Drop in Death Rates for Diseases Treated with Pharmaceuticals, 1965–1996

SOURCE: PhRMA 1998, based on Boston Consulting Group and U.S. National Center for Health Statistics, 1998.

pharmacology and molecular biology to target chronic degenerative diseases.

The twenty-first century beckons as the Biotechnology Century. Rapid scientific advances—in biochemistry, molecular biology, cell biology, immunology, genetics, and information technology—are transforming drug discovery and development, paving the way for unprecedented progress in developing new medicines to conquer disease.

In the 1980s, scientists identified the gene causing cystic fibrosis; this discovery took nine years. Last year, scientists located the gene that causes Parkinson's disease—in only nine days! Within a decade, gene chips will offer a road map for the prevention of illnesses throughout a lifetime.

Biotechnology offers new approaches to the discovery, design, and production of drugs, vaccines, and diagnostics. The new technology will make it possible to prevent, treat, and cure more diseases than is possible with conventional therapies; to develop more precise and effective new medicines with fewer side effects; to anticipate and prevent disease rather than just react to disease symptoms; to produce replacement human proteins on a large scale that would not otherwise be available in sufficient quantities, such as insulin for diabetics and erythropoietin for cancer patients; and to eliminate the contamination risks of infectious pathogens by avoiding the use of human and animal sources for raw materials, as with the use of recombinant Factor VIII for the treatment of hemophilia and human growth hormone for growth-deficient children.

With modern biological science, particularly genomics—the study of genes and their function—we better understand the underlying cause of disease, the ways in which drugs operate, and how to create new therapies. New technologies with such high-tech

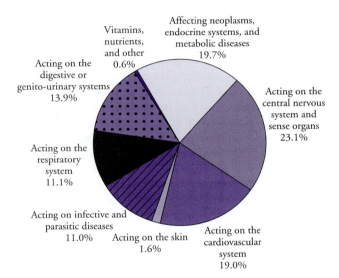

Figure 13.2. Share of U.S. Prescription Pharmaceutical Market by Product Class, 1998

SOURCE: PhRMA Annual Survey, 2000.

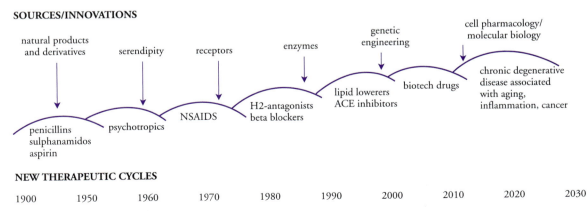

Figure 13.3. Chronology of Drug Innovation

SOURCE: Lehman Brothers Pharmaceutical Research

names as *combinatorial chemistry, high-throughput screening,* and *laboratories-on-a-chip* offer better ways to turn new knowledge into molecules—both conventional and biotech—for testing. And the use of genomics, coupled with modern information technology, is refining the processes by which diseases are defined and diagnosed, molecules are generated and tested, and data are analyzed and processed.

Among the sixty-three biologic products already on the market are treatments for heart attack, stroke, breast cancer, multiple sclerosis, human growth deficiency, rheumatoid arthritis, Crohn's disease, Gaucher's disease, anemia associated with chronic renal failure, diabetes, hairy cell leukemia, hemophilia A, and cystic fibrosis. Vaccines have been approved for hepatitis B, Haemophilus b with acellular pertussis, Haemophilus influenzae type b diseases (which include meningitis and hepatitis B virus), and for diphtheria, tetanus, and pertussis.

In the last three years alone, twenty-eight new biologic products were approved. They include the following:

- the first monoclonal antibody for one type of metastatic breast cancer
- the first recombinant clotting factor for hemophilia B, an inherited disorder that almost exclusively affects males and results in frequent hemorrhages
- the first biologic that promotes production of the body's platelet supply in patients undergoing chemotherapy for solid tumors or lymphoma
- the first monoclonal antibody for therapeutic use in cancer (non-Hodgkin's lymphoma)
- a genetically engineered injectable for rheumatoid arthritis
- the first humanized monoclonal antibody to help prevent acute kidney transplant rejection
- a bioengineered, non-naturally occurring recombinant type-1 interferon for chronic hepatitis C viral (HCV) infection
- a once-weekly injectable for relapsing forms of multiple sclerosis
- a thrombolytic agent for heart attacks
- a biologic to aid in the prevention of respiratory syncytial virus (RSV) disease in children under twenty-four months

Recent developments in genomics allow scientists to study genes on a very large scale—tens of thousands of new genes have been discovered each year since 1993—and build a catalogue that will one day encompass all human genes. By using this catalogue and the information the genes provide about the corresponding proteins, researchers are able to make biological discoveries in days that previously would have taken years.

Most drugs now work by binding to a specific protein, altering its activity to achieve the desired outcome (e.g., improve symptoms, eradicate infection). Proteins also can function as drugs themselves, not just as drug targets. Protein drugs are useful when the body makes too little of an important protein or when the presence of unusually large amounts of a protein can reverse or arrest a disease process. Protein drugs were made possible by the first biotechnology revolution: the industrial-scale production of proteins through genetic engineering. Patients who have had heart attacks and receive clot-dissolvers, patients with renal failure who receive anemia-combating erythropoietin, and patients with diabetes who receive human insulin are among the current beneficiaries of protein drugs. Through genomics, scientists have discovered many previously unknown proteins that can be explored for use as potential drugs. Among other uses, new genetic technology is being explored to develop vaccines to prevent or treat diseases that have eluded traditional vaccines, such as AIDS, malaria, tuberculosis, and cervical cancer.

Genetic research is being used to develop drugs for cancer, the second leading killer after heart disease. The major forms of therapy remain surgery, radiation therapy, and chemotherapy, but genetic research is offering increasing hope of more effective treatments. About 150 biologics are in development for cancer, including medicines for cancers of the breast, prostate, lung, colon, liver, ovary, pancreas, and kidney.

Most cancers are not inherited genetic diseases but result from mutations in a cell's genes, particularly those controlling cell growth, such as the tumor-suppressor genes. Mutation of the suppressor gene p53, for example, has been detected in nearly half of all human cancers. Tumors usually form after cells divide in an uncontrolled manner because growth-regulating proteins are overproduced or underproduced, and signals alerting the immune system to the problems are insufficient. New approaches with gene therapy—the introduction of genetic material into cells of the body—involve manipulating genes and using their properties to halt cancer or other diseases. This process is expected to be extended to fight diseases caused both by environmental factors and defective genes. Gene therapy also is being tested to induce the body's own cells to replace defective tissue or grow new, healthy organs or limbs.

DRUG RESEARCH

The pharmaceutical advances that have vastly improved life expectancy and health since World War II are the result of a steadily increasing investment in research. Research-based pharmaceutical companies invested $26.4 billion in R&D in 2000, a 10.1 percent increase over 1999. Over the past two decades, the percentage of sales allocated to R&D has increased from 11.9 percent in 1980 to an estimated 20.3 percent in 2000. Pharmaceutical manufacturers invest a higher percentage of sales in R&D than virtually any other industry, including high-tech industries such as electronics, aerospace, office equipment (including computers), and automobiles.

Approximately one-third of company-financed R&D in the United States is devoted to evaluation of promising drug compounds in human clinical trials. Phase I, II, and III trials, required for drug approval, account for 28.3 percent of R&D. An additional 5.8 percent of R&D is allocated to Phase IV clinical trials, which may occur after the product has been approved by the FDA. In addition, stringent manufacturing standards require 9.9 percent of R&D for process-development and quality-control functions.

The process of drug discovery begins with knowledge about disease. This knowledge is generally developed through basic research, which is financially supported primarily by the NIH and the major pharmaceutical companies. Basic research conducted in government, university, and industry laboratories reveals disease mechanisms or processes that become the target of pharmaceutical intervention.

Translational research is a transition between basic research and applied pharmaceutical research. Funded by pharmaceutical research companies and, in some areas, by NIH, academia, and private foundations, this research connects basic research with clinical practice. Translational research takes basic research into the first phases of product development and initial human trials, feeding back into the basic research library any findings that raise questions about safety and efficacy. This research adds to the body of basic research and increases scientists' knowledge about disease.

Applied research, or the actual development and testing of medicines, is supported primarily by pharmaceutical companies. It includes large-scale clinical trials, dosage testing, and research to determine information that should be included in product labeling. This research is conducted in the laboratories of companies, universities, and contract research organizations hired by pharmaceutical companies.

In 1950, the National Institutes of Health consisted of six component research institutes with a total appropriation of $43 million. By 1998, NIH had grown to twenty-four institutes, centers, and divisions with an appropriation of $13.6 billion. Although the NIH budget has more than doubled in the past ten years, its share of total health R&D expenditures in the United States has decreased from about thirty-five percent in the mid-1980s to about twenty-nine percent today. Over the same period, industry's share of total health R&D expenditures has increased from thirty-four percent to forty-three percent. According to NIH, public-private research collaboration has been a critical component of NIH's core research efforts.

The unprecedented pace of the development of new drugs to treat AIDS highlights the productive relationship between government and industry research. NIH scientists identified the AIDS virus in 1983. A pharmaceutical company brought the first drug treatment for AIDS to market just four years later, in 1987. Today, there are sixty-one approved products to treat AIDS and associated opportunistic infections, and another 102 products in clinical trials or awaiting FDA approval.

It costs a huge amount of money to discover and develop a new drug. The most recent estimate shows that the pre-tax cost of developing a drug is $500 million, including the cost of research failures as well as interest costs over the entire period of the investment. Since the late 1970s, major drivers of development costs, including the number of required clinical trials and patients in each trial, have more than doubled. During the 1990s, the average length of time required to develop a drug increased to nearly fifteen years. Lengthening development times dramatically increase the cost of bringing a new drug to market by increasing the cost of capital needed for R&D.

The development of thousands of new medicines over the past half-century has been fueled by growing R&D expenditures. Drug innovation is both high-cost and high-risk, and few drugs even recover average development costs. Companies rely on highly successful products to fund R&D. Without reasonable returns on R&D investments, companies will not attract the investment capital or generate the revenues needed to fund ongoing research to discover and develop new life-saving, cost-effective medicines.

REGULATORY AND LEGAL ISSUES

The drug discovery and development process is time-consuming, complex, and highly risky. At the same time, to ensure safety, the research-based pharmaceutical industry is one of the most heavily regulated in the country. The historic Food and Drug Administration Modernization Act of 1997 has enabled the agency to further reduce regulatory approval times (Kaitin, 1997). Manufacturers are able to make new cures and treatments available to patients about a year earlier than otherwise would have been possible.

The process of discovering and developing a new drug is long and complex. Of 5,000-10,000 chemically synthesized molecules screened, only one becomes an approved drug (DiMasi, 1995). In the discovery phase, pharmaceutical companies employ thousands of scientists to search for compounds capable of affecting disease. While this was once a process of trial and error and serendipitous discovery, it has become more rational and systematic through the use of more sophisticated technology. But safety remains the paramount concern.

From discovery through post-marketing surveillance, drug sponsors and the FDA share an overriding focus to ensure that medicines are safe and effective. The drug development and approval process takes so long—twelve to fifteen years on average—in large part because the companies and the FDA proceed extremely carefully and methodically to ensure that drug benefits outweigh any risks. More clinical trials are being conducted than ever before. More patients are participating in the trials than ever before. As a result, more information on benefits and risks is being developed than ever before. The companies and FDA cannot, however, guarantee that a drug will be risk-free. Drugs are chemical substances that have benefits and potential risks. The FDA does not approve a drug unless it determines that its overall health benefits for the vast majority of patients outweigh its potential risks. But there will always be some risks to some patients.

The FDA and the pharmaceutical industry follow elaborate scientific procedures to ensure safety in four distinct stages:

1. Preclinical safety assessment
2. Pre-approval safety assessment in humans
3. Safety assessment during FDA regulatory review
4. Post-marketing safety surveillance

The relative safety of newly-synthesized compounds is initially evaluated in both in vitro and in vivo tests. If a compound appears to have important biological activity and may be useful as a drug, special tests are conducted to evaluate safety in the major organ systems (e.g., central nervous, cardiovascular, and respiratory systems). Other organ systems are evaluated when potential problems appear. These pharmacology studies are conducted in animals to ensure that a drug is safe enough to be tested in humans. An important goal of these preclinical animal studies is to characterize any relationship between increased doses of the drug and toxic effects in the animals. Development of a drug is usually halted when tests suggest that it poses a significant risk for humans, especially organ damage, genetic defects, birth defects, or cancer.

A drug sponsor may begin clinical studies in humans once the FDA is satisfied that the preclinical animal data do not show an unacceptable safety risk to humans. The time ranges from a few to many years for a clinical development program to gather sufficient data to prepare an NDA seeking FDA regulatory review to market a new drug. Every clinical study evaluates safety, regardless of whether safety is a stated objective. During all studies, including quality-of-life and pharmacoeconomic studies, patients are observed for adverse events. These are reported to the FDA and, when appropriate, the information is incorporated in a drug's package labeling. The average NDA for a novel prescription drug is based on almost seventy clinical trials involving more than 4,000 patients—more than twice the number of trials and patients for the NDAs submitted in the early 1980s.

Clinical studies are conducted in three stages:

- **Phase I:** Most drugs are evaluated for safety in healthy volunteers in small initial trials. A trial is conducted with a single dose of the drug, beginning with small doses. If the drug is shown to be safe, multiple doses of the product are evaluated for safety in other clinical trials.
- **Phase II:** The efficacy of the drug is the primary focus of these second-stage trials, but safety also is studied. These trials are conducted with patients instead of healthy volunteers; data are collected to determine whether the drug is safe for the patient population intended to be treated.
- **Phase III:** These large trials evaluate safety and efficacy in groups of patients with the disease to be treated, including the elderly, patients with multiple diseases, those who take other drugs, and/or patients whose organs are impaired.

Investigators must promptly report all unanticipated risks to human subjects. Investigators also are required to report all adverse events that occur during a trial. A sponsor must report an adverse event that is unexpected, serious, and possibly drug-related to the FDA within fifteen days. Every individual adverse event that is fatal or life-threatening must be reported within seven days.

A sponsor submits an NDA to the FDA for approval to manufacture, distribute, and market a drug in the United States based on the safety and efficacy data obtained during the clinical trials. In addition to written reports of each individual study included in the NDA, an application must contain an integrated summary of all available information received from any source concerning the safety and efficacy of the drug. The FDA usually completes its review of a "standard" drug in ten to twelve months. One hundred and twenty days prior to a drug's anticipated approval, a sponsor must provide the agency with a summary of all safety information in the NDA, along with any additional safety information obtained during the review period. While the FDA is approving drugs more expeditiously, the addition of 600 new reviewers made possible by the user fees paid by pharmaceutical companies has enabled the agency to maintain its high safety standards. Over the years, the percentage of applications approved and rejected by the FDA has remained stable. Two decades ago, ten to fifteen percent of NDAs were rejected—the same as today.

Monitoring and evaluating a drug's safety become more complex after it is approved and marketed. Once on the market, a drug will be taken by many more patients than in the clinical trials and physicians are free to use it in different doses, different dosing regimens, different patient populations, and in other ways that they believe will benefit patients. This wider use expands the safety information about a drug. Adverse reactions that occur in fewer than one in 3,000-5,000 patients are unlikely to be detected in Phase I-III investigational clinical trials, and may be unknown at the time a drug is approved. These rare adverse reactions are more likely to be detected when large numbers of patients are exposed to a drug after it has been approved.

Safety monitoring continues for the life of a drug. Post-marketing surveillance is a highly regulated and labor-intensive global activity. Even before a drug is approved, multinational pharmaceutical companies establish large global systems to track, investigate, evaluate, and report adverse drug reactions (ADRs) for that product on a continuing basis to regulatory authorities around the world. As a condition of approval, the FDA may require a company to conduct a post-marketing study, or a company may decide on its own to undertake such a study to gather more safety information. A company may also undertake a study if it believes that the reports of ADRs it has received require such action. These studies may consist of new clinical trials or they may be evaluations of existing databases. For its part, the FDA sponsors a MedWatch Partners program to solicit, monitor, and assess reports of ADRs. Supported by more than 140 organizations including health professionals and the health industry, MedWatch Partners help to ensure that safety information is promptly collected and that new information is rapidly communicated to the medical community. The FDA collects reports of ADRs from companies (which submit more than ninety percent of the reports), physicians, and other health care professionals. The agency evaluates the reports for trends and implications and may require a company to provide more data, undertake a new clinical trial, revise a drug's labeling, notify health care professionals, or even remove a product from the market.

In addition to meeting regulatory requirements necessary to prove drug safety and efficacy, manufacturers must also comply with FDA regulations to ensure the quality of pharmaceutical manufacturing. These "Good Manufacturing Practice" (GMP) requirements govern quality management and control for all aspects of drug manufacturing. To enforce GMP requirements, the FDA conducts field inspections where trained investigators periodically visit manufacturing sites to ensure that a facility is in compliance with the regulations.

The FDA also regulates all aspects of pharmaceutical marketing. These regulations are to ensure that health care professionals and the public are provided with adequate, balanced, and truthful information and that all promotional claims are based on scientifically proven clinical evidence. Key aspects of marketing regulations include labeling, advertisements, promotional claims, investigational new drugs, and advertising in the form of Internet, television, and direct-to-consumer marketing.

Labeling

Labels and other written, printed, or graphic matter on a drug or its packaging (including all other promotional material such as brochures, slides, videotapes, and other sales aids) must not be false or misleading in any way. The labeling must include

adequate directions for use of a product, warnings when needed against use in children and people with certain conditions, dosage information, and methods and duration of use. Labeling must include a brief summary of a drug's side effects, contraindications, and effectiveness. Any deviation from labeling regulations is considered "misbranding," a serious violation of federal law.

Advertisements

All advertising is subject to the same requirements that apply to drug labeling. An ad must include a brief summary that gives a balanced presentation of side effects, contraindications, and effectiveness. It also must include information on all indications for which a drug is approved, but may not include any information on unapproved or "off-label" uses. All promotional claims must be in agreement with the most current information and scientific knowledge available. An ad may be cited by the FDA as false, misleading, or lacking in fair balance based on its emphasis or manner of presentation.

Promotional Claims and Comparisons

Claims of safety relate to the nature and degree of side effects and adverse reactions associated with a drug or the overall risk benefit ratio of the drug. Claims of effectiveness relate to the ability of a drug to achieve its indicated therapeutic effect. Any product claims relating to safety and effectiveness must be supported by adequate and well-controlled studies. The FDA Modernization Act allows promotion of economic claims to HMOs based on "competent and reliable scientific evidence."

Investigational New Drugs

Unapproved drugs under clinical development or approved drugs under investigation for a new indication can be discussed in scientific literature and at medical conferences, but cannot be promoted as safe or effective. The FDA may authorize distribution of an unapproved treatment investigational new drug to seriously ill patients who are not participating in clinical trials. In these cases, the FDA may allow manufacturers to advertise the availability of these drugs to physicians.

Internet, Television, and Direct-to-Consumer Advertising

For several years, the FDA prohibited manufacturers from identifying both the drug and the disease or condition it was approved to treat in the same advertisement unless a manufacturer provided extensive information about contraindications, side effects, and other matters. This "brief summary" is the fine print that appears on the back page of print advertisements in consumer-oriented magazines.

In 1997, the FDA modified the requirements for advertising to consumers. Commercials on television or radio now can mention a drug name in conjunction with the disease or condition for which the drug is approved. The broadcast ad must include the most important warnings and possible side effects, but does not have to include the entire "brief summary" as long as the ad directs consumers to a source for that information, such as a toll-free telephone number or an ad in a general-circulation magazine. The new requirements have led to an increase in television advertising directed to consumers. With the exception of the new requirements for broadcast advertising to consumers, the FDA's labeling and advertising requirements apply uniformly to all promotional materials, regardless of the medium in which they occur. As a result, communications on the Internet are subject to the same restrictions as communications in general-circulation magazines.

The Orphan Drug Act was passed to spur the development of "orphan drugs" to treat diseases that affect fewer than 200,000 patients. Ten to twenty million Americans suffer from about 5,000 orphan diseases for which there is no effective cure or treatment. The law was enacted only temporarily in 1983 and reenacted periodically thereafter. It expired in 1994 and was permanently reinstated three years later. One special difficulty in developing orphan products is that there are not many patients available for clinical trials, and the patients who are available often live far apart. To help these patients, the law provides two

principal incentives to try to make it commercially feasible to develop orphan drugs: (1) a seven-year period of market exclusivity following approval of an orphan drug by the FDA, and (2) a fifty percent tax credit for certain clinical research expenses involved in developing an orphan product. Although orphan exclusivity generally is regarded as the key incentive, it has limitations. A 1997 study noted that the exclusivity applies only to the approved orphan indication. Thus, one or more versions of the same drug may be approved for different indications, and these versions can then be prescribed off-label for the original orphan indication. In addition, any number of different drugs may be approved for an already-approved orphan indication prior to the expiration of the seven-year exclusivity period.

Health care liability in the United States is governed by a patchwork of different laws in each state and separate rules in the federal court system. Cases heard in different jurisdictions may operate under different theories and standards for establishing a pharmaceutical manufacturer's liability. Under the current liability system, damage awards can vary widely and may or may not be commensurate with the severity of the injury or degree of liability. Two common provisions of state law are punitive damages and joint and several liability.

In most states, a pharmaceutical company can be held liable for huge punitive damage awards even though all drugs meet the FDA's approval standards. Punitive damages are intended to punish a defendant for acting willfully, flagrantly, or maliciously in conduct that shocks the conscience of the community. Nonetheless, juries have held manufacturers responsible for punitive damages even though they have followed the FDA's requirements in developing and testing their products, provided all required warnings, reported patients' adverse reactions, and sought FDA approval to modify warnings when they learned of additional risks posed by a product.

Another common provision in state laws is that all defendants in a product liability case are jointly and severally liable for the damages. Under these provisions, it is possible for a manufacturer to pay the majority of damages even if other parties in the litigation were found more at fault. Vaccines provide a dramatic example of the chilling effect liability concerns can have on investment decisions. Because vaccines are administered to large numbers of healthy people, adverse reactions are both more likely and less tolerated than such reactions to therapeutic drugs. In the case of childhood vaccines, the potential for many decades of lost productivity results in greater liability exposure than from products administered to adults. Between 1966 and 1977, half of all private vaccine manufacturers stopped manufacturing and distributing vaccines, largely because of liability concerns. In 1986, the Vaccine Injury Compensation Program was created as a no-fault compensation system for children adversely affected by vaccines. Although lawsuits have decreased significantly under the program, manufacturers still face liability concerns because the program does not cover all vaccines.

DRUGS AND HEALTH SERVICES

Prescription drugs not only prolong life and improve the quality of life, they also frequently reduce or replace more expensive forms of medical treatment such as hospitalization, nursing care, and surgery. With the great potential for continued pharmaceutical breakthroughs, prescription drugs will continue to play an important role in containing costs, even as overall health care expenditures increase.

Prescription drug therapy is highly cost-effective. Other interventions such as surgery, hospitalization, physician visits, and nursing care are typically time-consuming and expensive. Prescription drug therapy often eliminates the need for these costly interventions. Until cures are discovered, incremental advances in drug therapies often reduce treatment costs by controlling symptoms and alleviating pain.

Ulcer therapy illustrates the progression of drug innovation and its ability to lower medical costs. Prior to the advent of H2 antagonist drug therapy in 1977, 97,000 operations were performed for ulcers each year. By 1987, the number of surgeries had dropped to 18,926. In the early 1990s, the annual cost of drug therapy per person amounted to about $900, compared to $28,000 for surgery. The discovery that the H. pylori bacterium is the principal cause of ulcers has led to the use of antibiotics in combination with H2 antagonists to treat duodenal ulcers. At a cost of about $140

per patient, combination therapies now eradicate the bacterial cause of most ulcers.

A study sponsored by the NIH found that treating stroke patients promptly with a clot-busting drug not only reduces disability, but also helps moderate health care costs (Fagan et al., 1998). The study showed that while it initially costs more to treat patients with the drug, the expense is more than offset by reduced rehabilitation and nursing home costs. Treatment with the clot-buster costs an additional $1.7 million per 1,000 patients. But reduced rehabilitation and nursing-home costs result in net savings of more than $6.1 million for every 1,000 patients.

Use of a cholesterol-lowering drug in patients with angina or who have had a heart attack increases life expectancy in men and women of various ages and varying cholesterol levels, according to a Scandinavian study (Johannesson et al., 1997). The Scandinavian researchers analyzed the direct costs saved by this therapy for people of different ages and cholesterol levels and found that savings ranged from $3,800 per year of life for seventy-year-old men with cholesterol levels over 300, to $27,400 per year of life for thirty-five-year-old women with cholesterol levels in the lower 200s. The 6,595-patient "West of Scotland Coronary Prevention Study" found that a cholesterol-lowering drug reduced the risk of heart attack by thirty-one percent and the risk of death from all cardiovascular causes by thirty-two percent in individuals who have elevated cholesterol levels, but have never had a heart attack (Shepherd et al., 1995). These findings showed for the first time that cholesterol-lowering drugs could prevent heart disease and reduce the risk of death.

Pharmaceutical manufacturers' sales are mainly to large drug wholesalers. Wholesalers, in turn, distribute the products to retail pharmacies, hospitals, HMOs, clinics, mail-order companies, and other organizations that fill prescriptions. In 1998, 80.0 percent of sales of human-use ethical pharmaceuticals flowed through wholesalers, up from 78.4 percent in 1997, 71.8 percent in 1990, and 57.3 percent in 1980. In 1998, the retail sector—including independent, chain, food store, and mass-merchandise pharmacies—dispensed more than 2.1 billion prescriptions. In terms of dollar sales, retail channels account for over seventy-three percent of dispensed prescription sales in the United States Sales by hospital pharmacies account for 10.5 percent of the market, mail-order pharmacies comprise 10.2 percent, clinics 6.1 percent, long-term care pharmacies 2.7 percent, and staff-model HMOs 1.1 percent. More than ninety percent of HMOs contract with retail pharmacies to fill prescriptions.

Unless patients take their medicines according to physicians' instructions and systems are in place to guard against adverse drug interactions, prescription drugs may not be used cost-effectively. It is estimated that only about half of all prescribed medicines are taken correctly. Noncompliance is a costly problem for employers, insurers, the health care system, and, of course, patients. The National Pharmaceutical Council (NPC), an industry research organization, estimates that noncompliance costs more than $100 billion a year due to increased hospital admissions, nursing-home admissions, lost productivity, and premature deaths. Noncompliance results in more hospital admissions, emergency-room care, physician visits, and, occasionally, surgeries. There are also serious personal consequences. For example, failure to take contraceptives can lead to unwanted pregnancies, failure to take estrogen-replacement medication can cause osteoporosis, and failure to take hypertension medicine can result in heart attack or stroke.

Noncompliance includes acts of omission and acts of commission. Acts of omission include never filling a prescription, taking less than a prescribed dosage, taking a medicine less frequently than prescribed, taking medicine "holidays," and stopping a regime too soon. Acts of commission include overuse, sharing medicines, and consuming food, drink, or other medicines that can interact with a prescribed drug.

THE PHARMACEUTICAL MARKETPLACE

The way health care is delivered and paid for in the United States has been undergoing rapid, market-driven change. These changes have had, and will continue to have, profound effects on the pharmaceutical industry. Managed-care organizations frequently use a variety of cost-containment techniques specifically for pharmaceutical expenditures (Horn et al., 1996). About ninety percent of HMOs now use formularies. A formulary is a list of prescription drugs approved for insurance coverage. Drugs are selected principally on the bases of therapeutic value, side effects, and cost. Formularies range in restrictiveness from "open," under which both listed and non-listed drugs are reimbursed, to "closed," under which only listed drugs are reimbursed.

In addition to formularies, HMOs also use a number of other techniques to limit expenditures on prescription drugs:

- Therapeutic Interchange: This practice involves the dispensing of a different drug having a different chemical composition than the one prescribed, usually, but not always, in the same therapeutic class. In some circumstances, pharmacists make this substitution without the knowledge of the prescribing physician. *[handwritten: illegal]*
- Step-care Therapy: Step-care therapy requires that physicians follow a sequence of treatments for a given condition, usually starting with the lowest-cost treatment and progressing to higher-cost treatments only if previous treatments are not effective.
- Drug Utilization Review (DUR): DUR programs involve retrospective monitoring of physicians' prescribing patterns. Historically, they have been used to ensure the appropriate, safe, and effective use of prescription drugs. More than ninety percent of HMOs now require DUR.
- Generic Substitution: In generic substitution, a brand-name drug is replaced with a generic copy. Switching patients from a brand-name to a generic copy can cause problems, particularly with illnesses such as heart failure, cancer, diabetes, and seizure disorder that are treated with drugs that have a narrow therapeutic index. Narrow therapeutic index is a narrow dosage range between an ineffective amount of a drug, a safe and effective amount, and an amount where the risks of the drug begin to exceed its benefits. *[handwritten: all false on...cost]*

The increasing trend toward managing drug benefits has spawned specialized companies called *pharmacy benefit managers* (PBMs). Virtually nonexistent until the late 1980s, these companies evolved from insurance claims-processing and mail-order prescription companies. PBMs now provide managed-pharmacy benefits for approximately half the insured population in the United States. PBMs manage pharmaceutical care only, marketing their services to employers, insurance companies, managed-care groups, and Medicaid. There are approximately 40 PBMs in the United States today, although the top five companies account for more than seventy-five percent of the market. Some managed-care organizations have found that disease-management programs are a good way to control costs while improving health outcomes. These programs attempt to improve care by integrating various treatment components. Most disease-management programs focus on chronic diseases, which account for sixty percent of U.S. medical costs. Under a typical program, a single health care provider will be responsible for the entire range of services needed by a patient. Such a program will usually try to monitor and coordinate physician-office visits, hospitalization, emergency-room visits, medical tests, the use of supplies, and patient compliance through the use of an integrated information system. Additional measures such as treatment guidelines, health-outcomes studies, and patient-education programs further systematize the provision of care.

Intensifying competition in the pharmaceutical marketplace also is demonstrated by the shrinking time during which the first drug in a therapeutic class is the sole drug in that class. For example, Tagamet, an ulcer drug introduced in 1977, had an exclusivity period of six years before another drug in the same class, Zantac, was introduced. In contrast, Recombinate, a genetically engineered clotting factor for hemophilia introduced in 1992, had less than one year of exclusivity before the introduction of a competitor product, Kogenate. Invirase, the first of a new class of anti-viral drugs known as protease inhibitors, was on the market only three months before a second protease inhibitor, Norvir, was approved. During the 1980s, the profitable lifetime for drugs—the time companies have to recoup development costs and build reserves for future drug development—was greatly shortened. This is due to passage of the Drug Price Competition and Patent Term Restoration Act of 1984, which allowed quick approval of generic copies of brand name drugs (Figure 13.4). Although this law increased the time between FDA approval of a drug and patent expiration, it virtu-

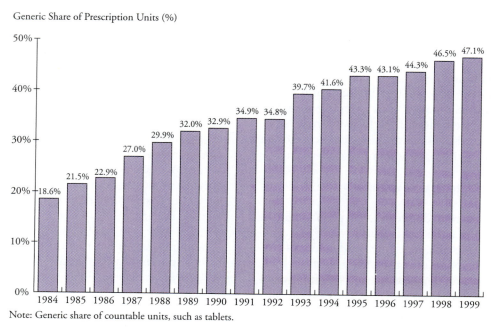

Generic Share of Prescription Units (%)

Note: Generic share of countable units, such as tablets.

Figure 13.4. Generic Share of Prescription Units (%)

SOURCE: MS Health, 2000.

ally eliminated the period between patent expiration and the entry of generic competitors into the market. The effect has been to reduce to less than twelve years the time available for research-based drug companies to recoup R&D investment. Increasing emphasis on generic substitution by managed-care organizations has led to more rapid market-share erosion for originator products once their patents expire.

Increasingly, companies have responded to shorter product life cycles, cost-containment pressures, and research opportunities by forming strategic alliances. These alliances are diverse in nature and may involve domestic and foreign pharmaceutical companies, biotech firms, university research centers, contract research organizations, or other parties. Strategic alliances often allow pharmaceutical companies to draw upon others' research expertise, bring products to market more rapidly, and more effectively commercialize products after approval by the FDA. For example, a biotech firm developing a new product may form a strategic alliance with a larger pharmaceutical company to gain venture capital, regulatory expertise, and establish market presence. Since the mid-1980s, the industry has also been characterized by larger and more frequent acquisitions and mergers.

THE ROLE OF GOVERNMENT

Both the federal and state governments are major purchasers of pharmaceuticals. The Defense Department (DoD) and the Department of Veterans Affairs (DVA) buy drugs for their own health-care institutions and for beneficiaries of their health-care programs. The U.S. Public Health Service (PHS) sponsors a variety of programs that include pharmaceutical assistance. Medicaid, a federal-state partnership that serves as the nation's principal public health-care program for low-income individuals, provides outpatient prescription drug coverage in all fifty states. In addition to participating in Medicaid, states operate separate pharmacy assistance programs for low-income individuals, particularly the elderly. However, most government programs that cover prescription drugs mandate various forms of price controls, including rebates, discounts, caps on prices, and limits on price increases. Various restrictions are also imposed on beneficiaries' access to drugs.

Federal and state governments affect the pharmaceutical market in many ways. Many programs require rebates or are imposing restrictions on the physicians' ability to prescribe drugs for their patients. Medicaid, state pharmaceutical assistance programs, and other federal drug-purchasing programs are experimenting with restrictive drug formularies, prior-authorization systems, and limits on the number of prescriptions or amount of any one drug that will be reimbursed. Cost-containment/quality-control techniques used in Medicaid programs include Drug Utilization Review (DUR) and Disease Management. Under DUR, physicians' prescribing habits are systematically reviewed and physicians and pharmacists are educated about common drug interaction problems. Disease-management programs are an attempt to manage high-risk disease populations by integrating all of the components of treatment to maximize their clinical outcome while controlling cost. In the private sector, managed-care programs have adopted such an approach in several disease areas. A number of states are considering this approach for such diseases as asthma, heart disease, mental illness, and AIDS, which account for a significant part of the overall Medicaid expenditures.

State Medicaid programs are increasingly turning to managed care, which offers both a means of controlling costs and the potential for achieving greater coordination and continuity of care. There are three basic types of Medicaid managed-care plans: full-risk capitation, partial capitation, and primary-care case management. Nearly half of Medicaid beneficiaries covered by managed care are in full-risk capitation plans, the fastest growing managed-care model. Under this model, states contract with HMOs or other managed care plans to provide health-care services to participating beneficiaries for a fixed amount per enrollee per month. The plan is at risk for all the services provided, but may negotiate with providers for discounts. Some Medicaid managed-care enrollees are in partial capitation plans. Under such programs, plans are paid for a limited number of services on a per-head basis and are reimbursed for other services on an actual-cost basis. Some Medicaid managed-care beneficiaries are in primary-care case management plans (PCCMs). Under this model, beneficiaries are assigned to case managers who provide basic medical care and act as gatekeepers, referring patients to specialists when considered appropriate. Managed-care plans provide pharmaceutical benefits to enrollees in either of two basic ways. In some plans, pharmaceutical benefits are fully integrated into the per-person rate the state pays to the managed-care group. In other cases, the pharmaceutical benefit is "carved out" and administered separately by the state. This strategy appeals to some states because it allows them to retain access to federally mandated Medicaid rebates. The first population groups targeted for enrollment in Medicaid managed care programs have been the younger, less costly populations: single-parent families eligible for welfare payments under Temporary Assistance to Needy Families (TANF) and low-income pregnant women and children.

States are moving more cautiously to include elderly and disabled Medicaid recipients and residents of nursing homes in managed care because these groups are high users of services. As a result, it is difficult for private- sector managed-care organizations to assume the risk of caring for them. Other groups that need special consideration include mentally ill individuals, substance abusers, AIDS patients, women with high-risk pregnancies, and individuals with chronic diseases such as diabetes.

Medicare is a nationwide federal program of health insurance for the elderly and certain disabled persons. On July 30, 1964, when President Lyndon B. Johnson signed the Medicare Act into law, there were approximately 20 million Americans sixty-five and older, about half the number today. Like the private-sector health care system of the day, Medicare was a fee-for-service program. Doctors, hospitals, and other providers were reimbursed for "reasonable and customary" charges. Outpatient prescription drugs, which were not covered by Medicare, were a relatively minor component of health care. The breakthrough drugs available today for heart disease, ulcers, depression, and other diseases had not yet been discovered. Surgery, lengthy hospitalizations, and doctor visits were the usual forms of care.

Since that time, health care has undergone a sea of changes. An estimated sixty-nine percent of Americans sixty-five and older have prescription drug insurance coverage, either through employer-provided retiree health plans, Medicare HMOs, "Medigap" insurance plans, or Medicaid state assistance programs. In addition, about 1.5 million people, including many seniors, receive medicines through pharmaceutical company patient-assistance programs. In 1987, Congress established the AIDS Drug Assistance Program (ADAP) to help uninsured or underinsured patients with AIDS who do not qualify for Medicaid gain access to medicines. ADAPs are funded through Title II of the Ryan White CARE Act. States may contribute additional funding to these programs, but are not required to do so.

The Vaccines for Children (VFC) program, enacted in 1994, expanded the federal government's already substantial role in purchasing childhood vaccines. Federal purchasing of childhood vaccines began with enactment of Section 317 of the Public Health Service Act of 1962. That provision initiated distribution, free of charge, of federally contracted vaccines to children at public-health clinics. Also, prior to the VFC program, twelve states had combined funds from Medicaid and the Section 317 program with state funds to offer free vaccines to all physicians to be distributed to all patients in their practices, including the fully insured. Through the VFC program, the federal government purchases vaccines to be distributed at participating physicians' offices to Medicaid-eligible children, Native Americans, uninsured children, and children whose insurance coverage does not include vaccines.

SUMMARY

The phenomenal progress in biotechnology that we are now experiencing will fundamentally alter medical practice and the delivery of services. Pharmaceuticals will lead the way in this change as illustrated in the discussions contained in this chapter. As with any huge and fundamental change in technology, and as has occurred many times in the past such as with the advent of the industrial revolution, the development of new transportation technologies such as the railroad and air travel, and advances in computers and electronics, change in one sector of our economy and society impacts many others. Advances in biotechnology and especially in pharmaceuticals will have a tremendous impact on government, society, and our daily lives as we live longer and better. At the same time, serious issues of paying for progress, litigation resulting from the testing and dissemination of this technology, and pressures to address the needs to provide such lifesaving and life improving technologies to those who cannot directly afford to pay for the technology, throughout the world, must be addressed. Progress never comes easily or cheaply, but few can argue that the path we are now pursuing, however fraught with danger, will result in a longer, better life for us all.

References

DiMasi, J. A. (1995). Success rates for new drugs entering clinical testing in the United States. *Clinical Pharmacology & Therapeutics, 58*(1): 1–14.

Fagan, S. C., Morgenstern, L. B., Petitta, A., Ward, R. E., Tilley, B. C., Marler, J. R., Levine, S. R., Broderick, J. P., Kwiatkowski, T. G., Frankel, M., Brott, T. G., & Walker, M. D. (1998). Cost-effectiveness of tissue plasminogen activator for acute ischemic stroke. *Neurology, 50,* 883–889.

Horn, S. D., Sharkey, P. D., Tracy, D. M., Horn, C. E., James, B., & Goodwin, F. (1996). Intended and unintended consequences of HMO cost-containment strategies: Results from the managed care outcomes project. *The American Journal of Managed Care, 2*(3), 253–264.

Johannesson, M., Jonnson, B., Olsson, A. G., Pedersen, T. R., & Weidel, H. (1997). Cost effectiveness of simvastation treatment to lower cholesterol levels in patients with coronary heart disease. *New England Journal of Medicine, 336,* 332–336.

Kaitin, K. I. (1997). FDA Reform: Setting the stage for efforts to reform the agency. *Drug Information Journal, 31,* 22–33.

Shepherd, J., Cobbe, S. M., Ford, I., Isles, C. G., Loyimer, A. R., MacFarlane, P. W., McKillop, J. H., & Packard, C. J. (1995). Prevention of coronary heart disease with Pravastatin in men with hypercholesterolemia. *The New England Journal of Medicine, 333*(20) 1301–1307.

Varmus, H. (1995). Special Report: Shattuck Lecture-biomedical research enters the steady state. *The New England Journal of Medicine, 333*(12), 811–815.

C H A P T E R

14

Health Care Professionals

Stephen S. Mick

Chapter Topics

- Employment Trends in the Health Care Sector
- The Expanding Supply of Physicians
- Osteopathy
- Dentistry: A Profession in Transition
- Public Health: New Roles, New Possibilities
- Nursing
- Pharmacists
- Physician Assistants and Nurse Practitioners
- The Changing Nature of Health Professionals
- The Impact of Managed Care
- Summary

Learning Objectives

Upon completing this chapter, the reader should be able to:

- Appreciate the growth and changes in the composition of the health profession workforce during the twentieth century and into the twenty-first century
- Understand the key role of physicians and osteopaths in the workforce, and account for the growth in physician supply
- Account for the various trends and changes in dentistry, public health, nursing, and pharmacy, and the forces affecting these health professionals
- Comprehend the importance and potential of physician assistants and nurse practitioners in the health care system
- Understand the various major transitions occurring in the health care workforce, with particular emphasis on the impact of managed care

Health care professionals play a key role in the provision of health services to meet the needs and demands of the population. This chapter highlights health care professional trends and discusses issues of provider supply, education and training, distribution, specialization, and the impact of managed care on the health professions workforce.

EMPLOYMENT TRENDS IN THE HEALTH CARE SECTOR

At the dawn of the twenty-first century, observers look back at the previous century and are struck by the dramatic growth in the number and types of personnel employed in the health care sector. Table 14.1 shows the large gains in health sector employment in the United States, starting with a pool of about 624,000 employed persons in 1920 and growing to almost 10 million by 1998. These figures primarily include those people with training and skills unique to the health care sector and exclude clerical staff, artisans, laborers, and others who have supporting roles in the delivery of health services. Although these several million non-clinical workers are not discussed in this chapter, they are important because they evidence the role the health care sector has played for new employment opportunities in the service-oriented economy that now characterizes the United States.

The health care sector has maintained a steadily increasing proportion of all persons employed, and it currently includes about 7.5 percent of the U.S. labor force. Thus, growth in employment in the health care sector (1,487 percent increase between 1920 and 1998) has outpaced growth in overall employment in the economy (216 percent increase) as well as total population growth (154 percent increase). This growth is underscored by the 525 percent increase in the rate of health care personnel per 100,000 population, from a low of 586 in 1920 to a high of 3,660 in 1998 (Table 14.1).

At least as extraordinary as the increased supply of health care personnel has been the emergence of a wide variety of new categories of personnel, including physicians' assistants (PAs), nurse practitioners

Table 14.1. The Health Sector as a Proportion of All Employed Persons, by Decade: 1920–1998

	1920	1930	1940	1950	1960	1970	1980	1991	1994	1998
Employment in health sector (thousands)[a]	624	859	972	1,394	1,966	3,130	5,030	6,981	8,001	9,904
Total number of persons employed (thousands)[b]	41,614	48,829	44,888	56,225	64,639	78,627	97,270	116,877	123,060	131,463
Health sector as a proportion of all occupations	1.5%	1.8%	2.2%	2.5%	3.0%	4.0%	5.2%	6.0%	6.5%	7.5%
Total U.S. population (millions)	106.5	123.1	132.6	152.3	180.7	205.1	227.7	252.7	260.7	270.6
Number of health personnel per 100,000 population	586	698	733	915	1,088	1,428	2,209	2,763	3,069	3,660

[a] These figures do not include secretarial and office workers, craftsmen, laborers, and other personnel such as cooks, janitors, and so on who work in supporting roles in the health care sector. Figure for 1998 reported under rubric "Health Services."
[b] Figures for 1980 and 1990 include employed persons 16 years of age and over; figures from 1940 to 1970 include employed persons 14 years of age and over; earlier data are based on persons 10 years of age and over.
SOURCES: Adapted from Mick, S. (1978). Understanding the persistence of human resources problems in health. *Milbank Memorial Fund Quarterly, 56,* 463–499, table 3; U.S. Bureau of the Census (1992). *Statistical Abstract of the United States: 1992* (112th ed.). Washington, D.C.: U.S. Government Printing Office; U.S. Bureau of the Census (1995). *Statistical Abstract of the United States: 1995* (115th ed.). Washington, D.C.: U.S. Government Printing Office; U.S. Bureau of the Census (1999). *Statistical Abstract of the United States: 1999* (119th ed.), Washington, D.C.: U.S. Government Printing Office.

(NPs), dental hygienists, laboratory technicians, nursing aids, orderlies, attendants, home health aides, occupational and physical therapists, medical records technicians, X-ray technicians, dietitians and nutritionists, social workers, and the like. The Department of Labor recognizes about 400 different job titles in the health sector. Some of the most rapid growth in the supply of health care personnel has occurred in these recently developed categories.

The traditional health care occupations of physician, dentist, and pharmacist have generally experienced declines—some dramatic—in their relative proportion of all health care personnel. For example, physicians (including osteopaths) constituted thirty percent of all persons in health occupations as the decade of the 1920s began, but declined to 7.5 percent by 1998. Over the same period, dentists declined from eight to 1.6 percent, and pharmacists from eleven to 1.8 percent. Registered nurses have fluctuated up, then down during this eighty-year period: about twenty percent in 1920 to a high of thirty-six percent in 1940, then a steady decline to 20.5 percent in 1998. The group of health care workers that has gained the largest share of the overall number includes allied health technicians, technologists, aides, and assistants: they composed a mere one to two percent in 1920, but in 1998, they made up over fifty percent. These figures should not mask the fact that *all* groups of health care personnel have increased in absolute number from year to year. What the data in this chapter emphasize is the higher rate of growth of nontraditional allied health and support personnel, who now constitute more than two-thirds of all personnel employed in the health care sector.

The primary reasons for the increased supply and wide variety of health care personnel in the previous century are the interrelated forces of technological growth, specialization, health insurance coverage, the aging of the population, and the emergence of the hospital as the central institution of the health care system. The hospital became the setting where new technology could be used and where medical, nursing, and other health professional students could be educated. The technological revolution has led to diagnostic and treatment procedures that, in turn, have led to an increased use of hospitals, with a corresponding concentration of health personnel. The rise of private health insurance in the 1940s, plus enactment of publicly funded insurance systems in the mid-1960s (Medicare and Medicaid), fueled hospital growth because reliable payment mechanisms provided hospitals with assured revenues.

However, current concerns with escalating health care costs have led to a substantial increase in the use of health care facilities outside the hospital. These facilities include urgent care centers, ambulatory surgery centers, hospices, freestanding diagnostic centers, and others. Furthermore, the number of people cared for in their own homes has increased, leading to a demand for such personnel as home health aides and inhalation or respiratory therapists as well as nursing personnel. Whereas demand has created new employment opportunities, a general emphasis on efficiency—often associated with managed-care systems—has created a counter pressure in favor of a more limited use of health professionals. What the net effect of these pressures will be is one of the unanswered questions of the early 2000s. Thus, the hospital sector, although critical to the growth in health care personnel throughout most of the twentieth century, is giving way to these systems, and they will probably do much to shape the size and structure of employment in health care well into this century, a topic addressed throughout this chapter.

Technological innovation has also led to increased specialization of health care personnel, primarily during the last forty years. This specialization has resulted in new categories of health care providers within the traditional professions (e.g., pediatric nephrologists and gastroenterologists in medicine, periodontists in dentistry, intensive care unit (ICU) specialists in nursing). In addition, new types of allied health professions (e.g., occupational and radiological technicians and speech pathologists) have emerged.

Health care personnel will be discussed in greater detail by focusing on five of the more traditional groups of professions—physicians and osteopaths, dentists, public health professionals, nurses, pharmacists—and two of the more recently developed categories of personnel: PAs and NPs.

THE EXPANDING SUPPLY OF PHYSICIANS

The Continuing Fear of a Surplus

The number of physicians in the United States has increased rapidly in the last thirty years, with an estimated 723,500 active physicians, including osteopaths (described more fully in a later section), practicing in 1997. Between 1970 and 1997, there was a 122 percent increase in the supply of active physicians, resulting in an average of approximately 270 physicians per 100,000 population. In 1980, the Graduate Medical Education National Advisory Committee (GMENAC) reported to the Secretary of the U.S. Department of Health and Human Services that there would be a surplus of physicians of 70,000 in 1990, and roughly 140,000 in 2000, underscoring the belief that the nation could substantially reduce its subsidization of medical education (Graduate Medical Education National Advisory Committee, 1980). In 1999, the Council on Graduate Medical Education (COGME), an advisory group to the Federal government, noted that despite the warning of a surplus made twenty years ago, only limited progress had been made in reducing the growth of the U.S. physician supply (Council on Graduate Medical Education, 1999).

Why has physician supply grown so much? To answer this question, one must understand that the U.S. physician workforce consists of two different groups: first, persons who are U.S. citizens and who are trained in U.S. medical schools; second, persons who are foreign-trained physicians, known as International Medical Graduates or IMGs.

As for U.S. medical graduates, Table 14.2 shows the substantial increase in both the number of medical schools and the number of medical students (first-year and total enrolled) over the last thirty-five years. By 1999–2000, the yearly number of graduates had more than doubled the 1965–1966 number. This increase can be directly attributed to massive federal outlays for training, research, and construction in the 1960s and 1970s. By the early 1970s, forty to fifty percent of medical school support came from federal sources. However, the retreat of the federal government from an active role in the financial support of medical education was initiated in the early 1980s as a result of pressures to reduce federal spending because of the perception that there was an adequate

Table 14.2. Number of Allopathic Medical Schools, Applicants, Students, Graduates, and Ratio of First-Year Students to Applicants: Selected Academic Years 1965–1966 through 1999–2000

Academic Year	Number of Schools	Number of Applicants	Number of Students		Number of Graduates	Ratio of First-Year Students to Applicants
			Total	First Year		
1965–1966	88	18,703	32,835	8,759	7,574	1:2.4
1970–1971	103	24,987	40,487	11,348	8,974	1:2.2
1975–1976	114	42,303	56,244	15,351	13,561	1:2.8
1980–1981	126	36,100	65,497	17,204	15,667	1.2.0
1985–1986	127	32,893	66,604	16,929	16,125	1:1.9
1990–1991	126	29,243	64,986	16,803	15,481	1:1.7
1995–1996	125	46,591	66,906	17,024	16,029	1:2.7
1999–2000	125	38,529	66,550	16,856	15,830	1:2.3

SOURCES: Adapted from the following: Undergraduate medical education. (1980). *Journal of the American Medical Association, 243,* 849–866; Jonas, H., Etzel, S., & Barzansky, B. (1991). Educational programs in U.S. medical schools. *Journal of the American Medical Association, 226,* 913–923; Barzansky, B., Jonas, H., & Etzel, S. (1996). Educational programs in US medical schools, 1995–1996. *Journal of the American Medical Association, 276,* 714–719; Barzansky, B., Jonas, H., & Etzel, S. (2000). Educational programs in US medical Schools, 1999–2000. *Journal of the American Medical Association, 284,* 1114–1120.

supply of physicians in the United States, and because of a conservative administrative ideology regarding federal intervention in medical education. By the early 1990s, the federal government provided about twenty to twenty-five percent of medical school financial support through direct subsidies and research, down from about forty-four percent in 1970. In short, dramatic growth in the domestically educated supply of physicians occurred between the mid-1960s and 1980s. Thereafter, the domestic supply of newly graduated physicians has been relatively constant, hovering around 16,000 new MDs annually.

The second important factor in the increased supply of physicians has been the influx of IMGs into the United States. In 1997, 164,900, or twenty-four percent of the total active physician population of 684,600 physicians were IMGs. The inflow of IMGs began after World War II, when the U.S. Congress passed legislation that made it relatively easy for professionals from foreign countries to come to this country to obtain advanced graduate training. This effort was in response to the need for skilled personnel in many developing countries and of other countries' rebuilding after the war's destruction to educate a new cadre of professional personnel. It was also an attempt to inculcate the values of democracy into a new generation of young professionals who were offered advanced education in former communist bloc countries and who were exposed to Communist ideological positions.

By the mid-1960s, favorable immigration policies for physicians had encouraged this movement; there was, in addition, an unceasing demand for interns and residents in U.S. hospitals as measured by the existence each year of unfilled house officer positions. By the early 1970s, IMGs accounted for more than forty percent of new physician licentiates, thirty percent of filled residency positions, and twenty percent of the active physicians in the United States. One-third of the growth in physician supply in the 1970s was due to increases in the number of physicians trained outside the United States.

As the 1980s began, the number of IMGs filling residency positions was in decline, having decreased from 18,395 in 1972–1973 to 12,259 in 1980–1981. Throughout the decade of the 1980s, the number of IMGs stabilized between 12,000 and 13,000. Then, most

unexpectedly, the number of IMGs begin to increase: in 1990, there were 14,914 IMGs undertaking residency training, a jump from 12,259 in the preceding year, or a growth of twenty-two percent. This compared to 73,071 and 67,988 USMGs in residency training in 1989 and 1990, respectively, an actual drop of nearly one percent. By 1999, the trend had continued: 20,965 IMGs were in residency training, a 40.6 percent increase over the 1990 figure.

Why are so many IMGs entering U.S. medicine when there is a supposed surplus of physicians according to the GMENAC in 1980 and reaffirmed by the important federal advisory group, the Council on Graduate Medical Education (COGME) in its various reports from the late 1980s to the present day (Council on Graduate Medical Education, 1999)? Although there is no clear answer to this question, there are a number of probable causes. First, although the United States may have a surplus of physicians (i.e., more physicians than there are requirements for their services), they have continued to be distributed too often in non-primary care specialties, in urban and suburban locations rather than rural and inner city locations, in practice settings that are desirable (e.g., group practices, well-established HMOs, and the like), and not in less desirable settings (e.g., public hospitals, state mental hospitals, and prison health services). Thus, IMGs who have entered the U.S. health care system "fill gaps" to some extent, frequently practicing in specialties, geographic locations, and employment settings avoided by U.S. medical graduates.

A second reason for the large IMG presence in the United States has been that teaching hospitals—those in which physicians, nurses, and most other health professionals are trained—have enjoyed relatively generous funding via the Medicare program to underwrite the costs of graduate medical education (Council on Graduate Medical Education, 1995a). The result has been that many more residency positions exist than there are U.S. medical graduates to fill them. This acts as a sort of "pull" factor to bring IMGs to the United States. Often, these hospitals serve large numbers of persons who are poor or without health insurance, or both, as well as those on Medicaid. Estimates of the number of hospitals that are "dependent" on IMG residents *and* that serve the poor vary between 77 and 276, many concentrated in New York, Texas, New Jersey, Michigan, and Illinois (Whitcomb & Miller, 1995). However, the actual number of hospitals falling into this category is probably greater because the authors used conservative criteria to determine "IMG dependence."

A third reason for the IMG presence is related to the increased market penetration of managed-care plans in urban areas. These plans generally are not linked to teaching hospitals and therefore do not train residents or any other health professionals. Nor do they incur the costs of research as do teaching hospitals. Managed-care plans can therefore charge lower premiums and offer lower-cost services to employers and other groups anxious to cut their rising health care costs. Teaching hospitals, in order to compete, have searched for lower cost substitutes, and residents—often IMGs—actually may provide a lower cost substitute than skilled nurse, NP, or PA services because the latter work fixed hours per week and are generally paid higher overtime rates. A resident works longer hours, is paid a fixed salary, and is a physician. Thus, as managed care has spread in urban markets where IMG residents are traditionally located, there has been more pressure on teaching hospitals to increase the residency complement.

Other factors undoubtedly have played a role in the recent increase of IMGs. Whatever the case, the medical community and groups such as the Institute of Medicine have evinced concern about the IMG situation. The Institute of Medicine (1996) has called for limits on the number of residency slots available each year. Such limits on residency positions, if somehow implemented, would make it exceedingly difficult for most new IMGs to compete for training opportunities in the United States, such that the international component of physician supply would be severely curtailed.

In summary, there was a marked increase in the supply of U.S. physicians in the 1970s and 1980s due to an increased number of U.S. medical schools and the number of U.S. medical graduates. The immigration of IMGs supplemented this increase during the 1970s, but contributed to an increasingly smaller proportion of this increase during the 1980s. In the 1990s and into the 2000s, a new cycle of IMG growth

is now the major factor contributing to the increase in physician supply.

An obvious question related to the dramatic increase in supply over the last thirty years is why it was necessary to use a dual—domestic and foreign—strategy to achieve this. The answer is twofold. First, before the 1970s, policy makers and medical experts strongly believed that there was a serious shortage of physicians in the United States, with several studies estimating the shortage in 1975 to be in the range of 10,000 to 50,000. This set in motion unprecedented public and private spending to increase the capacity of the nation's medical education establishment. Second, our nation has never had a coordinated physician personnel policy as has, for example, France or Canada; in particular, undergraduate and graduate medical education systems have operated largely independently of each other. Thus, the policy of increasing the number of U.S. medical schools and U.S. medical graduates has not been closely connected to the graduate medical training system. The result has been that students graduating from U.S. medical schools have filled a smaller proportion of available residency positions, often leaving—as noted earlier—the less desirable positions (both for residencies and permanent employment) for IMGs (Mick, 1992; Mick & Worobey, 1984).

As the physician shortage was perceived to turn into a surplus, the number and proportion of IMGs fell to lower levels. Specialties once heavily populated by IMGs gained appreciable numbers of U.S. medical graduates, and the number of unfilled residency positions almost disappeared. Most observers believed that IMGs were less able to compete against U.S. medical graduates for scarcer residency slots. However, the nation has witnessed a reversal of all these trends. The number of IMGs has soared, and these foreign-trained physicians continue to serve in areas that U.S. medical graduates continue to avoid. Furthermore, during most of the 1990s, the proportion of IMGs undertaking primary care residencies has generally been higher than the proportion of U.S. medical graduates training in primary care. The argument that IMGs have used primary care as a base from which to subspecialize is not evident: in each of the residency training years between 1991 and 2000, the proportion of IMGs in internal medicine subspecialties has hovered close to the comparable proportion of USMGs. Still, an overall primary care specialty shortage appears to exist, and we now turn to this topic.

Trends in Specialty Distribution

Simply increasing physician supply has not guaranteed the ready availability of necessary medical services to the general population. Of particular interest is the availability of primary care—the entry level into the health care system where basic medical services are provided. Primary care includes the diagnosis and treatment of common illness and disease, preventive services, home care services, uncomplicated minor surgery, and emergency care.

The increased supply of physicians has not resulted in major changes in the proportion of physicians in primary care specialties: general practice, family practice, general internal medicine, and general pediatrics (Table 14.3). There has been substantial growth in primary care specialties both in absolute numbers and in percent: from 1980 to 1995, the number of primary care physicians has grown to over 45,000, an increase of twenty-eight percent. However, growth in *other* spe-

cialty groupings has been greater: over the period 1986 to the year 2000, primary care increased by about 22 percent, but other specialties enjoyed greater growth: the specialties of internal medicine, 50 percent; general surgery and surgical subspecialties, 27 percent; and, all other specialties, 39 percent. Efforts in the 1970s to increase support for primary care residencies appear to have helped increase their proportion of all active physicians only slightly, to a little more than thirty-eight percent in 1980. Since then, however, the proportion in primary care fell to thirty-four percent in 1986, and then to 32.5 percent in 1995. On the other hand, although the proportion dropped to 32 percent by 2000, there was an increase over the period 1992–1997 in graduating medical students who planned to enter a primary care specialty (Council on Graduate Medical Education, 1999). This reversal is due to efforts by medical schools to modify their curricula to favor primary care, discussed later, as well as the sustained demand from managed care plans for primary care practitioners.

Despite these trends, there are those who argue that the nation is not in any urgent need for more primary care physicians or for any radical public policy effort to educate more (Whitcomb, 1995). The propo-

Table 14.3. Number of Active Physicians (MDs) and Percentage Distribution by Specialty Groups: Selected Years, 1980, 1986, 1995, 2000

Specialty	1980		1986		1995[b]		2000[b]		Percent Change 1986–2000
	Number	Percent	Number	Percent	Number	Percent	Number	Percent	
All specialties	414,916	100.0%	521,010	100.0%	630,670	100.0%	684,850	100.0%	31.4%
Primary care specialties[a]	159,922	38.5%	179,410	34.4%	205,200	32.5%	219,190	32.0%	22.2%
Other medical specialties	25,882	6.2%	62,530	12.0%	83,170	13.2%	93,940	13.7%	50.2%
Surgical specialties	110,778	26.7%	134,140	25.7%	158,970	25.2%	170,340	24.9%	27.0%
All other specialties	118,334	28.5%	144,930	27.8%	183,330	29.1%	201,380	29.4%	38.9%

[a]Includes general practice, family practice, general internal medicine, and general pediatrics.
[b]Estimated.
SOURCES: *Fifth report to the President and Congress on the status of health personnel in the United States* (DHHS Pub. No. [HRS]-P-OD-86-1). (1986, March). Washington, D.C.: U.S. Government Printing Office; *Seventh report to the President and Congress on the status of health personnel in the United States* (DHHS Pub. No. [HRS]-P-OD-90-1). (1990, March). Washington, D.C.: U.S. Government Printing Office; *Health personnel in the United States: Eighth report to Congress* (DHHS Pub. No. HRS-P-OD-92-1). (1992). Washington, D.C.: U.S. Government Printing Office.

sition that the United States should have fifty percent of all physicians in primary care specialties is challenged, and the rationale for the challenge is that, in the early 1990s, the United States already had a physician-to-population ratio of about sixty-nine per 100,000, which compared favorably with ratios in Canada, England, and Germany, countries in which experts believed that an adequate number of primary care physicians existed. One conclusion is that it is not so much the number of primary care physicians that is the problem, but rather the number of specialist physicians. Many assert that the latter group should be reduced in number while the former group should be left alone.

Observers of the managed-care phenomenon note that high market penetration of such plans is already producing change in the specialty composition of physicians in these markets. As managed-care plans use more primary care "gate-keeper" physicians to care for patients and to make referrals to specialists, the demand for the former grows and the latter decreases. Evidence of this is found in recruitment advertising for physicians. A study of seven medical journals from 1984 through 1995 revealed a doubling of advertised positions for family medicine physicians and declines in positions for internal medicine specialists, pediatric specialists, anesthesiologists, pulmonologists, and orthopedic surgeons, among others (Seifer, Troupin, & Rubenfeld, 1996). Furthermore, many specialists find it to their advantage to redefine themselves as primary care providers, abandoning their specialty practices and even going so far as to take "refresher" courses in basic patient care medicine. These market experiences have already sent signals to medical schools and residency training programs that a shift in training emphasis toward primary care is a major element in the ability of medical graduates to find employment opportunities.

Geographic Distribution of Physicians

One of the assumptions underlying federal health personnel policy in the 1960s and early 1970s was that a significant increase in the overall supply of physicians would both resolve the problem of a serious shortage and improve the geographic distribution of physicians. Although there is debate between adherents of the surplus and shortage hypotheses, there is less debate about the persistent chronic shortages in rural and inner-city areas.

With the output of physicians from medical schools outpacing the growth of the U.S. population, the population/physician ratio has steadily declined over the past forty years, from one physician per 840 people in 1960, one per 513 people in 1980, one per 415 people in 1990, and one per 370 people in 1997. From 1960 to 1970, the vast majority of these physicians located in urban and suburban areas. However, the supply of physicians increased in both metropolitan statistical areas (MSAs) and non-MSAs after 1970 to the present day. Among the total population living in both MSAs and non-MSAs, there was a twenty-eight percent decrease in the population/physician ratio during the period 1970–1983. Thus, there was some evidence in favor of the market "diffusion" theory that argued that an abundance of physicians in urban areas would cause the movement of physicians in these crowded areas to less densely populated rural areas, provided that the demand for medical services was present.

Policy makers have traditionally assumed that physicians, particularly specialists, would not locate in rural areas. Market forces have caused some change in the distribution of those specialists who were certified by one of twenty-three specialty boards, those medical societies that confirm via a number of procedures whether a physician is qualified to engage in his or her specialty. By the late 1970s, locales with populations of more than 20,000 had at least one board-certified physician in each of a variety of specialties. However, communities with populations of fewer than 20,000 were not as likely to have physicians such as these, and counties with smaller populations still had difficulties in attracting physicians of any kind, be they board-certified or not. Rural counties with the smallest populations have gained a few new physicians, but today in some states, counties without a primary care physician continue to exist.

The impact of specialization on geographic distribution is not surprising. Until recently, general practitioners were the majority of physicians in rural areas.

The supply of general practitioners has since almost disappeared, to be replaced in the late 1970s and 1980s by recently trained family medicine practitioners. Graduates of family medicine residency programs have located in non-MSA areas more frequently than other specialists, with, for example, twenty-seven percent of family medicine residents who graduated in 1991 locating in towns of 25,000 people or fewer that were not within twenty-five miles of a large city. When one adds those graduate family medicine residents in the same size towns but within twenty-five miles of a large city, the proportion jumps to forty-two percent (American Academy of Family Physicians, 1991). Family medicine practitioners appear to have become the new core of rural physician supply, particularly in smaller towns.

Physicians have been reluctant to locate in rural areas because of inadequate medical facilities; professional isolation; limited support services; inadequate organizational settings including lack of group practices; excessive workloads and time demands; limits on earnings; lack of social, cultural, and educational opportunities; and spousal influence (Gordon, Meister, & Hughes, 1992). Efforts to improve the distribution of physicians have tried to address some of these factors.

Federal efforts to improve the distribution of physicians have included loan forgiveness, the National Health Service Corps, Area Health Education Centers (AHECs), and extensive support for the development of family practice training programs, among others (Ricketts, 1994). These programs have experienced a number of difficulties over the last twenty years: many were severely cut back during the Reagan era and were only partially refunded during the Clinton administration. The Republican-dominated U.S. Congress has called for the abolition of most of these programs, including the successful AHECs. What the future holds for federal policy to improve physician distribution remains to be seen.

At the state level, there have been efforts to improve physician distribution through the authority of Offices of Rural Health in states like North Carolina, North Dakota, and Nevada. State-level policy has been aimed at increasing the recruitment and retention of health care providers in rural areas as well as on cooperative ventures of consortia of states to decentralize medical education programs and coordinate placement of graduates.

Despite the variety of approaches to alter the urban/rural location of physicians, unequal distribution persists. Market forces have altered distribution to some degree, but many rural communities still find it difficult to recruit and retain physicians. The same is true for inner-city locations. Often those locales with the greatest need continue to have the biggest problems attracting physicians. As mentioned earlier, national bodies like the Institute of Medicine (1996) have called for a cutback in IMGs, and others have even proposed a reduction in the number of U.S. medical schools. However, without specific programs aimed at increasing the number of physicians in underserved areas, it is difficult to see how a reduction in the overall number of physicians can do anything but worsen the historic problem of physician maldistribution.

Developing policies to alter physician distribution has therefore turned out to be a difficult undertaking. The limited impact of previous attempts suggests that broader policy options should be considered. The possibilities include changing reimbursement systems to provide a financial reward for physicians practicing in underserved areas. Another remedy might be to modify, even more than has been done, the admissions policies of medical schools so as to place more emphasis on applicants interested in primary care practice. Or, undergraduate and graduate medical education systems could be changed to ensure that the curriculum, counseling, clinical setting, and role models presented are better related to the health needs of the underserved. A revitalized and expanded National Health Service Corps might be one of the best short-term solutions to the distribution problem. Whatever steps are taken, a balance must be found between changing the size and composition of the physician workforce so that the goals of improving physician distribution are not forgotten.

Changes in Medical Education

The past thirty-year period has been one of change for both undergraduate and graduate medical education.

Change has occurred and is occurring in two general realms: the size and composition of classes and the organization of medical education itself. In the first case, the stereotype of the typical medical student—a white urban male who will eventually practice a medical or surgical specialty in a large urban setting—has changed. In the second case, the relationship of medical schools to the rest of the health care sector has changed.

On the undergraduate level, from 1970–1971 to the current time, the first-year medical school class size increased by over fifty percent, with the 1999–2000 entering class totaling 16,856. First-year enrollments hovered in the 17,000 range throughout the 1980s and 1990s. Compared to the early 1970s, there is no question that U.S. medical schools responded to the call to increase the supply of physicians.

The undergraduate medical curriculum remains broad-based, with the first two years consisting of lectures and laboratory work in the basic sciences, followed by two years of work in the clinical sciences through seminars and work in hospital wards and clinics. The role models and values in most medical schools continue to emphasize acute care for hospitalized patients. However, this is changing with the increase in ambulatory and non-institutional services. More and more medical students are experiencing out-of-hospital training experiences. The professional socialization of medical students shows signs of changing, with more emphasis on preceptorships in primary care settings and shifts in the focus of a growing number of medical school faculty from research to the provision of patient care. The latter has occurred due to changes in the distribution of medical school funding resulting from a de-emphasis on federal funding and greater reliance on state and local support as well as revenues from faculty practice plans.

Another important issue in the system of medical education concerns women and minority students. Concerted efforts to increase their enrollment have borne fruit: over the past thirty-year period, the first-year enrollment of female medical students has increased from 11.1 percent to 45.8 percent; total female enrollment increased from 9.6 percent to 43.9 percent. A more modest but still significant increase in minority students has been registered: from 1970–1971 to 1999–2000, the percentage of minority students in allopathic medical schools increased from about nine percent to nearly thirty-five percent of all first-year students. The greatest increase in minority students has been among Asian Americans, Native Americans, Hispanic Americans, and African Americans, in that order. For example, although African Americans increased their number by ninety-one percent over the thirty-year period just noted, Asian Americans increased over sixteenfold. The presence of minority physicians is extremely important because it has been shown that minority patients are four times more likely to receive care from minority physicians than non-minority ones. Low income, Medicaid recipients, and uninsured patients were also more likely to receive care from minority physicians (Moy & Bartman, 1995).

The graduate medical education "pipeline" has also undergone major changes in the last thirty years. The total number of residency positions increased significantly, from 65,615 in 1971 to 97,989 in 1999. The percentage of positions filled had increased until 1985, when only 1,696 posts, or two percent of the total, remained vacant. After 1986, however, there was an increasing percentage of unfilled posts to five percent in 1989. This figure stabilized through 1994 (5,408 unfilled positions, or five percent). As noted earlier, the declining proportion of IMGs in residency slots reversed itself about the same time as unfilled slots began to rise: the percent of IMGs in U.S. residency positions increased from sixteen percent to twenty-six percent.

Notable shifts have also occurred in the organization of medical schools and their relationship to the rest of the health care sector. First and foremost, medical schools and their affiliated hospitals have been forced to compete for patients—both ambulatory and in-patient—by managed-care plans. These plans, as noted earlier, do not bear the costs of medical education, nor do they sponsor basic clinical research; hence, they are able to under bid the prices that medical school-affiliated hospitals and health systems must charge to recover their costs. This phenomenon has resulted in both the downsizing of many medical schools and their affiliated hospitals as well as the merger of some others. For example, a number of medical school mergers have taken place in New York City and Philadelphia.

Another result of the increased competition felt by university medical centers is the willingness of some to affiliate with national for-profit hospital systems. For instance, in a number of states, medical schools have arranged leasing arrangements with for-profit systems to run teaching hospitals, to refurbish outdated facilities, to institute efficient management techniques, and generally to bring a new infusion of capital to hard-pressed teaching institutions. In return, the for-profit systems gain a foothold into the very heart of the U.S. medical education establishment. Observers view medical school and for-profit hospital system affiliations with mixed feelings. On the one hand, for-profit systems bring a wealth of management expertise to often antiquated organizational arrangements and procedures; they also provide a means of allowing medical centers to compete more effectively with the growing number of managed-care plans. In fact, teaching hospitals often become part of a preexisting managed-care plan that has already proven itself effective in the market. On the other hand, it was ninety years ago that the famous Flexner Report urged the medical education community to rid itself of institutions that were run on a for-profit basis, arguing that the for-profit motive was inconsistent with the thorough and scientific training of physicians (Flexner, 1910). The year 2000 is not the early part of the twentieth century, and conditions have changed so dramatically that the worry of the Flexner Report may be inappropriate today. However, there will probably be increasing discussion and debate about the propriety of for-profit organizations' involvement in medical education and to what degree the profit motive is compatible with the social welfare function of health care delivery.

In summary, undergraduate and graduate medical education has changed in the last thirty years. Even with a warning of a surplus of physicians, some of the recommendations of the final report of the GMENAC, such as a decrease in the size of medical school classes by ten percent by 1984, were largely ignored. It is therefore not surprising that, in 2000, there should once again be renewed calls for reductions in the number of physicians in training and a greater emphasis on primary care specialization. Managed care competition may end up producing the reduction in medical education capacity at both the undergraduate and graduate levels that numerous blue-ribbon committees with their downsizing recommendations have been unable to achieve. These issues, joined to the debate engendered by the presence of IMGs in U.S. residencies, promise to keep the fundamental problems of the training and deployment of the physician workforce a number one policy issue as the country moves toward the twenty-first century.

OSTEOPATHY

Often neglected in discussions of medical personnel is the small but significant number of osteopaths in the United States. Osteopathy differs from allopathic medicine in that osteopaths traditionally emphasize treatments that involve corrections of the position of joints or tissues, and they stress diet or environment as factors that might destroy natural resistance. Allopathic medicine views the physician as an active interventionist attempting to neutralize the effects of disease by using treatments that produce a counteracting effect. Despite these differences, osteopaths are licensed to practice medicine and perform surgery in all states, and are eligible for graduate medical education in either osteopathic or allopathic residencies. In fact, there were 3,869 osteopaths in accredited allopathic residency programs in 1999–2000. Finally, osteopaths are reimbursed by both Medicare and Medicaid, the two major federal financing programs.

The growth in osteopaths has been great, but this is partially due to the small base number to begin with: In 1970, there were 12,000 osteopaths; in 1997, there were about 38,900, an increase of about 224 percent. The ratio of osteopaths to population was 11.1 to 100,000. However, this figure is deceptive because osteopaths are unevenly distributed around the country. Four of five osteopaths were located in just sixteen states, led by Michigan, Pennsylvania, Ohio, Florida, Texas, and New Jersey, in descending order. Hence, in states like these, osteopaths make a contribution to health care disproportionate to their overall number. Finally, although there were only five doctors of osteopathy per 100,000 in metropolitan areas in 1986, the rate in rural areas was six times as great, or thirty per 100,000 in non-metropolitan areas. This is, of course, the opposite of allopathic physicians, whose ratio is larger in metropolitan than non-metropolitan areas.

There are now nineteen schools of osteopathy, up from fifteen schools in the early 1990s. These schools are located, for the most part, in the states with the largest number of osteopaths. From 1975–1976 to 1999–2000, there was an increase in first-year class size of 174 percent. There has been an increasing proportion of first-year female students (fourteen percent to thirty-four percent, from 1975–76 through 1990–1991), as well as an increase in minority first-year students (five percent to twenty percent over the same period). Since 1987, there have been more osteopaths in allopathic residency programs than in osteopathic programs, underlining the narrow difference between the two groups. Nearly forty percent of osteopaths train in the primary care specialties of general internal medicine and general practice, although in 1990, of those osteopaths in actual practice, about fifty-five percent were in primary care. Combining these facts with osteopaths' location in specific states underscores their importance to health care delivery of primary care medicine.

In short, osteopathic medicine is a small but important form of medical practice that shares the burden of care with allopathic physicians. It has experienced the same changes—increasing proportion of women and minorities, increasing number of applicants—as its larger cousin has undergone.

DENTISTRY: A PROFESSION IN TRANSITION

In 1997, there were approximately 138,435 dentists practicing in the United States. The supply of dentists increased during the 1990s, but has now gradually declined, as has the ratio of active dentists to population: in 1960, the ratio was 49.4 per 100,000 population, in 1991, 61.3 per 100,000, but in 1997, down to 51.7 per 100,000 (Table 14.4). As in medicine, the earlier increases that occurred can be attributed to federal legislation passed in the early 1960s and 1970s that directly attempted to remedy the perceived shortage. This legislation resulted in increases in the number of dental schools from forty-seven to sixty in the period 1960 to 1980, and an increase in the number of first-year dental students from 3,600 to more than 6,000 in the same period (Table 14.5). However, since 1980, the total number of dental schools and the first-year class dropped to 54 and 4,347, respectively, by 1997–1998.

Some of the recent trends that are descriptive of medical schools are also descriptive of dental schools.

Table 14.4.   Total and Active Dentists and Dentist/Population Ratios: Selected Years, 1960 through 1997

| Year | Number of Dentists[a] | | Total Population (Thousands) | Active Dentists per 100,000 Population |
	Total	Active		
1960	105,200	90,120	182,287	49.4
1970	116,250	102,220	206,466	49.5
1975	126,590	112,020	217,095	51.6
1980	147,280	126,240	228,831	55.2
1991	—	155,000	252,700	61.3
1997	—	138,435	268,000	51.7

[a]Includes dentists in federal service.
SOURCES: *Fourth report to the President and Congress on the status of health personnel in the United States* (DHHS Pub. No. [HRS]-P-0084.4). (1984, May). Washington, D.C.: U.S. Government Printing Office; *Seventh report to the President and Congress on the status of health personnel in the United States* (DHHS Pub. No. [HRS]-P-OD-90-1). (1990, March). Washington, D.C.: U.S. Government Printing Office; *Health personnel in the United States: Ninth report to Congress* (1993). Washington, D.C.: U.S. Government Printing Office; adapted from Brown, L.J., & Lazar, V. (1999). Trends in the dental health work force. *Journal of the American Dental Association, 130,* 1743–1749.

Table 14.5. Number of Dental Schools, Students, Including Female and Minority Students, and Graduates: Selected Academic Years, 1960–1961 through 1997–1998[a]

Academic Year	Number of Schools	Number of Students[b]		First-Year Female Students	Percent Female of First-Year Students	Total Minority Students	Percent Minority of Total Students	Total Number of Graduates[b]
		Total	First-Year					
1960-1961	47	13,580	3,616	—	—	—	—	3,290
1970-1971	53	16,553	4,565	94	2.1%	552[c]	3.3%	3,775
1980-1981	60	22,842	6,030	1,194	19.8%	2,453	10.7%	5,550
1990-1991	55	15,951	4,001	1,522	38.0%	4,766	29.9%	3,995
1997-1998	54	16,926	4,347	1,609	37.0%	5,888	34.8%	3,930

[a]Includes African, Hispanic, Native, Asian American, and, for 1970, "Other Minorities."
[b]Excludes graduates of the University of Puerto Rico for 1960–61 and 1970–71.
[c]Estimated minority enrollment.

SOURCES: *Minorities & women in the health fields, 1990 edition* (DHHS Pub. No. [HRSA]-P-DV-90-3). (1990). Washington, D.C.: U.S. Government Printing Office; *Health personnel in the United States: Eighth report to Congress, 1991* (DHHS Pub. No. HRS-P-OD-92.1). (1992). Washington, D.C.: U.S. Government Printing Office; *Health personnel in the United States: Ninth report to Congress, 1993.* Washington, D.C.: U.S. Government Printing Office; *Minorities & women in the health fields, 1994 edition* (DHHS Pub. No. [HRSA-P-DV-94-2). (1994). Washington, D.C.: U.S. Government Printing Office; Adapted from Brown, L.J., & Lazar, V. (1999). Trends in the dental health work force. *Journal of the American Dental Association, 130,* 1743–1749.

The percentage of female first-year students has soared from a mere two percent in 1970–1971 to thirty-seven percent in 1997–1998 (Table 10.5). The proportion of minority students has also increased dramatically, from three percent in 1970–1971 to thirty-five percent in 1997–1998. Dental schools have started to de-emphasize their support from federal sources and have increased their state support, dental clinic revenues, and fees from tuition. Also, as with medicine, there was a sizable decrease in the number of applicants to dental school in the 1980s, although the decline started earlier and was steeper for dentistry. Since 1975, when dental school applications peaked at 15,734, there was a steady decline until 1989 when 4,996 persons applied, yielding an applicant-admission ratio of 1:3. Since then, applications have increased so that for the 1991–1992 academic year, 5,632 persons applied for dental school. The decline, smaller class sizes, reductions in federal support, and increased costs have reduced the number of dental schools from sixty to fifty-four.

Unlike their physician counterparts, dentists typically work in solo or small group private practices. However, current economic pressures on the dental profession have initiated changes in the delivery of dental services. During the 1980s, a variety of nontraditional practice settings have emerged for dentists, including HMOs and retail locations in malls, stores, and plazas. Although only a small proportion of dental services are provided in these settings and the number of active private practitioners is expected to grow (Brown & Lazar, 1999), this organizational innovation is an indication of the more competitive environment dentistry is facing in the early 2000s.

The vast majority of dentists are in general practice. Only about one-seventh of all dentists are specialists, and the proportion of specialists has remained stable in recent years. Orthodontists comprise roughly one-third of all dental specialists, with oral surgeons totaling almost another one-fourth of the specialist population.

There is significant variation in the distribution of dentists across the regions of the United States and metropolitan versus non-metropolitan areas. This variation is caused by the same factors that have led to physician maldistribution, as well as by the lack of reciprocity in the licensing of dentists across states. More than one-half of all dentists practice in the state in which they were trained, yet at least eighteen states have no school of dentistry. Those portions of the country that are most rural have the lowest dentist/population ratios: for example, in 1992, an urban state like Massachusetts had 79.9 dentists per 100,000 population, whereas a rural state such as Alabama had 44.2 per 100,000. In the late 1980s, there were over 700 federally designated dental shortage areas, approximately three-quarters of which were in nonmetropolitan areas.

In addition to the traditional maldistribution of dentists, there is concern that there may be a growing gap between the availability of dentists and the need for their services, especially because the financing of dental services is on a much smaller scale than that of physician services. Currently, less than one-half of the U.S. population has dental insurance, and federal funds pay for less than two percent of all dental care (*Health Personnel in the United States: Ninth Report to Congress*, 1993). Three other factors contribute to this gap. First, whereas fluoridation of water has reduced the number of dental caries and fillings needing replacement, about seventy-five percent of dental caries in children are concentrated in about twenty-five percent of the population, with disease levels higher among minority populations. Second, minority populations where dental problems appear to be concentrated and that have little, if any, dental insurance are expected to grow between the mid-1990s and 2020, thus potentially widening the gap between the ability to pay and receipt of services. Third, the ever-growing adult population—at greater risk for gingivitis and adult-onset periodontis (a major contributor to tooth loss)—will need more dental services.

Auxiliary Personnel

The practice of dentistry has undergone major technological and organizational changes in the past several decades. Of particular importance has been the increased use of dental auxiliary personnel. Two major types of dental auxiliaries are dental hygienists and dental assistants. Dental hygienists provide oral prophylaxis services and dental health education and comprise the only group of auxiliaries that is licensed. Dental assistants have generally supported the dentist at chairside and have had the opportunity in some states to perform expanded functions under the dentist's supervision. In 1998, there were about 112,000 active dental hygienists, and roughly 230,000 dental assistants.

Most dentists employ some dental auxiliary on a full- or part-time basis. The government has supported the training of expanded-function dental auxiliaries (dental hygienists or dental assistants who receive additional education and training that enable them to perform a broader array of clinical functions), as well as the training of dental students to help improve their administrative and organizational skills in managing multiple auxiliary team practices. Support for the auxiliary concept has been due largely to an increase in the productivity of dental practices that employ such persons.

Increasing educational and professional requirements for dental hygienists (they must carry their own malpractice insurance) has made them able to practice without the physical presence of a dentist, something allowed in forty states. There is evidence that these hygienists can provide greater access to dental services in underserved areas at lower cost and without an overall reduction in the quality of care. However, state regulations and the opposition of professional dentists' organizations do not favor the use of dental hygienists, and there is currently a struggle between dentists and dental hygienists over self-regulation and autonomy. This controversy will continue as long as the maldistribution of dentists persists and evidence continues to appear that dental hygienists can perform a variety of functions independently and inexpensively with no loss of quality.

Thus, the dental professions are in transition. The growth in numbers of dentists will continue, but probably at a lower rate than other health professions. The financial condition of a number of the remaining fifty-four dental schools, especially private ones, is poor, and there may be more closures in the next several years, further reducing the growth of dentistry. The role of the expanded function dental auxiliary is still unclear. The demand for dental care is very sensitive to economic conditions (because dental insurance covers only two-fifths of the population and one-third of dental expenditures) and can decrease during periods of recession. Hence, a shortage one year can quickly turn into a surplus the next. Yet, these economic conditions mask the epidemiological and demographic changes that are slowly altering the need for services. How these many factors combine to affect the future of dentistry should be watched closely.

PUBLIC HEALTH: NEW ROLES, NEW POSSIBILITIES

Traditionally, health professionals trained in public health have been sharply demarcated from those involved in the direct delivery of personal health services. Even so, the Institute of Medicine, in its landmark publication, *The Future of Public Health*, stated that the goal of public health activities was nothing less than assuring the conditions for people to be healthy (Institute of Medicine, 1988). In theory, then, there is a natural affinity between health professionals in public health and those in direct health care delivery.

In practice, public health roles have centered on, among others, administration of local, state, and national public health agencies; on planning, implementing, and evaluating prevention; on screening and health education programs; on surveillance and control of environmental hazards and pollutants; and on the epidemiological description and explanation for the incidence and prevalence of disease and trauma in populations. In certain settings—municipal or county health departments, for example—public health professionals have worked closely with other health professionals in the delivery of primary care services to special populations such as indigent families, migrant workers, and groups of uninsured persons. In general, however, public health professionals have been a relatively unseen group of persons working to maintain a fundamental infrastructure allowing an understanding of and an implementation of health-promoting activities at the population level: safe drinking water, adequate sanitary systems, control of infectious diseases, and prevention of disease- and injury-producing behavior such as smoking, high speed driving, and the like.

The principal training programs for careers in public health are located in the twenty-nine accredited schools of public health as well as a small number of accredited health education programs, and eleven community medicine programs. Nearly 400 other non-accredited programs exist that offer training in the various subfields of public health such as health administration and environmental health. The primary academic degree is either the Master of Public Health (MPH) or the Master of Science in Public Health (MSPH). Other common avenues for careers in public health include the study of medicine with emphasis on, and board certification in, preventive medicine, the study of public health nursing, dentistry, nutrition, industrial hygiene, and social work, among others. Advanced graduate training in some of the fields of public health—epidemiology, environmental health sciences, health services research, health behavior and health education, and biostatistics—is normally obtained through accredited schools of public health, leading to the Doctor of Philosophy (Ph.D.), the Doctor of Public Health (Dr.P.H.), or the Doctor of Science (Sc.D.)

Total enrollment in schools of public health has nearly doubled over the period 1975–1976 to 1991–1992, growing from 6,461 to 12,032, respectively—an 86.2 percent increase. In 1990–1991, there were 3,903 graduates from these schools. Of the total of the students enrolled during the 1981–1982 academic year, 9.9 percent were members of underrepresented minority groups (African American, Hispanic, and Native Americans); by the 1991–92 academic year, this proportion had grown to 15.7 percent. The percent of women in the 1981–82 total enrollment was 55.4 percent, whereas this percent was 65.9 percent by 1991–1992 (Bureau of Health Professions, 1993). Thus, during a period of major expansion in the number of students studying public health (public health ranked fourth in total enrollment after allopathic medicine, pharmacy, and dentistry), there has been a significant growth of opportunity for historically underrepresented minorities (116 percent increase) and women (63 percent) during the decade of the 1980s.

New Roles for Public Health Professionals

The melding of public health functions with those of professionals in the direct delivery of personal health services is now underway with the expansion of managed-care plans. As explained in other chapters in this text, managed-care plans assume the responsibility for the health care of defined populations of enrollees within a budgetary system constrained by capitation arrangements (i.e., a prospectively fixed payment for each enrollee for a defined period of time, usually one year). Because the financing system no longer permits an open-ended, cost-based billing for services to insurers, the managed-care plan has clear incentives to find ways to deliver health care services efficiently, but more to the point here, to find ways to keep the covered population healthier in the first place.

This function is part of the fundamental mission of public health: collect information on and monitor disease incidence and prevalence of the plan's enrollees; monitor the outcome of the health care delivery process; develop, implement, and monitor programs of prevention and other forms of positive intervention into the health habits and behavior of the plan's enrollees (e.g., smoking and diet), receipt of prenatal care; immunization against infectious diseases; and the like. To the extent that managed-care plans emphasize these traditional public health roles, the plans may well be the catalysts for the integration of public health and personal health services that have long been called for in the United States. But because of traditional insurance schemes based on retrospective cost-based reimbursement, the deep professional fissures between some health professionals and public health professionals, and other reasons, this integration has proceeded very slowly.

In short, more than ever, future careers in public health promise to join community-based practice—the historical purview of public health—and the institutional practice of the healing arts. The task of disease prevention and health maintenance promises to force integration of these two domains. However, if universal entitlement to health care via a comprehensive health insurance program fails to materialize, there will continue to be a need for traditional community-based public health specialists involved in meeting the needs of disadvantaged groups.

NURSING

Registered nurses are the largest group of licensed health care professionals in the United States. The supply of registered nurses (RNs) grew from 1,662,382 in 1980 to over 2,033,032 in 1988, an increase of twenty-two percent. In 1994, the *active* (employed) supply of RNs was 1,887,055, a number considerably less than the overall figure six years earlier. This reflects a major feature of the nursing workforce: a substantial number of nurses not working in nursing or inactive in the economic workforce.

Profiles show that most nurses are women; less than five percent are male. About seven of ten nurses are married, and less than ten percent are from minority groups. Historically, over forty percent of RNs are diploma school graduates, usually from hospital-based programs. The shifting education pattern of RNs, with increasing emphasis on a four-year baccalaureate degree, is discussed in greater detail below.

Despite the overall absolute increase in the number of nurses employed in nursing, over the years there has been a recurrent cyclical pattern of too few nurses, then too many nurses, then too few once again. Data from the early 1990s indicated that the late 1980s shortage was easing: in 1991, for example, the national average RN vacancy rate in hospitals was 8.7 percent; the previous year it had been eleven percent (*Health Personnel in the United States: Ninth Report to Congress*, 1993). However, recent trends in many states, such as New York, suggest another round of too few nurses for positions offered. The number of nurses graduating between 1996 and 2000 in New York is expected to decline by twenty-five percent, which will probably worsen the shortage (Center for Health Workforce Studies, 2000). Understanding the causes of the apparently cyclical nature of the imbalance between supply and demand for nurses is not easy. Some have pointed to the large number of inactive nurses as the main reason for the fluctuation: economic forces cause nurses to enter and leave the workforce when required. However, the labor force participation of nurses is similar to that of women in comparable professions, and so the existence of a pool of inactive nurses may not in itself be the key reason. What may be more fundamental are the personal characteristics and the persistent position of women in society as influences on nurses' ability and desire to work. Only about eight percent of unemployed nurses actively seek nursing employment; the vast majority of unemployed nurses are over fifty years of age or are married with children at home (Levin & Moses,

1982). One job characteristic that does appear to influence nurse employment is salary (Aiken, 1982). Nurses are not paid well relative to their training and responsibilities, and thus, when there has been a shortage, it has been termed a shortage due to lagging salaries.

Approximately one-third of employed nurses work part-time, and the majority of these are married with children at home. Although concern has also been focused on nursing attrition due to "burn-out," poor working conditions, or both, surveys indicate that only a small number of nurses work in other professions. Thus, the shortages of nurses cannot simply be attributed to increases in the number of part-time workers or attrition from the profession. Another emerging factor that may account for current shortages is the fact that a growing proportion of new RNs has entered the workforce from associate degree programs, increasing from about forty percent in 1977 to about sixty percent in 1996, and new graduate RNs are also about five years older than the average from twenty years earlier (Auerbach, Buerhaus, & Staiger, 2000). Simultaneously, there has been a decline in the rate at which younger students (born after 1960) enter nursing school, usually into baccalaureate programs, with the net result that the rate of overall growth of the RN workforce is slowing down.

In short, whereas the nursing shortage was easing during the 1990s, it now appears to be worsening once again as older nurses who were both baby boomers and more recent entrants, just discussed, retire at a level that is not being replaced by younger RN entrants (Minnick, 2000). The total number of nursing graduates, while having fallen throughout the 1980s, registered increases in the 1990s.

Like most health care professionals, nurses are not distributed evenly throughout the United States. For example, in 1991, the RN to population ratio in the United States was 697 to 100,000 population. New York's state's ratio was 823 to 100,000, whereas that of Arkansas was 506 to 100,000. The maldistribution appears to be due to the geographic immobility of women who are married and second wage earners in a family, as well as the inability of rural and inner-city hospitals and other facilities to offer an adequate range of incentives (e.g., flexible working hours, increased salaries, and fringe benefits, safe working conditions) to attract nurses.

Rural institutions have found that urban-based education and training programs often have not been relevant to rural needs. Rural hospitals must frequently hire recent nursing graduates with limited skills and often resort to dependence on pool nurses from temporary employment agencies. This problem is of particular concern because of the increased responsibilities and range of skills needed by rural nurses. In the near future, rural providers are not likely to improve their chances of attracting well-trained nurses with a broad range of skills. Still, cooperative efforts by state government and local providers can often make a difference in the presence of RNs. South and North Dakota, rural states with traditional shortages of physicians, have managed to achieve nurse to population ratios well above the national average: 910 and 976 to 100,000, respectively.

Nursing Education and Role Changes

The federal government was largely responsible for the increases in nursing school class size over the period 1960–1980, having spent about $2.0 billion for nursing education. The more than doubling of the admissions to nursing schools over this period is eloquent testimony to this. The growth in admissions slowed considerably between 1980 and the early 1990s, but there continues to be growth nonetheless. Of particular interest, however, is the switch that has occurred in the control of nursing education from the hospital to nursing educators in colleges and universities.

Three forms of training lead to licensure as an RN: three-year diploma programs that are hospital-based, two-year associate degree programs that are generally in community colleges, and four-year baccalaureate nursing programs in universities or four year colleges. In 1995–1996, only 6,227 (five percent) of new nursing students were enrolled in diploma programs; in 1960–1961, the percentage had been seventy-eight. By contrast, the majority (sixty-one percent) of new nursing students are trained in associate degree programs, with baccalaureate at thirty-four percent of the total.

In contrast to the other health professions discussed in this chapter and for reasons that are not clear, the supply of RNs has not included as great a proportion of minority group members. Table 14.6 shows that, in recent years, from sixteen to seventeen percent of RN students were members of minority groups. The largest minority group—African Americans—grew from about seven percent in 1980 to about nine percent in 1994. Why the field of nursing should lack appeal to minorities that other health professions appear to have remains an unanswered question, deserving inquiry and remedy.

The major employment patterns now and in the future are shown in Table 14.6. The hospital is and will remain the major locus of employment for RNs, sectioning off about two-thirds of the nursing workforce. Nursing home employment is expected to increase in importance whereas other areas of employment will show stability over the period 1995–2005. These figures may appear to contradict the notion that non-hospital-based employment is gaining in popularity; however, because many hospitals are themselves involved in owning and operating non-hospital-based services (such as home health services and ambulatory care sites), these figures may not reveal the true picture. Within these settings, new roles have emerged for the RN. These include clinical nurse specialist, nurse practitioner, nurse anesthetist, and nurse clinician. These positions involve employment in new ambulatory care settings (e.g., managed-care plans, ambulatory surgery centers, free-standing urgent care centers, and the like),

nursing homes, and home care programs providing care for the elderly and others with chronic illness. Nurses are also finding opportunities in statewide, regional, and hospital-level utilization and quality review roles in which they participate in the inspection of clinical records describing patient care.

The nursing profession is attempting to change its broader role in the health care system, calling for an expansion of the *independent* role of the nurse within institutional settings and the creation of new professional roles outside them. Nurses are seeking to clarify their relationship to physicians, particularly within the context of clinical decision making in the hospital. They have developed new delivery modes, such as primary nursing, in which the nurse assumes direct responsibility for comprehensive care for a group of patients over a given period of time.

Nursing professionals want to control their future. They are trying to shed the traditional stereotype of the nurse as underpaid female hospital laborer. In the process, considerable controversy has been created both inside and outside the profession. This is often most visible when labor collective bargaining groups attempt to unionize nurses, forcing to the surface the ambivalence many nurses feel between being a highly skilled professional delivering personalized services versus an underpaid employee in a bureaucratic health care organization. Associate degree and diploma graduates want to continue to function in viable

Table 14.6. Estimated and Projected Requirements for Full-Time Equivalent Registered Nurses by Employment Setting, 1990, 1995, 2000, 2005

Field of Employment	Estimated 1990	Percent	Estimated 1995	Percent	Estimated 2000	Percent	Projected 2005	Percent
Registered Nurse Total	1,466,000	100.0%	1,610,200	100.0%	1,735,400	100.0%	1,854,300	100.0%
Hospital	1,009,700	68.9%	1,086,600	67.5%	1,155,700	66.6%	1,224,700	66.0%
Nursing Home	105,300	7.2%	130,300	8.1%	157,300	9.1%	183,100	9.9%
Home Health	53,000	3.6%	57,000	3.5%	60,900	3.5%	64,400	3.5%
Other Community/ Public Health	111,900	7.6%	136,700	8.5%	149,000	8.6%	157,600	8.5%
Ambulatory Care	101,200	6.9%	107,200	6.7%	111,500	6.4%	115,600	6.2%
Other	84,900	5.8%	92,400	5.7%	101,000	5.8%	108,900	5.9%

SOURCE: *Health personnel in the United States: Eighth report to Congress* (DHHS Pub. No. HRS-P-OD-92-1). (1992). Washington, D.C.: U.S. Government Printing Office.

roles within the nursing profession. Institutions want to employ combinations of nursing personnel suitable to their particular environments. These forces, as well as the current restrictive interpretation of state nurse practice acts, suggest that there will be no easy solutions to changing and, one hopes, strengthening the future relationships among nurses, physicians, and health care organizations.

PHARMACISTS

As is the case for all of the health professional groups discussed so far, pharmacists are also undergoing extensive change. Until recently, pharmacists performed the traditional role of preparing drug products and filling prescriptions. In the 1980s, 1990s, and into the 2000s, pharmacists expanded that role to include drug production education and acting as an expert for clients and patients about the effects of specific drugs, drug interactions, and generic drug substitutions for brand-name drugs. This role has even expanded to include selecting, monitoring, and evaluating appropriate drug regimens and to providing information not only to patients but also to other health care professionals. Finally, in their role as businessmen and women, pharmacists have had to learn more about the managerial and financial aspects of working in a retail trade.

There has been steady growth in the number of pharmacists during the last quarter-century, although the percentage of growth has not been as great as in other health care professions From 1973–1974 to 2000–2001, there has been a seventy-four percent increase in the overall number. First-year enrollment in pharmacy schools leveled off during the 1980s, although there was a major increase in the proportion of female first-year students, from about thirty percent in 1973–1974 to about sixty-three percent in 1991–1992. The growth of minorities in pharmacy, although not as great, has been steady, increasing from about twelve percent in 1980–1981 to twenty-one percent in 1991–1992. Another phenomenon of note is the popularity of Doctorate in Pharmacy programs, which lead not only to research and teaching positions, but also to levels of higher administrative responsibil-

ity, often in health care organizations and managed-care plans (Gershon, Cultice, & Knapp, 2000).

Pharmacists are employed in a number of settings, but the growth of chain drugstores has had a notable impact. As the 1990s began, about forty percent of all pharmacists were employed in chains. Over the decade of the 1980s, the proportion of new pharmacy graduates hired by chains increased from about twenty-seven percent to forty-two percent. About forty percent of the remainder of the graduates worked in hospitals and independent pharmacies.

Forces that may contribute to an increase in the need for pharmacists include the increased use of drugs, especially among the growing aged population, and pharmacy's expanded role under changes in the Medicaid program that require review of patient drug use and patient counseling. Nevertheless, making projections about the future supply of pharmacists in relation to future need or demand is difficult because of the rapidly changing employment circumstances in the field. Further, the aging of the American population would suggest that more medication prescriptions will be written and more work for pharmacists will result. At the same time, because pharmacists are expanding their role to include nontraditional activities, as mentioned, the amount of time an individual pharmacist might spent in traditional "druggist" activities will probably decline. With computerized information processing systems, assistance from pharmacy technicians, and mail order approaches that pharmacists will be using in increasing numbers, one would expect a positive gain in productivity, and perhaps a diminished need for an increased supply. In short, a number of factors make predicting the future balance of supply and demand difficult, and given the importance of drug therapies for modern medical care, policy makers should watch this important health profession closely.

PHYSICIAN ASSISTANTS AND NURSE PRACTITIONERS

The perceived shortage of physicians in the mid-1960s led to the development of two types of health care providers: physician assistants (PAs) and nurse practitioners (NPs). PAs are qualified by academic and practical training to provide patient services under the direct supervision of a licensed physician who is responsible for the performance of the PA. PAs are able to diagnose, manage, and treat common illnesses, provide preventive services, and respond appropriately to common emergency situations. Laws and regulations in all states (except Mississippi) and the District of Columbia now authorize the use of PAs under a physician's supervision. Over thirty states, as well as the District of Columbia, allow a physician to authorize the PA to prescribe certain medications. The typical PA training program consists of two-years of didactic study followed by clinical training. However, programs vary widely in terms of admission requirements, curriculum, and site of educational training. There were fifty-nine accredited PA programs in the early 1990s, and over 56,000 PAs were employed in 1994. Estimates are that more than 69,000 PAs will be employed by 2005 (Darnay, 1998).

The number of PA graduates has surged during the 1990s with 3,400 graduates projected in 2001, up from 1,360 graduates in 1992. There has been a tendency for PAs to serve in rural and medically underserved areas more often than physicians, with about thirty-four percent of PAs working in communities of less than 50,000. Although men represent more than one-half (fifty-eight percent) of practicing PAs, women now make up more than one-half of all newly graduating PAs. Most PAs are white, non-Hispanic (ninety-one percent), with the remainder consisting mostly of underrepresented minorities.

In 1983, there were 3,807 PAs employed in U.S. hospitals, and by 1994, there were 8,860, a 133 percent increase. Still, only about sixteen percent of PAs work in hospitals, with the majority located in ambulatory care settings (for example, in 1994, 55.8 percent worked in physicians' offices). However, the percentage of PAs in hospital settings varies widely by state. For example, Connecticut has over fifty percent of its PAs employed in hospitals, while California has nine percent in hospitals. Most PAs work in the private sector (eighty-one percent), and about twelve percent work for the federal government in the Veterans Administration, the Armed Forces, and the U.S. Public Health Service. Finally, the proportion of PAs working in primary care settings declined over the period 1978 to 1991, from sixty-seven percent to forty-three percent. General surgery, surgical subspecialties, orthopedics, and emergency medicine all registered increases. There appears to be a correlation between specialization of this sort and states that do not allow physician delegation of prescription writing to PAs.

NPs are registered nurses who have completed formal programs of study preparing them for expanded roles and responsibilities. These roles include obtaining comprehensive health histories, assessing health status, performing physician examinations, formulating and managing a care regimen for acute and chronically ill patients, teaching, and counseling (Abdellah, 1982). As of 1992, there were 48,200 NPs in the United States.

There is a range of training programs for NPs, including pediatric, nurse-midwife, family, adult, psychiatric, and geriatric programs. At the beginning of the 1990s, there were 212 NP training programs that graduated 1,500 NPs in 1992, and a projected graduating class of over 7,000 in 2001 (Cooper, Laud, & Dietrich, 1998). The growth of the NP workforce is expected to be nothing short of spectacular: numbering about 60,000 in 1995, the prediction is that there will be about 110,000 NPs by 2005 (Cooper, Laud, & Dietrich (1998). The focus of training for about sixty-three percent of students has been advanced clinical practice, with nearly one-fourth in medical surgical specialties, fifteen percent in maternal and child specialties, and the remainder in psychiatric-mental health, community health, and gerontological specialties. Of the thirty-seven percent not in advanced clinical practice, thirteen percent focused on teaching and nearly one-fourth on administration and management (Health Personnel, 1993).

There are important differences in the perceptions of the roles of PAs and NPs. PAs are viewed by the medical profession as physician "extenders" who can perform many of the usual functions completed by physicians. Nurses view NPs as registered nurses in an expanded role. This includes greater supervision of and responsibility for primary patient care, with extra emphasis on the traditional nursing values of prevention and counseling. Despite these perceptual differences, as well as differences in education, training, and outlook, many of the performance characteristics of PAs and NPs appear to be similar.

Issues in PA and NP Use

Among the issues that need to be resolved before PAs and NPs can be used to their full capacity and original promise are legal restrictions concerning practice, reimbursement policies, and relationships with physicians. The legal status of PAs and NPs varies considerably across states. As noted in the case of PAs, many states permit considerable delegation of tasks and responsibilities, including prescribing certain drugs. State legislation expanding medical delegation has been unduly restrictive with regard to the scope of practice of qualified nonphysicians, although progress is being made.

Laws and regulations governing the expanded role of the nurse practitioner are also changing rapidly but inconsistently. Although the majority of states have altered their nurse practice acts to facilitate expanded roles, the constraints on the scope of NP practice continue to vary from state to state. A particular barrier is whether an individual state will authorize prescription practices of NPs. Although more than forty states have explicit regulatory provision for limited prescriptive authority, these authorizations vary in the degree of independence and in the types of drugs and devices that may be prescribed. There may also be geographic limitations; for example, more NP discretion in rural than urban settings.

Third party reimbursement imposes another constraint on the use of PAs and NPs. Current policies generally link their reimbursement directly to the employing physician or institution. Since 1989, federal law requires direct Medicaid reimbursement for pediatric NPs and family NPs, whether or not the NP is directly supervised by a physician. Yet, many states are not yet in compliance with federal legislation. As for the private health insurance sector, some states have laws allowing reimbursement to NPs, but this coverage is usually optional and is not widespread. Some progress has been made in reimbursement of NPs and PAs through the Medicare program. For ex-

ample, in 1989, the U.S. Congress, in its mandate that a Resource-Based Relative Value Scale (RBRVS) fee schedule supplant the usual and customary schedule for physician payment under Medicare Part B, called for the study of including "nonphysician providers" in the fee schedule. Experimental programs are under review and may lead to a special reimbursement schedule.

A final area of concern is current and future relations with physicians. In the past, physicians were reasonably accepting of these personnel. Yet, about the time that these mid-level practitioners were becoming popular among those seeking a lower-cost substitute for physician services, the physician surplus was discovered, and physicians were wary of employing personnel who might take away their work. Further, as noted earlier in this chapter, there was a tendency for some physicians to move into previously medically underserved areas.

There has been an increase in the numbers of NPs and PAs, and much of the current demand has been generated by managed-care plans whose efforts to cut costs, to find flexibility in the deployment of caregivers, and to emphasize primary care and prevention coincide with the lower salaries, the broad skill set, and the training that are typical of NPs and PAs. In addition, there are many roles that these mid-level professionals have been filling and continue to fill: providing primary care to underserved populations often in underserved areas as well as care to the elderly and the mentally ill; providing preventive care and health education; and delivering specialty services in hospitals in lieu of house staff. New practice settings for NPs and PAs include schools, industrial settings, prisons, and nursing homes.

The outcome of the current debate about the physician surplus and the role of IMGs in the physician workforce will be consequential for PAs and NPs. If efforts are successful in reducing the growth of physician supply, the employment of these mid-level health professionals will be enhanced throughout the health care system. If the physician workforce is not reduced in number, the historic barriers to PAs and NPs will continue to provide difficulty for attainment of the full promise of PA and NP service delivery.

THE CHANGING NATURE OF HEALTH PROFESSIONALS

This chapter has summarized trends in the supply of health professionals. From the 1960s into the early 1980s, federal and state support resulted in large increases in the number of graduates of most health professional occupations. From the mid-1980s to the present time, the growth of some occupational groups (e.g., PAs and NPs), has probably been affected as much by the workforce requirements of managed-care plans as by any public policy effort. Simultaneously, women and minorities have greatly benefited from this overall growth. During much or part of the 1980s, there was stability and even decline in the number of applicants to various health professional training programs (e.g., medicine, nursing, and dentistry). Although these trends were reversed in many instances, with a new phase of growth in a number of fields, in the late 1990s, there was once again a decline in applications in some areas, notably medicine. By contrast, and in addition to the "standard" health professions discussed in this chapter, there has been steady growth—and popularity with the American public—in numerous less conventional health care occupations like chiropractors, acupuncturists, and naturopaths (Cooper, Laud, & Dietrich, 1998).

The federal and state investment in health care personnel improved access to health care and helped schools training health professionals to remain financially viable. The reduction of government spending for the health professions has been caused by the reallocation of these funds to other portions of federal and state budgets and by the belief that a surplus of many types of health professionals existed. Many of the major trends affecting the U.S. health care system, such as restrictive public and private sector reimbursement, growth of alternative delivery systems and managed-care plans, portend continuing pressures against health professions' growth. Thus, stories are becoming more common of hospitals having potential shortages in not only RNs, but also in pharmacists, among others (Steinhauer, 2000). Still, as noted, the demand for training in almost all the health professions has increased dramatically from the downturn of the mid- to late-1980s, all of which suggests a restrictive labor market with employment opportunities less abundant than in the past decade.

The increasing number of women in all of the health professions also suggests that, on balance, with the rise of single-parent households and the continued disproportionate household and child-rearing responsibilities that married or single working mothers bear, female health professionals—particularly physicians—will probably work fewer hours per week and fewer weeks per year than men. This could add up to a need for more personnel to make up desirable levels of full-time equivalent labor. For example, if the proportion of women entering medicine continues at the current pace, the effective full-time equivalent supply of physician services will decline by about four percent between 1986 and 2010, other things being equal (Kletke, Marder, & Silberger, 1990). On the other hand, the increase in managed-care plans with their efficient use of health care personnel will produce a countervailing force in relation to the overall numbers of health care professionals. Such conflicting forces make predicting the balance between need and demand versus supply of health professionals a very difficulty enterprise.

THE IMPACT OF MANAGED CARE

Managed care deserves the final comment in this chapter's conclusion. The rapid growth of managed-care plans and in the number of Americans enrolled in these plans has become a major force reshaping the size and composition of the health care professions workforce. In the immediate future, there are at least four important consequences of managed care on the workforce (Council on Graduate Medical Education, 1995b). First, more and more health professionals will have some sort of relationship with managed care. For example, most physicians are now involved in managed care either as full time employees or as contractors with one or more plans. Over three-fourths of all physicians are estimated to have at least one managed-care contract. This trend appears irreversible.

Second, many observers believe that continued managed care growth will only magnify and exacerbate the problem of a provider surplus, particularly among physicians. Furthermore, there is worry that the historical imbalance between primary care and specialization will be worsened. However, market pressures from the plans are already having an impact in favor of medical student and resident choice of primary care medicine and away from other specialties.

Third, many educational institutions will experience severe financial difficulty as managed-care plans erode their patient bases. That is, managed care plans, which historically have had little if any involvement with education and training, are underbidding educational institutions such as university medical schools, which have had higher per patient expenses because of the costs of training. What the impact of this pressure will be is hard to predict. Some likely results include lower clinical income for teaching organizations, and, hence, lower health professional income. There may be a reduction in the number of training sites for health professional students. Educational institutions will move to employ the lowest paid health professionals who can practice within a given level of patient care. The open-ended growth of clinical diagnostic and treatment capacity will surely be dampened.

Fourth, the education that health professionals receive will probably witness a shift to the kind of clinical practice that health plans require. Those educational institutions that have not already adapted to these new demands are showing themselves to be obsolete and are placing themselves at risk for organizational failure. This emphasis will consist of prevention, treatment of the whole person and not simply one or the other organ system, prudent exercise of diagnostic and treatment approaches in which efficiency and cost-effectiveness are key, emphasis on "evidence-based" care in which preferred treatment approaches will have predictably positive and clear cut outcomes, reliance on provider teams with more integration of different skill sets, and the like.

Until such education becomes the norm, some health professionals will be ill-equipped to provide services in managed-care plans. Further, the cost savings pressures on managed-care plans may lead some to overload primary care givers with more work than they can handle and to pressure primary care givers to accept clinical responsibilities that are beyond their purview and training. Taken together, the educational content and work requirements that managed-care plans demand will place a heavy challenge on health professional training programs of all types.

In the long run, these problems will probably be addressed by all the health professions because the market pressure that managed-care plans exert is perhaps stronger than even the combined lobbying ability of organized medicine, medical schools, nursing, and the like. Adaptation will occur, but its shape is hard to anticipate. One intriguing hypothesis that must be entertained is whether attempts already underway in the medical profession to limit the growth in physician supply will eventually work against managed-care plans as they are currently controlled. Steady growth in physician supply did not begin until the early 1970s, about the same time that steady growth in managed care began. Although certainly not the only factor that has spurred managed care growth, an increase in the supply of physicians has been a key component of managed care success: more physicians finding it difficult to start private practices and, once started, to attract sufficient patient bases have turned to managed care employment. If medicine reduces its growth and thus moves toward relative scarcity, it may well be able to exert its control over its employers.

Although this particular scenario is speculative, what is not is the interactive nature of all the health professions and the delivery organizations and the often surprising outcomes of that interaction. The future presents a vastly different possibility than that predicted at the beginning of the twenty-first century, and the trends that emerge will be of the greatest interest.

SUMMARY

Health care services depend on people. And the increasingly technological orientation of the health care system demands better-trained and more skilled individuals in all employment categories. The challenges of changing technology, the pressures of increasing costs, and the complexities of human interaction and motivation will pressure health care personnel for the foreseeable future.

References

Abdellah, F. (1982). The nurse practitioner 17 years later: Present and emerging issues. *Inquiry, 5,* 470–497.

Aiken, L. (1982). The impact of federal health policy on nurses. In L. Aiken (Ed.). *Nursing in the 1980s: Crises, opportunities, challenges.* Philadelphia: Lippincott.

American Academy of Family Physicians. (1991). *Report on survey of 1991 graduating family practice residents.* Washington, DC: American Academy of Family Physicians.

Auerbach, D. I., Buerhaus, P. I., & Staiger, D. O. (2000). Associate degree graduates and the rapidly aging RN workforce. *Nursing Economics, 18,* 178–184.

Brown, L. J., & Lazar, V. (1999). Trends in the dental health work force. *Journal of the American Dental Association, 130,* 1743–1749.

Bureau of Health Professions, Health Resources and Services Administration. (1993). *Factbook: Health personnel United States* (DHHS Pub. No. HRSA-P-AM-93-1). Washington, DC: U.S. Government Printing Office.

Center for Health Workforce Studies. (2000). *Meeting future nursing needs of New Yorkers: The role of the State University of New York.* Rensselaer, NY: Center for Health Workforce Studies, State University of New York at Albany.

Cooper, R. A., Laud, P., & Dietrich, C. L. (1998). Current and projected workforce of nonphysician clinicians. *Journal of the American Medical Association, 280,* 788–794.

Council on Graduate Medical Education. (1995a). *Seventh report to Congress and the Department of Health and Human Services Secretary: Recommendations for Department of Health and Human Services' Programs.* Washington, DC: U.S. Government Printing Office.

Council on Graduate Medical Education. (1995b). *Sixth report to Congress and the Department of Health and Human Services Secretary: Managed health care: Implications for the physician workforce and medical education.* Washington, DC: U.S. Government Printing Office.

Council on Graduate Medical Education. (1999). *COGME physician workforce policies: Recent developments and remaining challenges in meeting national goals.* Washington, DC: U.S. Government Printing Office.

Darnay, A. J. (Ed.). (1998). *Statistical record of health & medicine.* Detroit: Gale Research.

Flexner, A. (1910). *Medical education in the United States and Canada: A report to the Carnegie Foundation for the Advancement of Teaching.* Bulletin no. 4. New York: The Carnegie Foundation.

Gershon, S. K., Cultice, J. M., & Knapp, K. K. (2000). How many pharmacists are in our future? The Bureau of Health Professions Projects Supply to 2020. *Journal of the American Pharmaceutical Association, 40,* 757–764.

Gordon, R. J., Meister, J. S., & Hughes, R. G. (1992). Accounting for shortages of rural physicians: Push and pull factors. In W. M. Gesler & T. C. Ricketts (Eds.), *Health in rural North America: The geography of health care services and delivery.* New Brunswick, NJ: Rutgers University Press.

Graduate Medical Education National Advisory Committee. (1980). *Report to the Secretary, DHHS, Vol. I; GMENAC summary report* (DHHS Pub. No. [HRA] 81–653). Washington, DC: U.S. Government Printing Office.

Health personnel in the United States: Ninth report to Congress, 1993 Edition (DHHS Pub. No. P-OD-94-1). Washington, DC: U.S. Government Printing Office.

Institute of Medicine. (1988). *The future of public health.* Washington, DC: National Academy Press.

Institute of Medicine. (1996).*The nation's physician workforce: Options for balancing supply and requirements.* Washington, DC: National Academy Press.

Kletke, P. R., Marder, W. D., & Silberger, A. B. (1990). The growing proportion of female physicians: Implications for U.S. physician supply. *American Journal of Public Health, 80,* 300–304.

Levin, E., & Moses, E. (1982). Registered nurses today: A statistical profile. In L. Aiken (Ed.), *Nursing in the 1980s: Crises, opportunities, challenges.* Philadelphia: Lippincott.

Mick, S. S. (1992). *The 1987 career characteristics of foreign and U.S. medical graduates who entered the U.S. medical system between 1969 and 1982.* Report to the Educational Commission for Foreign Medical Graduates, Philadelphia, PA.

Mick, S. S., Lee, S.-Y. D., & Wodchis, W. (2000). Variations in geographical distribution of International Medical Graduates and U.S. medical graduates: "safety nets" or "surplus exacerbation?" *Social Science & Medicine, 50,* 185–202

Mick, S. S., & Worobey, J. L. (1984). Foreign and United States medical graduates in practice: A follow-up. *Medical Care, 22,* 1014–1025.

Minnick, A. F. (2000). Retirement, the nursing workforce, and the year 2005. *Nursing Outlook, 48,* 211–217.

Moy, E. & Bartman, B. A. (1995). Physician race and care of minority and medically indigent patients. *Journal of the American Medical Association, 273,* 1515–1520.

Ricketts, T. C. (1994). Health care professionals in rural America. In J. E. Beaulieu & D. E. Berry (Eds.), *Rural health services: A management perspective.* Ann Arbor, MI: AUPHA Press/Health Administration Press.

Seifer, S. D., Troupin, B., & Rubenfeld, G. D. (1996). Changes in marketplace demand for physicians: A study of medical journal recruitment advertisements. *Journal of the American Medical Association, 276,* 695–699.

Steinhauer, J. (2000, December 25). Shortage of health care workers keeps growing. *The New York Times,* p. A1–17.

Whitcomb, M. E. (1995). A cross-national comparison of generalist physician workforce data. *Journal of the American Medical Association, 274,* 692–695.

Whitcomb, M. E., & Miller, R. S. (1995). Participation of International Medical Graduates in graduate medical education and hospital care for the poor. *Journal of the American Medical Association, 274,* 696–699.

PART

5

Assessing and Regulating Health Services

CHAPTER
15

Health Policy and the Politics of Health Care

Philip Lee
A. E. Benjamin

Chapter Topics

- Dimensions of Policy Making in Health
- A Historical Framework: The Development of Health Policy from 1798 to 1988
- The Early Years of the Republic: A Limited Role for the Federal Government (1798–1862)
- The Evolution of Health Policy: The Emergence of Dual Federalism and the Transformation of American Medicine (1862–1935)
- The Evolution of Health Policy: From Dual Federalism to Cooperative Federalism (1935–1961)
- The Transformation of Health Policies: The New Frontier, the Great Society, and Creative Federalism (1961–1969)
- Health Policy in an Era of Limited Resources: From Creative Federalism to New Federalism and a Return to Dependence on Competition and the Private Sector (1969–1992)
- Health Policy: New Solutions, Old Problems (1993–Present)

Learning Objectives

Upon completing this chapter, the reader should be able to:

- Understand the impact of health policies on health care
- Understand the political system in the United States as it pertains to the development of health policy
- Gain knowledge of the development of health policy in the United States
- Appreciate the actual and potential roles of government in health care
- Appreciate the competing political, economic, and social goals of health policy objectives
- Understand political pressures between public and private forces in health care

Political considerations have significantly affected nearly all of the developments discussed in this book. However, the importance and central role of health care policy analysis and politics can best be highlighted by directly discussing these issues. That is the purpose of this chapter. While many of the topics mentioned here have been discussed from a variety of perspectives in other chapters, the policy and politics of changes in health care in the nation are the focus here, and examples of developments in health care serve as illustrations of the central role of political forces in shaping our health care system.

Government plays a major role in planning, directing, and financing health services in the United States. The significance of the public sector is apparent as one considers the following: public programs account for approximately forty percent of the nation's personal health care expenditures; most physicians and other health care personnel are trained at public expense; over fifty percent of all health research and development funds are provided by the government; and most nonprofit community and university hospitals have been built or modernized with government subsidies. The bulk of government expenditures are federal, with state and local governments contributing significant, but much smaller, amounts.

Health policies and programs of the United States government have evolved piecemeal, usually in response to needs that were not being met by the private sector or by states and local governments. The result has been a proliferation of federal categorical programs administered by more than a dozen government departments. Over the years, new programs have been added, old ones redirected, and numerous efforts made to integrate and coordinate services. In the 1980s, a major effort was made by the Reagan administration to significantly diminish the federal role in domestic social policy through the transfer of some programs to the states, reduced federal funding, or elimination of federal support entirely. The effort has been only partially successful and has not changed the basic configuration of publicly supported health programs, although the burden of financing now falls more heavily on state and local governments. Functions of the public and private sectors have become increasingly interrelated, and roles are often poorly delineated. There can be little argument that the primary function of most government programs in health has been to support or strengthen the private sector (for example, hospital construction, subsidy of medical student training, Medicare) rather than to develop a strong system of publicly provided health care.

Although United States government policies have evolved over a two-hundred-year period, most of those affecting health services have developed since the enactment of the Social Security Act of 1935. Many federal health programs evolved because of failures in the private sector to provide necessary support (for example, biomedical research); others arose because results of the free market were grossly inequitable (for example, hospital construction); and some programs, such as Medicare and Medicaid, developed because health care was so costly that many could not afford to pay for necessary health services. Some federal health programs, such as biomedical research, potentially benefit everyone, while others, such as the Indian Health Service, reach only a small but needy segment of the population. Some programs, such as poliomyelitis immunization and health personnel development, have been effective in achieving their goals; others, such as health planning, have probably not realized even limited objectives; still others, such as Medicare, have reached some goals, although at a much higher cost than originally anticipated.

The process by which health policy is made in this country can be best understood by considering a fundamental paradox in American health care: government spends more and more money to support a wide range of health programs, services, and agencies, yet the role of government in the reform of our health care system remains limited and halting. Government is faced with a crisis in health care, defined primarily in terms of rising costs to public treasuries, while proposed solutions are framed in terms that do not address in a comprehensive fashion the sources of demand on the public purse. Indeed, solutions to the cost crisis have combined withdrawing benefits from those very recipient populations whose health care needs justify government intervention with attempts to reduce costs by either stimulating competition or regulating (reducing) payment to hospitals, nursing homes, and physicians. While federal policies may move in one direction, state policies may move in another. To understand this paradox, it is necessary to consider several characteristics of public policy making and thus to explore the sources of the paradox and the nature of policy processes in health.

DIMENSIONS OF POLICY MAKING IN HEALTH

Policy making in health care crosses several levels of government and hundreds of programs and is complex; no single analytical scheme can do it sufficient justice. Still, public policy students have identified five dimensions of the policy process: (1) the relationship of government to the private sector, (2) the distribution of authority within a federal system of government, (3) pluralistic ideology as the basis of politics, (4) the relationship between policy formulation and administrative implementation, and (5) incrementalism as a strategy of reform. Each will be considered in detail.

Public and Private Sector Politics

Although the role of government in health care has grown considerably in recent years, that role remains relatively limited. The United States government is less involved in health care than are the governments of many other industrialized countries (Jonas & Banta, 1981). This circumstance derives primarily from a persistent ideology that identifies the market system as the most appropriate setting for the exchange of health services and from a related belief that private sector support for public sector initiatives can be acquired only through accommodation to the interests of health care providers. The persistence of doubts about the appropriate role of government is certainly apparent in the renewed vitality of neoconservatism, in which it is argued that the market can better respond to the economic and social problems of our time if it is unfettered by government intervention.

Uncertainty about the role of government in health care has numerous consequences. The primary concern is the absence of any design or blueprint for governmental reform. Instead, the public sector (with its immense capacity to raise revenues) is called on periodically to open and close its funding spigots to stimulate the health care market. Hospital construction and physician education are prominent examples of public activity. Not only is there no blueprint for public sector action, but governments in America harbor grave doubts about the appropriateness of regulation as a public sector activity. Dependence at the federal level on "voluntary approaches," such as the reduction of hospital costs in the late 1970s, delayed serious consideration of more stringent measures even as the costs to government of hospital care continued to rise dramatically (Pechman, 1979).

A Federal System

The concept of federalism has evolved dramatically in meaning and practice since the founding of the republic more than two hundred years ago. Originally, federalism was a legal concept that defined the constitutional division of authority between the federal government and the states. Federalism initially stressed the independence of each level of government from the other, while incorporating the idea that some functions, such as foreign policy, were the exclusive province of the central government, while other functions, such as education, police protection, and health care, were the responsibility of regional units— state and local government. Federalism represented a form of governance that differs both from a unitary state, where regional and local authority derive legally from the central government, and from a confederation, in which the national government has limited authority and does not reach individual citizens directly (Hale & Palley, 1981; Reagan & Sanzone, 1981).

Shifts in responsibilities assigned to various levels of government do not pose a serious problem for health policy if at least two conditions are met: (1) administrative or regulatory responsibilities and financial accountability are consonant, and (2) the various levels of government possess the appropriate capacities to assume those responsibilities assigned to them. Important questions can be raised regarding whether either of these conditions have been met in the development of health policy during the last three decades.

Analysis of federal-state relationships in programs as divergent as Medicaid, provider licensure, and family planning under Title X of the Public Health Service Act have suggested that the structure of these relationships produces outcomes widely held to be dysfunctional (for example, Medicaid cutbacks) because one level of government (for example, the states) can do nothing else under the conditions established by another (for example, the federal government). The disjunction between administrative responsibilities and financial accountability (that is, the term of federalistic arrangements) in these cases has yielded results for which governments and the recipients of health care ultimately have paid a price. What seems to matter most in the structure of relationships within federalism is not so much the distribution of activities but the relationships among levels of government.

For allocations of authority among levels of government to work, it is important that governments possess those capacities appropriate to the responsibilities they confront. Governments must possess the capacity to generate revenue, the capability to plan and manage policies and programs, and the political will to plan and implement needed reform. State and local governments have been found wanting in each of these respects. Because state governments do not tax as heavily as the federal government, and generally cannot accumulate deficit spending, their capacity for generating new revenues is limited. Some states, moreover, are viewed as having inadequate administrative infrastructures, lacking sufficient sophisticated management techniques, and having limited capabilities in the conduct of policy analysis and planning.

Finally, there is evidence that at times state and local governments may have had less political will to make decisions in the public interest than the federal government. Wide variations among states in program outputs (for example, Medicaid) suggest significant inequities. The argument is not that every state, if freed from federal constraints, would establish standards for health programs that are certain to fall below former federal standards. Rather, it is that some states will surely exceed some federal standards and others will fall far below what is generally considered adequate. At the heart of this problem, many argue, is the reputedly greater susceptibility of state governments to interest group pressures and narrow conceptions of the public good.

Perhaps the most significant instance of the failure of the states to provide their citizens equal rights and equal protection has been in the area of civil rights. In education, housing, health care, and virtually every area of domestic social policy, it has been necessary for the federal government, particularly the federal courts, to require compliance with federal laws and regulations.

There is some countervailing evidence that the capacity and will to govern is becoming more widely diffused within the federal system. States (taken as a group) have spent a higher percentage of their budgets on health care than the federal government has, even though absolute federal expenditures for health have grown to more than double state and local health expenditures combined. A considerable increase at the state level in the conduct of policy analysis and its use in policy deliberations is one indication that the state capacity to plan and manage is improving. Regarding inequities and political will, on the other hand, little counterevidence has emerged to challenge the argument that the states are more vulnerable to interest groups (for example, provider groups in health) and that the result is a wide program variation among states in response to provider, not consumer, interests. The structure of federalism enables provider groups to maximize their power at the expense of consumer interests (Estes, 1980; Vladeck, 1979).

In a monograph on federalism and the national purpose, Brizius (n.d.) groups the arguments favoring centralization into eight clusters of related principles: (1) national purpose, (2) national security, (3) equity, (4) guaranteeing rights, (5) efficiency, (6) competence, (7) uniformity, and (8) unity. In contrast to the principles tending toward centralization are those that support greater decentralization and the maintenance of a truly federal system. Brizius groups twelve arguments for decentralization into seven principles: (1) diversity, (2) political sovereignty, (3) guaranteeing rights, (4) limits on power, (5) accountability, (6) efficiency and competence, and (7) competition.

The argument regarding centralization and decentralization has not been settled, despite a vigorous debate in the past decade. No agreement has been reached on the vital question of the distribution of authority and responsibility among various levels of government. The federal government finances hospital and medical services for the elderly through Medicare; it contributes fifty percent of health care costs for Medicaid beneficiaries, is the major supporter of biomedical research, provides a limited amount of support for a variety of health services (for example, mental health, family planning, crippled children's services, AIDS, substance abuse), is the sole regulator of the entry of new drugs into the market, and plays a critical role in the regulation of environment and occupational health.

States spend a large portion of their general fund budgets on health care for the poor (Medicaid), on mental health services, on the support of a range of public health programs, and on the education and training of health professionals.

Local governments remain an important provider of health care, particularly hospital, outpatient, and emergency care for the poor, mental health and substance abuse services, and a variety of public health services. Both state and local governments are mandated by higher levels of government (by either regulation or court order) to provide services or implement various environmental health or occupational health and safety regulations.

Pluralistic Politics

Pluralism is a term used by political theorists to describe a set of values about the effective functioning of democratic governments. Pluralists argue that democratic societies are organized into many diverse interest groups that pervade all socioeconomic strata, and that this network of pressure groups prevents any one elite group from overreaching its legitimate bounds. As a theoretical framework for explaining the political context of policy making, this perspective has been criticized relentlessly and appropriately (Bachrach, 1967; Schattschneider, 1960). As an ideology that continues to influence the way elites and masses view government, pluralism becomes a basis for considering some essential elements of the process of public decision making in this country.

Interest groups play a powerful role in the health policy process. Most federal and state laws designed to address the health care needs of the population are shaped by the interaction among interest groups, key legislators, and agency representatives. Ginzberg (1977) identified four power centers in the health care industry that influence the nature of health care and the role of government: (1) physicians, (2) large insurance organizations, (3) hospitals, and (4) a highly diversified group of participants in profit-making activities within the health care arena.

The influence of these power centers is evident in policies at all levels of government. The development of Medicare and Medicaid policies reflects the powerful influence of physicians, hospitals, and nursing homes as well as their allies in the health insurance industry. For example, in enacting Medicare, Congress ensured that the law did not affect the physician-patient relationship, including the physician's method of billing the patient. The system of physician reimbursement adopted by Medicare was highly inflationary because it provided incentives to physicians to raise prices and to provide ancillary services, such as laboratory tests, electrocardiograms, and X-ray films. Hospital reimbursement historically has been based on costs incurred in providing care, creating strong incentives to provide more and more services. Despite the impact of steadily rising Medicare costs on the Social Security trust fund, on Social Security taxes (paid by employers and employees), and on the elderly, Congress for years steadfastly refused to alter Medicare's methods of payments to physicians and hospitals. It was not until 1989 that the United States Congress adopted a set of policies to reform payments for physicians' services in the Medicare program. Also, many features of the program, patterned on principles developed by the medical industry, have had remarkable staying power.

The passage of a hospital prospective payment system (PPS) for Medicare by Congress in 1983 signaled a potential shift in the power of key interest groups in health. History has made it clear that an apparent legislative defeat (for example, the passage of Medicare) can subsequently become an important source of benefits and power for ostensibly losing interests (for example, the medical lobby). The implementation of PPS has not been a fiscal disaster for hospitals, as some predicted, and it remains to be seen whether federal payment reforms will effect any fundamental alteration in the role of major power centers in health care.

As the case of Medicare suggests, health policy in the United States has largely been a product of medical politics (Silver, 1976a). Marmor, Wittman, & Heagy (1976) describe the political "market" in health (that is, institutional arrangements among actors in the political system) as imbalanced. In an imbalanced market, participants have unequal power, and those with concentrated rather than diffuse interests have the greater stake in the effects of policy. Provider interest groups often have had a far greater stake in shaping health policy than have consumer interests. Large employers have become increasingly important in the health policy debates at the federal and state levels, particularly on issues related to health care cost containment.

Some observers argue that the rising costs of health care may be changing the configuration of interest groups seeking to influence health policy. Steadily escalating costs have stimulated other interests, especially labor, business, and governments themselves, into giving greater attention to health policy and its implications. The public's interests may be shifting from diffuse to concentrated. The result may be that increased competition in the political marketplace from a more diverse set of participants will lessen the dominance of medical provider groups. The pluralist dream of effective interest groups that prevent any one group from overreaching its legitimate bounds continues to influence our thinking about health care.

Policy Implementation

The nature of the health process is determined not only by the balance between provider and consumer interests but also by the relationships of these interests to government actors. Public policy students have observed that policy making moves through at least three stages: (1) agenda setting, the continuous process by which issues come to public attention and are placed on the agenda for government action;

(2) policy adoption, the legislative process through which elected officials decide the broad outlines of policy; and (3) policy implementation, the process by which administrators develop policy by addressing the numerous issues unaddressed by legislation. An important element of the health policy process involves the relative roles of elected officials and professional administrators. As one moves from agenda setting to policy adoption and implementation, it can be argued that the role of elected officials becomes more remote and that of administrators more crucial.

No policy theorist has pressed this argument with more conviction than Lowi (1979). A central theme in what he calls "interest-group liberalism" is the growing role of administrators in politics. According to Lowi, in a period of resource richness and government expansion, such as the 1960s, government responded to a range of major organized interests, underwrote programs sought by those interests, and assigned program responsibility to administrative agencies. Through this process, the programs became captives of the interest groups because the administrative agencies themselves were captured. Interest groups dominate the policy process, he argues, not only through their influence on the legislative process (policy adoption) but also through control of administration (policy implementation). In effect, governments in the United States make policies without laws, and they leave the law making to administrators.

The study of policy implementation in health has received increased attention. Not surprisingly, the landmark legislation creating Medicare and Medicaid in 1965 has been the subject of much of this analysis. A study of Medicare by Feder is especially enlightening. She describes a number of crucial decisions related to the nature of the federal role that were not addressed by the legislation and discusses the process by which the Social Security Administration subsequently addressed these decisions. Feder argues that the agency could have pursued two fundamentally different strategies. Using a cost-effectiveness strategy, the agency could have assessed the impact of alternative approaches to a problem (for example, hospital payment) on cost and quality and selected a course that would achieve maximum health care value per dollar spent. As an alternative, with a balancing strategy, the agency could have sought to identify relevant political actors (for example, the American Hospital Association), weighed their capacity to aid or threaten program survival, and then selected those policies that would minimize political conflict (Feder, 1977).

Feder makes a persuasive argument that the Social Security Administration selected a balancing strategy. She traces the various consequences for the public interest of an approach that administratively transfers policy discretion to those provider groups with the greatest stake in the contents of that policy. For those directly involved in the implementation of the Medicare program, the primary motivation was not only to minimize political conflict but also to ensure access for elderly Social Security beneficiaries to hospital and physician services. At one point, access was jeopardized because of the vigorous enforcement of the Civil Rights Act by the United States Public Health Service and the Social Security Administration on instructions of the Secretary of Health, Education, and Welfare. When compliance with the Civil Rights Act was assured in hospitals, particularly in the South and Southwest, access barriers disappeared. Reimbursement policies followed the intentions of Congress and achieved the initial objective of ensuring high levels of hospital and physician participation in Medicare.

Incremental Reform

The powerful role of administrators in the implementation of policy is derived in part from the broad and ambiguous nature of much federal and state health legislation. Despite dramatic improvements in the capacity of congressional staff to conduct policy analysis, the constraints of politics are such that ambiguity is frequently employed to ensure the passage of legislation.

The public policy process in American government can best be described in terms of an incremental model of decision making (Lindblom, 1959; Wildavsky, 1964). Simply stated, this model posits that policy is made in small steps (increments) and that

policy is rarely modified in dramatic ways. Major actors in the political bargaining process, whether legislators, interest groups, or administrators, operate on the basis of certain rules, and these rules are founded in adherence to prior policy patterns. Because the consequences of policy change are difficult to predict and because unpredictability is risky in the political market, policy makers prefer reform in small steps to more radical change.

An example of incremental change was the gradual evolution of the National Institutes of Health from a small federal laboratory conducting biomedical research in the 1930s to a multibillion-dollar research enterprise. The addition of new institutes took place over a fifty-year period. Budgets also grew gradually, beginning after World War II. Even when major health policy initiatives such as Medicare and Medicaid were adopted, the change was in the source of funds to pay for medical care for the elderly and the poor, not in the organization or provision of medical care.

The incremental model was elaborated by decision theorists concerned with ways that policy makers manage a large information load and the uncertainty of their political environment. Quite a different view, but one that is compatible with this perspective, was developed by Alford (1975). Alford addressed the nature of reform in health care and its ideological basis. He identified three approaches to reform, including market reformers, who call for an end to government interference in health care delivery and the restoration of market competition in health care institutions, and bureaucratic reformers, who blame market competition for defects in the system and call for increased administrative regulation of health care. What these perspectives share, Alford noted, is that each leads to incremental reform and the extent to which they challenge fundamental patterns of policy is limited. A third approach, the structural interest perspective, begins with an analysis of the ways in which the other two accept and benefit from current arrangements in health care. This perspective is formulated to challenge the effective, institutional control exercised by dominant structural interests that benefit from continuance of the system in its present form. As Alford made clear, the market and bureaucratic approaches are descriptive of the limits of health care reform, and they underlie resistance to change in the health system.

Relatively little research in the United States has examined the institutional and class basis of public policy, including health policy (Estes, 1982). Those who hold that defects in health care are rooted deeply in the structure of a class society would radically alter the present health care system, creating a national health service, with decentralization of administration and community control over health care institutions and health professionals. Those who view defects in health care as having a class basis believe that tinkering with the health care system itself cannot achieve the desired outcomes, but that these will follow major structural changes in society.

European countries that practice a parliamentary rather than representative democracy can effect larger changes more swiftly. In the parliamentary form of government, party policies are implemented speedily because the winning party practices bloc voting. Delay is caused only by the inability to achieve power. In representative governments, the parties cannot manage the discipline necessary to enforce party loyalty to programs or policies because elected representatives owe more, or at least as much, to their personal appeal as to party designation. The party discipline of parliamentary government is replaced by the quest for consensus in representative government, and consensus is most readily achieved when proposed reforms involve only modest changes.

A HISTORICAL FRAMEWORK: THE DEVELOPMENT OF HEALTH POLICY FROM 1798 TO 1988

Although the federal system in the United States has evolved continuously, at certain periods in our history the relationship among the federal, state, and local governments has undergone dramatic change. The major shifts in intergovernment relations were often the result of a crisis (the Civil War, the Great Depression, civil rights issues) rather than the result of a critical examination of the issues (the Clinton efforts).

Public health and health care did not loom large in the policy debate about federalism until the late 1940s, when President Truman advocated a program of national health insurance, and again in the 1960s, when implementation of Medicare transformed the role of the federal government in health care. Over the years, however, health policy issues (for example, federal regulation of food and drugs, federal support for biomedical research, hospital construction, and health profession education) have raised critical issues about the role of government in health care, intergovernmental relations, and the role of the private sector.

The private sector in the United States has always maintained a larger role in health care than it has in most other industrial nations. This has been true in both the financing and delivery of services. While it is not possible to do full justice to the rich history of health care policy here, an effort is made to present highlights in the development of health policy that reflect the manner in which much has changed and much has stayed the same.

The slow emergence of public policies and programs related to health and health care in the United States has generally followed the pattern of other industrial countries, particularly those in western Europe (Lee & Silver, 1972). At least three stages in the process have been identified:

1. Private charity, including contracts between users and providers, and public apathy or indifference.
2. Public provision of necessary health services that are not provided by voluntary effort and private contract.
3. Substitution of public services and financing for private, voluntary, and charitable efforts.

Although these three stages have been identified within many nations, different patterns have been observed among industrial countries. Political parties in the United States have been more reluctant than those in European countries or Canada to challenge the medical profession, hospitals, and the health insurance industry to promote health care reform.

The role of government at the federal, state, and local levels in public health and health care evolved partly in response to changes occurring in the health care system. With the major changes in health care that have occurred over the past two hundred years, particularly those in the past fifty years, has come a transformation in the role of government.

THE EARLY YEARS OF THE REPUBLIC: A LIMITED ROLE FOR THE FEDERAL GOVERNMENT (1798–1862)

During the early years of the republic, the federal government played a limited role in both public health and health care, which were largely within the jurisdiction of the states and the private sector. Private charity shouldered the responsibility of care for the poor. The federal role in providing health care began in 1798, when Congress passed the Act for the Relief of Sick and Disabled Seamen, which imposed a twenty-cent-per-month tax on seamen's wages for their medical care. The federal government later provided direct medical care for merchant seamen through clinics and hospitals in port cities, a policy that continues to this day. The federal government also played a limited role in imposing quarantines on ships entering United States ports in order to prevent epidemics (Lee & Silver, 1972). It did little or nothing, however, about the spread of communicable diseases within the nation, a problem that was thought to lie within the jurisdiction of the individual states.

Through the eighteenth, nineteenth, and early twentieth centuries, the major diseases in the United States, as in Europe, were infectious diseases. Tuberculosis, pneumonia, bronchitis, and gastrointestinal infections were the major killers. As the sanitary revolution progressed in the nineteenth century, social and economic conditions advanced, nutrition improved, reproductive behavior was modified, the burden of acute infection declined, and the burden of chronic illness began to rise. National health policies during the eighteenth and nineteenth centuries were limited to the imposition of quarantines to prevent epidemics and the provision of medical care to merchant seamen and members of the armed forces. In laws beginning with the Act Relative to Quarantine of 1796, Congress preempted state and local authority and put an end to long-standing federal-state dis-

agreements regarding the authority to prevent and control epidemics of yellow fever and cholera, as well as recurring outbreaks of plague and smallpox (Lewis & Sheps, 1983).

States first exercised their public health authority through special committees or commissions. Most active concern with health matters was at the local level. Local boards of health or health departments were organized to tackle problems of sanitation, poor housing, and quarantine. Later, local health departments were set up in rural areas, particularly in the South, to counteract hookworm, malaria, and other infectious diseases that were widespread in the nineteenth and early twentieth centuries.

THE EVOLUTION OF HEALTH POLICY: THE EMERGENCE OF DUAL FEDERALISM AND THE TRANSFORMATION OF AMERICAN MEDICINE (1862–1935)

The Civil War brought about a dramatic change in the role of the federal government. Not only did the federal government engage in a war to preserve the union, but it also began to expand its role in other ways that significantly altered the nature of federalism in the United States. This changing federal role was reflected in congressional passage of the first program of federal aid to the states, the Morrill Act of 1862, which granted federal lands to each state. Profits from the sale of these lands supported public institutions of higher education, known as *land-grant colleges* (Hale & Palley, 1981). Toward the end of the nineteenth century, the federal government began to provide cash grants to states for the establishment of agricultural experiment stations. While the federal role was generally expanding, the change had little impact on health care. An important exception occurred in the late 1870s, when the Surgeon General of the Marine Hospital Service was given congressional authorization to impose quarantines within the United States.

While the first state health department was established in Louisiana in 1855, it was not until after the Civil War that the states began to assume a more significant role in public health. Massachusetts established the first permanent board of health in 1869. By

1909, public health agencies were established in all the states. During this period, there was also rapid development of local health departments; state and local governments based their policy changes and management practices on the rapid advances in the biological sciences. Drawing on these advances, state and local health departments moved beyond sanitation and quarantine to the scientific control of communicable diseases (Miller et al., 1981).

The basic policies that created both state and local health departments derived from the police power of state governments (Miller, Moos, Kotch, Brown, & Brainard, 1981). Thus, the states—not the federal government—were the key to translating the scientific advances of the late nineteenth century into public health policy and the dramatic improvements in public health that followed.

The most significant role played by state governments in personal health care during this period was in the establishment of state mental hospitals. These first developed as a result of a reform movement in the mid-nineteenth century led by Dorothea Dix. Over the next century, state mental institutions evolved into isolated facilities for custodial care of the chronically mentally ill. The development of these asylums reinforced the stigma attached to mental illness and placed the care of the severely mentally ill outside the mainstream of medicine for more than a century (Gollaher, 1995).

Hospitals began to evolve in the nineteenth century from almshouses that provided shelter for the poor. Hospital sponsorship at the local level was either public (local government) or through a variety of religious, fraternal, or other community groups. Thus, the nonprofit community hospital was born; this institution, rather than the local public hospital, gradually became the primary locus of medical care. Physicians provided voluntary services to the sick poor in order to earn the privilege of caring for their paying patients in the hospital (Silver, 1976b). Hospital appointments became important for physicians in order to conduct their practices. Hospitals increased in number in the late-nineteenth century and began to incorporate new medical technologies, such as anesthesia, aseptic surgery, and later, radiology. Although charity was the major source of care for the poor, pub-

lic services also began to grow in the nineteenth century. Gradually, local government assumed responsibility for indigent care.

After the Morrill Act, the next major change in the role of the federal government came more than forty years later in the regulation of food and drugs. After twenty years of debate and much public pressure, Congress enacted the Federal Food and Drug Act in 1906 to regulate the adulteration and misbranding of food and drugs, a responsibility previously exercised exclusively by the states. The law was designed primarily to protect the pocketbook of the consumer, not the consumer's health. While it provided some measure of control over impure foods, it had little impact on impure or unsafe drugs (Silverman & Lee, 1974). The legislation not only represented a major change in the role of the federal government but also provided the constitutional basis for present-day regulation of testing, marketing, and promotion of prescription and over-the-counter drugs.

A number of other important developments in the early decades of the twentieth century had a strong impact on health care and health policy. Among the most significant were reforms in medical education that transformed not only education but also professional licensing and, eventually, health care itself. The American Medical Association and the large private foundations (for example, Carnegie and Rockefeller) played a major role in this process. Voluntary hospitals also grew in number, size, and importance. Medical research produced new treatments. Infant mortality declined as nutrition, sanitation, living conditions, and maternal and infant care improved. Health care changed in significant ways, but it was little affected by public policy.

THE EVOLUTION OF HEALTH POLICY: FROM DUAL FEDERALISM TO COOPERATIVE FEDERALISM (1935–1961)

The Great Depression brought action by the federal government to save banks, support small businesses, provide direct public employment, stimulate public works, regulate financial institutions and businesses, restore consumer confidence, and provide Social Security in old age. The role of the federal government was transformed in the span of a few years. Federalism evolved from a dual pattern, with a limited role in domestic affairs for the federal government, to a cooperative one, with a strong federal role.

The Social Security Act of 1935 was certainly the most significant domestic social legislation ever enacted by Congress. This marked the real beginning of what has been termed "cooperative federalism." The act established the principle of federal aid to the states for public health and welfare assistance. It provided federal grants to states for maternal and child health and crippled children's services (Title V) and for public health (Title VI). It also provided for cash assistance grants to the aged, the blind, and destitute families with dependent children. This cash assistance program provided the basis for the current federal-state program of medical care for the poor, initially as Medical Assistance for the Aged in 1960 and then as Medicaid (Title XIX of the Social Security Act) in 1965. Both later programs linked eligibility for medical care to eligibility for cash assistance. More important, however, the Social Security Act of 1935 established the Old Age, Survivors', and Disability Insurance (OASDI) programs that were to provide the philosophical and fiscal basis for Medicare, a program of federal health insurance for the aged, also enacted in 1965 (Title XVIII of the Social Security Act). Passage of the Social Security Act of 1935 was significant, for it provided the basis for direct federal income assistance to retired persons and established the basis for federal aid to the states in health and welfare; however, this legislation did not include a program of national health insurance. This was due principally to the opposition of the medical profession to any form of health insurance, particularly publicly funded insurance.

In 1938, after the deaths of a number of children due to the use of Elixir of Sulfonamide, consumer protection became an important issue for policy makers. This disaster resulted in the enactment of the Food, Drug, and Cosmetic Act of 1938, which required manufacturers to demonstrate the safety of drugs before marketing. This law was a further extension of the federal role and was consistent with other major changes in that role that occurred during the 1930s. After the passage of this act, little change was made in

drug regulation law until the thalidomide disaster in the early 1960s.

Growing attention to maternal and child health, particularly for the poor, was reflected in grants to the states and in a temporary program instituted during World War II to pay for maternity care of wives of Army and Navy enlisted men. This means-tested program successfully demonstrated the capacity of the federal government to administer a national health insurance program. With rapid demobilization after the war and opposition by organized medicine, the program was terminated, but it was often cited by advocates of national health insurance, particularly those who accorded first priority to mothers and infants.

Introduction of the scientific method into medical research at the turn of the century and its gradual acceptance had a profound effect on national health policy and health care. The first clear organizational impact of the growing importance of research was the transformation of the United States Public Health Service Hygienic Laboratory, established in 1901 to conduct bacteriologic research and public health studies, into the National Institutes of Health (NIH) in 1930, with broad authority to conduct basic research. This was followed by enactment of the National Cancer Act of 1937 and the establishment of the National Cancer Institute within the framework of NIH. There followed multiple legislative enactments during and after World War II that created the present institutes, focused primarily on broad classes of disease, such as heart disease, cancer, arthritis, neurologic diseases, and blindness. In the fifteen years immediately after World War II, NIH grew from a small government laboratory to the most significant biomedical research institute in the world. NIH became the principal supporter of biomedical research, quickly surpassing industry and private foundations. Indeed, in the period after World War II until the 1960s, federal support for biomedical research represented one of the few areas of health policy in which the federal government was active. The influence of organized medicine was a critical factor in limiting the federal role in other areas during this period.

In addition to federal support for biomedical research, largely through medical schools and universities, and a limited program of grants to states for public health and maternal and child health programs, federal policy related to hospital planning and construction became of primary importance. After World War II, it was evident that many of America's hospitals were woefully inadequate, and the Hill-Burton federal-state program of hospital planning and construction was launched in response in 1942. Its initial purpose was to provide funds to states to survey hospital bed supply and develop plans to overcome the hospital shortage, particularly in rural areas. The Hill-Burton Act was amended numerous times as its initial goals were met. This legislation provided the stimulus for a massive hospital construction program, with federal and state subsidies primarily for community, nonprofit, and voluntary hospitals. Public hospitals, supported largely by local tax funds to provide care for the poor, received little or no federal support until the needs of private institutions were met. The program became a model of federal-state-private sector cooperation in the distribution of substantial federal resources. It was a prime example of cooperative federalism and the major force—until enactment of Medicare and Medicaid—behind modernization of the voluntary community hospital system.

After World War II, President Truman urged Congress to enact a program of national health insurance, funded through federal taxes. President Truman's efforts and those of his supporters in Congress and organized labor were thwarted, again largely as a result of opposition by the American Medical Association. No progress was made in extending the federal role in financing of medical care because the medical profession argued that voluntary health insurance, such as Blue Cross, and commercial insurance could do the job.

By 1953, when the Department of Health, Education, and Welfare (DHEW), now the Department of Health and Human Services, was created, the federal government's role in the nation's health care system, although limited, was firmly established. This role was primarily designed to support programs and services in the private sector. Biomedical research, research training, and hospital construction were the major pathways for federal support. The Food and Drug Administration also became part of DHEW and was its primary regulatory agency. Traditional public health programs, such as those for venereal disease

control, tuberculosis control, and maternal and child health, were supported at minimal levels through categorical grants to the states. Federal support for medical care was restricted to military personnel, veterans, merchant seamen, and Native Americans until 1960, when enactment of the Kerr-Mills law authorized limited federal grants to states for medical assistance for the aged. This program proved short-lived, but it highlighted the need for a far broader federal effort in medical care for the poor and the aged.

THE TRANSFORMATION OF HEALTH POLICIES: THE NEW FRONTIER, THE GREAT SOCIETY, AND CREATIVE FEDERALISM (1961–1969)

A number of major federal health policy developments took place between 1961 and 1969, during the presidencies of John F. Kennedy and Lyndon B. Johnson. Although federal support was extended directly to universities, hospitals, and nonprofit institutes conducting research, most federal aid in health was channeled through the states. The term *creative federalism* was applied to policies developed during the Johnson administration that extended the traditional federal-state relationship to include direct federal support for local governments (cities and counties), nonprofit organizations, and private businesses and corporations to carry out health, education, training, social services, and community development programs (Reagan & Sanzone, 1981). The primary means used to forward the goals of creative federalism were grants-in-aid. More than two hundred grant programs were enacted during the five years of the Johnson administration.

The first major health policy changes after the election of President Kennedy were again the result of a crisis. The thalidomide disaster in Europe had little direct impact in the United States because the Food and Drug Administration had not approved the drug for marketing here. The disaster nonetheless focused renewed attention on the problems of drug safety, efficacy, and promotion and led to the most sweeping reforms of federal drug laws in twenty-four years. The 1962 amendments to the Food, Drug, and Cosmetic Act specified that a drug must be demonstrated to be effective as well as safe before it could be marketed. Advertising also was strictly regulated, and more effective provisions for removal of unsafe drugs from the market were included (Silverman & Lee, 1974).

The categorical programs that developed during the period of creative federalism were numerous and varied. Some programs were based on disease (heart disease, cancer, stroke, and mental illness), some on public assistance eligibility (Medicaid), some on age (Medicare, crippled children), some on institutions (hospitals, nursing homes, neighborhood health centers), some on political jurisdiction (state or local departments of public health), some on geographic areas that did not follow traditional political boundaries (community mental health centers, catchment areas, the Appalachian Regional Commission), and some on activity (research, facility construction, health professionals training, and health care financing) (Lewis & Sheps, 1983).

Among the more important new laws enacted during the Johnson administration were the Health Professions Educational Assistance Act of 1963, which authorized direct federal aid to medical, dental, pharmacy, and other professional schools, as well as to students in these schools; the Maternal and Child Health and Mental Retardation Planning Amendments of 1963, which initiated comprehensive maternal and infant care projects and centers serving the mentally retarded; the Civil Rights Act of 1964, which prohibited racial discrimination, including segregated schools and hospitals; the Economic Opportunity Act of 1964, which provided authority and funds to establish neighborhood health centers serving low-income populations; the Social Security Amendments of 1965, particularly Medicare and Medicaid, which financed medical care for the aged and the poor receiving cash assistance; the Heart Disease, Cancer, and Stroke Act of 1965, which launched a national attack on these major killers through regional medical programs; and the Comprehensive Health Planning and Public Health Service Amendments of 1966 and the Partnership for Health Act of 1967, which reestablished the principle of block grants for state public health services (reversing a thirty-year trend of categorical federal grants in health). This legislation also created the first nationwide health planning system, which was dramatically changed in the 1970s to focus on the

regulation of health care as well as health planning (U.S. Department of Health, Education, and Welfare, 1976). It should be noted that not until the Nixon and Reagan administrations was the block grant concept widely applied to federal grants-in-aid to the states. Of the many new health programs initiated during the Johnson presidency, only Medicare was administered directly by the federal government.

The programs of the Johnson presidency had a profound effect on intergovernmental relationships, the concept of federalism, and federal expenditures for domestic social programs. Grant-in-aid programs alone (excluding Social Security and Medicare) grew from $7 billion at the beginning of the Kennedy and Johnson administration in 1961 to $24 billion in 1970, at the end of that era. In the next decade, the impact was to be even more dramatic as federal grant-in-aid expenditures for these programs grew to $82.9 billion in 1980. "Grants-in-aid," note Reagan and Sanzone (1981), "constitute a major social invention of our time and are the prototypical, although not statistically dominant, form of federal domestic involvement."

The programs of the Johnson administration not only had a significant effect on the nature and scope of the federal role in domestic social programs but also had important consequences for health care. Federal funds for biomedical research and training, health personnel development, hospital construction, health care financing, and a variety of categorical programs were designed primarily to improve access to health care and secondarily to improve its quality. Increased attention during this period was given to the notion of health care as a right, a concept similar to the principle of the "earned right" that underlies the Social Security System (Callahan, 1977; Lee & Jonsen, 1974).

Although there was a profound change in the role of the federal government, many policies adopted during this time reflected the interests of the medical profession, the hospitals, and the health insurance industry. Medicare and Medicaid hospital reimbursement policies were designed to ensure hospital participation. Adoption of the cost-based method of reimbursement proved a boon for hospitals but was very costly for the taxpayer. Policies designed to meet the physician shortage of the 1960s eventually developed full support from organized medicine. Designed to strengthen the capacity of the nation's medical schools to respond to a nationally perceived need, these policies also provided direct benefit to an interest group of growing power: medical schools.

HEALTH POLICY IN AN ERA OF LIMITED RESOURCES: FROM CREATIVE FEDERALISM TO NEW FEDERALISM AND A RETURN TO DEPENDENCE ON COMPETITION AND THE PRIVATE SECTOR (1969–1992)

During the 1970s, President Nixon coined the term *new federalism* to describe his efforts to move away from the categorical programs of the Johnson years toward general revenue sharing, through which federal revenues were transferred to state and local governments with as few federal strings as possible, and toward block grants, through which grants were allocated to state and local governments for broad general purposes. During the Nixon and Ford administrations (1969–1977), considerable conflict developed between the Republican-controlled executive branch and the Democrat-controlled Congress with respect to domestic social policy, including the new federalism strategy originally advocated by President Nixon. Congress strongly favored categorical grants, with their detailed provisions, and was opposed to both revenue sharing and block grants. This period also witnessed an erosion of trust between federal middle management and congressional committees and subcommittees (Walker, 1981).

President Nixon also differed sharply from President Johnson in his explicit support for private rather than public efforts to solve the nation's health problems. On this fundamental issue, the Nixon administration made its position clear:

> Preference for action in the private sector is based on the fundamentals of our political economy— capitalistic, pluralistic and competitive—as well as upon the desire to strengthen the capability of our private institutions in their effort to provide health services, to finance such services, and to produce the resources that will be needed in the years ahead. (Richardson, 1971)

Although Nixon was a strong advocate for private sector leadership, he did propose a national health insurance plan based on an employer mandate. The proposal lost in Congress because the liberals felt that they would soon be able to enact a single-payer program, based on the Medicare model.

Although the Nixon administration attempted to implement its new federalism across a broad front, progress was made primarily in the fields of community development, personnel training, and social services. Categorical grant programs in health continued to expand despite attempts by both the Nixon and Ford administrations to transfer program authority and responsibility to the states and to reduce the federal role in domestic social programs. During the period 1965–1975, more than seventy-five major pieces of health legislation were enacted by Congress, indicating continued support for the categorical approach by the legislative branch of the federal government (U.S. Department of Health, Education, and Welfare, 1976).

Although categorical health programs proliferated in the 1960s and 1970s, the expansion of two programs—Medicare and Medicaid—dwarfed the others. While those programs contributed to medical inflation, their growth was due largely to the rising costs of medical care. Federal and state governments became third parties that underwrote the costs of a system that had few cost-constraining elements, and the staggering expenditures had profound effects on health policy.

The federal government's response to skyrocketing health care costs (and thus government expenditures) assumed a variety of forms. Federal subsidies of hospitals and other health facility construction were ended and replaced by planning and regulatory mechanisms designed to limit their growth. In most cases, these proved to be short-lived and ineffective because they were not directly linked to Medicare or Medicaid. In the mid-1970s, health personnel policies focused on specialty and geographic maldistribution of physicians rather than physician shortage, and by the late 1970s concern was expressed about an over-supply of physicians and other health professionals. Direct subsidies to expand enrollment in health profession schools were cut back and then eliminated. Funding for biomedical research began to decline in real dollar terms when an abortive "war on cancer" launched by President Nixon appeared to produce few concrete results and when Medicare and Medicaid preempted most federal health dollars.

An additional regulatory initiative enacted during President Nixon's second term was the National Health Planning and Resources Development Act of 1974 (PL 93–641). This law incorporated some of the planning principles from the Partnership for Health Act of 1967 and the Heart Disease, Cancer, and Stroke Act of 1965, both of which were terminated with the enactment of PL 93–641. In addition to the health planning responsibility assigned to state health planning and development agencies (SHPDAs) and to local health systems agencies (HSAs), the law required that health care facilities obtain prior approval from the state for any expansion, in the form of a "certificate of need" (CON). The impact of this new approach to health planning and regulation was limited (Salkever & Bice, 1976), and the program was eliminated early in the Reagan administration.

More important than the constraints placed on resources allocated for health care were regulations instituted to slow the growth of health care costs in the Medicare and Medicaid programs. Two direct actions were taken by the federal government: (1) a limit on federal and state payments to hospitals and physicians under Medicare and Medicaid (included in the 1972 Social Security amendments), and (2) a period of wage and price control applied to the general economy when the Economic Stabilization Program was introduced to dampen increasing inflation. Wage and price controls on hospitals and physicians were continued after the general restrictions were removed. When controls were lifted in 1974, health care costs again began to climb.

Another regulatory initiative was designed to control costs through limiting the use of hospital care by Medicare and Medicaid beneficiaries. Although the original Medicare and Medicaid legislation required hospital utilization review committees, these appeared to have little effect on hospital use or costs. In 1972, amendments to the Social Security Act (PL 92–103) required the establishment of professional standards review organizations (PSROs) to review the quality and appropriateness of hospital services provided to beneficiaries of Medicare, Medicaid, maternal and child health, and crippled children programs (paid for under the authority of Title V of the Social Security Act). PSROs were composed of physicians who reviewed hospital records in order to determine whether length of stay and services provided were appropriate. Results of these efforts have been mixed. In only a few areas where PSROs have been in operation is there evidence that cost increases have been restrained, and in these areas, it is not clear that the PSRO has been a critical factor.

An attempt was also made to control costs through major changes in the organization of medical care. Efforts were made to stimulate the growth of group practice repayment plans, which provide comprehensive services for a fixed annual fee. These capitation-based prepayment organizations were defined in federal legislation enacted in 1973 as health maintenance organizations (HMOs). Studies had demonstrated that HMOs could provide comprehensive care at significantly less cost than fee-for-service providers, primarily because of lower rates of hospitalization (Luft, 1980). Predictably, the federal stimulus for development of HMOs encountered strong resistance from organized medicine. Nevertheless, the program successfully enhanced professional and public awareness of HMOs and assisted in the development of a number of small prepaid group practices.

Although the new federalism advocated by President Reagan was a dramatic departure from previous policies and trends because of the scope of his proposals, the roots of these policies were first evident in the comprehensive Health Planning and Public Health Service amendments enacted in 1966 during the presidency of Lyndon Johnson. They were increasingly evident in both the policy initiatives and the budgetary decisions of Presidents Nixon and Ford. Not only were Nixon and Ford's new federalism policies similar to those later advocated by President Reagan, but their fiscal and monetary policies were also designed to reduce the growth of federal spending and program responsibility.

During the presidency of Jimmy Carter (1977–1981), there were few health policy initiatives that were successful. The Carter administration tried without success to get Congress to enact hospital cost-containment legislation. Special interests, particularly hospitals and physicians, again prevailed. They were able to convince Congress that a voluntary effort would be more effective. Escalating health care costs did moderate during the debate in Congress, but when the threat of mandatory controls was no longer present, costs rose at a record rate. The picture in the late 1970s was one of frustration with efforts to control health care costs. Concern about access to care became a secondary consideration.

Following the Clinton effort at health care reform in 1993–1994, the most significant development of the 1990s was the rapid growth of managed care. Managed care has cast a wide net and means different things to different observers. Included under this umbrella is the integration of health insurance and the delivery of care. Health services can be provided either directly or through another entity, possibly including the management of that practice.

While growth in both public sector and private sector supporting HMOs was slow during the 1970s and 1980s, it was building the base for explosive growth in the 1990s. Medicare has been the slowest to take advantage of the potential savings in shifting from a payer to a purchaser. Beginning in 1972 (the year before the HMO Act passed), Medicare initiated a risk-sharing contract option for HMOs. The program did not begin, however, until 1978 with a five-site demonstration program. Because of the slow growth in the original risk-sharing demonstration, Congress authorized a managed care capitated-payment option based on prospective payment methodologies. This option was implemented in 1985. Medicare HMO enrollment has increased steadily since risk contracting began in 1985. Growth in the private sector, however, far outpaced the Medicare growth of managed care in the late 1980s and in the 1990s. The congressionally mandated Physician Payment Review Commission (PPRC), in its 1996 report to Congress, noted:

> The changes in managed care during the past three years have been extraordinary. What were once considered "alternative delivery systems" have emerged as mainstream methods of financing and delivering medical care in the U.S. (Physician Payment Review Commission, 1996)

The PPRC survey found three major types of managed care plans: (1) staff/group model HMOs;

(2) network/independent practice associations (IPAs); and (3) preferred provider organizations (PPOs). The plans are also offering a point of service (POS) option that permits an enrollee to seek care outside the plan network for an added charge.

Medicaid growth in managed care, driven largely by the states' desire to control rapidly rising costs, has been far more rapid than has Medicare's growth. The two mechanisms used by the states have been section 1915(b) and section 1115 waiver authority. In recent years, states have turned increasingly to the section 1115 waivers. The section 1115 waiver authority was enacted in 1962 to authorize research and demonstration projects that are "likely to assist promoting the objectives" of the Social Security program (including Medicaid since 1965). By the late 1990s, a total of thirty-three states were either developing, operating, or had applied for approval of statewide Medicaid waivers under section 1115 authority. The waivers have included expansion of eligibility, limited cost-sharing, mandatory enrollment in managed-care systems, eliminating provider reimbursement protections, program monitoring, and delivery systems innovations (Kaiser Commission on the Future of Medicaid, 1995).

In the private sector, growth in the numbers enrolled in managed care has been rapid in the past two decades. Often employers give their employees a limited choice of plans. By contrast, federal employees who are privately insured (for example, federal employees' health benefits) may choose from among a number of managed-care plans.

While there was initially a sharp drop in the rate of increase in medical care costs after the rapid growth of managed care, premiums are again escalating. Past savings were largely derived from dramatic reductions in hospital admissions, with a consequent reduction in hospital occupancy and hospital costs. As hospital length-of-stays are reduced, less and less savings can be gained in this area. At the same time, technology continues to advance and to be one of the primary drivers of lost increases.

The failure to pass national health care reform in 1993–1994, as well as the political trauma of the adoption and repeal of Medicare catastrophic coverage in 1988–1989, has produced much reflection about the political forces that doomed these efforts and about the prospects for substantial reform in the foreseeable future. Informed observers provide us with little ground for optimism. Many reasons are cited, among them a governmental system of separated institutions that routinely frustrates major policy change and the growing power of politics and ideology over health services research and policy analysis. Most daunting, perhaps, is the fact that policy making at the federal level has become budget-driven to a degree that opportunities for legislating new programs have all but vanished. Deficit pressures and the imperatives of the budget process have effectively driven out serious attention to substantive policy issues and focused policy making on cost-cutting revisions of existing programs (Mann & Ornstein, 1995). If 1993–1994 represented a rare window of opportunity for reform (and some argue that the window was barely ajar), then that opportunity has clearly passed, and the prospects for any major reform under President George W. Bush and a Congress without mandate are few.

As bleak as that scenario may seem, there is also reason to believe that government will remain deeply involved in the business of health care policy for the foreseeable future and that occasions for policy change will continue to emerge as the latest incremental policy solutions fall short of the mark and themselves generate new policy problems. The politics of health care reform and the continuing debate about managed care have significantly raised the awareness of the American public about issues in the organization and financing of health care. This new salience, combined with a stronger economy and some possible tempering of antigovernment sentiment, suggest that efforts at modest policy reform will continue and that universal coverage, while still a dream, has not disappeared from the American policy agenda.

The Reagan administration accelerated the degree of pace of change in policy that had been developing since the early Nixon years. The most prominent shifts in federal policy advanced by the Reagan administration that directly affected health care were (1) a significant reduction in federal expenditures for domestic social programs, including the elimination of the revenue-sharing program initiated by President Nixon; (2) decentralization of program authority and responsibility to the states, particularly through block grants; (3) deregulation and greater emphasis on market forces and competition to stimulate health care reform and more effective control of health care costs; (4) tax reductions, despite significant increases in the national debt, with a resulting decline in the fiscal capacity of the federal government to fund domestic social programs; and (5) Medicare cost containment through the implementation of a prospective payment system for hospitals based on costs per case, using diagnosis-related groups (DRGs) as the basis for payment.

An important consequence of the block grants enacted by Congress at the urging of the Reagan administration is that the wide discretion that these grants provide to the individual states fosters inequities in programs among the states. This, in turn, makes it impossible to ensure uniform benefits for target populations, such as the poor and the aged, across jurisdictions or to maintain accountability with so many varying state approaches (Estes, 1982). Because the most disadvantaged individuals are heavily dependent on state-determined benefits, they are especially vulnerable in periods of economic flux. These policies also have increased pressure on state and local governments to underwrite program costs at the same time that many states, cities, and counties are under mounting pressure to curb expenditures.

Although the Reagan administration strongly favored deregulation and stimulation of competitive market forces, this had little impact on federal health care policies except in the health planning area. The federal health planning legislation was not renewed in the 1980s, but a number of states continue to operate certificate of need programs in an attempt to control the proliferation of expensive technologies.

In contrast to eliminating health planning as a means of regulation, the Reagan and Bush administrations used regulations to limit hospital reimbursement and physician fees in the Medicare program.

At the state level, however, major changes were underway in the 1980s that responded to the growing influence of the free-market ideology. In California, major reforms were enacted in 1982 in an attempt to increase competition among hospitals and reduce the costs of Medicaid in that state. Private insurance companies were authorized to contract directly with hospitals through preferred provider contracts in an attempt to stimulate price competition among hospitals.

Congress has considered a number of procompetitive proposals related to Medicare, Medicaid, and private health insurance. Although the proposals differ in detail, several elements characterize the procompetitive approach: (1) changes in tax treatment for employers, employees, or both, regarding employer contributions to health insurance plans (not supported by Congress) in the 1980s or the 1990s even though costs continued to escalate; (2) establishment of incentives or requirements for employers to offer employees multiple choices of health insurance plans, subject to certain limitations with respect to coverage of services and cost sharing, including catastrophic illness benefits and preventive care (in many states, employers have provided employees with fewer choices of managed care plans in the 1990s); and (3) establishment of Medicare voucher systems under which elderly and disabled individuals would receive a fixed payment instead of a defined benefit.

The politics of limited resources in the 1970s continued into the 1980s and 1990s. The prolonged period of postwar economic growth, based on productivity gains, came to a halt in the early 1970s and was not reviewed until the mid-1990s. The additional resources needed in domestic social programs and defense were more and more constrained as a result. Controlling the costs of health care became a critical need at the federal and state levels. In the 1970s, policy efforts focused more on limiting federal and state expenditures in Medicare and Medicaid than they did on dealing with the root causes of the problem: the growing supply of physicians, the rapid growth in biomedical technologies in health care, and reimbursement incentives in Medicare, Medicaid, and private insurance mediated through the fee-for-service health system that has led to enormous inflation in health care costs.

Given a policy process characterized by limited government roles, federalism, pluralism, administrative bargaining, and incrementalism, prospects remain relatively dim for controlling expenditures in ways that protect vulnerable groups such as the poor and the elderly. It is increasingly evident that those groups whose needs originally inspired special programs are relinquishing the gains achieved in access to care.

The cost-containment strategies of past decades, particularly those since 1981, combined with the effects of the recessions of 1981–1982 and 1990–1992 on unemployment and access to private health insurance, contributed to the lower priority accorded to access to care for the poor, as did the growth of the undocumented alien, immigrant, and refugee populations and the diminishing commitment to provide for the near poor and the working poor with private health insurance through employment. This has led to a significant increase in the number of uninsured and underinsured. Despite the improved economy and low levels of unemployment, the number of uninsured, particularly among low-wage workers and their dependents, continues to grow.

Federal policies related to Medicare and Medicaid, taxes, and refugees and undocumented aliens, state policies related to health care cost containment and Medicaid, and the policies of private insurance companies and employers related to private health insurance, competition, and cost containment have all contributed to the rising number of uninsured and underinsured. Because the working poor, the disabled, refugees, new immigrants, undocumented aliens, and workers in small businesses do not have the influence of large employers, the insurance industry, physicians, hospitals, and other influential participants in health policy, it is unlikely that their voices will be heard unless the costs of their care impose such a burden on state and local governments and community hospitals (that is, bad debt and charity care) that these groups will gain allies willing to advocate on their behalf. Because the interests of these groups remain diffuse in terms of the potential for political action, it is unlikely that they can compete effectively in the policy process with the interest groups that have long influenced the shape of public policy in health.

The rise in health care costs continued as the dominant health policy issue of the 1990s. Between 1970 and 1990, the share of gross national product (GNP) spent on health care rose from 7.3 percent to 12.3 percent. Health insurance premiums are again rising.

For two decades, health care spending in the United States outpaced the growth of the rest of the economy, with consequences for workers (depressed wages), business (a growing share of profits to health care), families (rising out-of-pocket costs and rising taxes to pay for public programs), and government (increasing share of government expenditures for health care).

HEALTH POLICY: NEW SOLUTIONS, OLD PROBLEMS (1993–PRESENT)

As the Clinton administration took office in 1993, there was talk in health care circles of federally driven reform on the scale of that produced by the Social Security Act legislation of 1935 and 1965. To the surprise of most, the election campaign of candidate Bill Clinton in 1992 not only raised health care as a salient national issue but also set the stage for a major health care reform process in 1993–1994. President Clinton and his team proposed comprehensive financing reform based on a strategy he called "managed competition," orchestrated by government and designed to stimulate private sector decisions that would expand coverage and control costs. The president initiated an elaborate process that developed a plan that he presented to Congress and the American people in September 1993. The thirteen hundred pages that translated this plan into legislative specifics were introduced in Congress in early 1994. The essential elements included universal coverage, purchasing cooperatives, budget caps, employer-mandated coverage, and no tax increase to expand coverage. The proposal was translated by its opponents into limited choice for consumers, loss of benefits and increased costs for many of the insured, government interference with the market and consumer choice, the addition of new government bureaucracies, and limits on professional autonomy. The public was confused. Congress could not reach agreement on any reform, and the proposal died in the spring of 1994. The failure of health care reform was yet another example of "American exceptionalism" when compared to other industrialized democracies. Indeed, even Taiwan and Korea had enacted programs of universal health in-

surance while the United States failed again. It also illustrated the difficulty of enacting comprehensive, as opposed to incremental, reforms in the United States.

If this period began with the promise of comprehensive reform at the federal level, by late 1994, the tables were turned once again as policy attention shifted back to reliance on competitive forces and the market with selective interference from government. In the 1994 election, the Republicans gained control of both the United States House of Representatives and the United States Senate. The result was prolonged stalemate, with little accomplished in any area of health policy except for the enactment of the Kennedy-Kassenbaum bill, which extended health insurance protection for individuals who were changing jobs or were temporarily unemployed. In addition, the Ryan White CARE Act (AIDS services) was extended, but no other significant health legislation was even reauthorized. After the 1996 presidential and congressional elections, President Clinton was returned to office, but the Republicans strengthened their control in the Senate and maintained their majority, although somewhat diminished, in the House. The result was a dramatic shift from the confrontation and deadlock of 1995–1996 to a consensus on a play to balance the federal budget, including the most significant reforms in the Medicare program since 1965. The Balanced Budget Act of 1997 called for a reduction in Medicare spending increases of $115 billion by 2002 and a dramatic increase in the choice of managed-care plans, including HMOs, independent practice associations (IPAs), preferred provider organizations (PPOs), provider service organizations (PSOs), and even medical savings accounts. Medicare's basic fee-for-service option would continue.

Various forces affect health care policies: some, such as the aging of the population, are beyond the control of policy makers; others, such as the rapid increase in physician supply and the use of an increasing number of new technologies in health care, are amenable to more direct policy interventions. One of the keys will be to reach agreement on the nature and scope of cost containment. The Balanced Budget Act of 1997 was a major step forward in reaching consensus on health care cost containment in the future. It combined both managed care strategies and regulatory policies that focus on limiting provider payments rather than restricting consumer choice.

The difficult election process that led to the inauguration of President George W. Bush without a strong national mandate and the concurrent election of an extremely divided United States Congress created a difficult environment for national health policy initiatives. Even areas of relative agreement between the primary national parties, such as a drug benefit program under Medicare, became subject to intense political bickering and a difficult policy environment. Although there continues to be concurrence that the evolution of the nation's health care system currently falls short of the ideals embodied in the principles of access, fairness, and cost efficiencies, resolution of many long standing issues will continue to face difficult political and economic environments in the foreseeable future. Even recognizing the potential of significant national and state revenue surpluses, competing obligations for funds, and the failure to create clear national mandates in the health care arena will stymie any revolutionary approaches to the provision of health care, particularly the cost of pressures that continue to build in the system (Bilheimer & Colby, 2001; Blendon, Altman, Benson, & Brodie, 2001).

While two fundamentally different approaches to cost containment have been advocated and applied in the past fifteen years—regulation and competition—it appears that a mixed system will continue in the United States because of the strong role of the private sector, a federalist system of government, the dominance of pluralistic politics, and a penchant for incremental reform (Mann and Ornstein, 1995).

Incrementalism appears to be returning to the issue of extending coverage to the uninsured. Health care financing and cost containment are domestic social policy issues that are likely to remain on the national policy agenda until the process of incremental reform truly deals with the twin problems of rising health care costs and access to health insurance. The next chapters in health care reform will reflect the same factors that have affected health policy during the past sixty years.

References

Alford, R. R. (1975). *Health care politics: Ideological and interest group barriers to reform.* Chicago: University of Chicago Press.

Bachrach, P. (1967). *The theory of democratic elitism: A critique.* Boston: Little, Brown.

Bilheimer, L. T., & Colby, D. C. (2001). Expanding coverage: Reflections on recent efforts. *Health Affairs, 20,* 83–95.

Blendon, R. J., Altman, D. E., Benson, J. M., & Brodie, M. (2001). Health policy 2001: The implications of the 2000 election. *New England Journal of Medicine, 344,* 679–684.

Brizius, J. A. (n.d.). *Federalism and national purpose* (pp. 72–98). Working paper 2, Project on the Federal Social Role, National Conference on Social Welfare, Washington, DC.

Callahan, D. (1977). Health and society: Some ethical imperatives. *Daedalus, 106,* 1.

Estes, C. L. (1980). *The aging enterprise.* San Francisco: Jossey-Bass.

Estes, C. L. (1982). Austerity and aging in the United States: 1980 and beyond. *International Journal of Health Services, 12,* 573.

Feder, J. M. (1977). *The politics of federal hospital insurance.* Lexington, MA: Lexington Books.

Ginzberg, E. (Ed.). (1977). *Regionalization and health policy.* Washington, DC: U.S. Government Printing Office.

Gollaher, D. L. (1995). *Voice for the mad: The life of Dorothea Dix.* Free Press: New York, NY.

Hale, G. E., & Palley, M. L. (1981). *The politics of federal grants.* Washington, DC: Congressional Quarterly Press.

Jonas, S., & Banta, D. (1981). Government in the health care delivery system. In S. Jonas (Ed.), *Health care delivery in the United States.* New York: Springer.

Kaiser Commission on the Future of Medicaid. (1995, September). *Medicaid and the elderly, policy brief.* Washington, DC: Author.

Lee, P. R., & Jonsen, A. R. (1974). The right to health care. *American Review of Respiratory Diseases, 109,* 591–593.

Lee, P. R., & Silver, G. A. (1972). Health planning—A view from the top with specific reference to the USA. In J. Fry & W. A. J. Farndale (Eds.), *International medical care.* Oxford, UK: Medical and Technical Publishing.

Lewis, I., & Sheps, C. (1983). *The sick citadel: The American academic medical center and the public interest.* Cambridge, UK: Oelgeschlager, Gunn & Hain.

Lindblom, C. E. (1959). The science of "muddling through." *Public Administration Review, 10,* 79–88.

Lowi, T. J. (1979). *The end of liberalism: The second republic of the United States.* New York: Norton.

Luft, H. S. (1980). *Health maintenance organizations: Dimensions of performance.* New York: Wiley-Interscience.

Mann, T. E., & Ornstein, N. J. (Eds.). (1995). *Intensive care: How Congress shapes health policy.* Brookings Institute.

Marmor, T. R., Wittman, D. A., & Heagy, T. C. (1976). The politics of medical inflation. *Journal of Health Politics, Policy and Law, 1,* 69–84.

Miller, C. A., Moos, M. K., Kotch, J. B., Brown, M. L., and Brainard, M. P. (1981). Role of local health department in the delivery of ambulatory care. *American Journal of Public Health, 71,* (1 Suppl): 15–29.

Pechman, J. A. (Ed.). (1979). *Setting national priorities: The 1980 budget.* Washington, DC: The Brookings Institution.

Physician Payment Review Commission. (1996). *Annual report to Congress, 1996.* Washington, DC: Author.

Reagan, M. D., & Sanzone, J. G. (1981). *The new federalism* (2nd ed.). New York: Oxford University Press.

Richardson, E. L. (1971). *Towards a comprehensive health policy in the 1970s.* Washington, DC: U.S. Department of Health, Education, and Welfare.

Salkever, D. S., & Bice, T. W. (1976). The impact of certificate-of-need controls on hospital investment. *Milbank Memorial Fund Quarterly, 54,* 185–214.

Schattschneider, E. E. (1960). *The semisovereign people.* New York: Holt, Rinehart & Winston.

Silver, G. A. (1976a). Medical politics, health policy, party health platforms, promise and performance. *International Journal of Health Services, 6,* 331–343.

Silver, G. A. (1976b). *A spy in the house of medicine.* Germantown, MD: Aspen.

Silverman, M., & Lee, P. (1974). *Pills, profits, and politics.* Berkeley, CA: University of California Press.

U.S. Department of Health, Education, and Welfare. (1976). *Health in America 1776–1976* (DHEW Pub. No. HRA 76–616). Washington, DC: U.S. Government Printing Office.

Vladeck, B. C. (1979). The design of failure: Health policy and the structure of federalism. *Journal of Health Politics, Policy and Law, 4,* 522–535.

Walker, D. (1981). *Toward a functioning federalism.* Cambridge, MA: Winthrop.

Wildavsky, A. (1964). *The politics of the budgetary process.* Boston: Little, Brown.

CHAPTER
~16~

Assessing and Improving Quality of Care*

Scott Weingarten

Chapter Topics

- What Is Quality?
- Variations in Care
- Opportunities to Improve Care
- Framework for Measuring Quality
- Attempts to Standardize Quality Measures
- Cost Containment and Quality
- Managed Care and Quality
- Practice Guidelines
- Disease Management
- Clinical Pathways
- Information Technology and Quality
- Hazards of Quality Measurement
- Examples of Successful Quality Improvement Programs
- Further Recent Examples and Concerns
- Summary

Learning Objectives

Upon completing this chapter, the reader should be able to:

- Appreciate the complexity of defining and measuring the quality of care
- Understand how measuring and monitoring quality can result in improved outcomes
- Define how quality is assessed and assured
- Appreciate strategies that now exist for influencing physician behavior
- Review illustrative scenarios of quality improvement programs

*In part from "Implementing Clinical Practice Guidelines," by S. Weingarten and S. Deutsch, 1997, *Internal Medicine* (5th ed.), Chapter 6. Copyright 1997 by Mosby. Adapted with permission.

The debate on the quality of health care has taken center stage. On one hand, advances in medical care proceed at an astronomical pace. The populations' life span has been steadily increasing. New medical technologies and procedures abound. American medical care has produced some of the most sophisticated technologies in the world.

The paradox of health care, however, is that while there have been unprecedented advances in medical technology, concerns about quality of care not only continue but intensify. For example, recent studies have documented compromised outcomes for patients who have reduced access to medical care. Furthermore, there are concerns that the proliferation of managed care will promote the underutilization of necessary medical resources and compromise the quality of patient care.

WHAT IS QUALITY?

This debate on quality has forced us to ask some very basic questions. What is quality of patient care? Can quality of care be measured? Purchasers of health care are asking these questions about the quality of care provided by health plans, hospitals, and health care providers. As they spend an increasing amount of money on health care and public concern about health care quality receives greater attention, they are searching for objective information on the quality of care that patients are receiving.

An Illustration of Quality

An example of the difficulty of making judgments about quality of care could be illustrated through the experience of a patient undergoing coronary artery bypass surgery. A patient with significant coronary artery disease consults with a cardiac surgeon prior to surgery. The cardiac surgeon spends little time with the patient during the preoperative visit. She makes little effort to educate the patient about what will happen before, during, and after surgery. One week later, the surgery is performed without complications. The length of stay for the patient in the acute care hospital is eleven days, which is five days longer than the average length of stay for patients undergoing coronary

artery bypass surgery in that particular hospital. The total hospital costs for that patient are $10,000 more than for an average patient in that particular hospital. After adjusting the length of stay and cost for case complexity, the cost and length of stay is still much greater than for comparable cases in that hospital and region. The patient, however, survived the operation, had an uncomplicated hospital course, and was free from postoperative complications. Three months later, the patient's health is excellent, and he is able to enjoy tennis free from symptoms.

From a technical standpoint, the operation went flawlessly and the clinical outcome was excellent. The "art" of caring for the patient, however, was questionable, as the patient received little information about the care that he was going to receive before, during, and after surgery. The physician exhibited poor communication skills. And if utilization were considered a measure of quality, the prolonged length of stay and increased costs associated with the operation might be considered indicative of a suboptimal quality of care.

Did this patient receive excellent or poor quality medical care? Judgments of this type depend on many different factors, and the importance attached to each of those factors. Some patients might believe that the quality of care was excellent as evidenced by the clinical outcome (the patient had an uncomplicated hospital course and was able to resume an active lifestyle). Some patients, however, especially those who place a higher value on the "art" of care and desire a more personalized approach, might have a more negative opinion about the quality of care that they received. Finally, if one examines the economic outcome, the care would not have compared favorably to the care provided to other patients. To a certain extent, quality is in the eyes of the beholder, and it may not always be perfectly clear whether an individual patient received good or poor quality medical care. This principle can also apply to evaluating the care provided to populations of patients.

Measurement Issues

Competition and market forces have taken hold of health care delivery. In the past, competition in health care was largely based on cost. As in many other sectors of the economy, there is a strong desire to base competition on both quality and cost, or the value of care. To achieve this goal, it is necessary to have valid and reliable measures of quality of care that can be measured relatively cost-effectively.

In the past, physicians have often felt comfortable ordering tests, prescribing treatments, and advising patients relatively free from scrutiny regarding the care that they provided. The focus of providing care was on individual patients rather than populations of patients. Assessments of quality of care were usually made only in the most egregious of cases, such as by peer review committees and through medical malpractice litigation. Furthermore, research investigations question the ability of peer review committees to accurately assess quality of care; the validity of this method for assessing quality has been shown to be poor. Review of medical malpractice cases is also considered to be an insensitive and nonspecific measure of quality of care because poor quality of care may not be associated with litigation and not all medical malpractice cases are caused by poor quality of care.

As a result of quality measurement, "report cards" and other expressions of quality of care information have become commonplace. Physicians often are concerned that accountability and report cards intrude into the care that they provide to patients. However, physicians' and other health care providers' concern about this intrusion seems to be outweighed by the sentiments of the purchasers who are demanding to understand the care provided to their employees or beneficiaries through the inspection of objective data.

In many industries, purchasing decisions are made based on cost and quality. In health care, however, this has not been the case. Purchasing decisions have been largely based on the cost of care. Cost has been the predominant factor driving health care purchasing, in part because cost has been easier to measure than quality of care. Information on quality, if available, could be used to direct value-based purchasing decisions. The alternative is that competition in health care would be based entirely on the cost of care; this could lead to a downward price spiral where care is provided by those who offer medical care at the lowest cost. In the most extreme case, this could mean that clinicians and health care organiza-

tions providing the least care to patients would have the opportunity to care for the most patients.

One of the most notable attempts to measure quality of care provided at different hospitals is published annually by *U.S. News and World Report.* These reports, which have been published since 1990, are based on the opinion of physicians who have been identified as leaders in the field of medicine. The ratings are based on clinical expertise, technology, teaching status, experience, and outcome (mortality rates). Recent critiques of this effort, however, suggest that the data included in this analysis preclude valid and meaningful comparisons of quality. Furthermore, an analysis of the information suggests that the ratings reflect hospital reputation rather than objectively measured information about the quality of patient care.

Assuming that quality rankings are based on reputation rather than objective measures of quality, a hospital providing excellent quality of care, without a matching reputation, might not be publicly acknowledged as a high-quality institution. Furthermore, a hospital with an excellent reputation might continue to be regarded as high quality regardless of whether there are data that support or refute that finding.

VARIATIONS IN CARE

Variations in care have been demonstrated in different regions throughout the country, in different hospitals in the same region, and even among different physicians practicing at the same hospital. Increasingly, questions are being asked regarding the cause of these variations (Wennberg & Gittelsohn, 1973). One possible explanation is that many clinical decisions cannot be supported by scientific evidence and, instead, are determined by an individual physician's experience and training, along with the "art" of medicine. Of those clinical decisions that are based on scientific evidence, the scientific knowledge is at times inconsistent and difficult for physicians and other health care providers to access in real time while they are caring for patients. Variations in care may be further accentuated by differences in patient preferences, as patients may choose different options when informed about alternative treatments.

Another factor affecting variations in patient care is the explosion of available medical information. It has been said that there are more than 20,000 biomedical journals and more than 2,000,000 medically related articles published each year. The tremendous increase in the scope of progress in biomedical research perhaps is best illustrated by the release of the human genome, and the increasing elucidation of underlying biological mechanisms has led to an explosion of scientific knowledge related to all aspects of human biology and health, permanently altering the practice of clinical medicine. An individual physician could be expected to read and retain a relatively small fraction of the published medical literature. The proliferation of medical information has led to the concern that physicians will not be able to keep current with the latest medical literature. Without a method of organizing and summarizing available, current, and relevant clinical information, it may be impossible for an individual clinician to remain current and to apply available clinical information to each patient's care. Failure to remain current with the literature may lead to delays in translating important new medical advances into widespread clinical practice.

OPPORTUNITIES TO IMPROVE CARE

There are many reasons to measure quality of care. Perhaps the most compelling reason is to attempt to improve quality of care. It has been said, "If you cannot measure it, you cannot manage it." Measurement of quality can illuminate opportunities to improve quality of care. For example, one might discover missed opportunities to immunize children against infectious diseases and to offer mammograms to women. Measurement of quality is also important to determine whether there are gaps between actual medical practice and optimal medical practice as defined by review of the scientific literature. The measurement of quality may be particularly important when the scientific evidence demonstrates that there is a "best practice" or an optimal method of caring for patients. In this case, one could compare the actual provision of therapy with best practice. For example,

beta-blockers have been shown to improve the outcomes of patients with an acute myocardial infarction. Therefore, because there is a process (provision of beta-blockers) and outcome (survival) link, the discovery of underutilization of this treatment could be associated with compromises in patient care.

Additional research has disclosed a significant gap between optimal medical care (care that would lead to the best patient outcomes) and care that is being provided on a widespread basis (Ellerbeck et al., 1995; Krumholtz et al., 1995; Weiner, Parente, Garnick, Fowles, Lawthers, & Palmer, 1995). Whether examining influenza immunization of elderly patients, the performance of mammograms, or childhood immunizations, studies have consistently demonstrated opportunities to improve the quality of patient care. For example, the published literature demonstrated that thrombolytic therapy was associated with a reduction in mortality long before it was widely recommended for clinical practice for patients suffering with acute myocardial infarction. In addition, aspirin is an inexpensive, safe, and effective medication for treating patients with acute myocardial infarction. To determine the use of aspirin in patients with acute myocardial infarction, a retrospective study was performed on hospitalized patients sixty-five years of age and older (Krumholtz et al., 1995). Among those patients without contraindications to aspirin, more than one-third did not receive aspirin during the first two days of hospitalization. Those patients who received aspirin had a lower mortality rate than those who did not. Increasing the use of aspirin for elderly patients after acute myocardial infarction may be a cost-effective and simple strategy to improve quality of care and to reduce the mortality rates for elderly patients suffering from acute myocardial infarction (Krumholtz et al., 1995).

Research has also demonstrated a significant opportunity to improve the quality of care provided to elderly diabetic patients (Weiner et al., 1995). A majority of patients did not receive regular glycosylated hemoglobin levels (which is important for monitoring the control of blood sugar in diabetic patients). Furthermore, many patients did not receive cholesterol screening. These findings demonstrated a significant opportunity to improve quality of care provided to diabetic patients.

Health services researchers have discovered a significant rate of inappropriate care, including the use and application of invasive procedures (Brook, 1989). Inappropriate care can be determined using many different definitions, including the provision of care when risks are greater than the potential benefits. Furthermore, it is believed that the provision of inappropriate care may contribute to rising health care costs, and curbing this care may be an excellent method of reducing costs without sacrificing, and with possibly improving, quality of patient care.

Benchmarking

Many of the early efforts to measure quality were primitive and not felt to be reflective of quality of care by many clinicians. Some of these efforts included the measurement of hospital admission rates and hospital lengths of stay. "Benchmarking" was performed to compare a hospital's admission rate with admission rates at the best-performing hospitals. The problem with these analyses is the difficulty in achieving consensus about what constitutes an appropriate hospital admission rate. For example, a hospital with a higher admission rate may have a lower rate of discharging patients from the emergency department to their home inappropriately. Benchmarking has traditionally been based on utilization, rather than on quality of care or patient outcome. Furthermore, utilization data that cannot be linked to patient outcomes is of limited value. Utilization data have often come from administrative data systems that were not designed to collect information to evaluate the quality of care.

FRAMEWORK FOR MEASURING QUALITY

Donabedian was an early pioneer in developing a framework for evaluating the quality of care. He defined quality as having at least three dimensions, including structure, process, and outcome of care. He said that "it is possible to divide this management into two domains: technology of medicine, and of the other health sciences, to the management of a personal health problem. Its accompaniment is the management of the social and psychological interaction between client and practitioner. The first of these has been called the science of medicine and the second its art." He also defined "a third element in care which could be called its 'amenities.'" The Institute of Medicine later defined quality as the "degree to which health services for individuals and populations increase the likelihood of desired health outcomes and are consistent with current professional knowledge." Quality of care can be measured in patients who are ill and also in patients who are well.

The locus of quality measurement can vary. Quality of health care can be measured in a community health plan, physician organization (such as a medical group or independent practice association), hospital, or even care provided by an individual physician. Another key issue affecting outcome measurement has to do with the timing of measurement. For example, for patients discharged following hospitalization for community-acquired pneumonia, one month after discharge may be an adequate amount of time to assess patient outcome. However, for patients recovering after total hip replacement surgery, it may be necessary to wait one to two years after surgery to fully understand a patient's recovery (reduction in pain and improvement in physical functioning), and possibly five to ten years or longer to determine whether a repeat operation is required.

Assessment of quality can also be performed through implicit and explicit measurement. Explicit measurement entails comparing the quality of care against some predetermined standard; for example, the number of patients who sustained a myocardial infarction and who were treated with a beta-blocker. Implicit measurement is usually subjective, without a comparison with a predetermined performance criteria.

Quality of care studies have also been influenced by recent attempts to better understand the impact of patient preferences on clinical decision making and the role of shared medical decision making. Patient involvement in the care process has assumed greater importance in recent years.

Structure of Care

The dimensions of quality of care include structure, process, and outcome. The structure of care includes information on the facilities and people caring for patients. Information on the facilities may include hospital bed size or the procedures performed in a hospital. Information on the caregivers might include the percentage of doctors who are board-certified. Studies on the structure of care often show a weak correlation between these characteristics and the quality of care provided to patients and patient outcomes. Therefore, the evaluation of structure as a measure of quality is often not regarded as clinically meaningful.

Process of Care

In contrast, process of care relates to what is done to particular patients (such as diagnostic tests or procedures). Measuring the process of care is clinically credible when there is a proven link between process (performing that test or procedure) and a clinically important outcome measure (mortality, quality of life, patient satisfaction). If there is not a link between the process of care and outcome, process measurement may not yield meaningful results.

Attempts have been made to detect under-utilization of medical care by measuring the processes of care (for example, an individual patient either did or did not have a mammogram). Process of care measurement may also be applied to a population of patients. For example, the annual mammography rate for women fifty years of age and older is seventy-five percent. This is clinically meaningful because there are randomized controlled clinical trials that have shown that mammography can reduce long-term mortality from breast cancer in women of an appropriate age range. Other process measures might include Pap smear rates and childhood immunization rates.

There is some concern about attempting to utilize process measures to evaluate quality of care. For example, results of such analyses have shown that a health plan may score very well in one area while scoring poorly in another area, making overall judgments about quality of care difficult. If a health plan had a high mammography rate and a low Pap smear rate, would this health plan be considered a good or poor quality health plan? If a consumer considering the selection of a health plan had access to these data, how would these rates, if at all, influence his or her

decision? Finally, because health plans are not directly responsible for the performance of mammograms or Pap smears, would this information be considered a valid measure of the health plans' performance?

Outcome of Care

Patient outcome can be measured to evaluate quality of patient care. An outcome is the result of the care provided to patients. Inadequate process of care, however, may not always result in poor patient outcome. For example, many children who are not immunized will not die from communicable diseases. In this case, the outcome is favorable even though most clinicians would regard the care as being of poor quality.

In the past, quality of care has been largely measured through the examination of clinical and physiologic variables. Such measures might include whether a patient recovering after total hip replacement develops a postoperative infection. For a patient recovering from a total hip replacement, the patient's severity of pain and ability to physically function might also be considered very important measures of quality. And the rapidity with which a patient is able to return to work can potentially relate to the quality of care.

The following are examples of patient outcome measures. These measures include clinical (survival), patient-centered (quality of life), and satisfaction measures:

- the five-year mortality rate from breast cancer
- the mean quality-of-life score for patients with stage II breast cancer
- the percentage of patients receiving a mammogram who were very satisfied with the care that they received in the radiology suite

Mortality Rates

There is controversy regarding whether hospital mortality rates are a valid measure of quality of care. Validity is enhanced when the rates are adjusted for severity of illness and the volume and severity of comorbid conditions. There are some studies that indicate that hospitals with higher severity-adjusted mortality rates have more preventable deaths, which could imply that quality of care relates to mortality rates. Issues about the validity of this information, however, led to concerns about publishing hospital mortality rates as a measure of quality.

One of the most visible efforts to measure the quality of care provided by physicians has been measuring severity-adjusted mortality rates for physicians who perform coronary artery bypass surgery. Because mortality is an important outcome measure for patients, mortality rates—assuming that there has been adequate adjustment for case severity—may relate to quality of care. Mortality rates, however, would be an insensitive measure of the quality of care provided to patients undergoing cataract surgery or to patients in the outpatient setting.

The most significant concern about attempting to infer information about quality of care from mortality rates is that there must be adequate adjustment for the severity of patient illness. For example, if one hospital treats patients who are more severely ill than another hospital, a higher mortality rate may not reflect worse quality of care, but rather that patients in that hospital are more severely ill and therefore have a higher probability of dying. In order to use outcome information to judge quality of care, adjustment must be made for patient severity of illness. Severity-of-illness measures have been used to predict probability of death, morbidity, or a prolonged length of hospital stay. Severity measures can incorporate variables related to diagnosis, physiological variables, and laboratory variables.

Comorbidity

Comorbidity relates to the volume and severity of existing illnesses. Comorbidity may also be predictive of adverse outcomes. For example, a patient suffering an acute myocardial infarction with severe diabetes mellitus and chronic obstructive pulmonary disease may have a higher probability of an adverse outcome than patients with acute myocardial infarction without any comorbid illnesses. Therefore, understanding the volume and severity of comorbid illnesses may be essential for relating the results of outcome measurement studies to the evaluation of the quality of care rendered to individual patients.

Health Status

Recently, there has been increasing interest in measuring patient-centered outcomes such as health status (and health-related quality of life). Recent studies have shown that there are valid, reliable, and responsive instruments to measure outcomes from the patient's perspective. The acceptance of these measures has increased as they have been shown to correlate with physiological measures (for example, a patient's physical functioning score correlates with her ability to perform on a treadmill). Because many procedures are performed to reduce pain and improve functioning, such as total hip replacement and cataract surgery, measurement of health-related quality of life and health status may better reflect quality of care than many clinical measures. Research efforts in measuring patient-based outcomes have led to improvements in these measures, including instrument reliability (in test and retest studies), validity (the results correlate with physiological measures of health), and responsiveness (the measures change over time in a manner consistent with changes in physiological health).

Patient Satisfaction

Significant attention has been devoted to the measurement of patient satisfaction. Satisfaction relates to the quality of service provided to patients. The validity of patient satisfaction as a measure of technical quality of care (technical aspects of medical care) is uncertain. Employer groups, however, view patient (employee) satisfaction as an important indicator for assessing the performance of health plans, hospitals, and physician organizations. Furthermore, certain organizations have attempted to understand patient ratings of individual physicians. Physician reimbursement and other incentives have been linked to patient satisfaction ratings.

Access to Care

Another important measure of quality of care is access to necessary health care services. Access may relate to care provided by physicians and/or subspecialists or the availability of tests and procedures. The recent interest in measuring access to care reflects the public's concern that necessary and appropriate health care services may be under-utilized in a capitated environment (an environment that provides a financial incentive to provide less medical care).

ATTEMPTS TO STANDARDIZE QUALITY MEASURES

One of the most significant challenges in the field of quality improvement is the need to standardize performance measures. If physician organizations must respond frequently to multiple queries about quality of care, the financial burden of measurement may exceed the benefits. This could occur if the resource requirements necessary for reporting quality diverted significant resources away from caring for patients and negatively impacted quality of patient care. This would be especially true if efforts to measure quality do not result in documented benefits in patient care.

The National Committee for Quality Assurance (NCQA) is responsible for coordinating the development of HEDIS (Health Plan Employer and Data Information Set) as a measure of the quality of care provided by health plans. Employer groups helped sponsor the development of these measures to monitor the care provided to their employees. The measures, largely developed by clinical and methodological experts, initially emphasized outpatient process of care measures (such as childhood immunization rates, mammography rates, and Pap smear rates). HEDIS has been expanded to include the measurement of patient outcomes. The outcome measures in HEDIS 3.0 include patient satisfaction and health status.

COST CONTAINMENT AND QUALITY

Health care costs have been rising at an unsustainable pace. As concerns about rising health care costs escalate, numerous efforts have been initiated to curb costs. These efforts include shortening hospital lengths of stay, decreasing hospital admission rates, reducing the use of expensive tests and procedures, and decreasing referrals to specialists. Some cost-containment strategies probably maintain and possibly enhance quality of care. Some efforts, however, may compromise quality of care, especially when necessary and appropriate care is eliminated.

A number of studies have demonstrated that when access to medical care is reduced for poor patients, quality of care is compromised and patient outcomes may worsen. Furthermore, some efforts to control costs for specific aspects of care may lead to an increase in costs in other sectors. For example, an effort to limit the number of drugs made available to mentally ill patients was found to increase the number of emergency department visits and partial hospitalizations for psychiatrically related conditions. This effort to reduce costs was associated with an increase in overall health care costs (the reduction in drug costs was offset by an increase in costs associated with patient care visits).

MANAGED CARE AND QUALITY

Outcome studies have been conducted to compare quality of care in managed care and fee-for-service health systems. In the aggregate, no system consistently demonstrated better quality of care, although differences in care have been reported in some studies. No clear differences are seen when comparing most quality of care and outcome measures.

Quality of preventive care has been shown in some studies to be better in managed-care organizations than in fee-for-service medicine. Other studies have shown better patient satisfaction among patients cared for in a fee-for-service setting when compared with a managed-care organization. One study, which received considerable attention, showed a greater decline in physical functioning among elderly patients enrolled in managed-care organizations when compared to fee-for-service medicine (Ware, Bayliss, Rogers, Konsinski, & Tarlov, 1996). However, studies have not consistently documented this finding. Furthermore, not all managed care organizations are equal, and it is possible that quality of care may vary with the organization.

PRACTICE GUIDELINES

Health services research studies left a trail of observations regarding the delivery of medical care services, including unexplainable variations in medical care, the provision of inappropriate medical care, and gaps between optimal medical practice and widespread clinical practice (Wennberg & Gittelsohn, 1973). Some have promoted the idea that practice guidelines may remedy this situation. Medical practice guidelines, otherwise known as *practice parameters* or *protocols*, are a means of providing organized medical knowledge to clinicians that could potentially influence the care delivered to individuals and populations of patients. Practice guidelines have been defined as "systematically developed statements to assist practitioner decisions about appropriate health care for specific clinical circumstances." The guidelines are often derived from systematic reviews of scientific evidence, and the information is condensed into documents to assist clinicians and patients. The guidelines consolidate available scientific knowledge about the best and most appropriate treatments for patients with common diseases and conditions (Brook, 1989). The expression of guidelines may vary from relatively simple statements, such as mammography should be offered to all women over a certain age, to more comprehensive and complicated patient care management strategies.

Proponents of clinical guidelines believe that they have the potential to improve clinical decision making, decrease undesirable variations in medical care, improve quality of care, and decrease health care costs. Enthusiasm for guidelines, however, is tempered by concerns that guidelines oversimplify the practice of medicine, devalue the art of medicine, and infringe upon physician autonomy and clinical freedom. There is also a concern that they may be used in a punitive manner or by plaintiffs' attorneys against health care providers in medical malpractice cases. In addition, some clinicians believe that the primary motivation behind the development of practice guidelines is to contain costs rather than to improve quality of care.

There are a number of organizations either producing or sponsoring the development of practice guidelines. Those organizations include the United States federal government (United States Preventive Services Task Force, the Agency for Health Care Policy and Research), specialty societies (American College of Cardiology, American College of Physicians), academic medical centers, health plans, and commer-

cial organizations. As a testimonial to the number of organizations producing practice guidelines, the American Medical Association's Directory of Practice Parameters lists and catalogues more than two thousand different guidelines. These guidelines, however, are of variable quality, ranging from scholarly syntheses of the available scientific evidence (for example, American College of Physicians, Agency for Health Care Policy and Research) to guidelines that are less rigorous and comprehensive.

Although many different guidelines are in circulation, their impact on patient care is unknown. Furthermore, the acceptability, credibility, and quality of guidelines vary. Professional society guidelines receive a higher level of confidence from some physicians than guidelines produced by other sources. Practice guidelines developed by health plans may be viewed as less credible than guidelines developed by other organizations.

With the large number of guidelines in existence, it may be a daunting task for clinicians to decide which are most appropriate for their patients, and which offer the greatest opportunity to improve medical care. Guidelines vary widely in the method used to create them, the rigor with which the scientific evidence is reviewed and organized, the background of the individuals who created them, and the resources devoted toward their development.

For many conditions, there are multiple guidelines available on the same topic. Given the variability in the process used to create guidelines, it is not surprising that conflicts have been identified between different guidelines on the same topic. These conflicts can create confusion among clinicians contemplating using them to assist in the care of their patients. Furthermore, it may be perceived that some developers of guidelines have conflicts of interest that may influence guideline recommendations. An example of this concern is the development of guidelines with the perceived goal of promoting subspecialty consultation.

There are different methods of developing practice guidelines. A preferred method includes the rigorous integration of all available and relevant scientific evidence (for example, randomized controlled clinical trials and meta-analyses). Guidelines developed in this manner are often called "evidence-based" guidelines. Many guidelines, however, are based on expert opinion alone, unsubstantiated by higher levels of scientific evidence. Some people believe that evidence-based guidelines may be more acceptable to clinicians, most of whom were trained in the application of the scientific method. (The scientific method is a basic foundation for medical, nursing, and pharmacy training.)

Some desirable attributes of practice guidelines include the following:

1. The purpose of the guideline should be clearly expressed. For example, the guideline was developed to improve the appropriateness of providing mammography to women.
2. The content of guidelines must be frequently reviewed and updated regularly. For example, a two-year-old guideline to assist clinicians who are caring for patients with AIDS that does not incorporate the latest scientific evidence could lead to suboptimal medical care. Ideally, guidelines should have an expiration date.
3. The guidelines must be flexible enough to account for the nuances of clinical medicine. The clinical nuances of medicine are often subtle; therefore, it is unrealistic to expect to apply a guideline to every conceivable patient.
4. Guidelines should be easy to follow. Complicated guidelines with multiple branch points are often difficult to remember. These guidelines may not be adopted into practice in the absence of sophisticated information technology.
5. The guidelines should be applicable in a variety of geographic and health care settings.
6. Guidelines should be linked to demonstrable improvements in patient outcomes, which may include morbidity, mortality, health status, quality of life, satisfaction, and cost of care. Outcome validation is especially important when scientific support for the recommendations is uncertain. It is often easier to achieve clinician support for guidelines that have been shown to improve patient outcomes.

Although an evidence-based approach to guideline development is appealing for eventual physician acceptance of the guidelines, there are limitations to this approach. One of the most notable limitations is a paucity of scientific evidence to support many common clinical practices. In other cases, the available evidence may be incomplete, contradictory, or of insufficient quality or credibility to be used to develop a guideline.

Despite the explosive growth in the number of medical practice guidelines, until recently there has been relatively limited evidence that they have had an impact on medical care. There has been a disproportionate amount of time spent on their development as compared with time spent on their implementation and evaluation. A systematic review of the published literature on practice guidelines, however, demonstrated that guidelines have significant potential to improve patient care (Grimshaw & Russell, 1993). Of fifty-nine published studies on practice guidelines, fifty-five demonstrated at least one significant change in care associated with the introduction of a guideline. The magnitude of the effects was variable. Moreover, of the eleven studies that examined patient outcomes, nine demonstrated beneficial changes in patient care. A more recent update of this work continues to demonstrate that the majority of guideline studies demonstrate at least one improvement in care. Although the clinical significance is not always large, overall available research would suggest that there is continued reason to pursue practice guideline development, implementation, and evaluation.

If a guideline is not adopted into practice, it will have relatively little impact on patient care. Dissemination of guidelines alone will fail to produce widespread adoption. Many barriers to physician adoption of guidelines must be overcome for guidelines to have the opportunity to improve patient care, and a carefully crafted implementation plan is requisite for the adoption of guidelines; otherwise, there may be no sustained change in clinical practice.

Physician attitudes and beliefs about practice guidelines may influence their adoption. Physicians often believe that guidelines are used for disciplinary actions. Physicians also believe that guidelines will increase health care costs even though their development is motivated by a desire to reduce costs.

Many different implementation strategies have been employed to encourage clinician adoption of guidelines (Table 16.1). For example, any one of these strategies, or several of them, could be employed to implement the United States Preventive Services Task Force (USPSTF) guidelines regarding mammography. The USPSTF guidelines state that "routine screening for breast cancer every 1–2 years, with mammography alone or mammography and annual clinical breast examination (CBE), is recommended for women aged 50–69."

A systematic overview was performed to determine the relative effectiveness of different strategies in modifying physician behavior (Davis et al., 1995). The results showed that information dissemination and education alone usually fail to change physician practice or patient outcomes. However, more comprehensive and multifaceted implementation strategies (for example, use of physician opinion leaders, "academic detailing") were effective in producing change in physician practice. These strategies were accompanied by a twenty- to fifty-percent reduction in the provision of inappropriate care. This information should cause a loss of confidence in dissemination strategies that depend on education alone and call for renewed enthusiasm for strategies that include multiple, simultaneous approaches toward implementing guidelines.

Table 16.1. Implementation Strategies to Encourage Adoption of Practice Guidelines

   I. Traditional education
  II. Retrospective feedback
 III. Concurrent feedback (reminders)
 IV. Incentives
  V. Administrative solutions
 VI. "Academic detailing"
VII. Opinion leaders
VIII. Patient education
 IX. Application of information technology
  X. Physician (clinician) involvement in the development and implementation process

Implementation Strategies

Some of the implementation strategies used with practice guidelines include the following.

Traditional Education

Published studies have demonstrated that traditional continuing medical education programs fail to produce sustained changes in clinical practice (Davis, Thomson, Oxman, & Haynes, 1995; Oxman, Thomson, Davis, & Haynes, 1995). Although educational programs may appear to be a cost-effective method of gaining widespread acceptance of guidelines, available information on the effectiveness of education as a dissemination strategy suggests that expectations should be low, except when education is used in conjunction with other implementation strategies. A Grand Rounds or continuing medical education program could be used to inform clinicians about the USPSTF guidelines on mammography; however, little sustained change should be anticipated.

Retrospective Feedback

Results are mixed regarding the effects of retrospective feedback and physician profiling on physician practice (Balas, Austin Boren, Brown, Ewigman, Mitchell, & Perkoff, 1996). Although changes in patient care have been demonstrated in studies employing retrospective feedback and profiling, the magnitude of the effect is often small. Therefore, enthusiasm for physician profiling and retrospective feedback may not always be supported by proven changes in patient care.

Retrospective feedback could be used to provide clinicians with feedback about their mammography rates (for example, seventy-five percent compliance with USPSTF mammography guidelines). Also, each clinician's mammography rates could be compared with those of his or her peers.

Concurrent Feedback (Reminders)

Studies have demonstrated that real-time feedback of guideline information to physicians, while they are caring for patients, can be associated with a significant increase in their adoption of the guidelines (Mugford, Banfield, & O'Hanlon, 1991). Reminders enable physicians to decide whether a particular guideline is appropriate for their individual patient at the time they are providing care. However, some studies have shown that the effects of guidelines on clinical practice diminish when reminders are discontinued.

To encourage adherence to USPSTF mammography guidelines, checklists, written reminders, or cues could be used to prompt physicians to perform mammograms in appropriate patients at the time of the visit. (See also information technology.)

Incentives

Incentives, monetary and otherwise, may significantly influence clinical decision making. It stands to reason that incentives, or removal of disincentives, may promote adoption of practice guidelines. Linking physician reimbursement to adoption of USPSTF mammography guidelines would be considered a method of incentives for physicians to follow the guidelines.

Administrative Solutions

In general, administrative rules produce changes in physician practice. Therefore, administrative mandates may be used to enforce adoption of guidelines, although the safety of this approach is largely unproved. An administrative solution to promote the adoption of guidelines could best be illustrated by the exclusion of a particular drug from a formulary. An administrative fiat might be less appropriate for increasing adoption of USPSTF mammography guidelines.

"Academic Detailing"

"Academic detailing," a method involving one-on-one educational interactions, has been shown to change physician behavior (Soumerai & Avorn, 1990). Face-to-face sessions may prove to be successful when the message is brief and repetitive. During these encounters, the educator attempts to understand each clinician's approach to a particular clinical situation. The "detailer" explains the guideline to the physician, who then has the opportunity to raise questions and concerns about the application of the guideline to patient care. Although this approach has proven effective, it can be costly and labor-intensive.

Using the academic detailing model, the educator might schedule a meeting or series of meetings with each clinician to better understand their beliefs and attitudes about the USPSTF mammography guidelines. Using that information as background, the detailer could explain the potential benefits of following USPSTF mammography guidelines.

Opinion Leaders

Visible support of practice guidelines by "opinion leaders" may promote adoption of the guidelines. Using a social influence model of changing clinician behavior, local peer pressure and influence may affect practice patterns. Therefore, recruiting local and influential "physician champions" to promote guidelines may prove to be effective. Respected opinion leaders could be used to promote the USPSTF mammography guidelines.

Patient Education

Patient education and outreach programs can be used to promote patient understanding of the rationale behind guidelines. Patients may initiate questions with their physician that lead to adoption of the guideline. Patient education could be used to directly inform women about the potential benefits of mammography with the hope that women who are overdue for a checkup would contact their physician and request a mammogram.

Application of Information Technology

Technological advances in clinical information systems have been accompanied by studies examining the use of computerized reminders to implement practice guidelines (Pestotnik, Classen, Evans, & Burke, 1996). Real-time computer reminders can lead to increased adoption of guidelines. The desire to implement multiple practice guidelines and the application of guidelines to patients with multiple conditions and comorbid illnesses will also increase the potential benefits of using computerized reminders as an implementation strategy. Furthermore, when physicians interact with practice guidelines on a dynamic basis (such as with computerized order entry systems), computer technology may prove to be a cost-effective method of implementing several guidelines at the same time. Finally, information technology may enable the performance of cost-effective outcome studies. Internet-based strategies to disseminate guidelines will undoubtedly receive significant attention as integrated delivery networks refine their attempts to disseminate and implement guidelines.

Busy physicians and clinicians may be less likely to seek out guidelines if they either detract from the patient encounter or reduce time with patients. Time constraints may limit the adoption of paper-based guidelines, especially if they require a physician to search out guidelines while the patient waits in the office or in the examining room. In the future, practice guidelines and other clinical decision support tools may be embedded in clinical decision support software housed in an electronic medical record. The key decision points and the guidelines to support the most appropriate clinical decisions may be linked to diagnoses, diagnostic tests, treatments, symptoms, or signs. The widespread deployment of this type of system may significantly advance attempts to implement complicated guidelines and allow for the capture of patient outcome data and the use of this information to improve medical care. With each patient encounter, a clinical information system could be used to process the age, gender, date of last mammogram (if appropriate), breast cancer risk factors (if appropriate and available), and the date of the visit to determine if the patient is overdue for a mammogram. If the patient is overdue, the physician would be prompted to speak to the patient about the potential benefits of mammography.

Physician (Clinician) Participation in the Development and Implementation Process

Social influence models suggest that the involvement of key individuals in the development of guidelines, especially those individuals involved with patient care, may encourage the eventual adoption of guidelines. Therefore, many health care organizations encourage the involvement of a diverse group of health care practitioners to develop, adapt, and update guidelines. A multidisciplinary team might be assembled to review and adopt the USPSTF mammography guideline and to discuss possible strategies for effectively implementing the guideline.

The most effective guideline implementation efforts often involve several different approaches to implementation; the use of a single strategy may prove to be less effective. However, guidelines are imperfect and may not be relevant to many patients. In fact, preserving each physician's ability to override guidelines is important for maintaining the quality of patient care. Therefore, with very few exceptions, guidelines should be used to complement rather than substitute for clinical decision making. Coercive implementation strategies, such as tying compliance with guidelines to physician incentives, may become problematic when the scientific evidence supporting a guideline is uncertain.

After a guideline has been implemented, especially guidelines based on uncertain scientific evidence, the effects on patient care should be evaluated (Weingarten, Riedinger, Conner, Johnson, & Ellrodt, 1994). Although there have been many different evaluations of guidelines, unfortunately, there have been relatively few considering the large number of guidelines that have been disseminated as part of a comprehensive effort to evaluate guidelines. Measured effects could include the acceptance of the guidelines by physicians, the impact on clinical outcomes (for example, mortality, morbidity), the effect on patient-centered outcomes (for example, patient health status, patient satisfaction, return to work), and economic outcomes (for example, cost of outpatient care and inpatient care). Finally, there is a definable cost associated with developing, updating, implementing, and evaluating guidelines. The true economic impact of any guideline should account for the cost of the guideline program. The cost savings attributed to the guideline, if any, should be offset by the program costs.

The importance of evaluating certain practice guidelines in clinical practice cannot be overestimated. In a study of patients with congestive heart failure, it was hypothesized that providing physicians with information on the timing of transfer of patients with congestive heart failure and pulmonary edema out of the coronary care unit or intermediate care unit would lead to better quality and less costly medical care (Weingarten et al., 1994). This hypothesis was then tested in a controlled study. That study showed that although lengths of stay in intermediate care units for patients with congestive heart failure were reduced, total length of stay actually increased. Therefore, the failure to address the continuum of medical care resulted in a probable increase in total health care costs following implementation of a strategy designed to reduce health care costs.

The Importance of Practice Guidelines

In conclusion, practice guidelines and other systematic approaches to clinical decision making are being promoted to reduce undesirable variations in care, reduce health care costs, and improve the quality of medical care. There is early evidence to suggest that guidelines based on available scientific evidence and implemented in an effective manner may improve patient care. Some dissemination and implementation strategies, however, may prove to be effective while others may incur cost without benefit. Given the current enthusiasm for guidelines and the resources devoted to their development, the promise of guidelines may best be realized through careful attention to their implementation and evaluation in clinical practice. In this new era of physician accountability for clinical decisions and greater attention to improving the health of populations of patients, systematic approaches to clinical decision making, including the use of practice guidelines, are likely to continue to play an important role in the practice of medicine.

DISEASE MANAGEMENT

Disease management, also known as *health care management,* is a concept that has been promoted to address the comprehensive management of patients across the continuum of care. Disease management programs reduce the emphasis on treating acute episodes of care while seeking a more comprehensive approach to the total care of a patient. The approach emphasizes preventive care and care that prevents or delays complications from a disease. Practice guidelines and clinical decision support tools are often developed to identify the primary determinants of both the quality and cost of care for patients enrolled in a disease management program.

CLINICAL PATHWAYS

Clinical pathways have emerged as recent strategies for improving the quality and cost-effectiveness of medical care. Clinical pathways have been used in industry for decades, and their purpose is to sequence work to maximize efficiency of the work flow. Unfortunately, there are very few available data examining the effect of clinical pathways on patient care; most of the literature on this topic comes from outside of the health care field.

Clinical pathways have been developed and implemented at many hospitals across the United States in an effort to improve the quality of care and to reduce health care costs safely. Clinical pathways often include information about the most appropriate treatment and timing of treatment (as well as sequencing different forms of therapy). There are recent examples of using clinical pathways to improve patient care.

INFORMATION TECHNOLOGY AND QUALITY

Many processes of care measures, such as mammography rates, Pap smear rates, and childhood immunization rates, are easier to measure in a managed-care population with sophisticated information systems. Organizations with less sophisticated information systems may struggle to cost-effectively determine process measures.

Information technology is critical for measuring and improving the quality of patient care. First, in order to cost-effectively measure quality of patient care, patients must be identified accurately and efficiently. For example, to measure the quality of care provided to patients with diabetes (for example, the level of blood sugar control), one must be able to rapidly identify all patients with diabetes.

Second, the data must be gathered efficiently and cost-effectively. In order to monitor quality of care, data needs to be ascertained quickly and with little labor and cost involved. The use of information systems allows the rapid determination of the numerator and denominator for many different variables. This could be most efficiently performed by employing information technology. For example, glycosylated hemoglobin levels reflect the control of blood sugar in patients with diabetes. If glycosylated hemoglobin levels could be determined cost-effectively from clinical information systems, then cost-effective monitoring could occur.

Finally, patients who receive the greatest benefit from quality improvement projects, such as those with the highest probability of developing complications, could be rapidly identified. For example, patients with the poorest blood sugar control might derive the greatest benefit from being enrolled in a structured program for diabetic patients (the opportunity for improvement is greatest).

The Internet is used for a variety of medical applications. First, it is used by patients to gather medical information. Second, Internet technologies are used to disseminate practice guidelines and protocols by provider organizations and to cost-effectively disseminate clinical strategies to improve the quality of patient care. Information on quality of care is disseminated over the Internet to consumers and providers. Finally, Internet technology may be used to gather patient outcome data. For example, information on patient outcomes (health status, satisfaction, and return to work) presumably could be obtained by querying patients via the Internet.

HAZARDS OF QUALITY MEASUREMENT

A hazard of measuring quality of care is that the data could be misused and adversely affect health care providers. If a measure is purported to reflect quality, yet truly reflects factors unrelated to quality, the information could be potentially misleading. The Health Care Financing Administration (HCFA) previously disseminated information on hospital mortality rates publicly. Although detailed efforts were made to adjust mortality rates for case complexity (severity of

patient illness), there was sufficient concern about the validity of the data to cause concern that the rates provided little insight about the quality of care provided at hospitals.

EXAMPLES OF SUCCESSFUL QUALITY IMPROVEMENT PROGRAMS

Hypertension

Studies have examined whether the use of practice guidelines can improve the care provided to patients in the outpatient setting and to patients with chronic diseases such as hypertension (Aucott, Pelecanos, Dombrowski, Fuehrer, Laich, & Avon, 1996). The guidelines were implemented using a strategy that included education, a "clinical champion," a pharmacist intervention, and physician feedback. The use of guideline medications was greater in the intervention (guideline) group than in the control group. Moreover, blood pressure control was better in the intervention group. In conclusion, intensive implementation of hypertension guidelines probably reduced costs and improved quality of patient care.

Depression

Disease management has been promoted as a strategy to improve the care of patients with depression. In a disease management study, patients with major or minor depression, treated by primary care physicians, were randomized to receive intensive treatment based on guidelines and patient education or usual care (Katon et al., 1995). Patients with major depression in the disease management group were more adherent to medication, more likely to believe that their medications were beneficial, and more likely to be satisfied with their medical care. Moreover, for patients with major depression, the intervention improved their symptoms. Patients with minor depression also were more adherent to medications and more likely to believe that their medications were helpful. A disease management approach to the care of patients with depression (with education, attention to patient adherence, and guidelines) can improve the care of these patients.

Diabetes Mellitus

A study was performed to determine the effectiveness of a disease management approach to the care of patients with diabetes mellitus (Peters, Davidson, & Ossorio, 1995). Care was provided by physician-supervised nurse specialists who followed computer-assisted protocols. Dietary counseling and patient education was also provided. After implementation of this program, there was a significant reduction in glycosylated hemoglobin levels (studies have demonstrated that lower glycosylated hemoglobin levels are associated with improved patient outcomes). Moreover, the hospitalization rate for acute complications from diabetes mellitus was much lower than the national average. This study demonstrated that a systematic approach to the provision of preventive care for diabetic patients can improve patient care.

Congestive Heart Failure

Disease management is a comprehensive approach to patient care that addresses care for patients across the continuum (including the hospital, subacute, and outpatient settings). A study examined whether this approach could improve the quality of care for patients with congestive heart failure (Rich, Beckham, Wittenberg, Leven, Freedland, & Carney, 1995). A multidisciplinary approach (involving physicians, nurses, pharmacists, and other health care providers) of providing health care was studied in patients hospitalized for congestive heart failure. The care included an educational intervention by a nurse, instruction by a dietitian, review of medications, social service, and home visits. The intervention was associated with a statistically significant reduction in the hospital readmission rate. The cost of health care also was reduced by $460 per patient, and there was a greater improvement in quality of life in patients in the intervention group. The multidisciplinary approach to the care of patients with congestive heart failure improved quality of care and patient outcome, and reduced health care costs. Therefore, a disease management approach appears to have improved quality of care and outcome for patients with congestive heart failure.

Coronary Artery Bypass Surgery

There are a limited number of scientifically rigorous studies that have demonstrated objectives and improvements in patient outcome from quality improvement projects. In one report, cardiac surgeons performing coronary artery bypass surgery in New England proposed an intervention that included physician training in continuous quality improvement, site visits to "benchmark" hospitals, feedback of data, protocols, clinical pathways, and many other techniques (O'Connor et al., 1996). Following this intervention, there was a twenty-four percent reduction in the hospital mortality rate. This study shows an association between a well-organized quality improvement program and a reduction in hospital mortality. A more recent study, however, demonstrated reductions in mortality rates from coronary artery bypass surgery in a state without a planned quality improvement program.

FURTHER RECENT EXAMPLES AND CONCERNS

There are several areas where the quality of American health care is still falling short, including underuse, overuse, misuse, and variation in use of health care services.

Underuse of Services

The failure to provide a needed service can lead to additional complications, higher costs, and premature deaths. For example, a study of heart attack patients found that nearly eighty percent did not receive life-saving beta-blocker treatment, leading to as many as 18,000 unnecessary deaths each year. A survey of managed-care plans by the National Committee for Quality Assurance (NCQA) found that sixty percent of diabetics age 31 and older had not received a recommended eye exam in the previous year. The same survey reported that thirty percent of women age fifty-two to sixty-nine had not had a mammogram in the previous two years, and thirty percent of women between ages twenty-one and sixty-four had not had a Pap smear in the previous three years, despite the fact that early screening reduces mortality.

Overuse of Services

Unnecessary services add costs and can lead to complications that undermine the health of patients. For example, half of all patients diagnosed with a common cold are incorrectly prescribed antibiotics. Overuse of antibiotics has been shown to lead to resistance and as much as $7.5 billion a year in excess costs. Another study found that sixteen percent of hysterectomies performed in the United States were unnecessary.

Misuse of Services

Errors in health care delivery lead to missed or delayed diagnoses, higher costs, and unnecessary injuries and deaths (Kohn, Corrigan, Richardson, and Donaldson, 2000). A study of New York State hospitals found one in twenty-five patients were injured by the care they received and deaths occurred in 13.6 percent of those cases. Negligence was blamed for 27.6 percent of the injuries and 51.3 percent of the deaths. Based on this study, researchers estimated that preventable errors in hospital care led to 180,000 deaths per year (Richardson, Berwick, & Bisgard, 2000). Researchers estimate that as many as thirty percent of Pap smear test results were incorrectly classified as normal.

Variation of Services

There are significant variations in the practice of medicine across the United States, among regions, and even within communities. For example, hospital discharge rates are forty-nine percent higher in the Northeast than they are in the West. A person with diabetes is one-and-a-half times as likely to get a needed eye exam in New England than in a Southern state.

In the last decade, federal and state governments, private employers, health insurers, health plans, health care professionals, labor unions, and consumer advocates have developed successful strategies to measure and improve the quality of health care.

- The New York State Department of Health releases data on the quality of heart bypass surgeries at all of the hospitals in that state. Use of these data has helped reduce mortality in bypass cases by fifty percent in five years.
- A Michigan hospital has reduced complications due to drug reactions in their cardiac care unit by eighty percent. At the LDS Hospital in Salt Lake City, Utah, a quality improvement program decreased adverse drug reactions related to antibiotics by seventy-five percent.
- An asthma program in Boston has led to an eighty-six percent reduction in hospital visits and seventy-nine percent reduction in emergency room visits. In 1992, asthma led to 468,000 hospitalizations in the United States and an annual cost of $6.2 billion.
- The use of NIH guidelines has led to a 100% increase in the use of a drug to prevent death among premature babies.
- Minnesota hospitals have increased the use of beta-blocker therapy to prevent second, often fatal, heart attacks in patients by sixty-three percent through provider education and performance feedback.

Private employers and health plans have also used quality measurement and reporting to improve care and inform consumers.

- General Motors provides its employees with report cards rating health plans' quality of care. The reports include quality measures, satisfaction ratings, accreditation reports, and reports from site visits.
- The Pacific Business Group on Health requires health plans to set aside two percent of the premiums they receive and only allows high-performance plans to retain those funds.
- The United Auto Workers requires all health plans serving its members to be accredited by the NCQA.
- Kaiser Permanente of Southern California has launched its "Intervention for Employment Maintenance for Members with End State Renal Disease" to help patients cope with this life-threatening illness and continue to work during treatment. Workers in the Kaiser program were 2.8 times more likely to maintain employment.

Poor quality care leads to sicker patients, more disabilities, higher costs, and lower confidence in the health care industry. Consumers want understandable and reliable information to help them make critical decisions about their health care. Most Americans consider it very important to know how well their health plan cares for members who are sick, catches health problems at an early stage, and keeps members as healthy as possible (Hanes & Greenlick, 1998). Private and public purchasers also want more information about the quality of the care they purchase for their employees, their dependents, and their beneficiaries as well as new strategies to improve it (Bodenheimer & Sullivan, 1998).

SUMMARY

Efforts to measure quality of care have accelerated during the past decade. The race to measure quality is fueled by the belief that valid and reliable measures of quality could be used to base health care competition on value (quality and cost) rather than just cost. This would allow patients and purchasers to select health care providers, physician organizations, hospitals, and health plans by reviewing information including objective measures of quality of care.

Most important, there have been some very exciting efforts involving the use of quality measures to identify areas for improvement of patient care. These opportunities have been identified in almost every aspect of health care. Moreover, through the use of quality improvement tools and techniques such as practice guidelines, clinical pathways, disease management programs, and information technology, significant strides have been made that have resulted in demonstrable improvements in patient care. As the field of quality measurement and improvement matures, the opportunities to improve the health of individuals and populations may prove to be boundless and should result in significant improvements in the quality of care and outcomes for patients around the world.

References

Aucott, J. N., Pelecanos, E., Dombrowski, R., Fuehrer, S. M., Laich, J., & Avon, D. C. (1996). Implementation of local guidelines for cost-effective management of hypertension. A trial of the firm system. *Journal of General Internal Medicine, 11,* 139–146.

Balas, E. A., Austin Boren, S., Brown, G. D., Ewigman, B. G., Mitchell, J. A., & Perkoff, G. T. (1996). Effect of physician profiling on utilization. Meta-analysis of randomized clinical trials. *Journal of General Internal Medicine, 11,* 584–590.

Bodenheimer, T., & Sullivan, K. (1998). How large employers are shaping the health care marketplace. *New England Journal of Medicine, 338,* 1003–1007.

Brook, R. H. (1989). Practice guidelines and practicing medicine. Are they compatible? *Journal of the American Medical Association, 262,* 3027–3030.

Davis, D. A., Thomson, M. A., Oxman, A. D., & Haynes, R. B. (1995). Changing physician performance: A systematic review of the effect of continuing medical education strategies. *Journal of the American Medical Association, 274,* 700–705.

Department of Health and Human Services for the Domestic Policy Council. (1998). *The challenge and potential for assuring quality health care for the 21st century,* Publication No. OM 98-0009. Washington, DC: U.S. Department of Health and Human Services.

Ellerbeck, E. F., Jencks, S. F., Radford, M. J., Kresowik, T. F., Craig, A. S., Gold, J. A., Krumholz, H. M., & Vogel, R. A. (1995). Quality of care for Medicare patients with acute myocardial infarction. A four-state pilot study from the Cooperative Cardiovascular Project. *Journal of the American Medical Association, 273,* 1509–1514.

Grimshaw, J. M., & Russell, I. T. (1993). Effect of clinical guidelines in medical practice: A systematic review of rigorous evaluations. *Lancet, 342,* 1317–1322.

Hanes, P., & Greenlick, M. R. (1998). *Grading health care: The science and art of developing consumer scorecards.* San Francisco, CA: Jossey-Bass.

Katon, W., Von Korff, M., Lin, E., Walker, E., Simon, G. E., Bush, T., Robinson, P., & Russo, J. (1995). Collaborative management to achieve treatment guidelines: Impact on depression in primary care. *Journal of the American Medical Association, 273,* 1026–1031.

Kohn, L. T., Corrigan, J., Richardson, W. C., & Donaldson, M. S. (2000). *To err is human: Building a safer health system.* Washington, DC: National Academy Press.

Krumholtz, H. M., Radford, M. J., Ellerbeck, E. F., Hennen, J., Meehan, T. P., Petrillo, M., Wang, Y., & Jencks, S. F. (1995). Aspirin in the treatment of acute myocardial infarction in elderly Medicare beneficiaries. Patterns of use and outcomes. *Circulation, 92,* 2841–2847.

Mugford, M., Banfield, P., & O'Hanlon, M. (1991). Effects of feedback of information on clinical practice: A review. *BMJ, 303,* 398–402.

O'Connor, G. T., Plume, S. K., Olmstead, E. M., Morton, J. R., Maloney, C. T., Nugent, W. C., Hernandez, F., Clough, R., Leavitt, B. J., Coffin, L. H., Marrin, C. A., Wennberg, D., Birkmeyer, J. D., Charlesworth, D. C., Malenka, D. J., Quinton, H. B., & Kasper, J. F. (1996). A regional intervention to improve the hospital mortality associated with coronary artery bypass graft surgery. The Northern New England Cardiovascular Disease Study Group. *Journal of the American Medical Association, 275,* 841–846.

Oxman, A. D., Thomson, M. A., Davis, D. A., & Haynes, R. B. (1995). No magic bullets: A systematic review of 102 trials of interventions to improve professional practice. *Canadian Medical Association Journal, 153,* 1423–1431.

Pestotnik, S. L., Classen, D. C., Evans, R. S., & Burke, J. P. (1996). Implementing antibiotic practice guidelines through computer-assisted decision support: Clinical and financial outcomes. *Annals of Internal Medicine, 124,* 884–890.

Peters, A. L., Davidson, M. B., & Ossorio, R. C. (1995). Management of patients with diabetes by nurses with support of subspecialists. *HMO Practice, 9,* 8–13.

Rich, M. W., Beckham, V., Wittenberg, C., Leven, C. L., Freedland, K. E., & Carney, R. M. (1995). A multidisciplinary intervention to prevent the readmission of elderly patients with congestive heart failure. *New England Journal of Medicine, 333,* 1190–1195.

Richardson, W. C., Berwick, D. M., & Bisgard, J. C. (2000). The Institute of Medicine report on medical errors. *New England Journal of Medicine, 343,* 663–664.

Soumerai, S. B., & Avorn, J. (1990). Principles of educational outreach ("academic detailing") to improve clinical decision making. *Journal of the American Medical Association, 263,* 549–556.

Ware, J. E., Jr., Bayliss, M. S., Rogers, W. H., Konsinski, M., & Tarlov, A. R. (1996). Differences in 4-year health outcomes for elderly and poor, chronically ill patients treated in HMO and fee-for-service systems. Results from the Medical Outcomes Study. *Journal of the American Medical Association, 276*(13), 1039–1047.

Weiner, J. P., Parente, S. T., Garnick, D. W., Fowles, J., Lawthers, A. G., & Palmer, R. H. (1995). Variation in office-based quality. A claims-based profile of care provided to Medicare patients with diabetes. *Journal of the American Medical Association, 273,* 1503–1508.

Weingarten, S., Riedinger, M., Conner, L., Johnson, B., & Ellrodt, A. G. (1994). Reducing lengths of stay in the coronary care unit with a practice guideline for patients with congestive heart failure. Insights from a controlled clinical trial. *Medical Care, 32,* 1232–1243.

Wennberg, J., & Gittelsohn, A. (1973). Small area variations in health care delivery. *Science, 182,* 1102–1108.

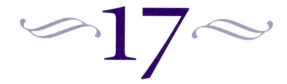

C H A P T E R
17

Ethical Issues in Public Health and Health Services*

Pauline Vaillancourt Rosenau
Ruth Roemer

Chapter Topics

- Overarching Public Health Principles: Our Assumptions
- Ethical Issues in Developing Resources
- Ethical Issues in Economic Support
- Ethical Issues in Organization of Services
- Ethical Issues in Management of Health Services
- Ethical Issues in Delivery of Care
- Ethical Issues in Assuring Quality of Care
- Mechanisms for Resolving Ethical Issues in Health Care

Learning Objectives

Upon completing this chapter, the reader should be able to:

- Appreciate the central role of public health ethical concerns in health policy and management
- Understand ethics issues with regard to the development and distribution of, and payment for, services, and with regard to the organization, management, assessment, and delivery of services
- Acquire a framework for ethical analysis of issues within health services systems
- Be a humanistic as well as technically adept participant in the health services field

*From *Changing the U.S. Health Care System* (pp. 503–535), by R. M. Anderson, T. H. Rice, and G. F. Kominski, 2001, San Francisco: Jossey-Bass. Copyright 2001 by Jossey-Bass. Reprinted with permission.

The cardinal principles of medical ethics—autonomy, beneficence, and justice—apply in public health ethics but in somewhat altered form (Beauchamp & Childress, 1989; Beauchamp & Walters, 1999). Personal autonomy and respect for autonomy are guiding principles of public health practice as well as of medical practice. In medical ethics, the concern is with the privacy, individual liberty, freedom of choice, and self-control of the individual. From this principle flows the doctrine of informed consent. In public health ethics, autonomy, the right of privacy, and freedom of action are recognized insofar as they do not result in harm to others. Thus, from a public health perspective, autonomy may be subordinated to the welfare of others or of society as a whole (Burris, 1997).

Beneficence, which includes doing no harm, promoting the welfare of others, and doing good, is a principle of medical ethics. In the public health context, beneficence is the overall goal of public health policy and practice. It must be interpreted broadly, in light of societal needs, rather than narrowly, in terms of individual rights.

Justice—whether defined as equality of opportunity, equity of access, or equity in benefits—is the core of public health. Serving the total population, public health is concerned with equity among various social groups, with protecting vulnerable populations, with compensating persons for suffering a disadvantage in health and health care, and with surveillance of the total health care system. As expressed in the now-classic phrase of Dr. William H. Foege, "Public health is social justice (1987)."

This chapter concerns public health ethics as distinguished from medical ethics. Of course, some overlap exists between public health ethics and medical ethics, but public health ethics, like public health itself, applies generally to issues affecting populations, whereas medical ethics, like medicine itself, applies to individuals. Public health involves a perspective that is population-based, a view of conditions and problems that gives preeminence to the needs of the whole society rather than exclusively to the interests of single individuals.

Public health ethics evokes a number of dilemmas, many of which may be resolved in several ways, de-pending on one's standards and values—that is, one's normative choices. Ours are indicated. Data and evidence are relevant to the normative choices involved in public health ethics. We refer the reader to health services research wherever appropriate.

To illustrate the concept of public health ethics, we raise several general questions to be considered in different contexts in this chapter.[1]

- What tensions exist between protection of the public health and protection of individual rights?
- How should scarce resources be allocated and used?
- What should the balance be between expenditures and quality of life in the case of chronic and terminal illness?
- What are appropriate limits on using expensive medical technology?
- What obligations do health care insurers and health care providers have in meeting the right-to-know of patients as consumers?
- What responsibility exists for the young to finance health care for older persons?
- What obligation exists for government to protect the most vulnerable sectors of society?

We cannot give a clear, definitive answer that is universally applicable to any of these questions. Context and circumstance sometimes require qualifying even the most straightforward response. In some cases, differences among groups and individuals may be so great, and conditions in society so diverse and complex, that no single answer to a question is possible. In other instances, a balance grounded in a public health point of view is viable. Sometimes there is no ethical conflict at all because one solution is optimal for all concerned: for the individual, the practitioner,

---

[1]Another public health question is how threats to the environment should be reconciled with the need for employment. We acknowledge that issues in environmental control have an enormous impact on public health. Here, however, our focus is on the ethical issues in policy and management of personal health services. For a discussion of equity and environmental matters, see Paehlke, R., and Vaillancourt Rosenau, P. "Environment/Equality: Tensions in North American Politics." *Policy Studies Journal*, 1993, 21(4), 672–686.

the payer, and society. For example, few practitioners would want to perform an expensive, painful medical act that was without benefit and might do damage. Few patients would demand it, and even fewer payers would reimburse for it.

A likely societal consensus would suggest that public health is better served if scarce health resources are used for better purposes.[2] But in other circumstances, competition for resources poses a dilemma, as with a new, effective, but expensive drug of help to only a few on the one hand; and use of a less-expensive but less-effective drug for a larger number of persons on the other. The necessity for a democratic, open, public debate about rationing in the future seems inevitable; seven countries in the Organisation for Economic Co-operation and Development (OECD) have already implemented such plans (Maynard & Bloor, 1998).

Even in the absence of agreement on ethical assumptions, and facing diversity and complexity that prohibit easy compromises, we suggest mechanisms for resolving the ethical dilemmas in health care that do exist. We explore these in the concluding section of this chapter.

A word of caution: space is short and our topic complex. We cannot explore every dimension of every relevant topic to the satisfaction of all readers. We offer here, instead, an introduction whose goal is to awaken readers—be they practitioners, researchers, students, patients, or consumers—to the ethical dimension of public health. We hope to remind them of the ethical assumptions that underlie their own public health care choices. This chapter, then, is limited to considering selected ethical issues in public health and the provision of personal health services. We shall examine our topic by way of components of the health system as outlined by Roemer (1991): (1) development of health resources, (2) economic support, (3) organization of services, (4) management of services, (5) delivery of care, and (6) assurance of the quality of care.

OVERARCHING PUBLIC HEALTH PRINCIPLES: OUR ASSUMPTIONS

We argue for these general assumptions of a public health ethic.

- Provision of care on the basis of health need, without regard to race, religion, gender, sexual orientation, or ability to pay
- Equity in distribution of resources, giving due regard to vulnerable groups in the population (ethnic minorities, migrants, children, pregnant women, the poor, the handicapped, and others)
- Respect for human rights—including autonomy, privacy, liberty, health, and well-being—keeping in mind social justice considerations

Central to the solution of ethical problems in health services is the role of law, which sets forth the legislative, regulatory, and judicial controls of society. The development of law in a particular field narrows the discretion of providers in making ethical judgments. At the same time, law sets guidelines for determining policy on specific issues or in individual cases.[3]

ETHICAL ISSUES IN DEVELOPING RESOURCES

When we talk about developing *resources*, we mean health personnel, facilities, drugs and equipment, and knowledge. Choices among the kinds of personnel trained, the facilities made available, and the commodities produced are not neutral. Producing and acquiring each of these involves ethical assumptions, and they in turn have public health consequences.

The numbers and kinds of personnel required and their distribution are critical to public health. We need to have an adequate supply of personnel and facilities for a given population in order to meet the ethical requirements of providing health care without discrimination or bias. The proper balance of primary care

---

[2]See Eddy, D. "Rationing Resources While Improving Quality." *Journal of the American Medical Association*, 1994, 272, 818–820, for some examples.

[3]For an example of the symbiotic relationship between ethics and law, see Annas, G. J. *Some Choice: Law, Medicine, and the Market.* New York: Oxford University Press, 1998. The work analyzes ethical issues in public health by weaving together the ethical, legal, and health service aspects of each problem discussed.

physicians and specialists is essential to the ethical value of beneficence so as to maximize health status (Cooper, 1994).[4] The ethical imperative of justice requires special measures to protect the economically disadvantaged, such as primary care physicians working in health centers. The imperfect free market mechanisms employed in the United States to date have resulted in far too many specialists relative to generalists. Canada has achieved some balance, but this has involved closely controlling medical school enrollments and residency programs.

At the same time, the ethical principle of autonomy urges that resource development also be diverse enough to permit consumers some choice of providers and facilities. Absence of choice is a form of coercion. It also reflects an inadequate supply. But it results, as well, from the absence of a range of personnel. Patients should have some—though not unlimited—freedom to choose the type of care they prefer. Midwives, chiropractors, and other effective and proven practitioners should be available if health resources permit it without sacrificing other ethical considerations. The ethical principle of autonomy here might conflict with that of equity, which would limit general access to specialists in the interest of better distribution of health care access to the whole population. The need for ample public health personnel is another ethical priority, necessary for the freedom of all individuals to enjoy a healthful, disease-free environment.

Physician assistants and nurses are needed, and they may serve an expanded role, substituting for primary care providers in some instances to alleviate the shortage of primary care physicians, especially in underserved areas.[5] But too great a reliance on these providers might diminish quality of care if they are required to substitute entirely for physicians, partic-

ularly with respect to differential diagnosis (Roemer, 1977). The point of service is also a significant consideration. For example, more effective and expanded health care and dental care for children could be achieved by employing the school as a geographic point for monitoring and providing selected services (U.S. General Accounting Office, 1994).

Health personnel are not passive commodities, and freedom of individual career choice may conflict with public health needs. Here autonomy of the individual must be balanced with social justice and beneficence. In the past, the individual's decision to become a medical specialist took precedence over society's need for more generalists. A public health ethic appeals to the social justice involved and considers the impact on the population. A balance between individual choice and society's needs is being achieved today by restructuring financial compensation for primary care providers.

Similarly, in the United States an individual medical provider's free choice as to where to practice medicine has resulted in underserved areas, and ways to develop and train health personnel for rural and central city areas are a public health priority (Braden, 1994; Helms, 1991; USDHHS, 1989). About twenty percent of the U.S. population lives in rural communities, and four in ten do not have adequate access to health care. Progress has been made in the complex problem of assuring rural health clinics. The Health Resources and Services Administration's Rural Hospitals Flexibility Program, which grants funding to improve services, is a step in the right direction, but more needs to be done (Fogel & MacQuarrie, 1994). For example, one option is to increase funds for the National Health Service Corps (Wolfe, 1991). If needs and preferences of the NHSC doctors and their families are taken into consideration, they remain at their posts longer and have better morale (Pathman, Konrad, & Ricketts, 1994). A second option is to develop quality standards that are appropriate to rural areas and that are practical, useful, and affordable (Moscovice & Rosenblatt, 1999).

An important issue in educating health professionals is the need to assure racial and ethnic diversity in both the training and practice of health professionals. In several cases, the U.S. Supreme Court has invalidated

---

[4]See Ayanian, J., and others. "Knowledge and Practices of Generalist and Specialist Physicians Regarding Drug Therapy for Acute Myocardial Infarction." *New England Journal of Medicine,* Oct. 27, 1994, p. 1136.

[5]State regulation has a significant impact on the success of such programs. See Sekscenski, E., and others. "State Practice Environments and the Supply of Physician Assistants, Nurse Practitioners, and Certified Nurse-Midwives." *New England Journal of Medicine,* Nov. 10, 1994, p. 1266.

affirmative action programs (as in the *Bakke* case in 1978 and *Hopwood* in 1996). Nevertheless, there are several grounds for a strong legal and ethical case for restoring affirmative action programs in education for the health professions. Writing about affirmative action in medical education, De Ville (1999) points out that three facts may constitute a compelling state interest justifying diversity: (1) that diversity increases the number of physicians in underserved areas and in primary care, (2) that it promotes an effective exchange of ideas in medical education, and (3) that it results in improved care for minority patients.

Similar ethical public health dilemmas are confronted with respect to health facilities. From a public health point of view, the need for equitable access to quality institutions and for fair distribution of health care facilities takes priority over an individual real estate developer's ends or the preferences of for-profit hospital owners. Offering a range of facilities to maximize choice suggests the need for both public and private hospitals, community clinics and health centers, and inpatient and outpatient mental health facilities, as well as long-term care facilities and hospices. At the same time, not-for-profit providers seem to do a better job than the for-profit institutions, at least to date. They have lower disenrollment rates, offer more community benefits, feature more preventive services, and provide hospital care at lower cost and better overall quality (Born & Geckler, 1998; Claxton, Feder, Shactmann & Altman, 1997; Dallek & Swirsky, 1997; Himmelstein, Woolhandler, Hellander, & Wolfe, 1999; Silverman, Skinner, & Fisher, 1999).[6] How long this can continue to be the case in the highly competitive health care market is unknown because not-for-profits must adopt for-profit business practices to survive (Melnick, Keeler, & Zwanziger, 1999).

The financial crisis facing public hospitals throughout the nation poses an ethical problem of major proportions (Sack, 1995). At stake is the survival of facilities that handle an enormous volume of care for the poor, that train large numbers of physicians and other health personnel, and that make available specialized services—trauma care, burn units, and others—for the total urban and rural populations they serve.

Research serves a public health purpose too. It has advanced medical technology, and its benefits in new and improved products should be accessible to all members of society. Public health ethics also focuses on the importance of research in assessing health system performance, including equity of access and medical outcomes. Only if what works and is medically effective can be distinguished from what does not and is medically ineffective are public health interests best served. Health care resources need to be used wisely and not wasted. Health services research can help assure this goal. This is especially important in an era in which market competition appears, directly or indirectly, to be having a negative influence on research capacity.

Research is central to developing public health resources. Equity mandates a fair distribution of research resources among the various diseases that affect the public's health because research is costly, resources are limited, and choices have to be made (Dionne, 1999; Light, 1999; Pear, 1998; Varmus, 1999). Research needs both basic and applied orientation to assure quality (Comroe & Dripps, 1976). There is a need for research on matters that have been neglected in the past, as has been recognized in the field of women's health.[7] Correction of other gross inequities in allocating research funds is urgent. Recent reports indicate that younger scientists are not sufficiently consulted in the peer review process, and they do not receive their share of research funds. Ethical implica-

---

[6]Taylor, D. H., Jr., Whellan, D. J., and Sloan, F. A. "Effects of Admission to a Teaching Hospital on the Cost and Quality of Care for Medicare Beneficiaries." *New England Journal of Medicine*, 1999, 340(4), 293–299; Woolhandler, S., and Himmelstein, D. U. "When Money Is the Mission—The High Costs of Investor-Owned Care." *New England Journal of Medicine*, 1999, 341(6), 444–446.

[7]Hafner-Eaton, C. "When the Phoenix Rises, Where Will She Go? The Women's Health Agenda." In P. Vaillancourt Rosenau (ed.), *Health Care Reform in the Nineties*. Thousand Oaks: Calif.: Sage, 1994; Council on Ethical and Judicial Affairs, American Medical Association. "Gender Disparities in Clinical Decision Making." *Journal of the American Medical Association*, 1991, 266, 559–562; U.S. Public Health Service. *Women's Health: Report of the Public Health Service Task Force on Women's Health Issues*. Washington, D.C.: U.S. Department of Health and Human Services, 1985.

tions involving privacy, informed consent, and equity affect targeted research grants for AIDS, breast cancer, and other special diseases. The legal and ethical issues in the human genome project involve matters of such broad scope—wide use of genetic screening, information control, privacy, and possible manipulation of human characteristics—that Annas (1989) has called for "taking ethics seriously." The orphan drug law, through tax exemption, focuses enormous resources on diseases that affect a very few individuals.[8] This law may be an instance of society assuming that beneficence takes precedence over equity and social justice. Apparent exaggerations in pricing and profitability have led to regulatory efforts to limit abuse (Coster, 1992). By contrast, in some instances discoveries made while researching diseases that have an effect on only a few individuals, as with basic research, can lead to findings that benefit broader populations.

Federal law in the United States governs the conduct of biomedical research involving human subjects. Ethical issues are handled by ethics advisory boards, convened to advise the Department of Health and Human Services on the ethics of biomedical or behavioral research projects, and by institutional review boards of research institutions seeking funding of research proposals. Both kinds of boards are charged with the responsibility for reviewing clinical research proposals and for ensuring that the legal and ethical rights of human subjects are protected.[9] Among the principal concerns of these boards is assurance of fully informed and unencumbered consent, by patients competent to give it, in order to assure the autonomy of subjects. They are also concerned with protecting the privacy of human subjects and the confidentiality of their relation to the project. An important legal and ethical duty of researchers, in the

event that a randomized clinical trial proves beneficial to health, is to terminate the trial immediately and make the benefits available to the control group and to the treated group alike.

The ethical principles that should govern biomedical research involving human subjects are a high priority, but criticism has been leveled at the operation of some institutional review boards as lacking objectivity and as being overly identified with the interests of the researcher and the institution (Annas, 1991). Recommendations to correct this type of problem include appointing patient and consumer advocates to review boards, in addition to physicians and others affiliated with the institution and along with the sole lawyer who is generally a member of the review board; having advocates involved early in drawing up protocols for the research; having third parties interview patients after they have given their consent to make sure that they understood the research and their choices; requiring the institution to include research in its quality assurance monitoring; and establishing a national human experimentation board to oversee the four thousand institutional review boards in the country (Hilts, 1995).

Correction of fraud in science and the rights of subjects are important ethical considerations in developing knowledge. Ethical conflict between the role of the physician as caregiver and as researcher is not uncommon inasmuch as what is good for the research project is not always what is good for the patient. Certainly, in some instances society stands to benefit at the expense of the research subject, but respect for the basic worth of the individual means that he or she has a right to be informed before agreeing to participate in an experiment. Only when consent is informed, clear, and freely given can altruism, for the sake of advancing science and humanity, be authentic. Still, exceptions to informed consent are sometimes justified. For example, because of the need for medically trained emergency personnel, a convincing case can be made for using deceased patients to teach resuscitation procedures. There is "no risk to the dead person, and families could not realistically be expected to discuss consent at such a difficult time (Burns, Reardon, & Truog, 1994; Orlowski, Kanoti, & Mehlman, 1988).

[8]See special issue of the *International Journal of Technology Assessment in Health Care* on orphan technologies, J. Wagner guest editor, 1992, *8*(4).

[9]422 USCS Secs. 289, 289a-1–6, 1994, 21 CFR Secs. 56–58, 1994. See Ladimer, I., & Newman, R. W. (eds.). *Clinical Investigation in Medicine: Legal, Ethical and Moral Aspects, An Anthology and Bibliography.* Boston: Law-Medicine Research Institute, Boston University, 1963.

Policy makers concerned with developing resources for health care thus confront tensions between protecting public health and protecting the rights of individual patients and providers. They face issues concerning allocation of scarce resources and use of expensive medical technology. We trust that in resolving these issues their decisions are guided by principles of autonomy, beneficence, and justice as applied to the health of populations.

ETHICAL ISSUES IN ECONOMIC SUPPORT

Nowhere is the public health ethical perspective clearer than on issues of economic support. Personal autonomy and respect for privacy remain essential, as does beneficence. But a public health orientation suggests that the welfare of society merits close regard for justice. It is imperative that everyone in the population have equitable access to health care services with dignity, so as not to discourage necessary utilization; in most cases, this means universal health insurance coverage (Light, 1999). Forty-four million Americans lack health insurance, which makes for poorer medical outcomes even though individuals without health insurance do receive care in hospital emergency rooms and community clinics (Dionne, 1999; Haas, Udvarhelyi, & Epstein, 1993; Weissman & Epstein, 1994). Most of the forty-four million are workers in small enterprises whose employers do not offer health insurance for their workers or dependents (Schauffler, Brown, & Rice, 1997).

From a public health perspective, financial barriers to essential health care are inappropriate. Yet they exist to a surprising degree.[10] If each and every human being is to develop to his or her full potential, to participate fully as a productive citizen in our democratic society, then preventive health services and alleviation of pain and suffering due to health conditions that can

be effectively treated must be available without financial barriers.[11] Removing economic barriers to health services does not mean that the difference in health status between the rich and poor will disappear. But it is a necessary, if not sufficient, condition for this goal.

Economic disparity in society is a public health ethical issue related to justice. Increasing evidence suggests that inequality in terms of income differences between the rich and the poor has a large impact on a population's health.[12] This may be due to psychosocial factors, a weakened societal social fabric, loss of social capital, or a range of other factors. Whatever the cause, as Lynch, Kaplan, and Shema (1997) assert, "Income inequality together with limited access to health care has serious consequences for the working poor."

From a public health point of view, the economic resources to support health services should be fair and equitable. Any individual's contribution should be progressive, based on his or her ability to pay. This is especially important because the rise of managed care has made it increasingly difficult to provide charity care (Cunningham, Grossman, St. Peter, & Lesser, 1999; Preston, 1996; Winslow, 1999). This may be because of funding restrictions for a defined population. Although some individual contribution is appropriate—no matter how small—as a gesture of commitment to the larger community, it is also ethically befitting for

[10]Flores, G., Bauchner, H., Feinstein, A. R., and Nguyen, U. S. "The Impact of Ethnicity, Family Income, and Parental Education on Children's Health and Use of Health Services." *American Journal of Public Health*, 1999, 89(7), 1066–1071; Brown, E. R., Wyn, R., and Ojeda, V. "Noncitizen Children's Rising Uninsured Rates Threaten Access to Health Care." Los Angeles: Center for Health Policy Research, UCLA June 1999. [http://www.healthpolicy.ucla.edu]

[11]The state medical boards are only now coming to sanction doctors who undertreat pain. Foubister, V. "Oregon Doctor Cited for Negligence for Undertreating Pain." *American Medical News*, Sept. 27, 1999. [http://www.ama-assn.org/sci-pubs/amnews/pick_99/prfa0927.htm] In addition, underuse of preventive services is increasingly a public health problem; see Center for the Evaluative Clinical Services. "The Quality of Medical Care in the United States." *Dartmouth Atlas of Health Care*, 1999.

[12]Wilkinson, R. G. *Unhealthy Societies: The Afflictions of Inequality.* London: Routledge, 1996; Kawachi, I., Kennedy, B. P., Lochner, K., and Prothrow-Stith, D. "Social Capital, Income Inequality, and Mortality." *American Journal of Public Health*, 1997, 87, 1491–1498. Kawachi, I., and Kennedy, B. P. "Income Inequality and Health: Pathways and Mechanisms." *Health Services Research*, 1999, 34(1), 215–228; Wilkinson (1996). Putnam, R. D. "Bowling Alone: America's Declining Social Capital." *Journal of Democracy*, 1995, 6(1), 65–78; Evans, R. G., Barer, M. L., and Marmor, T. R. *Why Are Some People Healthy and Others Not? The Determinants of Health of Populations.* Hawthorne, N.Y.: Aldine de Gruyter, 1994.

the nation to take responsibility for a portion of the cost. The exact proportion may vary across nation and time, depending on the country's wealth and the public priority attributed to health services (Roemer, 1991).

Similarly, justice and equity suggest the importance of the ethical principle of social solidarity in any number of forms.[13] By definition, social insurance means that there is wisdom in assigning responsibility for payment by those who are young and working to support the health care of children and older people no longer completely independent. A public health orientation suggests that social solidarity forward and backward in time, across generations, is ethically persuasive. Those in the most productive stages of the life cycle today were once dependent children, and they are likely to one day be dependent older persons.

Institutions such as Social Security and Medicare play a moral role in a democracy. They were established to attain common aims and are fair in that they follow agreed-upon rules. The alternatives to social solidarity between the young and the elderly are simply unacceptable. As members of a society made up of overlapping communities, our lives are intricately linked together. No man or woman is an island; not even the wealthiest or most "independent" can exist alone. The social pact that binds us to live in peace together requires cooperation of such a fundamental nature that we could not travel by car (assuming respect for traffic signals) to the grocery store to purchase food (or assume it is safe for consumption) without appealing to social solidarity. These lessons apply to health care as well.

In 1983, the President's Commission for the Study of Ethical Problems in Medicine and Biomedical and

Behavioral Research made as its first and principal recommendation on ethics in medicine that society has an obligation to assure equitable access to health care for all its citizens. Equitable access, the commission said, requires that all citizens be able to secure an adequate level of care without excessive burden. Implementation of this principle as an ethical imperative is even more urgent all these years later, as an increasing number of people become uninsured and as the prices of pharmaceuticals dramatically increase (Freudenheim, 1999; Soumerai & Ross-Degnan, 1999).

ETHICAL ISSUES IN ORGANIZATION OF SERVICES

The principal ethical imperative in organization of health services is that services be organized and distributed in accordance with health needs and the ability to benefit. The problem with rationing on the basis of ability to pay is that it encourages the opposite (Maynard & Bloor, 1998). The issues of geographic and cultural access also illustrate this ethical principle.

To be fair and just, a health system must minimize geographic inequity in distributing care. Rural areas are underserved, as are inner cities. Any number of solutions have been proposed and tried to bring better access in health services to underserved areas, be they rural or inner-city. They include mandating a period of service for medical graduates as a condition of licensure, loan forgiveness, expansion of the National Health Service Corps, rural preceptorships, creating economic incentives for establishing a practice in a rural area, and employing physician assistants and nurse practitioners (Lewis, Fein, & Mechanic, 1976). Telemedicine may make the best medical consultants available to rural areas in the near future, but the technology involves initial start-up costs that are not trivial (Smothers, 1992; Wheeler, 1994). Higher Medicare payments to rural hospitals also ensure that they will remain open (Moscovice, Wellever, & Stensland, 1999).

Similarly, the principles of autonomy and beneficence require health services to be culturally relevant to the populations they are designed to serve (Marin & Van Oss Marin, 1991). This means that medical care professionals need to be able to communicate in the language of those they serve and to understand the

---

[13]For an explanation of the communitarian form of social solidarity, see "The Responsive Communitarian Platform: Rights and Responsibilities: A Platform." *Responsive Community,* Winter 1991/1992, 4–20. Robert Bellah, Richard Madsen, William Sullivan, Ann Swindler, and Steven Tipton take a similar view in *Habits of the Heart* (New York: HarperCollins, 1985). See also Minkler, M. "Intergenerational Equity: Divergent Perspectives." (Paper presented at the annual meeting of the American Public Health Association, Washington, D.C., Nov. 1994); also Minkler, M., and Robertson, A. "Generational Equity and Public Health Policy: A Critique of 'Age/Race War' Thinking." *Journal of Public Health Policy,* 1991, *12*(3), 324–344.

cultural preferences of those for whom they seek to provide care (Maher, 1993; Rafuse, 1993). The probability of success is enhanced if needed health professionals are from the same cultural background as those they serve. This suggests that schools of medicine, nursing, dentistry, and public health should intensify their efforts to reach out and extend educational and training opportunities to qualified and interested members of such populations. To carry out such programs, however, these schools must have the economic resources required to offer fellowships and teaching assistant positions.

The development of various forms of managed care—health maintenance organizations, prepaid group practices, preferred provider organizations, and independent practice associations—raises another set of ethical questions. As experienced in the United States in recent years, managed care is designed more to minimize costs than to ensure that health care is efficient and effective. If managed care ends up constraining costs by depriving individuals of needed medical attention (reducing medically appropriate access to specialists, for instance), then it violates the ethical principle of beneficence because such management interferes with doing good for the patient.[14] If managed care is employed as a cost-containment scheme for Medicaid and Medicare without regard to quality of care, it risks increasing inequity. It could even contribute to a two-tiered health care system in which those who can avoid various forms of managed care by paying privately for their personal health services will obtain higher-quality care.

Historically, the advantages of staff-model managed care are clear: team practice, emphasis on primary care, generous use of diagnostic and therapeutic outpatient services, and prudent use of hospitalization. All contribute to cost containment. At the same time, managed care systems have the disadvantage of restricted choice of provider. Today's for-profit managed care companies run the risk of underserving; they may achieve cost containment through cost shifting and risk selection (Luft, 1981; Rice, 1998).

The ethical issues in the relationships among physicians, patients, and managed-care organizations include denial of care, restricted referral to specialists, and gag rules that bar physicians from telling patients about alternative treatments, which may not be covered by the plan, or from discussing financial arrangements between the physician and the plan, which may include incentives for cost containment (Miller & Sage, 1999). Requiring public disclosure of information about these matters has been proposed as a solution, but there is little evidence that disclosure helps the poor and illiterate choose a better health plan or a less-conflicted health care provider.

The ethical issues in managed care are illustrated most sharply by the question of who decides what is medically necessary: the physician or others, the disease management program, the insurer, the employer, or the state legislature (Bodenheimer, 1999; Mariner, 1994; Rosenbaum, Frankford, Moore, & Borzi, 1999). This question is not unique to managed care; it has also arisen with respect to insurance companies and Medicaid (*Pinneke v. Preisser*, 1980). On the one hand, the physician has a legal and ethical duty to provide the standard of care that a reasonable physician in the same or similar circumstances would. On the other hand, insurers have traditionally specified what is covered or not covered as medically necessary in insurance contracts. The courts have sometimes reached different results, depending on the facts of the case, the character of the treatment sought (whether generally accepted or experimental), and the interpretation of medical necessity (Mariner, 1994). With the rise of managed care, the problem becomes even more of an ethical dilemma because, as even those highly favorable to managed care agree, there is a risk of too little health care (Danzon, 1997).

[14]There is no evidence that HMOs, prior to 1992, offered reduced quality of care. Miller, R. H., and Luft, H. S. "Does Managed Care Lead to Better or Worse Quality of Care?" *Health Affairs*, 1997, *16*(5), 7–25. The evidence on HMOs and quality of care in the context of today's market competition is still out. The not-for-profit HMOs seem to provide better quality than do the for-profit HMOs. "How Good Is Your Health Plan?" *Consumer Reports*, Aug., 1996, pp. 40–44; Kuttner, R. "Must Good HMOs Go Bad? The Commercialization of Prepaid Group Health Care." *New England Journal of Medicine*, 1998, *338*(21), 1558–1563; Kuttner, R. "Must Good HMOs Go Bad? The Search for Checks and Balances." *New England Journal of Medicine*, 1998, *338*(22), 1635–1639; Himmelstein, Woolhandler, Hellander, and Wolfe (1999).

In the past, malpractice suits against managed-care organizations in self-insured plans have been barred by the provision in the Employee Retirement Income Security Act that preempts or supersedes "any and all state laws insofar as they may now or hereafter relate to any employee benefit plan."[15] As a result of the preemption, employees covered by such plans have been limited to the relief provided by ERISA—only the cost of medical care denied—with no compensation for lost wages and pain and suffering.[16] Self-insured health insurance plans that cause injury by denying care or providing substandard care have had *de facto* immunity from a suit because of legal interpretation of ERISA, but the situation appears to be changing.

In recent years, the interpretation of the ERISA preemption has been somewhat narrowed to bar only suits for denial of care but to allow suits relating to quality of care.[17] In 1995, further restriction of the ERISA preemption occurred in a unanimous decision of the U.S. Supreme Court holding that a New York statute imposing surcharges on hospitals and HMO fees for some health care payers, including ERISA plans, in order to create a pool of funding to cover the uninsured, was not preempted by ERISA because the statute had only an indirect economic effect.[18] This decision may signal a change in the legal climate of opinion on the right of employees in self-insured plans to sue their plans for denial of care.

In view of the fact that 140 million people receive their health care through plans sponsored by employers and covered by ERISA, it is a serious matter of equity to allow them access to the courts for medical malpractice (Rosenbaum et al., 1999). In fact, several states have recently adopted legislation that permits patients to hold managed care companies responsible for health care decisions imposed by the plan.[19] Experience suggests that according patients the right to hold their HMO liable generates little additional cost (Page, 1999). Federal courts appear to be moving in this direction as well (Pear, 1999).

But in June 2000, the U.S. Supreme Court held that a patient cannot sue a health maintenance organization under ERISA for giving physicians a financial incentive to cut treatment costs (*Pegram v. Herdrich*, 2000). "No H.M.O. organization could survive without some incentive connecting physician reward with treatment rationing," Justice Souter wrote. The Court held that mixed treatment-eligibility decisions by physicians are not fiduciary acts within the meaning of ERISA, which stipulates that fiduciaries shall discharge their duties solely in the interest of the participants and beneficiaries. In absolving the HMO of liability for breach of fiduciary responsibility, the Court left open the question of whether a decision on eligibility, as distinguished from a treatment decision, is a fiduciary matter for which the HMO would be liable, and it suggested that a health maintenance organization might be liable under ERISA for failure to disclose financial incentives to physicians.

This decision denying relief under ERISA emphasizes the urgency of state legislation granting patients the right to sue their HMOs for malpractice. Any state legislation, however, needs to guarantee the opportunity to sue a managed-care organization for denied or delayed care. Such legislation will compel the courts to address issues thus far ignored.

As more and more integrated health care delivery systems are formed, as more mergers of managed-care organizations occur, as pressure for cost containment increases, ethical issues concerning conflict of interest, quality of care choices, and patients' rights attain increasing importance. The principles

---

[15]29 U.S.C. Sec. 1144 (a)-(b), 1994.

[16]*Shaw* v. *Delta Airlines*, 463 U.S. 85, 1983; *Corcoran* v. *United Healthcare, Inc.*, 965 F.2d 1321 (5th Cir.), cert. denied 506 U.S. 1033, 1992. See Kilcullen, J. K. "Groping for the Reins: ERISA, HMO Malpractice, and Enterprise Liability." *American Journal of Law and Medicine*, 1996, 22(1), 7.

[17]See, for example, *Dukes* v. *U.S. Healthcare Inc.*, 57 F.3d 350 (3rd Cir. 1995), cert. denied, 116 S. Ct. 564, 1995.

[18]*New York State Conference of Blue Cross and Blue Shield Plans* v. *Travelers Ins. Co.*, 115 S. Ct. 1671, 1995.

[19]Rundle, R. H. "California's Managed-Care Legislation Generally Draws Industry's Support." *Wall Street Journal*, Sept. 13, 1999; Ingram, C., and Morain, D. "Ambitious Plan to Reform HMOs Nears Completion." *Los Angeles Times*, Sept. 10, 1999; Sterngold, J. "California Law to Let Patients Sue HMOs." *New York Times*, Sept. 28, 1999, pp. A1, A18; Johnson, D. "Illinois Court Lets Patients Sue HMOs." *New York Times*, Oct. 2, 1999, pp. A7. See Tex. Civ. Proc. & Rem. Code, Chapter 88; Marquis, J., Rubin, A. J., and Ingram, C. "Broad Health Care Reform Package Signed into Law." *Los Angeles Times*, Sept. 28, 1999, pp. 1, 18.

of autonomy, beneficence, and justice are severely tested in resolving the ethical problems facing a complex, corporate health care system.

If medicine is "for-profit," as seems to be the case today and for the near future in the United States, then the ethical dilemma between patients' interests and profits will be a continuing problem (Emanuel, 1999). Sometimes the two can both be served, but it is unlikely to be the case in all instances. Surveys of business executives admit and point out the presence of numerous generally accepted practices in their industry which they consider unethical (Baumhart, 1961). As Fisher and Welch conclude, "Stakeholders in the increasingly market-driven U.S. health care system have few incentives to explore the harms of the technologies from which they stand to profit" (Fisher & Welch, 1999; Deyo, 1997). That both consumers and employers are concerned about quality of care is clear from Paul Ellwood's statement expressing disappointment in the evolution of HMOs because "they tend to place too much emphasis on saving money and not enough on improving quality—and we now have the technical skill to do that" (Noble, 1995).

ETHICAL ISSUES IN MANAGEMENT OF HEALTH SERVICES

Management involves planning, administration, regulation, and legislation. The style of management depends on the values and norms of the population. Planning involves determining the population's health needs (with surveys and research, for example) and then ensuring that programs are in place to provide these services. A public health perspective suggests that planning is appropriate to the extent that it provides efficient, appropriate health care (beneficence) to all who seek it (equity and justice). Planning may avoid waste and contribute to rational use of health services. But it is also important that planning not be so invasive as to be coercive and deny the individual any say in his or her health care unless such intervention is necessary to protect public health interests. The ethical principle of autonomy preserves

the right of the individual to refuse care, to determine his or her own destiny, especially when the welfare of others is not involved. A balance between individual autonomy and public health intervention that affords a benefit to the society is not easy to achieve. But in some cases, the resolution of such a dilemma is clear, as in the case for mandatory immunization programs. Equity and beneficence demand that the social burdens and benefits of living in a disease-free environment be shared. Therefore, for example, immunization requirements should cover all those potentially affected.

Health administration has ethical consequences that may be overlooked because they appear ethically neutral: organization, staffing, budgeting, supervision, consultation, procurement, logistics, records and reporting, coordination, and evaluation (Roemer, 1991). But all these activities involve ethical choices. Faced with a profit squeeze, the managed-care industry is pressuring providers to reduce costs and services (Kuttner, 1999). The result has been downsizing, which means more unlicensed personnel are hired to substitute for nurses (Shindul-Rothschild, Berry, & Long-Middleton, 1996). California is the first state to mandate nurse-to-patient staffing ratios (Rundle, 1999). Surveys of doctors suggest patients do not always get needed care from HMOs. Denial of appropriate needed health care is an ethical problem related to beneficence. In addition, the importance of privacy in record keeping (to take an example) raises once again the necessity to balance the ethical principles of autonomy and individual rights with social justice and the protection of society.[20]

Distribution of scarce health resources is another subject of debate. The principle of first come, first served may initially seem equitable. But it also incorporates the "rule of rescue," whereby a few lives

---

[20]See, for example, *Whalen* v. *Roe*, 429 U.S. 589, 1977, upholding the constitutionality of a state law requiring that patients receiving legitimate prescriptions for drugs with potential for abuse have name, address, age, and other information reported to the state department of health.

are saved at great cost, and this policy results in the "invisible" loss of many more lives. The cost-benefit or cost-effectiveness analysis of health economics attempts to apply hard data to administrative decisions. This approach, however, does not escape ethical dilemmas because the act of assigning numbers to years of life, for example, is itself value-laden. If administrative allocation is determined on the basis of the number of years of life saved, then the younger are favored over the older, which may or may not be equitable. If one factors into such an analysis the idea of "quality" years of life, other normative assumptions must be made as to how important quality is and what constitutes quality. Some efforts have been made to assign a dollar value to a year of life as a tool for administering health resources. But here, too, we encounter worrisome normative problems. Does ability to pay deform such calculations?

Crucial to the management of health services are legal tools—legislation, regulations, and sometimes litigation—necessary for fair administration of programs. Legislation and regulations are essential for authorizing health programs; they also serve to remedy inequities and to introduce innovations in a health service system. Effective legislation depends on a sound scientific base, and ethical questions are especially troubling when the scientific evidence is uncertain.

For example, in a landmark decision in 1976, the Court of Appeals for the District of Columbia upheld a regulation of the Environmental Protection Agency restricting the amount of lead additives in gasoline based largely on epidemiological evidence (*Ethyl Corporation v. E.P.A.*, 1976). Analysis of this case and of the scope of judicial review of the regulatory action of an agency charged by Congress with regulating substances harmful to health underlines the dilemma the court faced: the need of judges trained in the law, not in science, to evaluate the scientific and epidemiological evidence on which the regulatory agency based its ruling (Silver, 1980). The majority of the court based its upholding of the agency's decision on its own review of the evidence. By contrast, Judge David Bazelon urged an alternative approach: "In cases of great technological complexity, the best way for courts to guard against unreasonable or erroneous administrative decisions is not for the judges themselves to scrutinize the technical merits of each decision. Rather, it is to establish a decision making process that assures a reasoned decision that can be held up to the scrutiny of the scientific community and the public.

The dilemma of conflicting scientific evidence is a persistent ethical minefield, as reflected by a 1993 decision of the U.S. Supreme Court involving the question of how widely accepted a scientific process or theory must be before it qualifies as admissible evidence in a lawsuit. The case involved the issue of whether a drug prescribed for nausea during pregnancy, Bendectin, causes birth defects. Rejecting the test of "general acceptance" of scientific evidence as the absolute prerequisite for admissibility, as applied in the past, the Court ruled that trial judges serve as gatekeepers to ensure that pertinent scientific evidence is not only relevant but reliable. The Court also suggested various factors that might bear on such determinations (*Daubert v. Merrell Dow Pharmaceuticals, Inc.*, 1993).

It is significant for the determination of ethical issues in cases where the scientific evidence is uncertain that epidemiological evidence, which is the core of public health, is increasingly recognized as helpful in legal suits (Ginzburg, 1986). Of course, it should be noted that a court's refusal (or an agency's) to act because of uncertain scientific evidence is in itself a decision with ethical implications.

Enactment of legislation and issuance of regulations are important for management of a just health care system, but these strategies are useless if they are not enforced. For example, state legislation has long banned the sale of cigarettes to minors, but only recently have efforts been made to enforce these statutes rigorously through publicity, "stings" (arranged purchases by minors), penalties on sellers, threats of license revocation, and banning cigarette sales from vending machines (Roemer, 1993; USDHHS, 1989). A novel case of enforcement involves a Baltimore ordinance prohibiting billboards promoting cigarettes in areas where children live, recreate, and go to school, enacted in order to enforce the minors' access law banning tobacco sales to minors.[21]

Thus, management of health services involves issues of allocating scarce resources, evaluating scientific evidence, measuring quality of life, and imposing mandates by legislation and regulations. Although a seemingly neutral function, management of health services must rely on principles of autonomy, beneficence, and justice in its decision-making process.

ETHICAL ISSUES IN DELIVERY OF CARE

Delivery of health services—actual provision of health care services—is the end point of all the other dimensions just discussed. The ethical considerations of only a few of the many issues pertinent to delivery of care are explored here.

Resource allocation in a time of cost containment inevitably involves rationing. At first blush, rationing by ability to pay may appear natural, neutral, and inevitable, but the ethical dimensions for delivery of care may be overlooked. If ability to pay is recognized as a form of rationing, the question of its justice is immediately apparent. The Oregon Medicaid program is another example. It is equitable by design and grounded in good part in the efficacy of the medical procedure in question, thus respecting the principle of ethical beneficence. It is structured to extend benefits to a wider population of poor people than those entitled to care under Medicaid. The plan does not qualify as equitable and fair, however, because it does not apply to the whole population of Oregon, but only to those on Medicaid. It denies services to some persons on Medicaid in order to widen the pool of

beneficiaries. It presents significant ethical problems in this respect (Annas, 1993; Rosenbaum, 1992).

Rationing medical care is not always ethically dubious; rather, it may conform to a public health ethic. In some cases, too much medical care is counterproductive and may produce more harm than good. Canada, Sweden, the United Kingdom, and the state of Oregon, among others, have rationing of one sort or another (Maynard & Bloor, 1998). For example, Canada rations health care, pays one-third less per person than the United States, and offers universal coverage; yet health status indicators do not suggest that Canadians suffer. In fact, on several performance indicators Canada surpasses the United States (Anderson & Poullier, 1999). If there were better information about medical outcomes and the efficacy of many medical procedures, rationing would actually benefit patients if it discouraged the unneeded and inappropriate treatment that plagues the U.S. health system (Greenberg, 1999; Schuster, McGlynn, & Brook, 1999).

Rationing organ transplants, similarly, is a matter of significant ethical debate. The number of organs available for transplant is less than the need. Rationing, therefore, must be used to determine who is given a transplant. Employing tissue match makes medical sense and also seems ethically acceptable. But to the extent that ability to pay is a criterion, ethical conflict is inevitable. It may, in fact, go against scientific opinion and public health ethics if someone who can pay receives a transplant even though the tissue match is not so good as it would be for a patient who is also in need of a transplant but unable to pay the cost. Rationing on this basis seems ethically unfair and medically ill advised.[22]

One solution would be to make more organs available through mandatory donation from fatal automobile accidents without explicit consent of individuals

---

[21]*Penn Advertising of Baltimore, Inc.* v. *Mayor of Baltimore,* 63 F.3d 1318 (4th Cir. 1995) aff'g 862 F.Supp. 1402 (D. Md. 1994), discussed by Garner, D. W. "Banning Tobacco Billboards: The Case for Municipal Action." *Journal of the American Medical Association,* 1996, 275(16), 1263–1269. On Sept. 1, 1999, the U.S. Court of Appeals for the 7th Circuit ruled that Chicago's cigarette and alcohol sign ordinance was not federally preempted. If the ordinance is found not in violation of the First Amendment (as the 4th Circuit determined for a similar ordinance), the way will be open for local boards of health to regulate tobacco advertising. *Federation of Advertising Industry Representatives, Inc.* v. *City of Chicago,* nos. 98–3191, 99–1115, and 99–1516, 1999.

[22]Sale of organs is unethical as well as scientifically unsound as a means of rationing, and yet it exists and persists. See Fox, R., and Swazey, J. *Spare Parts: Organ Replacement in American Society.* Oxford University Press, 1992; U.S. General Accounting Office. *Organ Transplants: Increased Effort Needed to Boost Supply and Ensure Equitable Distribution of Organs* (GAO/HRD-93-56). Washington D.C.: General Accounting Office, 1993.

and families. A number of societies have adopted this policy because the public health interest of society and the seriousness of the consequences are so great for those in need of a transplant that it is possible to justify ignoring the individual autonomy (preferences) of the accident victim's friends and relatives. Spain leads other nations regarding organ donation by interpreting an absence of prohibition to constitute a near-death patient's implicit authorization for organ transplantation (Bosch, 1999). This has not been the case in the United States to date.[23]

Delivery of services raises conflict-of-interest questions for providers that are of substantial public health importance. Criminal prosecution of fraud in the health care sector increased threefold between 1993 and 1997 (Defino, 1999). In today's market-driven health system, hospitals pressed by competitive forces strain to survive and in some cases do so only by less-than-honest cost shifting—and even direct fraud. A recent survey of hospital bills finds that more than ninety-nine percent included "mistakes" that favored the hospital.[24]

Class action suits claim that HMOs are guilty of deceiving patients because they refuse to reveal financial incentives in physician payment structures (Pear, 1999). Physicians have been found to refer patients to laboratories and medical testing facilities that they co-own to a far greater extent than can be medically jus-

tified.[25] As the trend to make medicine a business develops, the AMA's Council on Ethical and Judicial Affairs has adopted guidelines for the sale of nonprescription, health-related products in physicians' offices. The purpose is to "help protect patients and maintain physicians' professionalism (Prager, 1999). The public health ethic of beneficence is called into question by unnecessary products and inappropriate medical tests.

The practice of medicine and public health screening presents serious ethical dilemmas. Screening for diseases for which there is no treatment, except where such information can be used to postpone the onset or prevent widespread population infection, is difficult to justify unless the information is explicitly desired by the patient for personal reasons (life planning and reproduction). In a similar case, screening without provision to treat those discovered to be in need of treatment is unethical. Public health providers need to be sure in advance that they can offer the health services required to provide care for those found to be affected. This is the ethical principle of beneficence and social justice.

The tragic epidemic of HIV/AIDS has raised serious ethical questions concerning testing, reporting, and partner notification. The great weight of authority favors voluntary and confidential testing, so as to encourage people to come forward for testing, counseling, and behavior change.[26] All states require

[23]Roels, L., and others. "Three Years of Experience with a 'Presumed Consent' Legislation in Belgium: Its Impact on Multiorgan Donation in Comparison with Other European Countries." *Transplantation Procedures*, 1991, 23, 903–904; Associated Press. "Bill Would Allow Automatic Donation." *American Medical News*, Mar. 22–29, 1993, p. 10.

[24]The GAO estimate quoted is in Rosenthal, E. "Confusion and Error Are Rife in Hospital Billing Practices." *New York Times*, Jan. 27, 1993; see also Kerr, P. "Glossing over Health Care Fraud." *New York Times*, Apr. 5, 1992, p. F17; U.S. General Accounting Office. *Health Insurance: Remedies Needed to Reduce Losses from Fraud and Abuse—Testimony* (GAO/T-HRD-9308.) Washington, D.C.: General Accounting Office, Mar. 8, 1993. Alan Hillman, director of the Center for Health Policy at the University of Pennsylvania, suggests that hospital records are so deformed and manipulated for billing and reimbursement purposes that they are no longer of any use for outcomes research (quoted in *New York Times*, Aug. 9, 1994, p. A11.)

[25]Hillman, B., and others. "Physicians' Utilization and Charges for Outpatient Diagnostic Imaging in a Medicare Population." *Journal of the American Medical Association*, Oct. 21, 1992, 268, 2050–2054; Mitchell, J., and Scott, E. "Physician Ownership of Physical Therapy Services: Effects on Charges, Utilization, Profits, and Service Characteristics." *Journal of the American Medical Association*, Oct. 21, 1992, 268, 2055–2059; Kolata, G. "Pharmacists Help Drug Promotions; Pharmacists Paid by Companies to Recommend Their Drugs." *New York Times*, July 29, 1994, pp. A1, D2; Hilts, P. J. "FDA Seeks Disclosures by Scientists: Financial Interests in Drugs Are at Issue." *New York Times*, Sept. 24, 1994, p. 7; Winslow, R. "Drug Company's PR Firm Made Offer to Pay for Editorial, Professor Says." *Wall Street Journal*, Sept. 8, 1994, p. B12; U.S. General Accounting Office. "Medicare: Referrals to Physician-Owned Imaging Facilities Warrant HCFA's Scrutiny" (GAO/HEHS-95-2.) Washington, D.C.: General Accounting Office, 1994.

[26]*WHO Consultation on Testing and Counseling for HIV Infection* (WHO/GPA/NF/93.2.). Geneva, Switzerland: Global Programme on AIDS, World Health Organization, 1993; Field, M. A. "Testing for AIDS: Uses and Abuses." *American Journal of Law and Medicine*, 16(1 and 2), 33–106; Fluss, S. S., and Zeegers, D. "AIDS, HIV, and Health Care Workers: Some International Perspectives." *Maryland Law Review*, 1989, 48(1), 77–92.

confidential reporting of AIDS cases by name. The need to improve the tracking of the epidemic caused twenty-eight states, as of January 1998, to adopt confidential names-based reporting of HIV as well. A study by the U.S. Centers for Disease Control and Prevention (CDC) concludes that confidential names-based reporting of HIV has not deterred testing and treatment. Nevertheless, concern about violation of privacy and possible deterrence of testing and treatment with confidential names-based reporting of HIV persists. In California, it led to an agreement between the California Medical Association and AIDS advocacy groups to support a unique identifier system, that is, using a number to link the test and the patient (Marquis, 1998).

This issue raises sharply the ethical conflict between the individual's right to confidentiality and the needs of public health. Some guidance for resolving ethical questions in this difficult sphere is presented by Stephen Joseph, former commissioner of health for New York City, who states that the AIDS epidemic is a public health emergency involving extraordinary civil liberties issues—not a civil liberties emergency involving extraordinary public health issues (Joseph, 1992).

Partner notification was at first generally disapproved on grounds of nonfeasibility and protection of privacy, but in accordance with CDC guidelines, some states have enacted legislation permitting a physician or public health department to notify a partner that a patient is HIV-positive if the physician believes that the patient will not inform the partner.[27]

With the finding that administration of AZT during pregnancy to an HIV-positive woman reduces the risk of transmission of the virus to the infant (from approximately twenty-five percent to eight percent if administered in the later stages of pregnancy and during labor and to infants in the first six weeks of life), CDC recommends that all pregnant women be offered HIV testing as early in pregnancy as possible because of the available treatments for reducing the likelihood of perinatal transmission and maintaining the health of the woman. CDC also recommends that women should be counseled about their options regarding pregnancy by a method similar to genetic counseling.

The field of reproductive health is a major public health concern, affecting women in their reproductive years. Here the principles of autonomy, beneficence, and justice apply to providing contraceptive services, including long-acting means of contraception, surgical abortion, medical abortion made possible by the development of Mifepristone, sterilization, and use of noncoital technologies for reproduction. The debate on these issues has been wide, abrasive, and divisive. Twenty-two years after abortion was legalized by the U.S. Supreme Court's decision in *Roe v. Wade*, protests against abortion clinics have escalated. Violence against clinics and murders of abortion providers threaten access to abortion services and put the legal right to choose to terminate an unwanted pregnancy in jeopardy. The shortage of abortion providers in some states and in many rural areas restricts reproductive health services. The mergers of Catholic hospitals with secular institutions and the insistence that the merged hospital be governed by the Ethical and Religious Directives for Catholic Health Care Services means that not only abortion services are eliminated but also other contraceptive and counseling services, sterilization procedures, infertility treatments, and emergency postcoital contraception (even for rape victims).[28]

We state our position as strongly favoring the pro-choice point of view in order to ensure the autonomy of women, beneficence for women and their families faced with unwanted pregnancy, and justice in society. In the highly charged debate on teenage pregnancy, we believe that social realities, the well-being

---

[27]"1998 Guidelines for Treatment of Sexually Transmitted Diseases." *Morbidity and Mortality Weekly Report,* Jan. 23, 1998, 47(RR-1). See California Health and Safety Code, sec. 199.25 (1990) and the insightful analysis of Bayer, R. "HIV Prevention and the Two Faces of Partner Notification." *American Journal of Public Health,* Aug. 9, 1992, *82,* 1156–1164.

[28]Lagnado, L. "Their Role Growing, Catholic Hospitals Juggle Doctrine and Medicine." *Wall Street Journal,* Feb. 4, 1999, pp. 1, 8; Dressler, T. "Rise of Religious Hospitals Seen as Threat to Reproductive Rights." *Los Angeles Daily Journal,* Feb. 5, 1999, pp. 1, 8; O'Donnell, J. "Catholic Hospital Deals Limit Access, Activists Say." *USA Today,* Apr. 8, 1999, pp. B1, B2.

of young women and their children, and the welfare of society mandate access to contraception and abortion and respect for the autonomy of young people. The ethics of parental consent and notification laws, which often stand as a barrier to abortions needed and wanted by adolescents, is highly questionable.

Many other important ethical issues in delivering health care have not been discussed extensively in this chapter because of space limitations. There are three such issues that we want to mention briefly.

First, the death debate is generally considered a matter of medical ethics involving the patient, his or her family, and the physician. But this issue is also a matter of public health ethics because services at the end of life entail administrative and financial dimensions that are part of public health and management of health services.[29]

Second, in the field of mental health, the conflict between the health needs and legal rights of patients on the one hand and the need for protection of society on the other illustrates sharply the ethical problems facing providers of mental health services. This conflict has been addressed most prominently by reform of state mental hospital admission laws to make involuntary admission to a mental hospital initially a medical matter, with immediate and periodic judicial review as to the propriety of hospitalization—review in which a patient advocate participates.[30] The *Tara-*

soff case presents another problem in providing mental health services: the duty of a psychiatrist or psychologist to warn an identified person of a patient's intent to kill the person, despite the rule of confidentiality governing medical and psychiatric practice (*Tarasoff v. Regents of the University of California*, 1976). In both instances, a public health perspective favors protection of society as against the legal rights of individuals.

Third, basic to public health strategies and effective delivery of preventive and curative services are records and statistics. The moral and legal imperative of privacy to protect an individual's medical record gives way to public health statutes requiring reporting of gunshot wounds, communicable diseases, child abuse, and AIDS (Grad, 1990). More generally, the right of persons to keep their medical records confidential conflicts with society's need for epidemiological information to monitor the incidence and prevalence of diseases in the community and to determine responses to this information.

At the same time, it is essential, for example, that an individual's medical records be protected from abuse by employers, marketers, and other unauthorized persons (Starr, 1999). A common resolution of this problem is to make statistics available without identifying information. Congress has promised medical privacy legislation but, as of this writing, has failed to act. Health and Human Services, under instructions from Presidents Clinton and Bush, have been concerned about federal rules to protect the privacy of medical records, but the extent of police access to medical records has become an issue.

Ethical problems in delivering services will surely increase in number and kind in a period of great change in the health service system as private, fee-for-service, solo practice is being replaced by new ways of financing and providing health care. The most prominent problem is the question of who decides the appropriateness of services—the payer or the provider, the managed care plan or the physician—and what role the consumer has in the new system that is evolving.

[29]Scitovsky, A. A. "Medical Care in the Last Twelve Months of Life: The Relation between Age, Functional Status, and Medical Care Expenditures." *Milbank Memorial Fund Quarterly*, 1988, *66*(4), 640–660; Temkin-Greener, H., Meiners, M. S., Petty, E. A., and Szydlowski, J. S. "The Use and Cost of Health Services Prior to Death: A Comparison of the Medicare-only and the Medicare-Medicaid Elderly Populations." *Milbank Quarterly*, 1992, *70*(4), 679–701. For an insightful analysis of how a society's cultural beliefs, concept of autonomy, and informed consent laws influence resource allocation at the end of life, see Annas, G. J., and Miller, F. H. "The Empire of Death: How Culture and Economics Affect Informed Consent in the U.S., the U.K., and Japan." *American Journal of Law and Medicine*, 1994, *20*(4), 359–394.

[30]See, for example, N.Y. Mental Hygiene Law, Article 9, Secs 9.01–9.59, 1988 and Supp. 1995); Special Committee to Study Commitment Procedures of the Association of the Bar of the City of New York, in cooperation with the Cornell Law School. *Mental Illness and Due Process: Report and Recommendations on Admission to Mental Hospitals Under New York Law*. Ithaca, N.Y.: Cornell University Press, 1962.

ETHICAL ISSUES IN ASSURING QUALITY OF CARE

If a public health ethic requires fair and equitable distribution of medical care, then it is essential that waste and inefficiency be eliminated. Spending scarce resources on useless medical acts is a violation of a public health ethic.[31] To reach this public health goal, knowledge about what is useful and medically efficacious is essential.

As strategies for evaluating the quality of health care have become increasingly important, the ethical dimensions of peer review, practice guidelines, report cards, and malpractice suits—all methods of quality assurance—have come to the fore. Established in 1972 to monitor hospital services under Medicare to ensure that they were "medically necessary" and delivered in the most efficient manner, professional standards review organizations came under attack as overregulatory and too restrictive.[32] Congress ignored the criticism and in 1982 passed the Peer Review Improvement Act, which did not abolish outside review but consolidated the local peer review agencies, replaced them with statewide bodies, and increased their responsibility.[33] In 1986, Congress passed the Health Care Quality Improvement Act, which established national standards for peer review at the state and hospital levels for all practitioners regardless of source of payment.[34] The act also established a national data bank on the qualifications of physicians and provided immunity from suit for reviewing physicians acting in good faith.

The functions of peer review organizations (PROs) in reviewing the adequacy and quality of care necessarily involve some invasion of the patient's privacy and the physician's confidential relationship with his or her patient. Yet beneficence and justice in an ethical system of medical care mandate a process that controls the cost and quality of care. Finding an accommodation between protection of privacy and confidentiality on the one hand and necessary but limited disclosure on the other has furthered the work of PROs. Physicians whose work is being reviewed are afforded the right to a hearing at which the patient is not present, and patients are afforded the protection of outside review in accordance with national standards.

Practice guidelines developed by professional associations, health maintenance organizations and other organized providers, third-party payers, and governmental agencies are designed to evaluate the appropriateness of procedures. Three states—Maine, Minnesota, and Vermont—have passed legislation permitting practice guidelines to be used as a defense in malpractice actions under certain circumstances.[35] Defense lawyers are reluctant to use this legislation, however, because they fear their case will be caught up in a lengthy constitutional appeal. Such a simplistic solution, however, avoids the question of fairness: whose guidelines should prevail in the face of multiple sets of guidelines issued by different bodies, and how should accommodation be made to evolving and changing standards of practice?[36]

---

[31]McGlynn, E. A., and Brook, R. H. "Ensuring Quality of Care." In R. M. Andersen, T. H. Rice, and G. F. Kominski (eds.), *Changing the U.S. Health Care System.* San Francisco: Jossey-Bass, 1996; Chassin, M. R., and Galvin, R. W. "The Urgent Need to Improve Health Care Quality: Institute of Medicine National Roundtable on Health Care Quality." *Journal of the American Medical Association,* 1998, *280*(11), 1000–1005; Detsky, A. S. "Regional Variation in Medical Care." *New England Journal of Medicine,* 1995, *333*(9), 589–590; Leape, L. L. "Error in Medicine." *Journal of the American Medical Association,* 1994, *272,* 1851–1857.

[32]For a thoughtful discussion of peer review organizations under the law as it existed in November 1979, see Price, S. J. "Health Systems Agencies and Peer Review Organizations: Experiments in Regulating the Delivery of Health Care." In Roemer and McKray (1980). For a more recent analysis, see Luce, G. M. "The Use of Peer Review Organizations to Control Medicare Costs." *ALI-ABA Course Materials-Journal 10,* 1986; Pear, R. "Clinton to Unveil Rules to Protect Medical Privacy." *New York Times,* Oct. 27, 1999, p. A1.

[33]42 U.S.C. Sec. 1320c et seq.

[34]42 U.S.C. Sec. 11101 et seq.

[35]U.S. Congress, Office of Technology Assessment. *Impact of Legal Reform on Medical Malpractice Costs.* (OTA-BP-H-19.) Washington, D.C.: U.S. Government Printing Office, 1993.

[36]For analysis of various aspects of practice guidelines, see Capron, A. M. "Practice Guidelines: How Good Are Medicine's New Recipes?" *Journal of Law, Medicine and Ethics,* 1995, 23(1), 47–56; Parker, C. W. "Practice Guidelines and Private Insurers." *Journal of Law, Medicine and Ethics,* 1995, 23(1), 57–61; Kane, R. L. "Creating Practice Guidelines: The Dangers of Over-Reliance on Expert Judgment." *Journal of Law, Medicine and Ethics,* 1995, 23(1), 62–64; Pauly, M. V. "Practice Guidelines: Can They Save Money? Should They?" *Journal of Law, Medicine and Ethics,* 1995, 23(1), 65–74; Halpern, J. "Can the Development of Practice Guidelines Safeguard Patient Values?" *Journal of Law, Medicine and Ethics,* 1995, 23(1), 75–81.

Beneficence and justice are involved in full disclosure of information about quality to patients. Health plan report cards aim to fulfill this role. Employers, too, could use report cards to choose health plans for their employees, though some studies suggest that many employers are far more interested in cost than quality (McLaughlin & Ginsburg, 1998; Weinstein, 1999). How well reports actually measure quality is itself subject to debate (Hofer, 1999). There are major problems with those that currently exist (Poole, 1997).

Malpractice suits constitute one method of regulating the quality of care, although an erratic and expensive system. The subject is fully discussed elsewhere in this volume. Here we raise only the ethical issue of the right of the injured patient to compensation for the injury and the need of society for a system of compensation that is more equitable and more efficient than the current system.

The various mechanisms for ensuring quality of care all pose ethical issues. Peer review requires some invasion of privacy and confidentiality to conduct surveillance of quality, although safeguards have been devised. Practice guidelines involve some interference with physician autonomy but in return afford protection for both the patient and the provider. Malpractice suits raise questions of equity, since many injured patients are not compensated. In the process of developing and improving strategies for quality control, the public health perspective justifies social intervention to protect the population.

MECHANISMS FOR RESOLVING ETHICAL ISSUES IN HEALTH CARE

Even in the absence of agreement on ethical assumptions, and in the face of diversity and complexity that prohibit easy compromise, mechanisms for resolving ethical dilemmas in public health do exist. Among these are ombudsmen, institutional review boards, ethics committees, standards set by professional associations, practice guidelines, financing mechanisms, and courts of law. Some of these mechanisms are voluntary. Others are legal. None is perfect. Some, such as financing mechanisms, are particularly worrisome.

Although ethics deals with values and morals, the law has been very much intertwined with ethical issues. In fact, the more that statutes, regulations, and court cases decide ethical issues, the narrower is the scope of ethical decision making by providers of health care (Grad, 1978). For example, because the *Cruzan* case defines the conditions for terminating life support for persons in a persistent vegetative state (clear and cogent evidence of a prior statement by the patient, when competent, of her desire not to be kept alive by artificial means in a persistent vegetative state), the scope of decision making by physicians and families is constrained (*Cruzan v. Missouri Department of Health*, 1990). A court of law, therefore, is an important mechanism for resolving ethical issues.

The law deals with many substantive issues in numerous fields, including that of health care. It also has made important procedural contributions to resolving disputes by authorizing, establishing, and monitoring mechanisms or processes for handling claims and disputes. Such mechanisms are particularly useful for resolving ethical issues in health care because they are generally informal and flexible and often involve the participation of all the parties. Administrative mechanisms are much less expensive than litigation and in this respect potentially more equitable.

Ombudsmen in health care institutions are a means of providing patient representation and advocacy. They may serve as channels for expression of ethical concerns of patients and their families.

Ethics committees in hospitals and managed-care organizations operate to resolve ethical issues involving specific cases in the institution. They may be composed solely of the institution's staff, or they may include an ethicist specialized in handling such problems.

Institutional review boards, discussed earlier, are required to evaluate research proposals for their scientific and ethical integrity.

Practice guidelines, also discussed earlier, offer standards for ethical conduct and encourage professional behavior that conforms to procedural norms generally recognized by experts in the field.

Finally, financing mechanisms that create incentives for certain procedures and practices have the economic power to encourage ethical conduct. At the same time, they may function to encourage the opposite behavior.

As the health care system continues to deal with budget cuts, greater numbers of uninsured persons, and restructuring into managed-care and integrated delivery systems, ethical questions loom large. Perhaps their impact can be softened by imaginative and rational strategies to finance, organize, and deliver health care in accordance with the ethical principles of autonomy, beneficence, and justice.

Ethical issues in public health and health services management are likely to become increasingly complex in the future. New technology and advances in medical knowledge challenge us and raise ethical dilemmas. In the future they will need to be evaluated and applied in a public health context and submitted to a public health ethical analysis. Few of these developments are likely to be entirely new and without precedent, however. Already, current discussions, such as those presented here, may inform these new developments.

References

Anderson, G. F., & Poullier, J. P. (1999). Health spending, access, and outcomes: Trends in industrialized countries. *Health Affairs, 18*(3).

Annas, G. J. (1989). Who's afraid of the human genome? *Hastings Center Report, 19*(4), 19–21.

Annas, G. J. (1991). Ethics committees: From ethical comfort to ethical cover. *Hastings Center Report,* 18–21.

Annas, G. J. (1993). *The standard of care: The law of American bioethics.* New York: Oxford University Press.

Anonymous. (1999). Rural hospitals receive means to improve care. *Nation's Health,* 24.

Baumhart, R. C. (1961). How ethical are businessmen? *Harvard Business Review,* 6–19, 156–176.

Beauchamp, T. L., & Childress, J. F. (1989). *Principles of biomedical ethics.* New York: Oxford University Press.

Beauchamp, T. L., & Walters, L. (1999). Contemporary issues in bioethics. Belmont, CA: Wadsworth.

Bodenheimer, T. (1999). Disease management: Promises and pitfalls. *New England Journal of Medicine, 340*(15), 1202–1205.

Born, P., & Geckler, C. (1998). HMO quality and financial performance: Is there a connection? *Journal of Health Care Finance, 24*(2), 655–77.

Bosch, X. (1999). Spain leads the world in organ donation and transplantation. *Journal of the American Medical Association, 282,* 17–18.

Braden, J. (1994). *Health status and access to care of rural and urban populations.* Rockville, MD: U.S. Department of Health and Human Services.

Burns, J., Reardon, F., & Truog, R. (1994). Using newly deceased patients to teach resuscitation procedures. *New England Journal of Medicine, 331,* 1653.

Burris, S. (1997). The invisibility of public health: Population-level measures in a politics of market individualism. *American Journal of Public Health, 87*(10), 1607–1610.

Centers for Disease Control and Prevention. (1997). *HIV/AIDS surveillance report.* Atlanta: Centers for Disease Control and Prevention.

Claxton, G., Feder, J., Shactman, D., & Altman, S. (1997). Public policy issues in nonprofit conversions: An overview. *Health Affairs, 16*(2), 9–27.

Comroe, J. H., Jr., & Dripps, R. D. (1976). Scientific basis for the support of biomedical science. *Science, 192,* 105–111.

Cooper, R. A. (1994). Seeking a balanced physician workforce for the 21st century. *Journal of the American Medical Association, 272*(9), 680–687.

Coster, J. M. (1992). Recombinant erythropoietin: Orphan product with a silver spoon. *International Journal of Technology Assessment in Health Care, 8,* 635, 644–646.

Cruzan v. Missouri Department of Health, 497 U.S. 261, 1990.

Cunningham, P. J., Grossman, J. M., St. Peter, R. F., & Lesser, C. S. (1999). Managed care and physicians' provision of charity care. *Journal of the American Medical Association, 281*(12) 1087–1092.

Dallek, G., & Swirsky, L. (1997). *Comparing Medicare HMOs: Do they keep their members?* Washington, DC: Families USA Foundation.

Danzon, P. M. (1997). Tort liability: A minefield for managed care? *Journal of Legal Studies, 26*(2), 491–519.

Daubert v. Merrell Dow Pharmaceuticals, Inc. 509 U.S. 579, 113 S. Ct. 2786, 125 L.Ed 2d 469, 1993.

De Ville, K. (1999). Defending diversity: Affirmative action and medical education. *American Journal of Public Health, 89*(8), 1256, 1258.

Defino, T. (1999). Mediscare. *Healthcare Business, 2*(30), 60–70.

Deyo, R. A. (1997). The messenger under attack: Intimidation of researchers by special-interest groups. *New England Journal of Medicine, 336*(16), 1176–1180.

Dionne, E. J. (1999, June 17). 44 million uninsured and counting. *Washington Post,* p. A25.

Eddy, D. (1994). Rationing resources while improving quality. *Journal of the American Medical Association, 272,* 818–820.

Emanuel, E. J. (1999). Choice and representation in health care. *Medical Care Research and Review, 56*(1), 113–140.

Ethyl Corporation v. Environmental Protection Agency, 541 F.2d 1, 1976.

Fisher, E. S., & Welch, H. G. (1999). Avoiding the unintended consequences of growth in medical care: How might more be worse? *Journal of the American Medical Association, 281*(5), 452.

Foege, W. H. (1987). Public health: Moving from debt to legacy. *American Journal of Public Health, 77*(10), 1276–1278.

Fogel, L. A., & MacQuarrie, C. (1994). Benefits and operational concerns of rural health clinics. *Health Care Financial Management,* 40–46.

Freudenheim, M. (1999, January 25). Patients are facing sharp rise in costs for drug purchases. *New York Times,* p. A11, A18.

Ginzburg, H. M. (1986). Use and misuse of epidemiologic data in the courtroom: Defining the limits of inferential and particularistic evidence in mass tort litigation. *American Journal of Law and Medicine, 12*(3,4), 423–439.

Grad, F. P. (1978). Medical ethics and the law. *Annals of the American Academy of Political and Social Science, 437,* 19–36.

Grad, F. P. (1990). *The public health law manual* (2nd ed.). Washington, DC: American Public Health Association.

Greenberg, D. S. (1999, September 1). Snapshots of substandard health care. *Washington Post,* p. A23.

Haas, J., Udvarhelyi, S., & Epstein, A. (1993). The effect of health coverage for uninsured pregnant women on maternal health and the use of caesarean section. *Journal of the American Medical Association, 270*(1), 61–64.

Helms, D. (1991). *Delivering essential health care services in rural areas.* Rockville, MD: U.S. Department of Health and Human Services.

Hilts, P. J. (1995, January 15). Conference is unable to agree on ethical limits of research: Psychiatric experiment helped fuel debate. *New York Times,* p. 12.

Himmelstein, D. U., Woolhandler, S., Hellander, I., & Wolfe, S. M. (1999). Quality of care in investor-owned vs. not-for-profit HMOs. *Journal of the American Medical Association, 282*(2), 159–163.

Hofer, T. P. (1999). The unreliability of individual physician 'report cards' for assessing the costs and quality of care of a chronic disease. *Journal of the American Medical Association, 281*(22), 2098–2105.

Joseph, S. C. (1992). *Dragon within the gates: The once and future AIDS epidemic.* New York: Carroll and Graf.

Kaiser Family Foundation and Harvard University School of Public Health. (1999). *Survey of physicians and nurses: Randomly selected verbatim descriptions from physicians and nurses of health plan decisions resulting in declines in patients' health status.* Menlo Park, CA: Kaiser Family Foundation.

Kuttner, R. (1999). The American health care system: Wall Street and health care. *New England Journal of Medicine, 340,* 664–668.

Lewis, C. E., Fein, R., & Mechanic, D. (1976). *The right to health: The problem to access to primary medical care.* New York: Wiley.

Light, D. W. (1999). Good managed care needs universal health insurance. *Annals of Internal Medicine, 130,* 686–689.

Luft, H. S. (1981). *Health maintenance organizations: Dimensions of performance.* New York: Wiley.

Lynch, J. W., Kaplan, G. A., & Shema, S. J. (1997). Cumulative impact of sustained economic hardship on physical, cognitive, psychological, and social functioning. *New England Journal of Medicine, 337*(26), 1889–1895.

Maher, J. (1993). Medical education in a multilingual and multicultural world. *Medical Education, 27,* 3–5.

Marin, G., & Van Oss Marin, B. (1991). *Research with Hispanic populations.* Thousand Oaks, CA: Sage.

Mariner, W. K. (1994). Patients' rights after health care reform: Who decides what is medically necessary? *American Journal of Public Health, 84*(9), 1515–1519.

Marquis, J. (1998, October 28). Use of names won't lessen HIV testing, study says. *Los Angeles Times,* pp. A3, A14.

Maynard, A., & Bloor, K. (1998). *Our certain fate: Rationing in health care.* London: Office of Health Economics.

McLaughlin, C. G., & Ginsberg, P. B. (1998). Competition, quality of care, and the role of the consumer. *Milbank Quarterly, 76*(4), 737, 743.

Melnick, G., Keeler, E., & Zwanziger, J. (1999). Market power and hospital pricing: Are nonprofits different? *Health Affairs, 18*(3), 167–173.

Miller, T. E., & Sage, W. M. (1999). Disclosing physician financial incentives. *Journal of the American Medical Association, 281*(15), 1424–1430.

Moscovice, I., & Rosenblatt, R. (1999). Quality of care challenges for rural health [On-line]. Available: http://www.hsr.umn.edu/centers/rhrc/rhrc.html.

Moscovice, I., Wellever, A., & Stensland, J. (1999). Rural hospitals: Accomplishments and present challenges [On-line]. Available: http://www.hsr.umn,edu/centers/rhrc/rhrc.html.

Noble, H. B. (1995, July 3). Quality is focus for health plans. *New York Times*, pp. 1, 7.

Orlowski, J. P., Kanoti, G. A., & Mehlman, J. J. (1988). The ethics of using newly dead patients for teaching and practicing intubation techniques. *New England Journal of Medicine, 319*, 439–441.

Page, L. (1999). Texas law on HMO liability generates little cost—so far. *American Medical News*, 13.

Pathman, D., Konrad, T., & Ricketts, T. (1994). The National Health Service Corps experience for rural physicians in the late 1980s. *Journal of the American Medical Association, 272*, 1341.

Pear, R. (1998, July 9). Health agency is urged to re-evaluate spending priorities. *New York Times*, pp. 1, 19.

Pear, R. (1999, August 15). Series of rulings eases constraints on suing HMOs. *New York Times*, pp. 1, 19.

Pear, R. (1999, October 9). Stung by defeat in House, HMOs seek compromise. *New York Times*, p. A9.

Pegram v. Herdrich, U.S. 29 S. Ct. 2143 (2000).

Pinneke v. Preisser, 623 F.2d 546 (8th Cir. 1980).

Poole, W. (1997). The rating game. *California Medicine*, 18.

Prager, L. O. (1999, July 12). Selling products OK—but not for profit. *American Medical News*, p. 1.

President's Commission for the Study of Ethical Problems in Medicine and Biomedical and Behavioral Research. (1983). *Securing access to health care: The ethical implications of differences in the availability of health services* (Vol. 1). Washington, DC: U.S. Government Printing Office.

Preston, J. (1996, April 14). Hospitals look on charity care as unaffordable option of the past. *New York Times*, pp. A1, A15.

Rafuse, J. (1993). Multicultural medicine. *Canadian Medical Association Journal, 148*, 282–284.

Rice, T. (1998). *The economics of health reconsidered*. Chicago: Health Administration Press.

Roemer, M. I. (1977). Primary care and physician extenders in affluent countries. *International Journal of Health Services, 7*(4), 545–555.

Roemer, M. I. (1991). *National health systems of the world* (Vol. 1). New York: Oxford University Press.

Roemer, R. (1993). *Legislative action to combat the world tobacco epidemic* (2nd ed.). Geneva, Switzerland: World Health Organization.

Rosenbaum, S. (1992). Mothers and children last: The Oregon Medicaid experiment. *American Journal of Law and Medicine, 18*(1,2), 97–126.

Rosenbaum, S., Frankford, D. M., Moore, B., & Borzi, P. (1999). Who should determine when health care is medically necessary? *New England Journal of Medicine, 340*, 229–232.

Rundle, R. L. (1996, October 12). California is the first state to require hospital-wide nurse-to-patient ratios. *Wall Street Journal*, p. B6.

Sack, K. (1995, August 20). Public hospitals around country cut basic service. *New York Times*, p. A1.

Schauffler, H. H., Brown, E. R., & Rice, T. (1997). The state of health insurance in California. Berkeley: University of California.

Schuster, M. A., McGlynn, E. A., & Brook, R. H. (1999). How good is the quality of health care in the United States? *Milbank Quarterly, 76*(4), 517+.

Shindul-Rothschild, J., Berry, D., & Long-Middleton, E. (1996). Where have all the nurses gone? Final results of our patient care survey. *American Journal of Nursing, 96*, 25–39.

Silver, L. (1980). An agency dilemma: Regulating to protect the public health in light of scientific uncertainty. In R. Roemer & G. McKray (Eds.), *Legal aspects of health policy: Issues and trends*. Westport, CT: Greenwood Press.

Silverman, E., Skinner, J., & Fisher, E. (1999). The association between for-profit hospital ownership and increased Medicare spending. *New England Journal of Medicine, 341*(6), 420–426.

Smothers, R. (1992, September 16). 150 miles away the doctor is examining your tonsils. *New York Times*, p. C14.

Soumerai, S. B., & Ross-Degnan, D. (1999). Inadequate prescription drug coverage for Medicare enrollees—a call to action. *New England Journal of Medicine, 340*, 722–728.

Starr, P. (1999). Health and the right to privacy. *American Journal of Law and Medicine, 25*(2,3), 193–201.

Tarasoff v. Regents of the University of California, 17, Cal. 3d 425, 551 P. 2d 334, 131 Cal. Rptr. 14, 1976.

U.S. Department of Health and Human Services. (1989). *Reducing the health consequences of smoking: 25 years of progress* (USDHHS Publication No. CDC 89-8411). Washington, DC: U.S. Department of Health and Human Services.

U.S. General Accounting Office. (1994). *Health care: School-based health centers can expand access for children* (GAO/HEHS-95-35). Washington, DC: General Accounting Office.

Varmus, H. (1999). Evaluating the burden of disease and spending the research dollars of the National Institutes of Health. *New England Journal of Medicine, 340*, 1914–1915.

Weinstein, M. M. (1999, August 19). Economic scene: The grading may be too easy on health plans' report cards. *New York Times*, p. C2.

Weissman, J. S., & Epstein, A. M. (1994). *Falling through the safety net: Insurance status and access to health care.* Baltimore: Johns Hopkins University Press.

Wheeler, S. V. (1994). Telemedicine. *BioPhotonics,* 34–40.

Winslow, R. (1999, March 24). Rise in health-care competition saps medical research funds, charity care. *Wall Street Journal,* p. B6.

Wolfe, L. (1991). The National Health Service Corps: Improving on past experience. *Journal of the American Medical Association, 266,* 2808.

INDEX

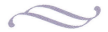

AARP (American Association of Retired Persons), 242
Abortion, 66–67, 406–407
Academic detailing, 384
Academic medical centers, 24, 220, 330–331
Access to health care, 84–88, 379–380, 398–399
Accreditation Manual for Hospitals, 231
Acquired immune deficiency syndrome (AIDS), 6, 80–81, 83, 241–242, 315, 405–406. *See also* Human immunodeficiency virus (HIV)
Act for the Relief of Sick and Disabled Seamen, 360
Act Relative to Quarantine, 360
Action for Mental Health Report, 287
Active medical staff, 230
Activities of daily living (ADL), 239, 256
Acute myocardial infarction, 376, 377, 388, 389
Administration for Children, Youth, and Families, 169
Administration on Aging, 169
Adult day services, 259–262
Adverse drug reactions, 317–318
Adverse selection, 98
Aetna, 145, 158
AFDC (Aid to Families with Dependent Children), 105, 120
Affective disorders, 294
Affirmative action, 395–396
Aged, long-term care, 240
Agency for Health Care Policy and Research, 381
Aid to Families with Dependent Children (AFDC), 105, 120
AIDS (acquired immune deficiency syndrome), 6, 80–81, 83, 241–242, 315, 405–406. *See also* HIV (human immunodeficiency virus)
AIDS Drug Assistance Program (ADAP), 324
Alcohol abuse, 84, 151
Alcohol/Drug Abuse/Mental Health Administration, 169
Almshouses, 204–205
Alzheimer's disease, 239
AMA. *See* American Medical Association (AMA)

Ambulatory health care services, 177–201
　ambulatory practice settings, 186–194
　continuum of care, 244
　government programs, 196–197
　group practice, 187–194
　history, 178–179
　institutionally based, 194–196
　levels, 179–180
　and managed care, 199–200
　mental health services, 294
　middle-income patients, 21
　military personnel, 27
　noninstitutional and public health services, 197–198
　office setting services, 183–186
　organization of ambulatory care systems, 198–199
　poor patients, 24
　settings, 180–186
　solo practice, 186–187
　surgery centers, 51, 195–196
　use of, 180–183
　veterans, 29
American Association of Homes and Services for the Aged, 253, 264
American Association of Retired Persons (AARP), 242
American College of Cardiology, 381
American College of Health Care Administrators, 253, 264
American College of Physicians, 381
American Health Care Association, 253, 264
American Hospital Association, 98, 250, 358
American Medical Association (AMA)
　Council on Ethical and Judicial Affairs, 405
　Directory of Practice Parameters, 381
　group practice, 187–188, 189
　health care reform, 118–119
　health insurance, 98, 100, 165, 363

American Medical Association (AMA)—*(cont.)*
  medical education, 209, 361
    surveys, 63
American Psychiatric Association, 282, 283, 287, 291, 298
American Psychological Association, 298
American Public Health Association, 172
Americans with Disabilities Act, 287
Analytic psychology, 284
Anesthesia, 206
Antibiotics, 6, 9–10, 311–312, 389
Antisocial disorders, 294
Antiviral therapies, 49
Anxiety disorders, 294
Applied pharmaceutical research, 315. *See also* Research
Area Health Education Centers, 334
Arteriosclerotic heart disease, 8
Aspirin, 376
Assistant Secretary for Health, Office of the, 169
Assisted Living Facilities of America, 264
Associate medical staff, 230
Autonomy, 393

Balanced Budget Act, 252, 254, 255, 267, 268, 272, 370–371
Base/major medical plans, 141, 152, 153
Basic research, 315. *See also* Research
Baylor Hospital (Dallas), 142
Bazelon, David, 403
Behaviorism, 284
Bellevue Hospital (New York), 3, 9, 208
Benchmarking, 377
Bendectin, 403
Beneficence, 393
Best practices, 376
Beta-blockers, 376, 377, 388, 389
Beth Israel Hospital (Boston), 34
Biomedical research, 362, 397. *See also* Research
Biotechnology medicines, 312–314
Bipolar disorders, 294
Birth defects, 403
Blind and visually impaired, 242
Block grants, 364, 368
Blood, artificial, 58–59
Blue Cross/Blue Shield, 145–146
  development, 13, 20, 209–210
  origins, 4, 98, 99, 142, 145
  premiums, 98
  tax status, 144, 146
Blue Cross and Blue Shield Association, 145
Blue Cross and Blue Shield of Massachusetts, 32, 33, 35
Blue Cross of California, 38

Board of Maternity and Infant Hygiene, 165
Boston, Mass., 32–36
Boston City Hospital, 34
Boston Medical Center, 32, 34, 35
Boston State Hospital, 287
Boston University Medical Center, 34
Boyd v. Albert Einstein Medical Center, 304
Brigham and Women's Hospital, 32, 33–34
Bristol Park Medical Group (Orange County, Calif.), 37
Bush, George, 118, 119, 288, 368, 407
Bush, George W., 120, 274, 368, 371
Bylaws, hospital staff, 229–230

California, 38, 171, 406
California Medical Association, 38, 406
California Medical Society, 98
California Public Employees Retirement Program (CalPERS), 119, 120
CalOPTIMA, 40–41
Cambridge Hospital (Mass.), 35
Canada, 121, 211, 404
Cancer
  drugs, 314
  incidence rates, 79–80, 81
  mortality rates, 77–78, 79
  prophylactic vaccination, 57–58
  survival rates, 78–79, 80
  therapy, 56, 57
Capitation
  and data collection, 130
  full-risk, 323
  HMOs, 100, 109, 127–128, 132, 151
  managed care, 132, 134
  Orange County, Calif., 36–37, 38, 39, 40
  partial, 323
  and public health, 174–175
  underutilization of services, 110, 131
Cardiologists, 52
Cardiovascular mortality, 74, 77
Care coordination, 247, 268–271
Caregivers, 242–243
CareGroup, 32, 33, 34, 35
Carnegie Foundation for the Advancement of Teaching, 9, 361
Carter, Jimmy, 118, 288, 366–367
Carter, Rosalyn, 288
"Carve-out" benefits, 153, 154, 324
Case management, 153, 268–271
Case-mix payment system, 252, 255
Categorical grants, 365

Centers for Disease Control and Prevention (CDC), 169, 170, 406

Cerebrovascular disease-related mortality, 77

Certificate of need (CON) programs, 207, 208, 210, 366

Charity Organization Societies, 299

Chief executive officers, hospitals, 228–229

Chiefs of staff, 230

Children, usual source of health care, 86

Children's Bureau, 165

Children's Hospital of Orange County, 40–41

Cholera, 5

Cholesterol-lowering drugs, 320

Chronic diseases, 6–8, 73, 74, 167, 236–237, 238, 239

Cigarette sales to minors, 403–404

Cigarette smoking, 83–84

CIGNA, 158

Civil commitment laws, 286

Civil Rights Act, 358, 364

Civilian Health and Medical Program of the Uniformed Services (CHAMPUS), 28

Client-centered therapy, 285

Clinical pathways, 386

Clinton, Bill
distribution of physicians, 334
health-care reform, 119–120, 158, 179, 274, 366, 370
privacy of medical records, 407

Clinton, Hillary Rodham, 119

Clot-busting drugs, 320

COBRA (Consolidated Omnibus Budget Reconciliation Act), 150

Cognitive impairment, severe, 294, 295

Coinsurance, 97, 99, 100, 102, 104, 153, 154

Combinatorial chemistry, 49

Commission for the Accreditation of Rehabilitation Facilities (CARF), 260

Committee on the Costs of Medical Care, 188

Community Health Association Program (CHAP), 255, 256

Community hospitals, 205–206, 215–219, 225–232, 248. *See also* Hospitals

Community Mental Health Center program, 197

Community psychiatry, 298

Community rated health insurance, 98, 146, 148

Comorbidity, 379

Composite International Diagnostic Interview, 281, 293

Comprehensive Health Planning and Public Health Service Amendments, 364

Comprehensive Health Planning legislation, 31

Concurrent feedback, 383–384

Confidentiality, 287, 304, 405–406, 407

Conflicts of interest, 405

Congestive heart failure, 388

Consolidated Omnibus Budget Reconciliation Act (COBRA), 150

Constitution (U.S.), 166, 168–169, 170

Consulting medical staff, 230

Continental Casualty Company, 153

Continuing Care Retirement Communities (CCRCs), 273

Continuum of care, 244–247. *See also* Long-term care

Cooperative federalism, 362

Copayments, 97, 153, 154

Coronary angioplasty, 52

Coronary artery disease, 163

Cost containment, 110, 380

Cost control continuum, 126–127

Council on Graduate Medical Education (COGME), 329, 330

Court of Appeals for the District of Columbia, 403

Courtesy medical staff, 230

Creative federalism, 363

Credential committees, 230

Cruzan v. Missouri Department of Health, 409

CT scanning, 50, 51

Cultural psychiatry, 285, 298

Cultural relevance, 399–400

Data, 62–63, 130–131, 377

Daubert v. Merrell Dow Pharmaceuticals, Inc., 403

Dawson Report, 179

Deaconess Hospital (Boston), 34

Death
causes of, 7, 44, 45, 72–82
debate concerning, 407
in hospitals, 378–379, 387
trends in U.S., 67–72

Decade of the Brain, 284

Deductibles, 97, 99, 100, 102, 103, 153

Defense, Department of, 323

Deficit Reduction Act, 103

Defined-benefit, 155

Defined-contribution, 155

Delta Dental plans, 153

Demographic transition, 66

Dental assistants, 339

Dental HMOs, 153. *See also* HMOs

Dental hygienists, 339

Dental plans, 153

Dental services, 87, 88, 337–340

Dependency ratio, 65

Depression, 387

Diabetes mellitus, 376, 387, 388, 389

Diagnosis-related groups (DRGs)
   case-mix index, 111
   cost containment, 108, 210, 368
   criticism of, 115
   hospital discharges, 225
   hospital inpatient services, 112–113
   and managed care, 104, 211
   mental health services, 302
   rural hospitals, 219
   teaching hospitals, 220
Diagnostic and Statistical Manual (DSM-IV), 282, 285, 294, 295
Diagnostic Interview Schedule (DIS), 282, 293, 294
Dietary behaviors, 84
Disabilities, 237, 239, 240–241
Disability Adjusted Life Years (DALYs), 43–46
Disability insurance, 155–156
Discharge planning, 225
Disease management, 323, 386
Diseases of the Heart (MacKenzie), 9
Dix, Dorothea, 208, 361
Donaldson v. O'Connor, 286–287
DRGs. *See* Diagnosis-related groups (DRGs)
Drug design, rational, 48–49
Drug Price Competition and Patent Term Restoration Act, 322–323
Drug research, 315–316. *See also* Research
Drug use, illicit, 84
Drug utilization review, 321, 323
Drugs. *See* Pharmaceuticals
Durable medical equipment, 257–258

Ebola virus, 73, 83
Economic market forces, 4–5
Economic Opportunity, Office of, 14
Economic Opportunity Act, 364
Education, continuing, 383
Electron-beam CT scanning, 50
Elizabethan Poor Laws, 283
Ellwood, Paul, 146, 402
Emergency medical services, 195, 196
Emergency rooms, 24, 25, 196
Emotional illness, 22, 25, 27–28. *See also* Mental illness
Employee assistance programs (EAPs), 301
Employee Retirement Income Security Act (ERISA), 151, 158, 401
Employers and long-term care, 243
Environmental Protection Agency, 403
Epidemiologic Catchment Area (ECA) Program, 281, 282, 293, 294, 295

Epidemiological evidence, 403
"Equal contribution" rule, 146
Equicor, 158
ERISA (Employee Retirement Income Security Act), 151, 158, 401
Ethical and Religious Directives for Catholic Health Care Services, 406
Ethics committees, 409
Ethyl Corporation v. Environmental Protection Agency, 403
"Etiology of Deficiency Diseases" (Funk), 9
Evidence-based guidelines, 381–382
Ex vivo approach to gene therapy, 55, 56
Exclusive provider organizations (EPOs), 118
Executive committees, hospital, 230
Experience rated health insurance, 98, 146, 148, 151

Farmer's Union Cooperative Health Association, 98
FASB (Financial Accounting Standards Board) regulation 106, 155, 158–159
Federal Food and Drug Act, 361
Federal government
   ambulatory health care services, 196–197
   health care, 12–13
   health care funding, 13–14, 15
   health care planning, 14
   public health, 165–166, 168–170, 171, 172
Federalism, 354–356
Fee for service, 108–109, 127, 128, 132, 134
Fertility trends, 65–67
FHP/Pacificare, 158
Financial Accounting Standards Board regulation (FASB 106), 155, 158–159
Financing, integrated, 247, 271–273
First-dollar insurance coverage, 141–142, 152–153. *See also* Health insurance
Fixed fees, 109
Fleming, Alexander, 6
Flexner, Abraham, 9, 209, 336
Food, Drug, and Cosmetic Act, 362, 363–364
Food and Drug Administration (FDA), 169, 311, 315, 316–319, 322–323, 363
Food and Drug Administration Modernization Act, 316, 318
For-profit institutions, 217–219, 386
Ford, Gerald, 365, 366
Formularies, 321
Foundation Health Corporation/Health Systems International, 158
FPA Medical Management, Inc., 38, 40
Franklin Health Insurance Company, 142
Free clinics, 197

Freud, Sigmund, 283–284, 299
Fromm, Erich, 284
Functional ability, 239
Functional imaging, 51
Funk, Casimir, 9
Future of Public Health, 167–168, 340

Gene therapy, 54–57, 314–315
General medical/nursing home sector, 293, 294, 295
General Motors, 389
Generic substitution, 321
Genetic mapping and testing, 53–54
Genetic marking, 56
Genometrics, 54
Genomics, 313–314
Geriatric research, education, and clinical centers (GRECCs), 248
Germ theory of disease, 206–207
Germany, 121
Global Burden of Disease study, 42, 281
"Good Manufacturing Practice" (GMP), 318
Government role in hospital industry, 211–212. *See also* Federal government; Local governments; State governments
Graduate Medical Education National Advisory Committee, 329, 330, 336
Great Britain, 109, 179, 188, 211. *See also* United Kingdom
Group coverage, 150. *See also* Health insurance
Group Health Cooperative of Puget Sound, 147, 148, 188, 223
Group practice, 187–194
Grouper Program, 113, 114, 115

Halsted, William, 6
Harmonic imaging, 50
Harvard Community Health Plan, 33, 148
Harvard Pilgrim Health Care, 32, 33, 35
Harvard University, 281
Harvard Vanguard, 33, 35
HCFA. *See* Health Care Financing Administration (HCFA)
Health, Education, and Welfare, Department of, 15, 166, 358, 363
Health and Human Services, Department of, 101, 169–170, 329, 363, 397, 407. *See also* Health Care Financing Administration (HCFA)
Health care
    administration, 402
    finance initiatives, 110–118
    inflation, 110
    issues, 3

professionals, 327–328, 347–348, 394–396, 402
public involvement, 3, 15–17
reform, 15, 118–121
services, 3–5, 62
social organization, 3, 4, 12–15
systems, 19–20, 30–32
Health Care Financing Administration (HCFA). *See also* Health and Human Services, Department of
    and Blue Cross and Blue Shield of Massachusetts, 33
    health insurance programs, 169–170
    hospice programs, 259
    hospitals, 250, 387
    Medicare, 101, 111, 113, 116, 135
    mental health services, 303
    nursing homes, 253, 254
    social HMOs, 271–272
Health Care Quality Improvement Act, 408
Health expenditures, 93–96
Health facilities, 396
Health insurance, 96–102
    comprehensive plan, 153
    consolidation among providers, 133–134
    contracts, 133
    development of, 14–15, 20, 96–97
    education/preparation in managed care, 130
    employers' cost, 152
    first-dollar coverage, 141–142, 152–153
    group coverage, 150
    growth of, 13
    history in U.S., 142–144
    and hospitals, 209–210
    individual coverage, 149–150
    industry, 145, 157–159, 158, 220–221
    personal health care expenditures, 95–96
    reimbursement policies, 4
    risk distribution, 97–98
    taxonomies, 144–145
    universal coverage, 31, 118, 174, 362, 363, 370, 398
Health Insurance Plan of New York, 148, 180
Health Insurance Portability and Accountability Act, 154, 158, 370
Health maintenance organizations. *See* HMOs
Health Plan Employer Data and Information Set (HEDIS), 130, 159, 219, 380
Health plan report cards, 389, 409
Health Planning and Public Health Service amendments, 366
Health Planning and Resource Development Act, 166
Health planning approach, 31
Health policy
    dimensions, 354–359

Health policy—(cont.)
  federal system, 354–356
  history, 360–371
  implementation, 357–358
  incremental reform, 358–359
  pluralistic politics, 356–357
  public and private sector politics, 354
Health Professions Educational Assistance Act, 364
Health promotion, 153
Health-related insurance programs, 149–151
Health Resources and Services Administration, 169, 170, 395
Health resources distribution, 30, 402–403
Health Security Act, 120
Health status, 379
Healthy People 2000, 173
Healthy People 2010, 173
Heart Disease, Cancer and Stroke Act, 364, 366
HEDIS (Health Plan Employer Data and Information Set), 130, 159, 219, 380
Hemoglobin products, 58–59
Hepatitis B, 312
High-risk state insurance pools, 150
Hill-Burton Act, 4, 211, 219, 363
Hitchcock Medical Center (New Hampshire), 33
HIV (human immunodeficiency virus), 55, 58, 73, 80–81, 287, 405–406. *See also* AIDS (acquired immune deficiency syndrome)
HMO Act, 51, 100, 146, 147, 148, 367
HMOs, 146–148. *See also* Managed care
  benefit structure, 153
  Boston, 32, 33, 35–36
  capitation, 100, 109, 127–128, 132, 151
  claims data, 130
  continuum of care, 271
  contracts, 175–176
  cost control, 110, 127
  dental, 153
  enrollment, 128
  ethical issues, 401–402
  fixed fees, 109
  group, 147
  growth of, 146–147
  as health insurance, 144
  health promotion and disease prevention, 174–176
  IPA-model, 147
  as managed care, 4, 127–128, 129
  Medicare, 104, 367
  mental health services, 303
  Orange County, Calif., 37, 39
    origins, 98
    pharmaceuticals, 321
    position payment structures, 405
    premiums, 98
    social, 271–272
    staff model, 147, 158
Home health services, 197, 245, 253–258
Honorary medical staff, 230
Hôpital Générale, 283
Horizontal integration, 221
Hospice de Bicetre, 283
Hospices, 258–259
Hospital indemnity plans, 99
Hospital Survey and Construction Act, 4, 211, 219, 363
Hospitals
  accreditation, 231
  admission rates, 377
  ambulatory surgery centers, 195
  city/county, 19, 24
  clients, 250
  community, 205–206, 215–219, 225–232, 248
  competition and cost-containment pressures, 224–225
  continuum of care, 247–250
  development, 206–213
  emergency medical services, 196
  and health insurance, 209–210
  and health systems, 220–225
  history, 3–4, 204–206
  industry characteristics, 213–220
  information sources, 250
  length of stay statistics, 213–214, 215
  long-term, 247
  and managed care, 128
  and Medicare, 14, 102–103, 217, 219, 225, 249, 356–357
  middle-income patients, 21
  military personnel, 27
  mortality rates, 378–379, 387
  national profile, 250
  operating characteristics, 249
  Orange County, Calif., 39–40
  outpatient and ambulatory care clinics, 194–195
  ownership, 212–213
  poor patients, 24
  private/not-for-profit, 216
  psychiatric, 247
  public, 216–217, 386
  and public involvement in health care, 16
  quality of care, 230–232
  rehabilitation, 247

small and rural, 219–220
state, 19
state mental hospitals, 19, 22, 361
teaching, 24, 220, 330–331
and technology, 9–10
types, 247–248
veterans, 29
Housing, 246, 262–264
Housing and Urban Development, Department of, 264
Human Genome Project, 53, 397
Human immunodeficiency virus (HIV), 55, 58, 73, 80–81, 287, 405–406. *See also* Acquired immune deficiency syndrome (AIDS)
Hybrid fee-based systems, 109
Hypertension, 387

Imaging, 49–51
IMGs (International Medical Graduates), 329, 330–332, 334, 335, 336, 346
Immigrants, 41
Immunizations. *See* Vaccines
Impairments, 237
In vivo approach to gene therapy, 55
Incentives, 384
Income tax, 168–169
Indemnity benefits, 97, 99, 108, 146, 153, 154
Independent practice associations (IPAs), 109, 128, 129, 131, 132, 190
Indian Health Service, 30, 170, 197, 353
Indigenous healers, 300–301
Individual coverage, 149–150. *See also* Health insurance
Inequality, 30–31
Infant mortality, 69, 71, 72
Infectious diseases, 5, 9, 73, 74, 83, 167
Information systems, integrated, 247, 268, 269
Information technology, 384–385, 386–387
Inpatient care, 244, 295
Institute of Medicine, 167–168, 252, 331, 334, 340, 377
Institutional review boards, 409
Institutionalization of health care, 3–4
Instrumental activities of daily living (IADL), 239, 256
Insulin, 6
Insurance concepts, 141–142. *See also specific types of insurance*
Integrating mechanisms, 246–247
Interagency Council on the Homeless, 291
Interentity structures, 247, 267–268
Intermediate care facilities, 250. *See also* Nursing homes

International Medical Graduates (IMGs), 329, 330–332, 334, 335, 336, 346
Internet, 387
Interventional MRI, 52
IPAs (independent practice associations), 109, 128, 129, 131, 132, 190

JCAHO (Joint Commission on Accreditation of Healthcare Organizations), 231, 250, 252, 255, 267
John Hancock (company), 158
Johns Hopkins Hospital, 6
Johns Hopkins University, 4
Johnson, Frank, 286
Johnson, Lyndon B., 324, 363, 364, 365, 366
Joint Commission Model, 231
Joint Commission on Accreditation of Healthcare Organizations (JCAHO), 231, 250, 252, 255, 267
Joint conference committees, 230
Joint ventures, 5
Joseph, Stephen, 406
Jung, Carl, 284
Justice, 393

Kaiser Foundation Health Plan, 39, 147, 148, 158, 188, 223
Kaiser Foundation Hospitals, 147
Kaiser Permanente, 126, 146, 147, 272, 389
Kennedy, John F., 287, 363, 364
Kennedy-Kassenbaum bill, 154, 158, 370
Kerr-Mills Act, 101, 104, 362, 363

Labor, Department of, 328
LaGuardia, Fiorello, 188
Lahey Clinic, 33, 34
Laparoscopy, 52
LDS Hospital (Salt Lake City), 389
Lead additives in gasoline, 403
Legal tools, 403–404, 409
Life expectancy, 67–69
Lifespan (company), 33
Lifestyle patterns and disease, 83–84
Lincoln, Abraham, 208
Liposomes, 55
Local governments, 171–172, 354–356, 360
Long-term care, 234–279
   availability and accessibility, 275
   definition, 236
   financing, 264–267, 274
   fragmentation, 275
   future of, 276–277

Long-term care—(*cont.*)
  insurance, 96, 154, 266, 272–273
  integrating mechanisms, 267–273
  and Medicaid, 107, 265, 266, 274, 275
  middle-income patients, 21–22
  military personnel, 27
  organization of, 243–247
  poor patients, 24–25
  public policy issues, 273–276
  service categories, 247–264
  staffing and expertise, 275–276
  users, 236–243
  veterans, 29
Long-term disability insurance, 156
Long-term hospitals, 247. *See also* Hospitals
Los Angeles County, Calif., 41–46
Loss, 141

MacKenzie, James, 9
Maine, 408
Malaria, 5
Malpractice suits, 401, 408, 409
Mammography, 86–87, 378, 383, 384, 385, 388
Managed care, 4, 124–139. *See also* HMOs
  access to health care, 87
  ambulatory health care services, 199–200
  Boston, 32, 33
  and chronic illness, 8
  components, 125–126
  concepts and principles, 130–133
  conflicts of interest, 136–137
  contracts, 133
  definition, 125
  ethical issues, 400–402
  and group practice, 190–191
  and health care professionals, 134–135, 347–348
  International Medical Graduates, 331
  issues, 133–139
  and medical education, 335–336
  mental health services, 136, 289, 302–304
  middle-income patients, 23
  objectives, 125
  Orange County, Calif., 36, 39, 40–41
  process, 126–130
  public health role, 174–176
  public involvement, 17
  public protection, 137–138
  and quality, 380
  regulation and oversight, 158
  types of plans, 127–130

Management service organizations (MSOs), 34
Mandated benefits, 151, 158
Massachusetts, 33, 35–36, 164, 360
Massachusetts General Hospital, 3, 32, 33–34, 206, 208
MassHealth, 35
Maternal and Child Health and Mental Retardation
      Planning Amendments, 364
Maternal mortality, 72
Mayo Clinic, 146, 188
McLean Hospital (Waverly, Mass.), 298
Medi-Cal, 40, 116–118
Medicaid
  access to health care, 87
  administration, 106–107
  adult day services, 260
  benefits, 106–107
  Boston, 35–36
  Bush proposal, 119
  California, 40, 116–118
  development, 4, 20, 107–108
  eligibility, 104–106, 121
  expenditures, 15, 93, 95, 105–106
  financing, 94, 101, 110, 169
  fixed fees, 109
  long-term care, 107, 265, 266, 274, 275
  managed care, 25–26, 40–41, 135–136, 367
  and Medicare, 102–103
  mental health services, 288, 289, 301–302, 303
  nursing homes, 96
  Orange County, Calif., 40–41
  Oregon, 404
  pharmaceuticals, 323–324
  poor patients, 25–26
  program structure, 104–106
  prospective payments, 210, 211–212
  providers, 107
  public hospitals, 217
  recipients, 105–106
  reform, 120
  services, 106
  skimming and dumping, 114
  state governments, 107–108, 171
  as welfare medicine, 101–102, 104–105
Medical Assistance for the Aged, 101, 104, 362, 363
Medical directors, 230
Medical education, 4, 8–9, 10, 209, 329–330, 334–336, 348
Medical Education in the United States and Canada (Flexner),
      9, 209, 336
Medical ethics, 393, 407. *See also* Public health ethics
Medical Group Management Association, 63, 187–188

Medical plans, 152–153
Medical records, 407
Medical research, 10. *See also* Research
Medical Savings Accounts (MSAs), 120
Medical science advances, 206–207
Medical Services for the Indigent (MSI), 41
Medical technology. *See* Medicine and technology
Medicare
    access to health care, 87
    and active employees, 154
    adult day services, 260
    catastrophic coverage, 103
    development of, 4, 13–14, 15, 20, 357–358
    diagnosis-related groups (*See* Diagnosis-related groups
        (DRGs))
    expenditures, 15, 93, 95
    financing, 65, 94, 101, 102, 110, 169
    HMOs, 104, 367
    home health, 254, 255, 256
    hospice benefit, 258, 259
    hospitals, 14, 102–103, 217, 219, 225, 249, 356–357
    indexes, 111, 112, 115, 117
    long-term care, 265, 266, 272
    and managed care, 8, 135
    medical education funding, 330–331
    mental health services, 289, 301, 302
    middle-income patients, 23
    nursing homes, 96
    physicians, 103–104
    political debate, 16
    poor patients, 26
    population age group projections, 65
    prescription drugs, 120, 324
    and private insurance, 154
    prospective payments, 103, 104, 111, 112–115, 118, 210,
        211, 219, 220, 356–357
    provider reimbursement, 4, 103–104, 115–116, 346, 356
    reasonable costs per discharge, 111
    service benefits, 108
    as social health insurance, 100–101
    Supplementary Medical Insurance (SMI), 103
    target rates, 111–112
    utilization, 104
Medicare Act, 324
Medicare Catastrophic Care Act, 274
Medicine and technology
    artificial blood, 58–59
    development of, 207–208
    gene therapy, 54–57
    genetic mapping and testing, 53–54
    imaging advances, 49–51
    rational drug design, 48–49
    surgery, minimally invasive, 51–53
    vaccines, 57–58
    xenotransplantation, 59–60
Medigap insurance, 99, 102
MedPartners, 33, 38, 39
MedWatch Partners program, 318
Mental Health Parity Act, 158, 289
Mental health personnel, 297–301
Mental health policy, 285–289
Mental health services
    ambulatory services, 294
    changes in, 291–293
    deinstitutionalization of, 285–286, 289, 290
    delivering, 289–291
    ethical issues, 407
    financing, 301–303
    inpatient services, 295
    and managed care, 136
    utilization patterns, 293–297
Mental Health Systems Act, 288
Mental illness. *See also* Emotional illness
    diagnosing, 282
    early views on, 282–284
    homeless, 290–291
    incidents and prevalence of, 281–282
    long-term care, 242
    poor patients, 24
    rational drug design, 49
    in the U.S., 284–285
Mental Retardation, 282
Mental Retardation Facilities and Community Mental
        Health Centers Construction Act, 287–288
MetraHealth, 158
Metropolitan Insurance Company, 145, 158
Metropolitan Jewish Geriatric Center (Brooklyn, N.Y.), 272
Metropolitan Life Insurance Co. v. Massachusetts, 151
Microchip technology, 54
Middle-income patients, 20–23
Military medical care, 12–13, 16, 19–20, 26–28
Mills v. Rogers, 287
Minimum premium plans, 151
Minnesota, 275, 408
Misuse of services, 389
Molecular modeling, 48–49
Monarch IPA, 37
Monetary flow, 94–96
Moral hazard, 97
Morrill Act, 360

Mortality. *See* Death
Moutin, Joseph, 165
MRI, 50, 51
Multiline insurers, 145
Mutual insurance companies, 145

National Adult Day Services Association, 260, 262
National Alliance for Caregiving, 242
National Ambulatory Medical Care Survey, 63, 183–186
National Association of Home Care, 258, 259
National Association of Psychiatric Health Systems, 303
National Association of Social Workers, 300
National Cancer Act, 362
National Cancer Institute, 362
National Center for Health Statistics, 250, 258, 259
National Chronic Care Consortium, 267
National Committee for Quality Assurance, 380, 388, 389
National Comorbidity Survey, 281, 293
National Council on Aging, 262
National health insurance, 31, 118, 174, 362, 363, 370, 398
National Health Interview Survey, 63, 236, 237, 240–241
National Health Planning and Resources Development Act, 14, 31, 366
National Health Service Corps (U.S.), 197, 334, 395, 399
National Health Service (Great Britain), 109, 179, 188
National health service model, 118, 119, 121
National Hospice and Palliative Care Organization, 258, 259
National Hospital Discharge Survey, 63
National Institute of Mental Health (NIMH), 281, 286, 288, 293
National Institute on Alcohol Abuse and Alcoholism (NIAAA), 291
National Institute on Drug Abuse (NIDA), 291
National Institutes of Health (NIH)
    guidelines, 389
    history, 362
    mental health, 281
    research, 169
    research funding, 4, 10, 11, 220, 315, 358
National League of Nursing, 256
National Mental Health Act, 286
National Mental Health Study Act, 287
National Pharmaceutical Council, 321
NDA (New Drug Application), 317
Neighborhood health centers, 14, 196
Neighborhood Health Plan (NHP), 33
Neuroradiologists, 52
New Deal, 12, 165
New Drug Application (NDA), 317
New England Medical Center, 33

New federalism, 365
New Haven Hospital, 206, 208
New Jersey State Nurses Association, 299
New York Hospital, 206
New York State Department of Health, 389
Nightingale, Florence, 208
Nightingale School for Nursing, 208
NIH. *See* National Institutes of Health (NIH)
NIMH (National Institute of Mental Health), 281, 286, 288, 293
Nixon, Richard, 146, 364, 365–366, 368
Noncompliance, 321
Northern Pacific Railroad, 188
Not-for-profit providers, 216, 386
Nurse practitioners, 344–346
Nurses
    development of profession, 208–209
    ethical issues, 395, 402
    statistics, 341–342
    training, 8–9, 10, 208, 298–299, 342–343
Nursing Home Reform Act, 252
Nursing homes
    clients, 252–253
    continuum of care, 250–253
    information sources, 253
    mental health services, 289–290
    national profile, 250–251
    operating characteristics, 251–252
    poor patients, 24–25

OBRA (Omnibus Budget Reconciliation Act), 252, 268, 290
Old Age, Survivors' and Disability Insurance (OASDI), 362
Ombudsmen, 409
Omnibus Budget Reconciliation Act (OBRA), 252, 268, 290
Omnibus Deficit Reduction Act, 154
On-Lok (program), 272
Opinion leaders, 384
Orange County, Calif., 36–41
Oregon, 404
Organ transplants, 404–405
Organisation for Economic Co-operation and Development (OECD), 394
OrNda, 36
Orphan Drug Act, 319, 397
Osteopathy, 336–337
Outcome of care, 378
Outpatient and ambulatory care clinics, 194–195. *See also* Ambulatory health care services
Outreach programs, 245
Overuse of services, 389

PACE (Program of All-Inclusive Care for the Elderly), 272
Pacific Business Group on Health, 389
Pacificare Health Systems, 135
Partners (health care system), 32, 33–34, 35
Partnership for Health Act, 364, 366
Patient education, 384
Patient satisfaction, 379
Payment monitoring, 109–110
Peer Review Improvement Act, 408
Peer review organizations (PROs), 408, 409
Pegram v. Herdrich, 401
Penicillin, 6
Pennsylvania Hospital (Philadelphia), 205–206
Pepper Commission, 274
Per capita form of reimbursement. *See* Capitation
Permanente Medical Groups, 147. *See also* Kaiser
        Permanente
Personal health care, 95–96
Pest houses, 205
Pew Health Professions Commission, 331, 334
Pharmaceuticals, 310–325
    adverse reactions, 317–318
    advertisements, 318, 319
    exclusivity period, 322–323
    government role, 323–324
    and health services, 320–321
    history, 311–315
    investigational new drugs, 318–319
    labeling, 318
    marketplace, 321–323
    product liability, 319–320
    promotional claims and comparisons, 318
    regulatory legal issues, 316–320
    research, 48–49, 315–316
    structure-based design, 48
    utilization review, 321, 323
Pharmacists, 344
Pharmacy benefit managers, 321–322
PhyCor, 38
Physician assistants (PAs), 344–346, 395
Physician-hospital consortia (PHCs), 40
Physician-hospital organizations (PHOs), 231
Physician Payment Review Commission (PPRC), 367
Physician practice management companies (PPMCs), 36,
        37–38, 40
Physicians
    geographic distribution, 333–334
    health promotion and disease prevention, 173–174
    managed care, 128–129, 131
    practice guidelines, 385–386

private practice, 21, 22
    reimbursement, 108–110
    salaried, 109, 110, 129
    specialty distribution trends, 332–333
    supply, 329–336, 346, 347–348
    and technology, 10
    training, 8, 9, 10
Pinel, Philippe, 283
Pinneke v. Preisser, 400
Pluralism, 356–357
Pneumonia, 6
Point-of-service (POS) plans, 127
Population size and composition, 63–65
PPMCs (physician practice management companies), 36,
        37–38, 40
PPOs (preferred provider organizations), 97–98, 109, 118,
        127, 128–129
Practice guidelines, 380–386, 408, 409
Predominant health problems, 3, 5–8
Preferred provider organizations (PPOs), 97–98, 109, 118,
        127, 128–129
Premium-equivalents, 145
Premiums, insurance, 145
Prepaid health plans, 100
Prepayment. *See* Capitation
Prescription drug plans, 154
President's Commission for the Study of Ethical Problems
        in Medicine and Biomedical and Behavioral
        Research, 399
President's Commission on Mental Health, 281, 288
Prevention levels, 163–164
Preventive medicine, 27, 246
Primary care, 180
Primary-care case management plans (PCCMs), 323–324
Primary care physicians (PCPs), 131–132, 175–176, 332–333
Primary prevention, 163, 179–180
Privacy of medical records, 407
Private health insurance, 142, 144, 148–149. *See also* Health
        insurance
Private/not-for-profit hospitals, 216. *See also* Hospitals
Private sector, 14–15
Pro-competition, 110–111
Probability surveys, national, 63
Professional Standards Review Organizations (PSROs),
        110, 366, 408
Program of All-Inclusive Care for the Elderly (PACE), 272
Protein drugs, 314
Provider-sponsored organizations (PSOs), 157
Prudential, 145
Psychiatric hospitals, 247. *See also* Hospitals

Psychiatric nurses, 298–299
Psychiatrists, 297–298
Psychologists, 298
Psychopharmacology, 285–286
Public assistance, 96–97, 101–102, 104–105
Public health, 162–176
    acute infectious diseases, 167
    agencies, 21, 23, 24, 198
    evolution in U.S., 164–167
    federal government, 165–166, 168–170, 171, 172
    government role, 167–168, 172–173
    HMOs' role, 174–176
    local government, 171–172
    managed care role, 174–176
    organized efforts in U.S., 167–173
    physicians' role, 173–174
    primary care physician role, 175–176
    private sector role, 173–176
    professionals, 340–341
    screening, 405
    state government, 165, 166, 170–171
Public health ethics, 392–413
    care delivery, 404–407
    economic support, 398–399
    health services management, 402–404
    issue resolution mechanisms, 409–410
    quality of care, 408–409
    resource development, 394–398
    service organization, 399–402
Public Health Service, 170, 173, 323, 358, 362
Public Health Service Act, 355
Public hospitals, 216–217, 386. See also Hospitals
Public welfare health care programs, 96–97, 101–102,
        104–105
Pussin, Jean Baptiste, 283

Quality of care, 373–391
    care variations, 375–376, 389–390
    clinical pathways, 386
    concerns, 388–390
    and cost containment, 380
    and disease management, 386
    ethical issues, 408–409
    examples of successful programs, 387–388
    hospitals, 230–232
    improvement opportunities, 376–377
    and information technology, 386–387
    and managed care, 380
    measurement framework, 377–380
    measurement hazards, 387

    measurement issues, 374–375
    measurement standardization, 380
    practice guidelines, 380–386

Radiology diagnosis, 9
Rand Corporation study, 210
Rational drug design, 48–49
Rationing health care, 404
Reagan, Ronald
    block grants, 364
    cost containment, 110, 118
    health policy, 353, 366, 368
    Medicare physician reimbursement, 115
    mental health services, 288
    physician distribution, 334
Red Cross, 16
Rehabilitation hospitals, 247. See also Hospitals
Report cards for health plans, 389, 409
Reproductive health, 406–407
Research, 10, 315–316, 362, 386–397
Residential treatment centers, 292
Residents (staff), 230
Resource-based relative values, 115–116, 117, 118, 302, 346
Retirees, 154–155, 158–159
Retrospective feedback, 383
Retroviruses, 55, 60
Right to refuse treatment, 287
Right to treatment, 286–287
Rightsizing, 223
Risk, 34–35, 132–133, 141
Rockefeller Foundation, 9, 361
Roe v. Wade, 406
Rogers, Carl, 285
Roosevelt, Franklin, 12, 100, 165
Ross-Loos Clinic, 98, 146
Rotavirus, 58
Rouse v. Cameron, 286
Rural Health, Office of, 334
Rural health care, 197–198, 219–220, 333–334, 395, 399
Rural Hospitals Flexibility Program, 395
Rush, Benjamin, 283
Ryan White CARE Act, 242, 324, 370

Salary continuation benefits, 156
Sanitation, 164, 166
SASI (Self-Assessment for Systems Integration), 267
Saunders, Cecily, 258
Schizophrenia, 284, 294
Scientific evidence, conflicting, 403
Scientific method, 4

Secondary care, 180
Secondary prevention, 163
Section 223 limits, 111
Secure Horizons Medicare, 33, 135
Selective contracting, 116–118
Self-Assessment for Systems Integration (SASI), 267
Self-funding (health insurance), 144–145, 150–151
Senior Health Action Network (SCAN), 272
Service benefits, 97, 108, 146
Sexual behaviors, 84
Shattuck, Lemuel, 164
Sheppard-Towner Act, 165
Short-term disability insurance, 156
Sick leave benefits, 156
Simian virus 40 (SV40) viral vector, 55–56
Single-line insurers, 145
Sixteenth Amendment, 168–169
Skilled nursing facilities (SNFs), 102, 103, 250, 252. *See also* Nursing homes
Smoking, 83–84
Social health insurance, 96, 100–101, 102, 399
Social HMOs, 271–272. *See also* HMOs
Social psychiatry, 297–298, 299
Social Security, 102, 105
Social Security Act
   amendments, 112, 364, 366, 370
   health policy, 353, 362, 370
   and Medicaid, 101, 104, 106
   and Medicare, 100
   mental health services, 288
   and national health insurance, 100, 118
   public health, 165
Social Security Administration, 169, 357–358
Social Security disability programs, 156, 289
Social workers, 299–300
Solo practice, 186–187
Somatic gene therapy, 55
Somatization disorders, 294
Somatogen, 59
Souter, David, 401
Spain, 405
Specialty mental health and addictive disorders (SMA), 293, 294
St. Joseph's Health System (Calif.), 39, 40, 41
St. Luke's Hospital (New York), 9
St. Mary's Hospital (London), 6
State Children's Health Insurance Program (SCHIP), 120
State Comprehensive Mental Health Services Plan Act, 288
State governments, 165, 166, 170–171, 354–356, 360–361
State Health Planning and Development Agency, 166

State mental hospitals, 19, 22, 361. *See also* Hospitals
Stensuad v. Reivil, 287
Step-care therapy, 321
Stock insurance companies, 145
Stop-loss insurance, 151
Strategic business units, 224–225
Stress, societal, 84
Stroke patients, 320
Substance Abuse and Mental Health Services Administration (SAMHSA), 281
Substance abuse disorders, 294, 295
Sullivan, Harry, 284
Supplemental Security Income (SSI), 105, 120, 289
Supreme Court, 151, 395–396, 401, 403, 406
Surgeon General's Report on Mental Health, 281
Surgery, 51–53, 388, 389
Surveys, 63, 85
Sweden, 404

Taft-Hartley funds, 145
TANF (Temporary Assistance to Needy Families), 105, 324
Tarasoff v. Regents of the University of California, 407
Target rate ceiling, 111–112
Tax Equity and Fiscal Responsibility Act (TEFRA), 104, 111, 154, 210
Tax Reform Act, 144
Teaching hospitals, 24, 220, 330–331. *See also* Hospitals
Technology, 3, 8–12
Teenage pregnancy, 406–407
TEFRA (Tax Equity and Fiscal Responsibility Act), 104, 111, 154, 210
Temporary Assistance to Needy Families (TANF), 105, 324
Tenet Healthcare Corp., 36, 39–40
Tenth Amendment, 170
Tertiary care, 180
Tertiary prevention, 163
Therapeutic interchange, 321
Third-party administrators, 145
Thrombolytic therapy, 376
"Toward a National Plan for the Chronically Mental Ill," 288
Traditional healers, 300–301
Transcultural psychiatry, 285, 298
Translational research, 315. *See also* Research
Travelers and disease, 164
Travelers Insurance Company, 142, 158, 243
Triage process, 136
Truman, Harry S., 359, 363
Tuberculosis, 311–312
Tufts Associated Health Plan, 32, 33, 35

UCR (usual, customary, and reasonable) fees, 108, 109
Ulcer therapy, 320
Ultrasonography, 50, 51
Underuse of services, 388
Uninsured, 23–26, 121, 143–144, 174, 398
Unions, 145
United Auto Workers, 389
United HealthCare, 145, 148, 158
United Kingdom, 404. *See also* Great Britain
United States Census of Population, 63–64
Universal health insurance coverage, 31, 118, 174, 362, 363, 370, 398
University of California at Irvine Medical Center, 40, 41
Urban Institute, 291
U.S. Healthcare (company), 145, 158
U.S. News & World Report, 375
U.S. Preventive Services Task Force (USPSTF), 173, 381, 383, 384, 385
Usual, customary, and reasonable (UCR) fees, 108, 109
Utilization, plan/provider control of, 131–132
Utilization data, 377
Utilization review, 118, 153

Vaccine Injury Compensation Program, 320
Vaccines, 56, 57–58, 164, 166, 311–312, 319–320
Vaccines for Children programs, 324
Vascular institutes, 52
Vermont, 408
Vertical integration, 221, 222–224
Veterans, 19–20, 241
Veterans Administration, 28–30, 170, 197, 286, 292, 298
Veterans Affairs, Department of, 241, 248, 251, 323
Viral vectors, 55–56

Virtual reality modeling, 49
Vision plans, 153
Visiting nurses associations, 254
Vital statistics data, 62–63
Vitamins, 9
Voluntary health insurance, 96, 98–100
Voluntary hospitals, 205–206, 215–219, 225–232, 248. *See also* Hospitals
Voluntary support network, 293, 294, 295

Wagner, Murray, Dingell National Health Insurance Bill, 100
War on Poverty, 4, 14, 16
Watson, John B., 284
Welfare medicine, 96–97, 101–102, 104–105
Wellness programs, 27, 246
WellPoint Health Networks, 158
"West of Scotland Coronary Prevention Study," 320
White House Conference on Mental Health, 281
Wickline v. State, 304
Williams v. HealthAmerica, 304
Winslow, C.E.A., 164
Wisconsin, 275
Workers' compensation, 100, 102, 156–157
World Bank, 281
World Health Organization, 281
Wyatt v. Stickney, 286

Xenotransplantation, 59–60

Yale University, 111
Years Lived with Disability (YLDs), 42, 43
Years of Life Lost (YLLs), 42–45
Yellow fever, 5